Essential Manual of

Preclinical Prosthodontics

Essential Manual of Preclinical Prosthodontics

Second Edition

Paranjay Prajapati BDS MDS
Professor
Department of Prosthodontics and Crown and Bridge
KM Shah Dental College and Hospital
Sumandeep Vidyapeeth Deemed to be University
Vadodara, Gujarat, India

Sneha Kulkarni BDS
Private Practitioner
Vadodara, Gujarat, India

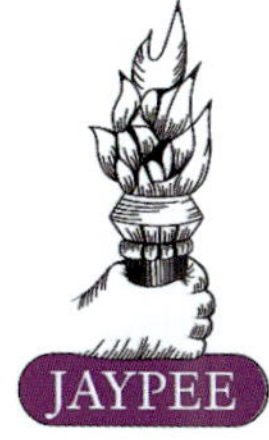

JAYPEE BROTHERS MEDICAL PUBLISHERS
The Health Sciences Publisher
New Delhi | London

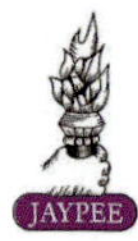

Jaypee Brothers Medical Publishers (P) Ltd

Headquarters
EMCA House
23/23-B, Ansari Road, Daryaganj
New Delhi - 110 002, India
Landline: +91-11-23272143, +91-11-23272703
+91-11-23282021, +91-11-23245672
E-mail: jaypee@jaypeebrothers.com

Corporate Office
4838/24, Ansari Road, Daryaganj
New Delhi - 110 002, India
Phone: +91-11-43574357
Fax: +91-11-43574314
E-mail: jaypee@jaypeebrothers.com

Overseas Office
J.P. Medical Ltd
83 Victoria Street, London
SW1H 0HW (UK)
Phone: +44 20 3170 8910
E-mail: info@jpmedpub.com

EU GPSR Authorised Representative
Logos Europe, 9 rue Nicolas Poussin
17000, La Rochelle, France
Phone: +33 (0) 6 67 93 73 78
E-mail: contact@logoseurope.eu

Website: www.jaypeebrothers.com
Website: www.jaypeedigital.com

Essential Manual of Preclinical Prosthodontics

First Edition: 2019

Second Edition: 2025, *Reprint:* **2026**

ISBN: 978-93-6616-100-6

Printed at: Samrat Offset Pvt. Ltd.

Contributors

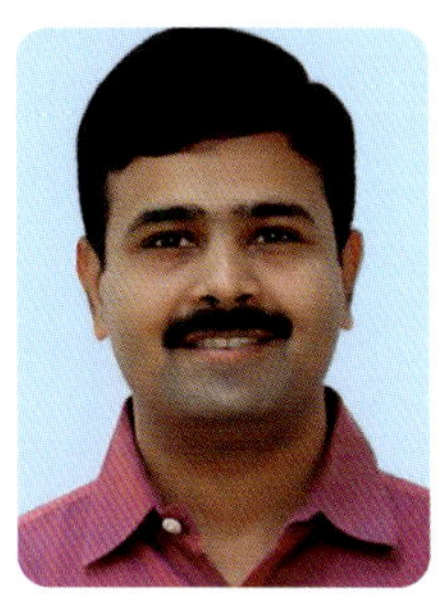

Rajesh Sethuraman
Professor and Head
Department of Prosthodontics and
Crown and Bridge
KM Shah Dental College and Hospital
Sumandeep Vidyapeeth
Deemed to be University
Vadodara, Gujarat, India

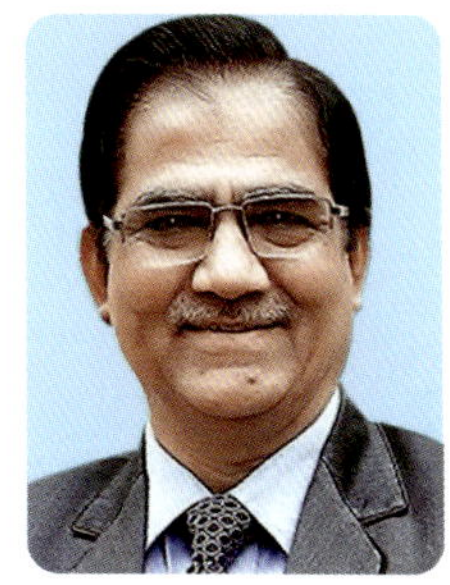

JR Patel
Professor Emeritus
Narsinhbhai Patel Dental College
and Hospital
Director Health Sciences
Sankalchand Patel University
Visnagar, Gujarat, India

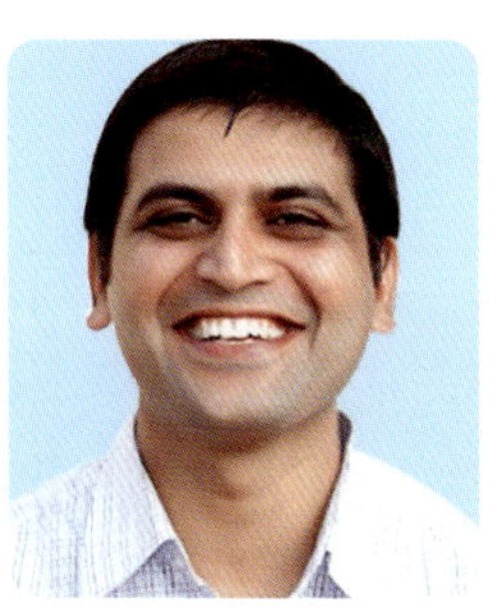

Jignesh Chaudhari
Reader
Department of Prosthodontics and
Crown and Bridge
Karnavati School of Dentistry
Gandhinagar, Gujarat, India

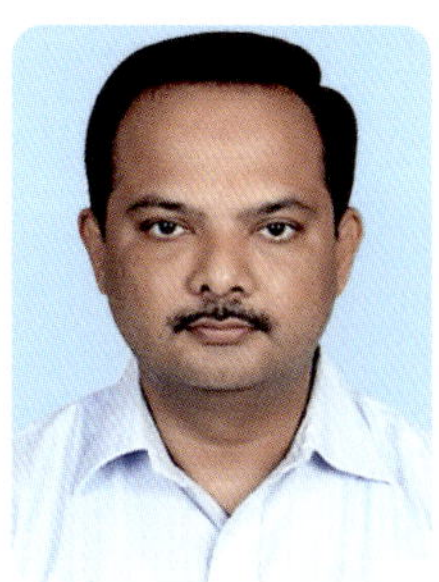

YG Naveen
Professor and Head
Department of Prosthodontics and
Crown and Bridge
Subbaiah Institute of Dental Sciences
Shimoga, Karnataka, India

Preface to the Second Edition

The preclinical education and training is different from other subjects in dental education. Skill developed and knowledge gained during these years are the building blocks for future prosthodontic art and science. The preclinical-level book should be easy and should provide ready reference for first- and second-year BDS students. Preclinical training aims at presenting a blend of instrumentation, scientific rationale, manual dexterity, and dental material knowledge. Encompassing such a multifold number of objectives, it often becomes difficult for an undergraduate student to grasp and perform solely with the best guidance of a prosthodontic instructor in clinic. A ready reference manual with simplified teaching and coherent revision was always felt a need during our academic career. It was out of this need that the writing of *Essential Manual of Preclinical Prosthodontics* began.

This book consists of 55 chapters divided into seven sections.

Section I: Deals with to-the-point description of theory and practical aspect for complete denture.

Section II: Explains about the basic of removable partial denture and fabrication of the same.

Section III: Provides principles and preparations of crown prosthesis and fixed partial denture.

Section IV: Deals with introduction to special prosthodontics, which includes treatment modalities with implant prosthodontics, maxillofacial prosthodontics, and restoration of endodontically treated tooth with post and core.

Section V: Provides information about all instruments and equipment used for preclinical and clinical exercises. Special notes provided for cleaning and caring of instruments and equipment.

Section VI: Explains briefly about all dental materials used during preclinical and clinical procedures for various treatments.

Section VII: Covers commonly asked viva questions with answers for ready reference and examination-oriented preparation. It also introduces OSCE/OSPE type of questions and methodology to write the answers for the same.

This book contains more than 1,100 high-quality color illustrations, flowcharts, schematic diagrams, and tables to improve understanding and reproducibility. Key points are provided for easy and quick recapitulation.

We wish first- and second-year BDS students a wonderful experience with preclinical prosthodontics that will be made easy by this must-have book.

Paranjay Prajapati
Sneha Kulkarni

Preface to the First Edition

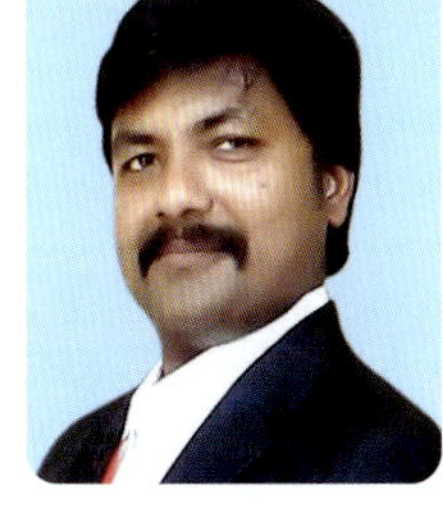

The dental curriculum is designed to educate students to achieve a necessary level of clinical competence in order to provide successful dental treatment. In prosthodontic training, preclinical exercises are the building blocks for sound prosthodontic art and science. Preclinical training should not only focus on preclinical expertise but also relate to real-time clinical situations and the role that laboratory work plays in successful completion of a treatment plan.

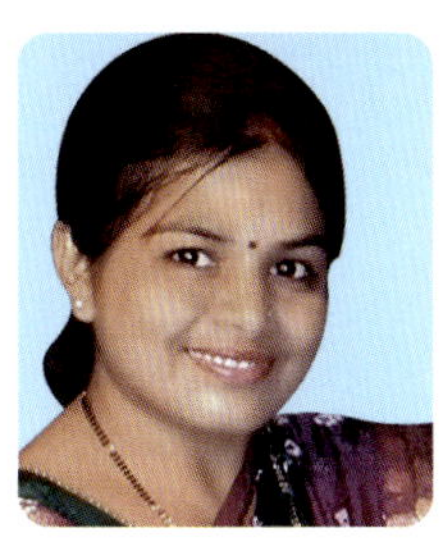

Preclinical training aims at presenting blend of instrumentation, scientific rationale, manual dexterity and dental material knowledge. Encompassing such a multifold number of objectives, it often becomes difficult for an undergraduate student to grasp and perform solely with the best guidance of a prosthodontic instructor in clinic. A ready-reference manual with simplified teaching and coherent revision was always felt a need during our academic career. It was out of this need that the writing of *Essential Manual of Preclinical Prosthodontics* began.

This book consists of 54 chapters divided into 07 sections.

- *Section 01:* Complete denture deals with to-the-point description of theory and practical aspect for complete denture.
- *Section 02:* Explains about basics of removable partial denture and fabrication of the same.
- *Section 03:* Provides principles and preparations of crown prosthesis and fixed partial denture.
- *Section 04:* Deals with introduction to special prosthodontics which includes treatment modalities with implant prosthodontics, maxillofacial prosthodontics, restoration of endodontically treated tooth with post and core.
- *Section 05:* Provides information about all instruments and equipment used for preclinical and clinical exercises. Special notes provided for cleaning and caring of instruments and equipment.
- *Section 06:* Explains briefly about all dental materials used during preclinical and clinical procedures for various treatment.
- *Section 07:* Covers commonly asked viva questions with answers for ready reference and examination-oriented preparation.

This book contains more than 1,100 high quality color illustrations, flowcharts, schematic diagrams and tables to improve understanding and reproducibility. Key points are provided for easy and quick recapitulation.

We wish 1st and 2nd year BDS students a wonderful experience with preclinical prosthodontics that will be made easy by this must-have book.

Paranjay Prajapati
Sneha Kulkarni

Acknowledgments

First and foremost, we would like to thank almighty GOD for giving us the strength, knowledge, ability, and opportunity to undertake this project and to persevere and complete it satisfactorily. Without his blessings, this achievement would not have been possible.

We acknowledge our contributors, Drs JR Patel (Professor and Dean, Narsinhbhai Patel Dental College and Hospital, Visnagar, Gujarat), Rajesh Sethuraman (Professor and Head and Additional Dean, Department of Prosthodontics and Crown and Bridge, KM Shah Dental College and Hospital, Vadodara, Gujarat), YG Naveen (Professor, Department of Prosthodontics, Sharavathi Dental College, Shimoga, Gujarat), and Jignesh Chaudhari (Reader, Department of Prosthodontics, Karnavati School of Dentistry, Gandhinagar, Gujarat), for their contribution in shaping this manual. Their suggestions, knowledge, and valuable guidance helped us to complete this book successfully.

We express our profound feeling of gratitude, respect, and indebtedness to Dr Rajesh Sethuraman (Head, Department of Prosthodontics and Crown and Bridge, KM Shah Dental College and Hospital) for giving us freedom to work and execute this project in our department. We thank all the teaching faculties of our department for their encouragement and support.

We thank all the postgraduate students of our department, especially Drs Rajkumar Chapla, Pritesh, Ketan, Sameer, Sweta, Bhagyashree, Sonali, Krishna, Shikha, Bindal, and Venu, for their unconditional help. Very special thanks go to Drs Rutvik, Jatin, Shreya, Mansi, and Mrugnayani, for their prompt help in photography and image editing for this manual.

My sincere appreciation extends to the entire team of Jaypee Brothers Medical Publishers, New Delhi, for their tremendous effort and unwavering support—Shri Jitendar P Vij (Group Chairman), Mr Ankit Vij (Managing Director), Mr MS Mani (Group President), Dr Madhu Choudhary (Director—Educational Publishing), Ms Pooja Bhandari [Director—Production (Books and Journals)], Dr Upma Tomar (Senior Development Editor), Ms Sunita Katla (Executive Assistant to Group Chairman and Publishing Manager), Ms Samina Khan (Executive Assistant to Director—Educational Publishing), Mr Ajay Kumar Sharma [Deputy General Manager (Books and Journals)], Mr Vijay Kumar Bhatia (Production Manager), Ms Seema Dogra (Cover Visualizer), Ms Neha Verma (Graphic Designer—Cover), Mr Dilip Kumar Jha (Quality Analyst), Mr Jagvir Singh Tomar (Typesetter), Mr Sumit Kumar (Team Lead–Graphic Designer). Without their cooperation, I could not have completed this project.

We are indebted to our parents Mr GH Prajapati, Mrs Kamalaben Prajapati, Mr RH Kulkarni, and Mrs Chandrika Kulkarni, for their unfailing love and support. Special love and hugs go to our little son Shrey Prajapati for his understanding and cooperation during making of this manual.

We appreciate the help of Mr Kanubhai Parmar, C/o Vishal Graphics, Vadodara, Gujarat, India, for designing all the line diagrams for this manual. We are also thankful to Mr Neeravbhai Darji for his help and professional tips on photography for this manual.

We once again thank all our teachers, colleagues, students, family, and friends for their unconditional help and support for shaping this manual.

Contents

Section III: Fixed Partial Denture

Section VI: Dental Materials

SECTION VII: OSCE/OSPE/ Spotter Section

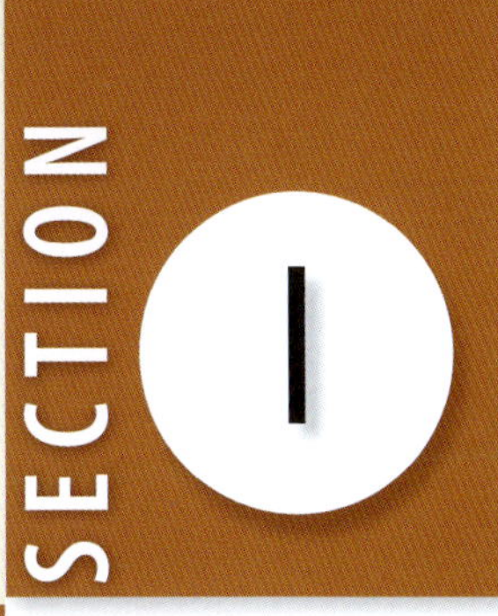

Complete Denture

Section Outline

CHAPTER 1

Overview of Prosthodontics

Paranjay Prajapati, Sneha Kulkarni

INTRODUCTION

Prosthodontics is branch of dentistry which deals with replacement of missing teeth and associated structure. Sub-branch of this specialty known as maxillofacial prosthodontics pertaining with replacement of missing oral and extraoral tissue or facial structure-like eye, nose, ear, etc. with artificial substitutes.

DEFINITION

Prosthesis: An artificial replacement of any part of the human body.

Prosthodontics: Prosthodontics is the dental specialty pertaining to the diagnosis, treatment planning, rehabilitation and maintenance of the oral function, comfort, appearance and health of patients with clinical conditions associated with missing or deficient teeth and/or maxillofacial tissues using biocompatible substitutes.

Masticatory Apparatus

The organs and structures involved in chewing and deglutition process are collectively known as masticatory apparatus. They are maxillary and mandibular jaws, teeth of maxillary and mandibular arches, muscles of mastication, temporomandibular joint, tongue, oral mucosa, lips and cheeks.

During mastication the jaw movements along with movement of tongue, lips and cheeks are important to move the food bolus inside oral cavity to place the bolus on the occlusal table of teeth to chew it effectively.

Some muscles are actively involved in mastication by guiding the movement of mandible. This group of muscles is known as "Muscles of Mastication". They are masseter, temporalis, lateral pterygoid, medial pterygoid, digastric, mylohyoid, and geniohyoid.

Temporomandibular joint (TMJ) is joint which connects the mandible jawbone with the skull. This joint is formed between condyle of mandible and temporal bone of skull so named as temporomandibular joint. Equilibrium among these structures is very important for effective mastication.

AIMS

- Restoration of missing tooth/teeth along with associated structures
- Restoration of maxillofacial defects/missing tissue
- Maintenance of masticatory apparatus (maintenance of jawbone and jaw joint with muscles)
- Restoration and maintenance of function, health comfort and appearance of patient
- Preservation of residual oral structures.

BRANCHES OF PROSTHODONTICS

There are four branches of prosthodontics which deals with replacement of missing structure.

Removable Prosthodontics

This branch of prosthodontics dealing with replacement of teeth and adjacent structures for complete edentulous or partially edentulous patients by artificial substitutes that are readily removed from the mouth.

(These prostheses are not fixed in mouth and patient can remove and reinsert it at his/her will).

Fixed Prosthodontics

The branch of prosthodontics dealing with the replacement and/or restoration of teeth by artificial substitutes that are not readily removed from the mouth.

(These prostheses are fixed in mouth with cementing medium and patient cannot remove it, but dentist can remove it if needed).

Maxillofacial Prosthodontics

The branch of prosthodontics dealing with the restoration and/or replacement of the stomatognathic and craniofacial structures with prosthesis that may or may not be removable.

[This prosthesis mainly replace missing facial structure (nose, ear, eye, etc.) and restores intraoral defects].

Implant Prosthodontics

The branch of prosthodontics dealing with the replacement of missing teeth and/or associated structure by restorations that are attached to dental implants.

Temporomandibular Disorders

There is emergence of new subspecialty which treats disorders related to temporomandibular joint and associated structures with non-surgical treatment approach. The disorders related to temporomandibular joint and associated structures are collectively known as temporomandibular disorders or TMDs. These disorders are treated with various occlusion splints and occlusal therapy.

PROSTHESIS: TYPES AND CLASSIFICATION (FLOWCHART 1.1)

- Removable prosthesis **(Figs. 1.1 and 1.2)**
- Fixed prosthesis **(Figs. 1.3 to 1.5)**
- Maxillofacial prosthesis **(Figs. 1.6 to 1.9)**
- Implant supported prosthesis **(Figs. 1.10 and 1.11)**.

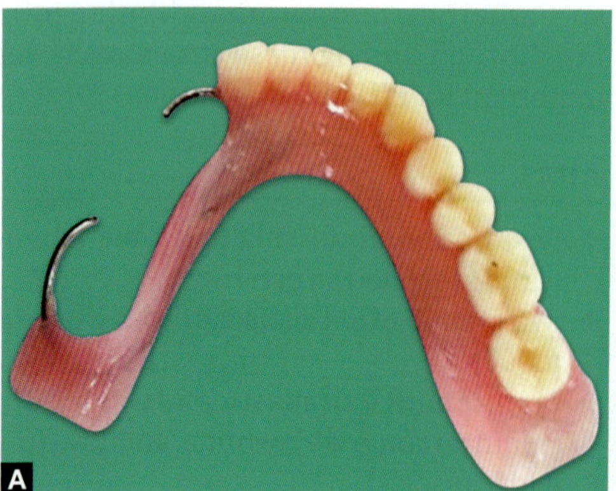

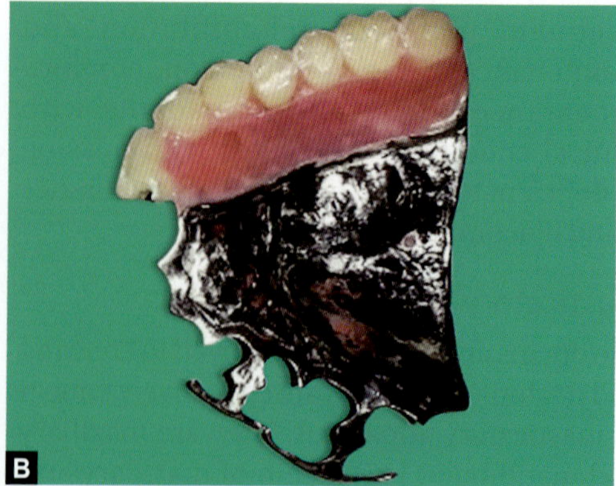

Figs. 1.1A and B: Removable partial denture.

Flowchart 1.1: Classification and types of prosthesis.

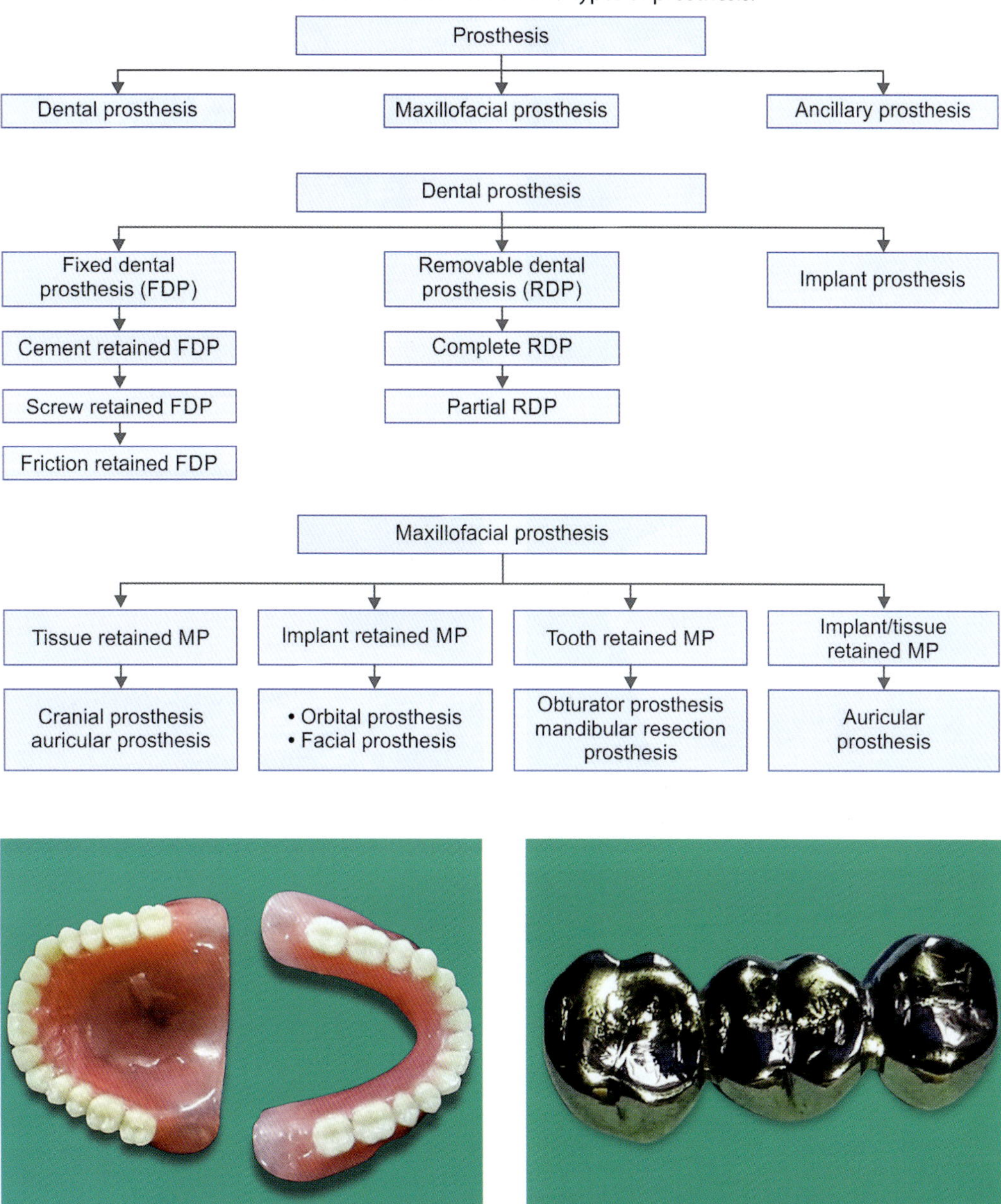

Fig. 1.2: Complete dentures.

Fig. 1.3: All metal fixed partial denture.

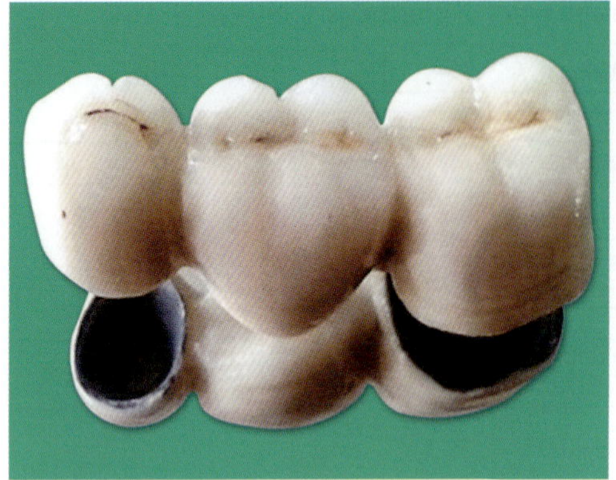

Fig. 1.4: Porcelain fused to metal (PFM) fixed partial denture.

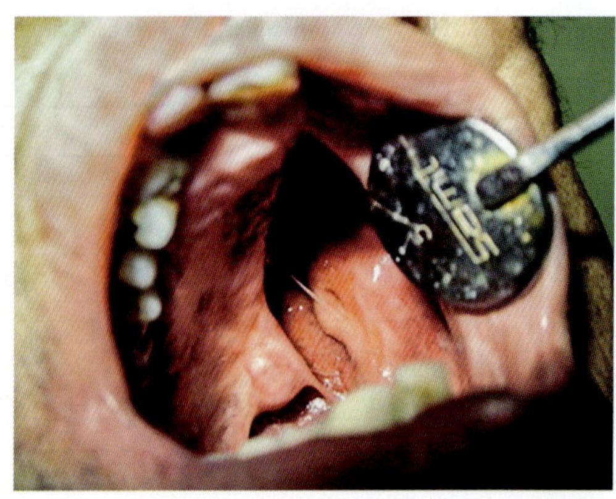

Fig. 1.6: Palatal defect.

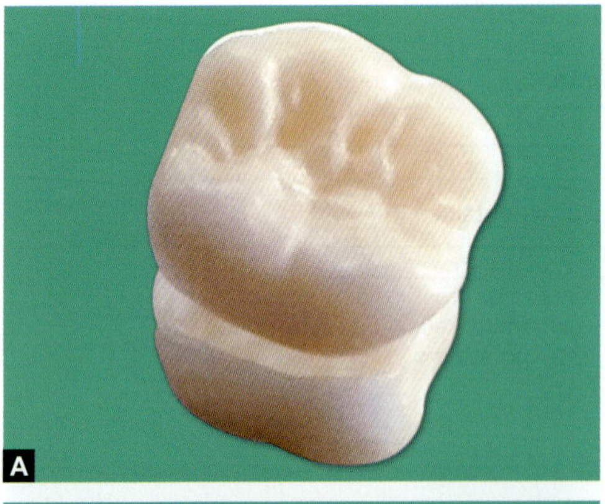

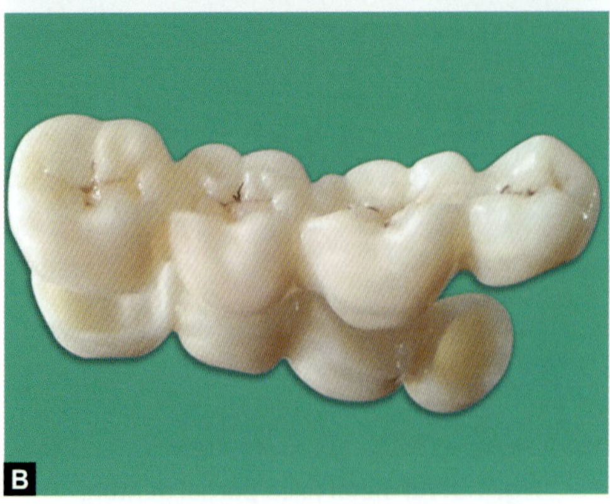

Figs. 1.5A and B: All ceramic crown and fixed partial denture.

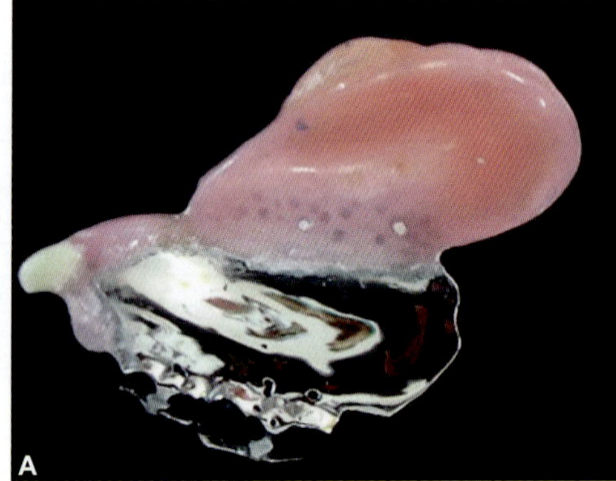

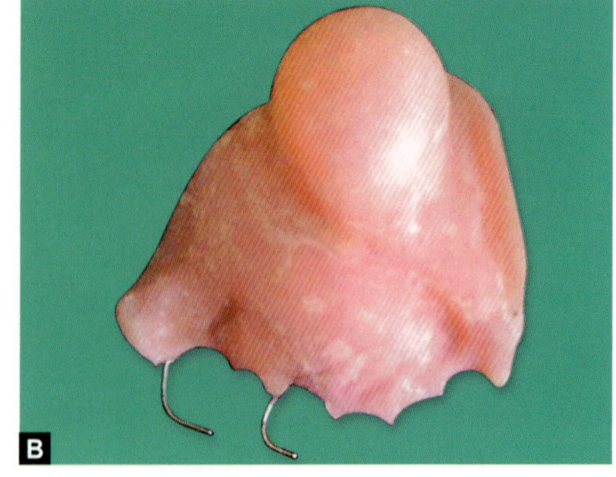

Figs. 1.7A and B: Obturator.

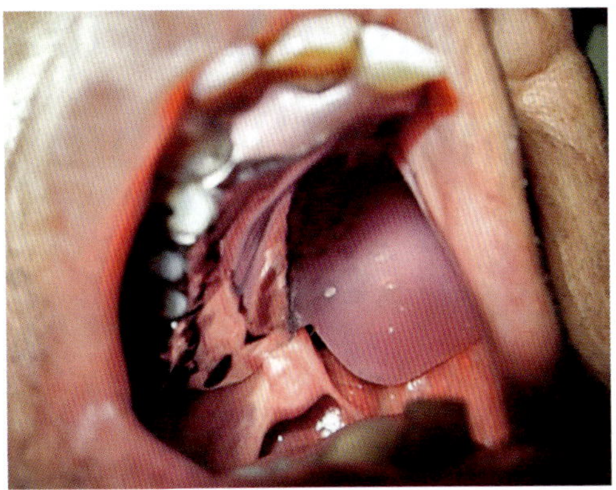

Fig. 1.8: Obturator in oral cavity.

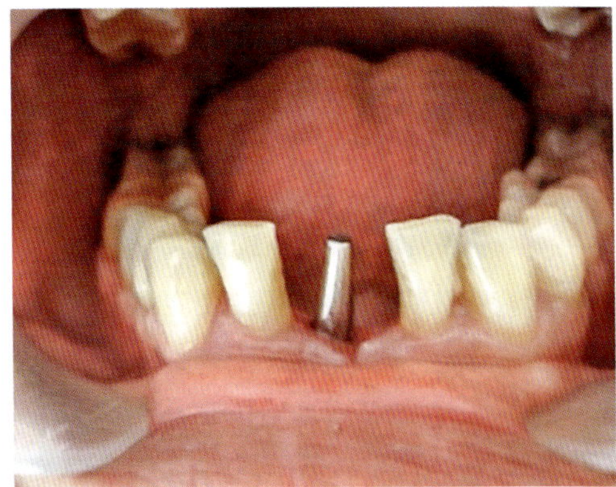

Fig. 1.10: Implant placed in mandibular anterior region.

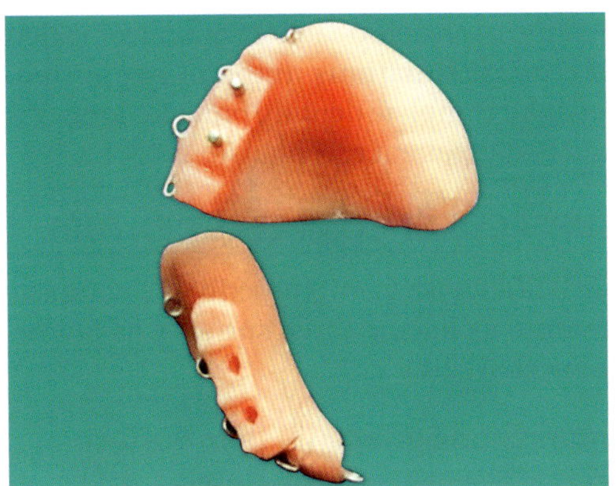

Fig. 1.9: Gunning splint.

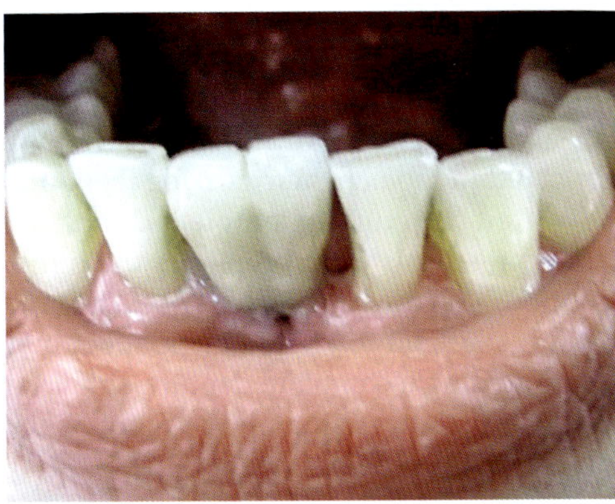

Fig. 1.11: Prosthesis retained by implant.

Introduction to Complete Denture

Sneha Kulkarni, Paranjay Prajapati

INTRODUCTION

Patients with no teeth in the oral cavity are known as completely edentulous patients. For such patients complete dentures are fabricated to replace their missing teeth and associated structures. Complete denture is dental prosthesis which replaces the entire dentition. They are usually set of maxillary and mandibular dentures. Sometime patient may need only single complete denture either for maxillary arch or for mandibular arch when only one arch is edentulous.

DEFINITION

Complete Denture

A removable dental prosthesis that replaces the entire dentition and associated structures of the maxillae or mandible.

Aim and Scope of Complete Denture

Complete denture replaces all the missing teeth in oral cavity and restores the function. Large number of world population is edentulous and facing difficulties in chewing and maintenance of general health due to poor nutrition. Complete denture fabrication involves several steps which are crucial for successful treatment. Various complete denture occlusal schemes and concepts make the complete denture a versatile treatment option for variety of clinical situations. Implant supported/retained complete denture provides longevity and better patient acceptance.

SURFACES OF COMPLETE DENTURE

Sir Wilfred Fish (1948) described a complete denture as having three surfaces as follows (**Flowchart 2.1**):

Impression Surface/Intaglio Surface

The portion of the denture surface that has its contour determined by the impression. This surface of complete denture is in contact with foundation area. Fit of denture depends on accuracy of impression surface. It contributes to retention, stability, support, and comfort of prosthesis **(Fig. 2.1)**.

Flowchart 2.1: Surfaces of complete denture.

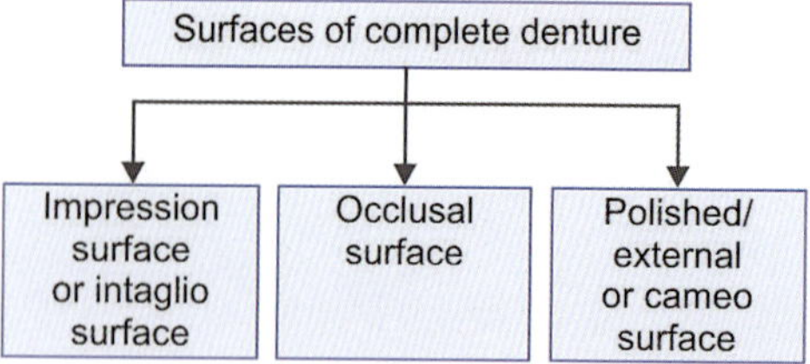

Occlusal Surface

It is occluding surface of denture which establishes contact with opposite denture while chewing and swallowing. This is actually occluding surfaces of artificial teeth of denture. It helps in mastication and directs the masticatory forces to edentulous foundation **(Fig. 2.2)**.

Polished Surface/External Surface/ Cameo Surface

The external surface of the denture which is typically polished and includes buccal, lingual, and labial surface of artificial teeth. This surface of denture is in contact with mucosa of cheek, lips, and tongue. It contributes in retention and stability of the denture **(Figs. 2.3 and 2.4)**.

PARTS OF A COMPLETE DENTURE

Complete denture has four parts in **Flowchart 2.2**.

Denture Base

That part of denture which rest on foundation area (residual alveolar ridge) and stabilize the denture on the foundation. It helps in distribution of masticatory forces over

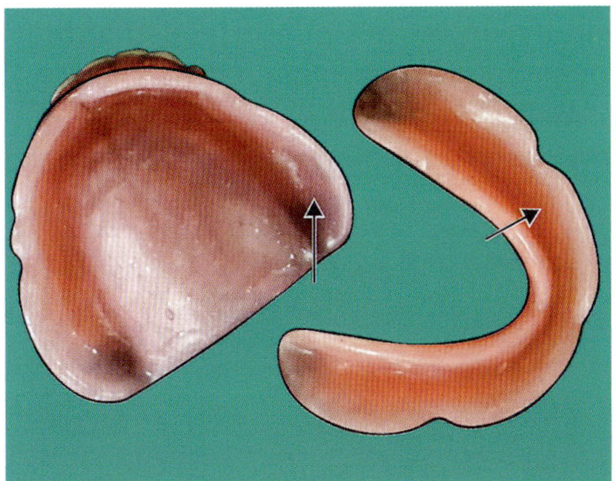

Fig. 2.1: Impression surface of maxillary and mandibular dentures.

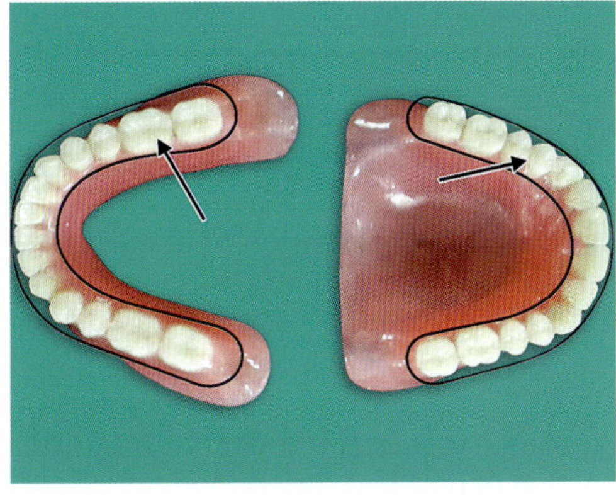

Fig. 2.2: Occlusal surface of denture.

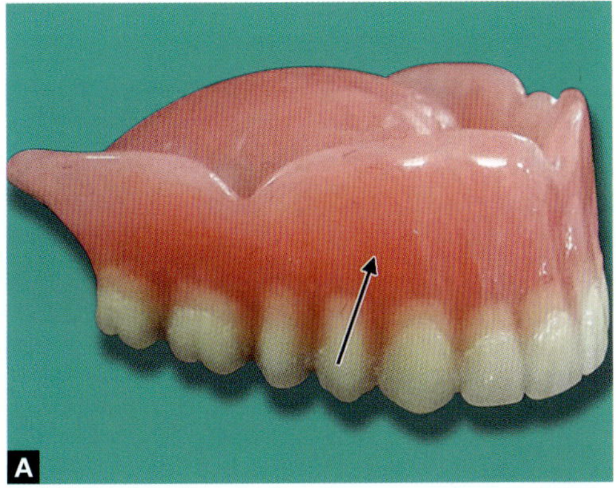

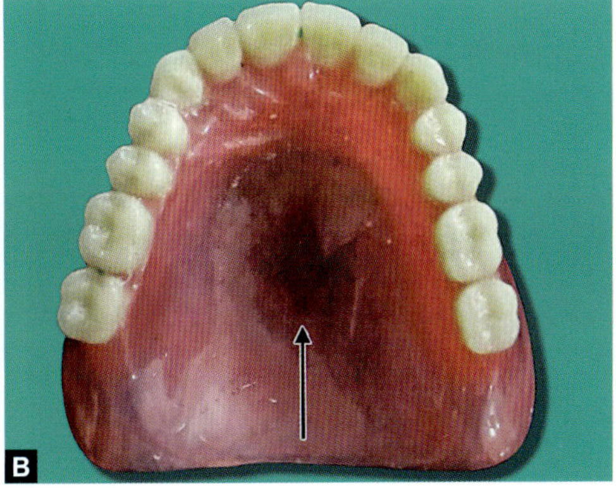

Figs. 2.3A and B: Polished surface of maxillary denture.

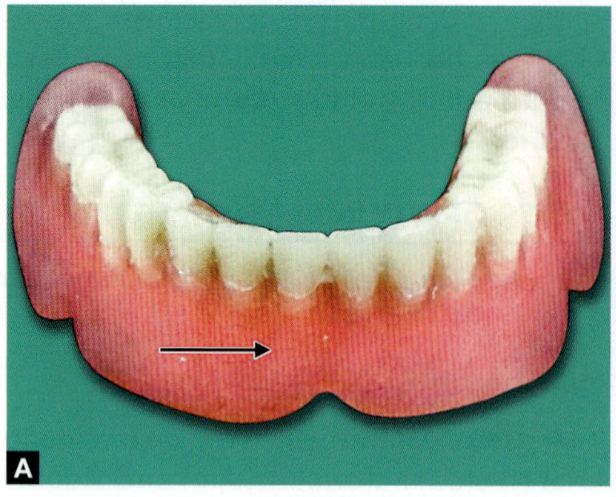

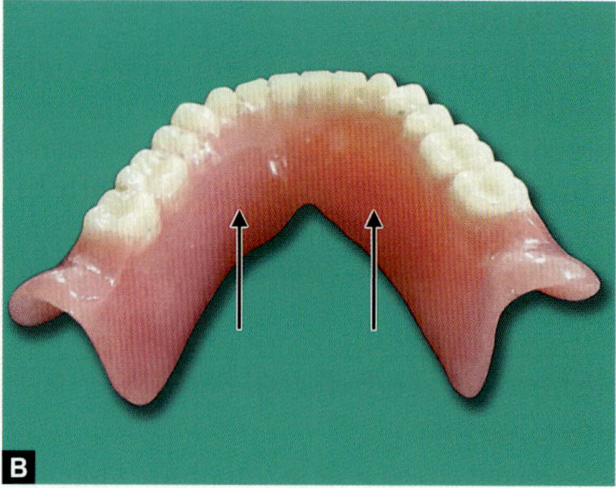

Figs. 2.4A and B: Polished surface of mandibular denture.

Flowchart 2.2: Parts of a complete denture.

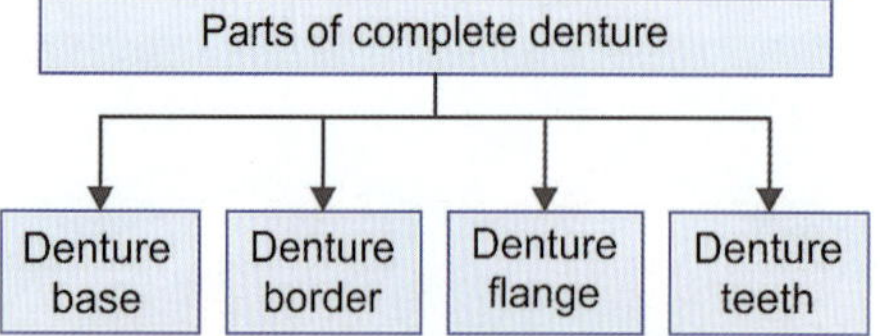

foundation area. Extension of denture base determines retention and support for the prosthesis **(Fig. 2.5)**.

Denture Borders

The margin (border) of the denture base at the junction of polished surface and impression surface. They are responsible for peripheral seal and retention of complete denture. If border is overextended, it may cause ulceration and hyperplasia. Underextended borders compromise the retention and peripheral seal **(Figs. 2.6A and B)**.

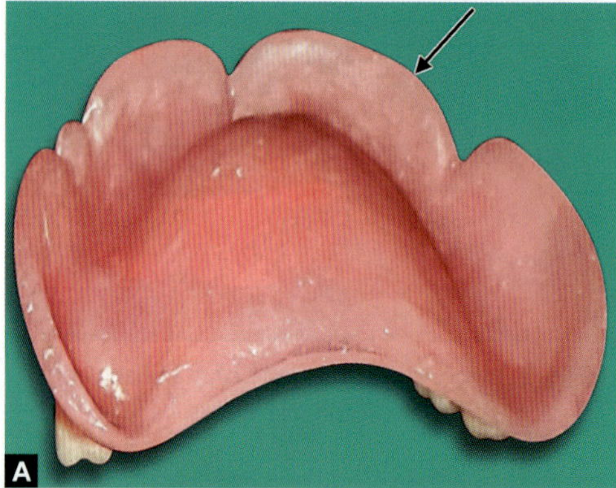

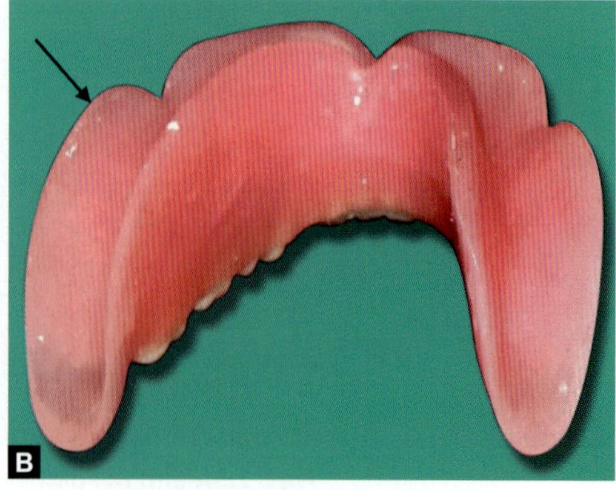

Figs. 2.6A and B: Denture borders.

Fig. 2.5: Denture base of maxillary and mandibular dentures.

Denture Flange

Part of the denture base that extends from the cervical ends of the teeth to the denture border. It contributes in denture stability. It is classified according to the matching vestibule.

Labial Flange

The portion of denture flange which extends in labial vestibule. It provides lip support and aids in esthetic. A notch is created in the midline to house the labial frenum **(Figs. 2.7A and B)**.

Buccal Flange

The portion of denture that extends in buccal vestibule. It provides cheek support. A wide notch is provided for the buccal frenum **(Figs. 2.8A and B)**.

Lingual Flange

It is present only in mandibular denture. It forms the portion of mandibular denture that extends in alveololingual sulcus. A notch is created for relief of lingual frenum. It should be in contact with tissue of oral floor **(Fig. 2.9)**.

Denture Teeth

These are artificial teeth of denture. They are made up of different materials like acrylic, porcelain, interpenetrating polymer network (IPN), composite resin, and metal. They are available in different designs of occlusal surface, i.e., anatomical, semianatomical, and nonanatomical **(Figs. 2.10A and B)**.

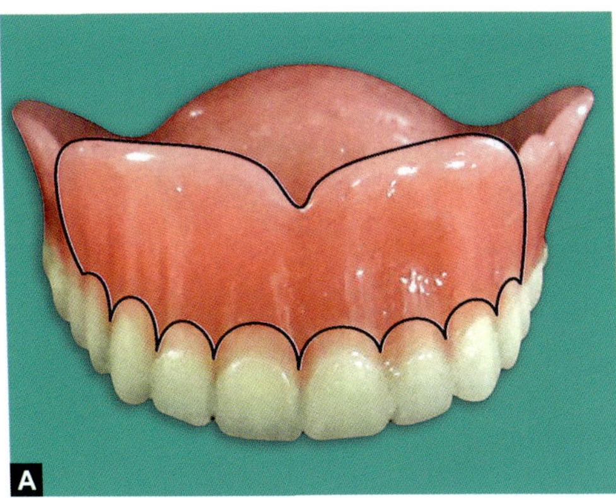

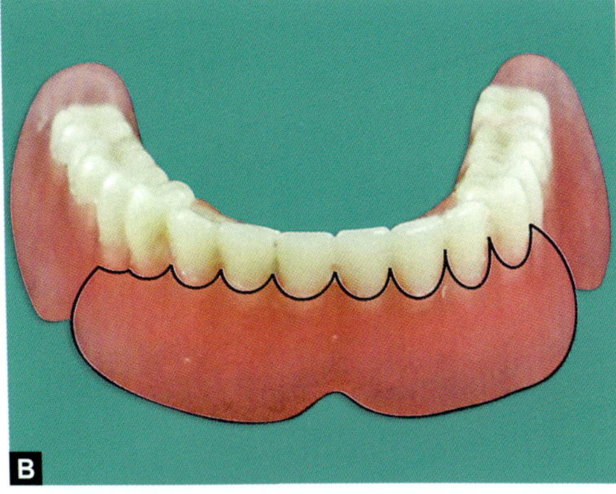

Figs. 2.7A and B: Labial flanges of maxillary and mandibular dentures.

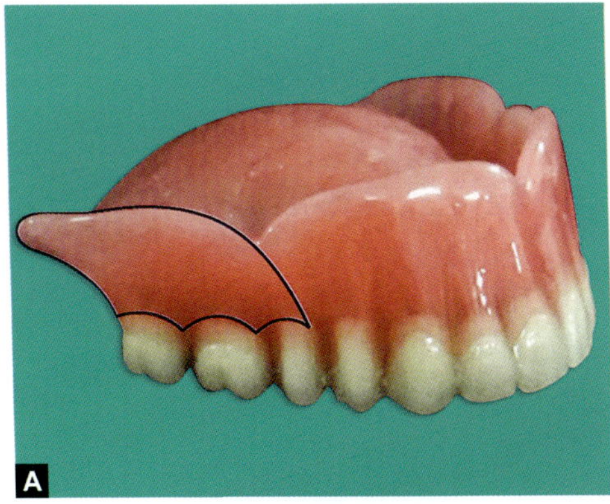

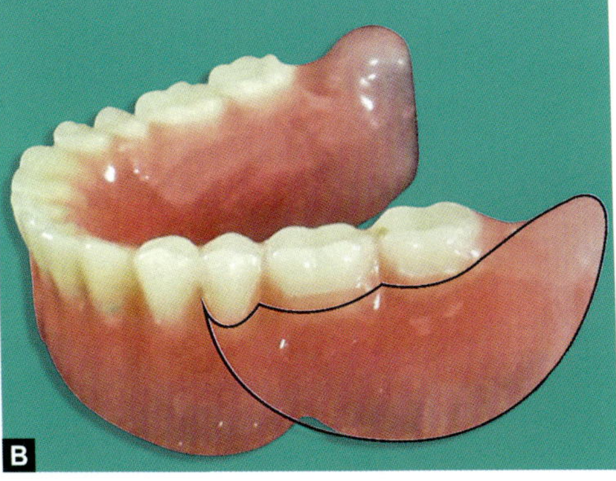

Figs. 2.8A and B: Buccal flanges of maxillary and mandibular dentures.

STEPS IN FABRICATION OF COMPLETE DENTURE

Fabrication of complete denture involves clinical and laboratory steps. The clinical steps and laboratory steps are as given in **Table 2.1**.

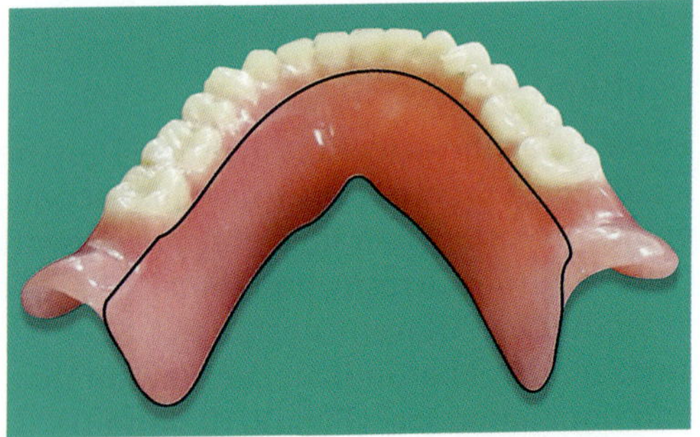

Fig. 2.9: Lingual flange of mandibular denture.

Table 2.1: Clinical and laboratory procedures to fabricate complete denture.

Clinical procedures	*Laboratory procedures*
❑ Diagnosis and treatment planning ❑ Mouth preparation ❑ Primary impression ❑ Final impression ❑ Recording jaw relations ❑ Try-in appointment ❑ Clinical remounting ❑ Denture insertion and postinsertion instructions ❑ Follow-up and maintenance	❑ Making diagnostic casts ❑ Making primary cast ❑ Fabrication of custom tray ❑ Making master cast ❑ Fabrication of occlusal rims ❑ Articulation (mounting) ❑ Arrangement of artificial teeth ❑ Processing of try in denture ❑ Laboratory remounting

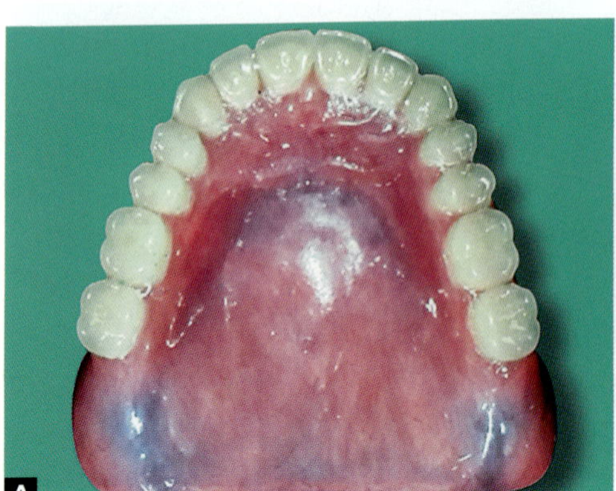

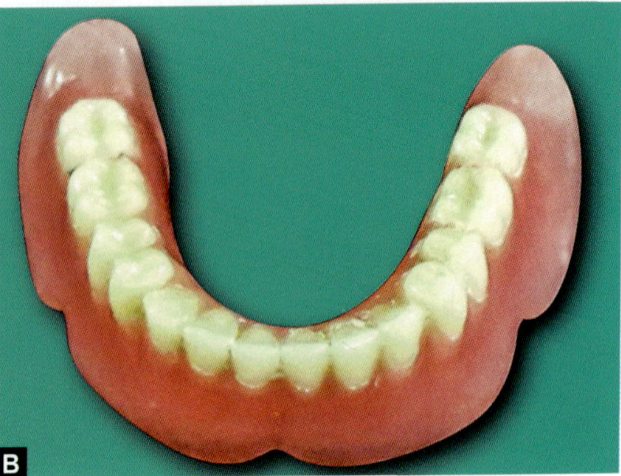

Figs. 2.10A and B: Denture teeth.

CHAPTER 3

Anatomical Landmarks

Paranjay Prajapati, Sneha Kulkarni

INTRODUCTION

A dentist must be aware of orofacial anatomy that is associated with the making of prosthesis before fabricating the prosthesis. This chapter is about the characteristics of anatomical landmarks of maxillary and mandibular denture foundations.

DEFINITION

Anatomical Landmark

A recognizable anatomic structure used as a point of reference.

OBJECTIVES OF KNOWING THE ANATOMIC LANDMARKS

- To find out the anatomic structures which provide a good denture support
- To know the structures limiting the periphery of dentures
- To ascertain the structures that will permit application of additional pressure
- To ascertain the structures which require relief
- To know vital structures to be taken care during implant placement
- To correlate the anatomic structures with the impression or landmarks produced on denture
- To estimate denture flange extension.

CLASSIFICATION

Anatomical landmarks are classified into three categories:

Supporting Structures (Stress Bearing Areas)

Support is resistance to vertical forces of mastication and to occlusal or other forces applied in a direction toward the denture foundation. The areas of support are divided into primary stress bearing areas (primary supporting area) and secondary stress bearing area (secondary supporting area).

Primary Stress Bearing Areas (Primary Supporting Areas)

Areas of edentulous ridges that are at right angles to occlusal forces and usually do not resorb easily. These areas are lined with grayish pink mucosa which is dense, keratinized and have minimal vascularity.

Secondary Stress Bearing Areas (Secondary Supporting Areas)

Areas of edentulous ridge that are at greater than right angles to occlusal forces or are parallel to them; also, areas of edentulous ridges that are at right angles to occlusal forces but tends to resorb under load, e.g., anterior ridge and ridge slopes. They appear deep pink due to increased vascularity.

Valve Producing Structures (Limiting Structures)

It is important to know the structures that will limit the extension of the dentures. The dentures should extend as far as possible within the limits of physiological health and function of the tissues and structures that surround and support them.

Relief Areas

Along with supporting and limiting areas some areas which cannot take up masticatory loads should be relieved. These areas are relieved due to presence of vital anatomical structures in that part of denture foundation, or bone and soft tissue is not of that quality which can withstand the masticatory force.

Anatomical Landmarks: Edentulous Maxillary Arch

Paranjay Prajapati, Sneha Kulkarni

INTRODUCTION

Maxillary landmarks are divided into three categories as supporting areas (stress bearing area), valve forming areas (limiting areas), and relief areas. All landmarks are discussed in this chapter with their anatomical position, identification, and clinical significance. Each landmark is shown on dental cast as well as in oral cavity for easy identification.

CLASSIFICATION

Supporting Areas (Stress Bearing Areas)

Primary Supporting Areas (Primary Stress Bearing Areas)

- Hard palate (on either side of palatal raphe)
- Firm maxillary tuberosity.

Secondary Supporting Areas (Secondary Stress Bearing Areas)

- Palatine rugae
- Maxillary alveolar ridge.

Valve Forming Areas (Limiting Areas)

- Labial frenum
- Labial vestibule
- Buccal frenum
- Buccal vestibule
- Hamular notch
- Posterior palatal seal area
- Coronomaxillary pouch.

Relief Areas

- Mid palatine raphe
- Incisive papilla
- Torus palatinus*
- Canine eminence*
- Bony protuberance on alveolar ridge*
- Opening of greater palatine foramen in severely resorbed cases.*

PRIMARY STRESS BEARING AREAS (PRIMARY SUPPORTING AREAS)

Hard Palate

The horizontal portion of the palate lateral to midline is primary stress bearing area. Trabecular pattern in the bone is perpendicular to the direction of force thus withstanding masticatory force. Serve as main supporting area for maxillary denture **(Figs. 4.1A and B)**.

*These structures are bony prominences or foramen opening which should be relieved to prevent discomfort to patient. You may not come across with these structures in each and every case of edentulous patient. Wherever needed provide relief accordingly.

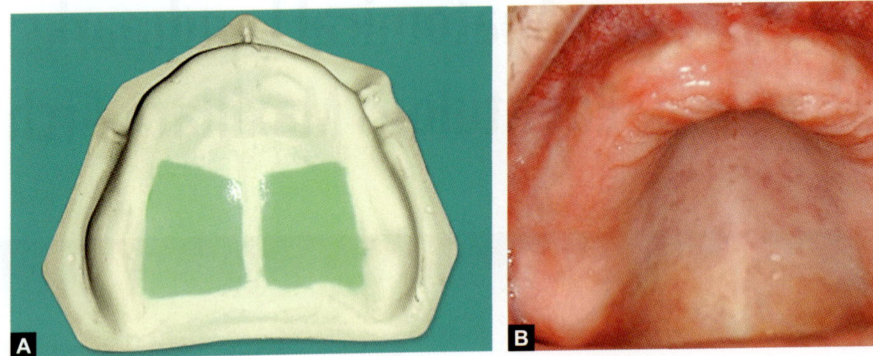

Figs. 4.1A and B: Hard palate.

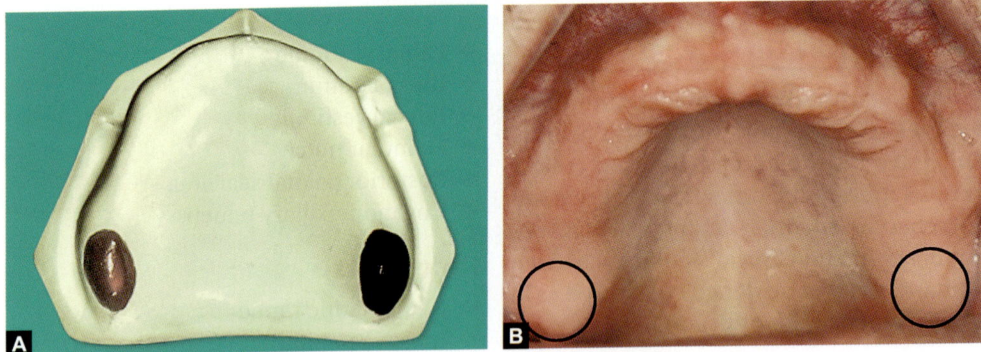

Figs. 4.2A and B: Maxillary tuberosity.

Maxillary Tuberosity (Figs. 4.2A and B)

This is bulbous extension of residual ridge in last molar region. It is covered with dense fibrous connective tissue which has minimal compressibility. Sometimes they show overgrowth and need surgical correction before fabrication of denture. Considered as primary stress bearing area as resorption in this area is very less.

SECONDARY STRESS BEARING AREAS (SECONDARY SUPPORTING AREAS)

Palatine Rugae (Figs. 4.3A and B)

Mucosal folds located in the anterior region of palatal mucosa. It is firmly attached to the bone and is keratinized. These folds are important for proper speech. They should not be distorted during impression making. They should be reproduced in denture. Rugae area is covered with mucosal folds and established at an angle with residual alveolar ridge, these two features prevent anterior displacement of denture hence considered as secondary stress bearing area.

Residual Alveolar Ridge

Portion of alveolus remaining after loss of teeth is called residual alveolar ridge. Alveolar ridge has firmly attached mucosa over it which is resilient enough to support denture. Mainly the posterolateral portion of residual ridge is the primary stress bearing area **(Figs. 4.4A and B)**.

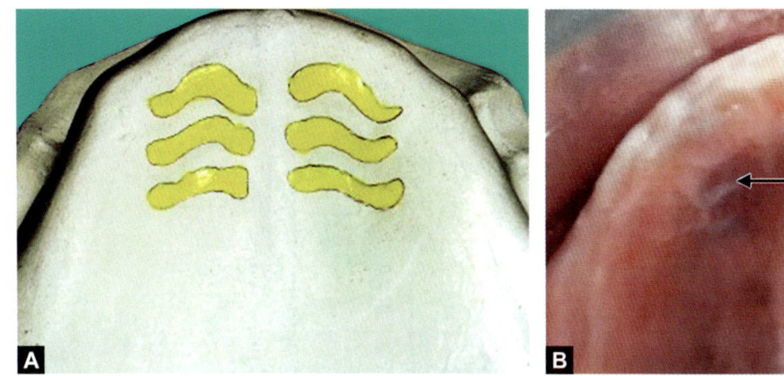
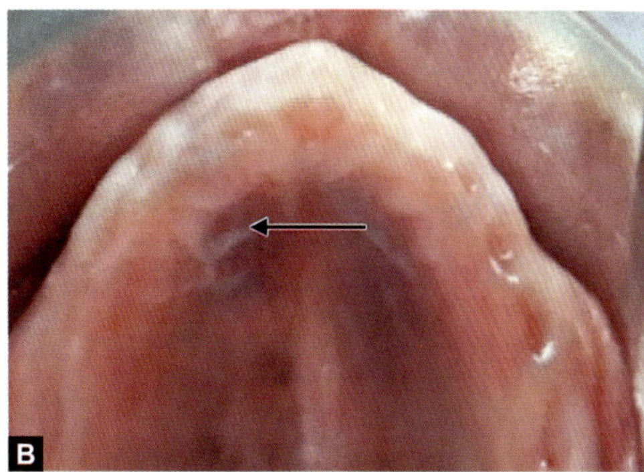

Figs. 4.3A and B: Palatine rugae.

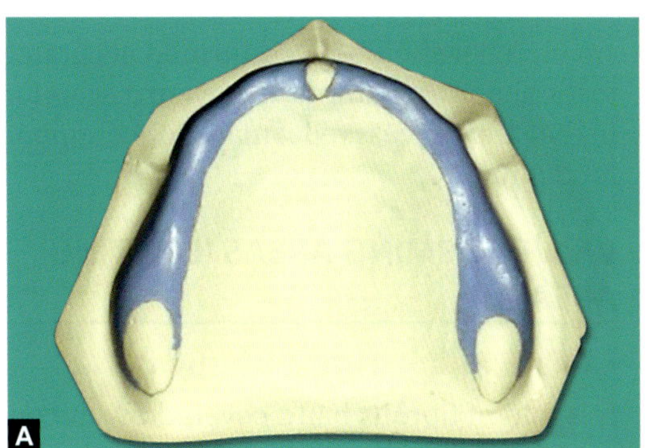
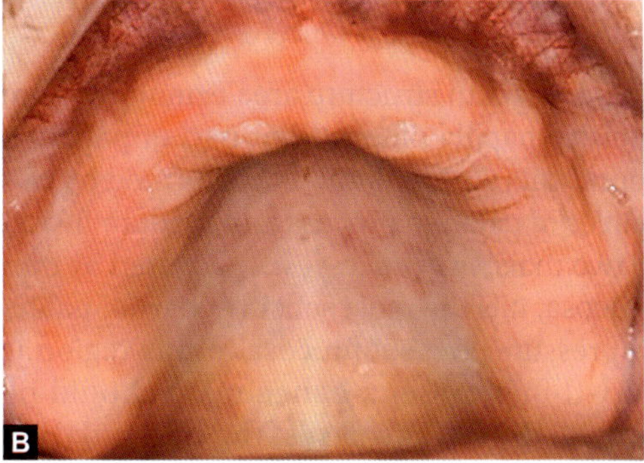

Figs. 4.4A and B: Posterior lateral slopes of residual alveolar ridge.

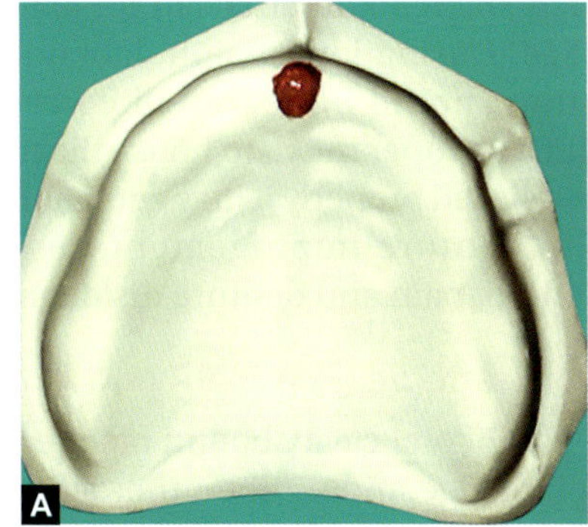
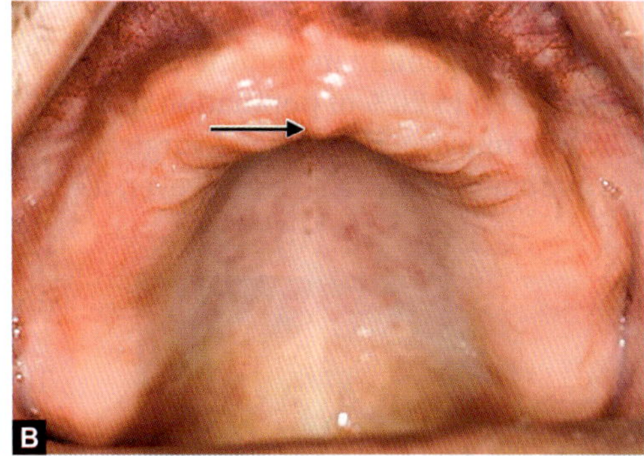

Figs. 4.5A and B: Incisive papilla.

RELIEF AREAS

Incisive Papilla (Figs. 4.5A and B)

It is a pad of fibrous connective tissue. It is located on midline (8–10 mm) behind the maxillary central incisor and so serves as guide during teeth arrangement. It covers incisive foramen which is exit point of nasopalatine nerve and vessels. If not relieved, the denture will compress the vessels and nerve and may lead to pressure ischemia and necrosis of distributing area and paresthesia of anterior palate.

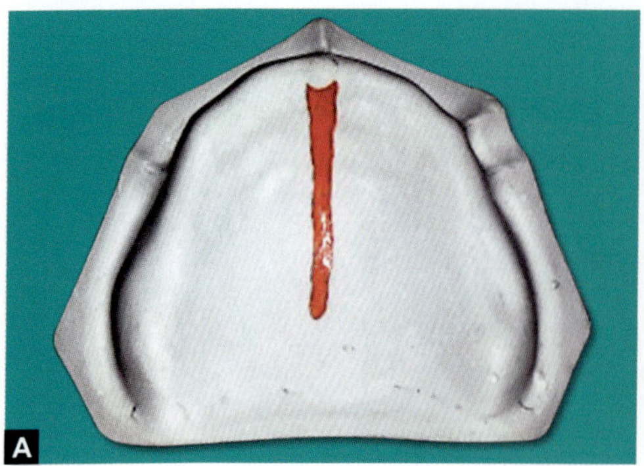

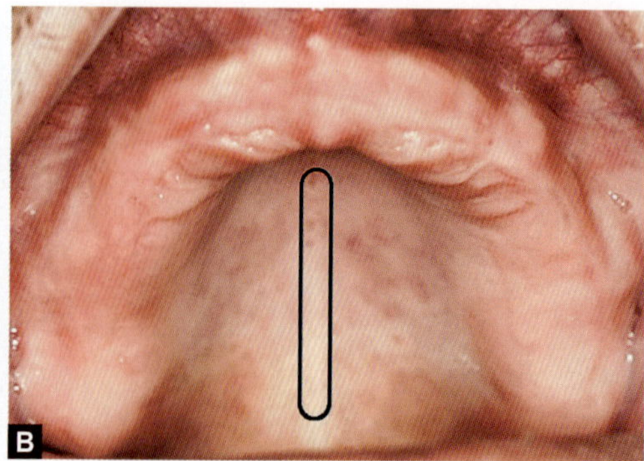

Figs. 4.6A and B: Median palatine raphe.

Median Palatine Raphe (Figs. 4.6A and B)

This is median structure area extending from incisive papilla till posterior part of palate. It represents area of bony suture formed by two halves of palatine process and median fusion of two maxillary processes. As covered by thin mucosa, it is the most sensitive part of palate to pressure. The submucosa in this region is very thin or absent, hence relief should be provided. In some cases, the mid palatine raphe is prominent.

Torus Palatinus (Fig. 4.7)

It is hard bony enlargement in midline region of palate. It is seen in 20% of population and covered by thin mucosa. It may need surgical removal if extremely large in size. However, if small, relief should be confirmed accurately to the shape of the torus to prevent discomfort in that area. Excess relief may reduce support for denture.

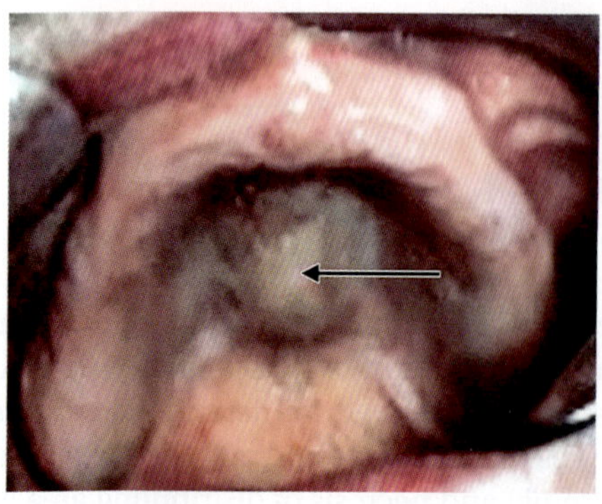

Fig. 4.7: Torus palatinus.

VALVE FORMING AREAS (LIMITING AREAS)

Labial Frenum (Figs. 4.8A and B)

It is fold of fibrous band covered by mucous membrane at the midline. It contains no muscle fiber so performs no particular action. It is fan-shaped and attached on labial side of ridge. During impression, labial frenum position should be recorded correctly to produce a proper notch to house the frenum. If not relieved properly it may get traumatized due to denture impingement, results in ulceration, pain and denture dislodgment.

Labial Vestibule (Figs. 4.9A and B)

That part of oral cavity bound on one side by alveolar ridge and on the other side by lip. Vestibule is covered by nonkeratinized lining mucosa. Submucosa is thick and contains loose areolar tissue and elastic fibers. Labial vestibule extends from labial frenum to buccal frenum (bilaterally). Labial flange corresponding to labial vestibule provide lip support and aids in peripheral seal.

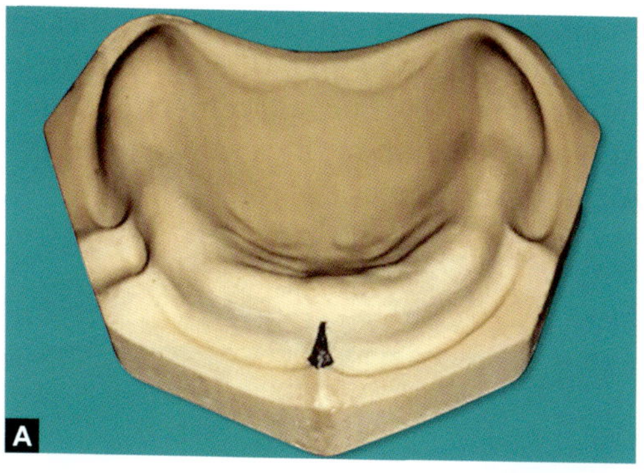
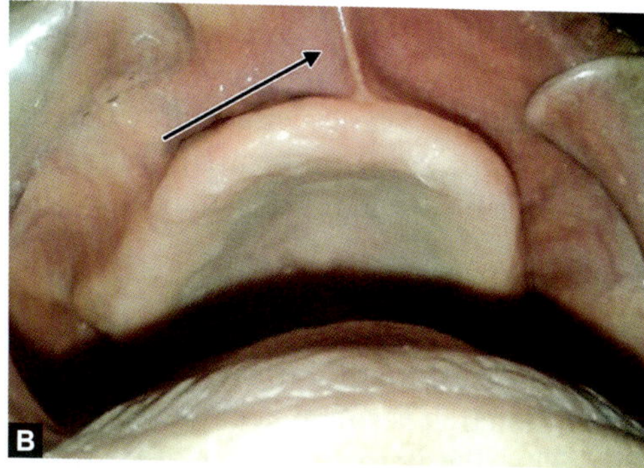

Figs. 4.8A and B: Labial frenum.

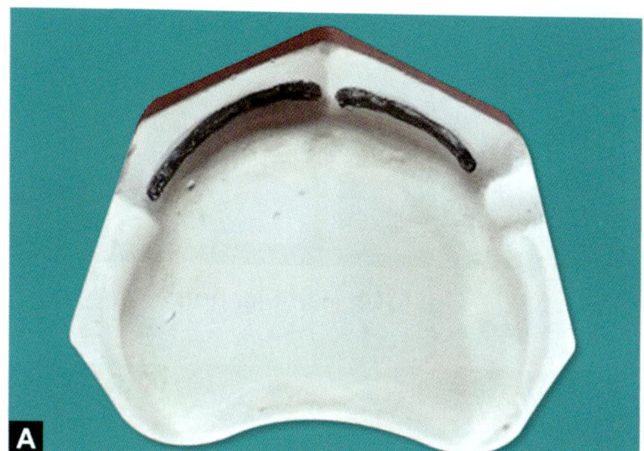
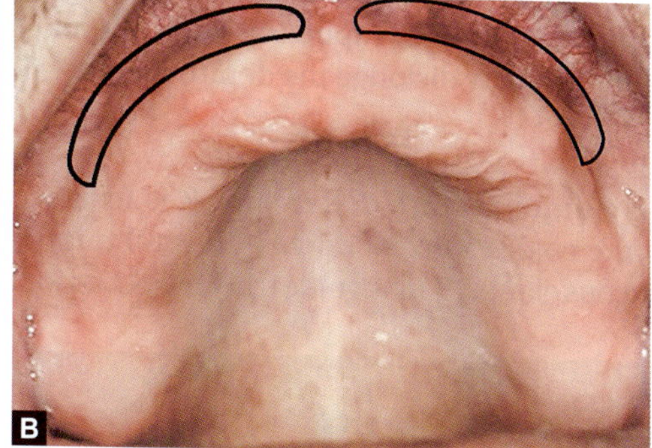

Figs. 4.9A and B: Labial vestibule.

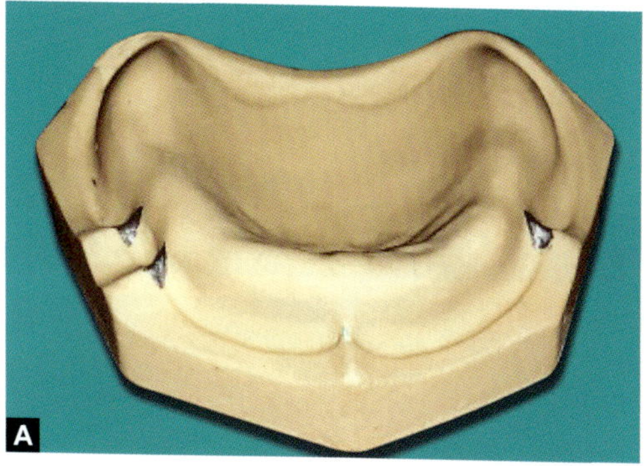
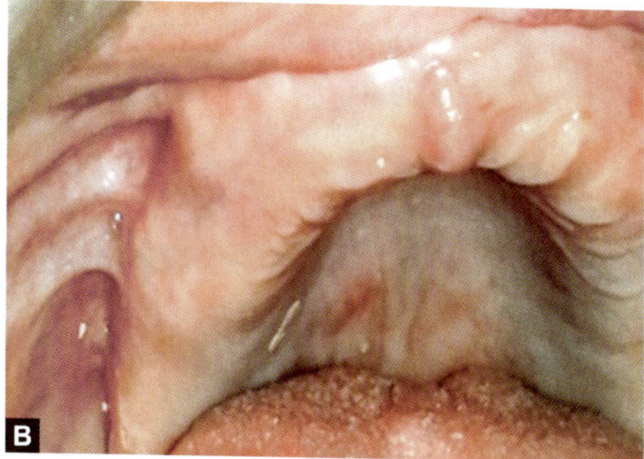

Figs. 4.10A and B: Buccal frenum.

Buccal Frenum (Figs. 4.10A and B)

It divides labial and buccal vestibule. It may be a single or double fold of mucous membrane. It is broad and fan-shaped and moves with muscles during speech and mastication thus active frenum. The muscles attached with it are orbicularis oris (OO), levator anguli oris (LAO), and buccinator (B). Adequate clearance should be provided in denture to allow muscle movements in buccal frenum area without compromising denture retention.

Buccal Vestibule (Figs. 4.11A and B)

It extends from buccal frenum to hamular notch posteriorly. Its size varies with contraction of the buccinator, position of mandible, and amount of bone lost in maxilla in that area.

Hamular Notch (Fig. 4.12)

A depression between the maxillary tuberosity and hamulus of medial pterygoid plate is hamular notch. It is soft area of loose areolar tissue. The distolateral border of denture rests in the hamular notch. If denture is over extended in this area, the forward pulling of pterygomandibular raphe (on wide opening of mouth) may dislodge the denture.

Fovea Palatine (Figs. 4.13A and B)

It is unique feature of humans. It is formed by the coalescence of ducts of several minor mucous glands. It may guide to locate posterior border of denture. In patient with thick and ropy saliva, fovea palatine should be left relieved to prevent displacement of denture due to collection of thick saliva in between denture and mucosa.

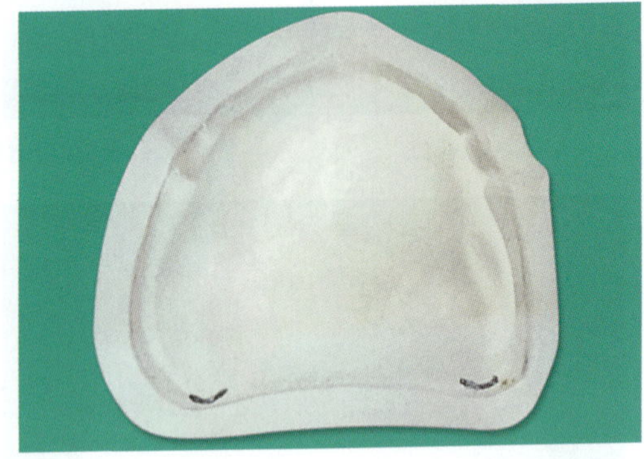

Fig. 4.12: Hamular notch.

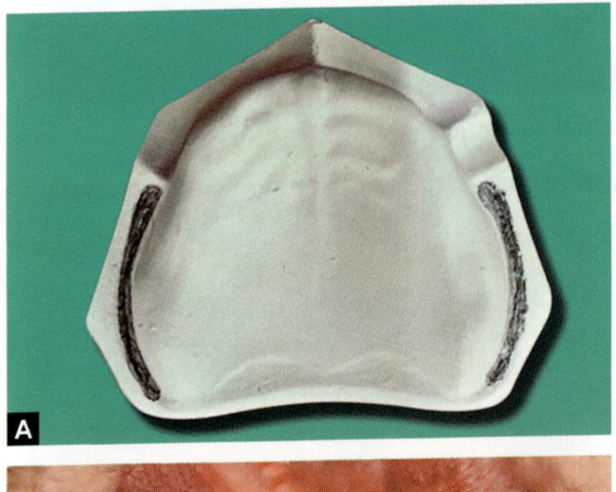

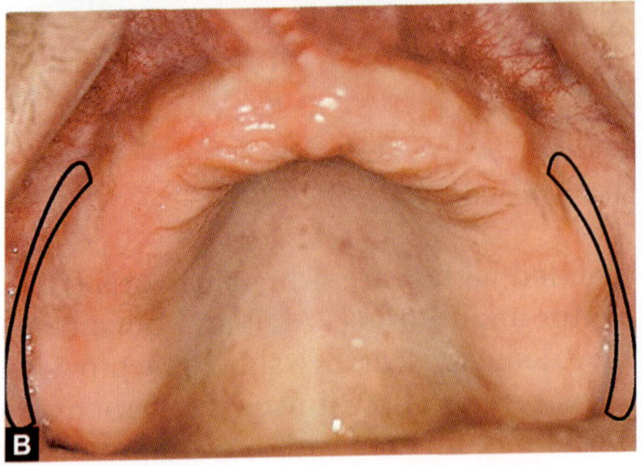

Figs. 4.11A and B: Buccal vestibule.

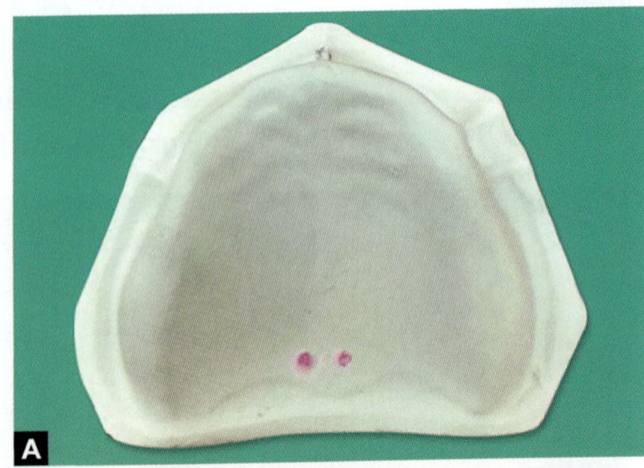

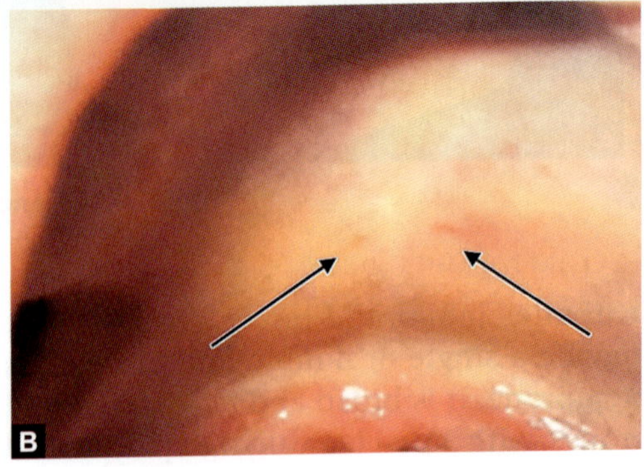

Figs. 4.13A and B: Fovea palatine.

Posterior Palatal Seal Area (Box 4.1)

It is junction of hard and soft palate on which pressure within physiological limits can be applied by denture to aid in its retention. It is area bounded anteriorly and posteriorly by two imaginary lines namely anterior vibrating line and posterior vibrating line **(Fig. 4.14)**.

Anterior vibrating line can be located by asking patient to perform *Valsalva maneuver*. Close patients' nostrils and ask him to blow slowly through nose, look at the posterior part of the palate you can see elevation of mucosa in cupid bow shape. This elevation is attachment of soft tissue with palatal bone indicating anterior vibrating line. From this point soft palate start its movements but in very slow burst (rhythms) **(Fig. 4.15)**.

Box 4.1: Boundaries of posterior palatal seal area.

- Anteriorly by anterior vibrating line
- Posteriorly by posterior vibrating line
- Medially from one tuberosity to the other
- Laterally extends through the pterygomaxillary notch continuing for 3–4 mm anterolateral approximating the mucogingival junction

As we go even posterior from this line we can observe clear demarcation of areas, i.e., one showing slow movement and the other one is showing vigorous or more movement of soft palate. The demarcation between slow and vigorous movement is done by posterior vibrating line, which runs from one hamular notch to the other one. Posterior vibrating line decides posterior limit of maxillary complete denture **(Fig. 4.16)**. Area bounded by anterior and posterior vibrating lines is posterior palatal seal area **(Fig. 4.17)**.

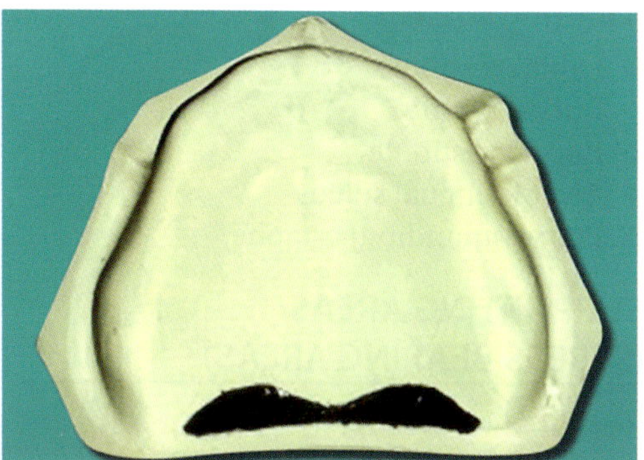

Fig. 4.14: Posterior palatal seal area.

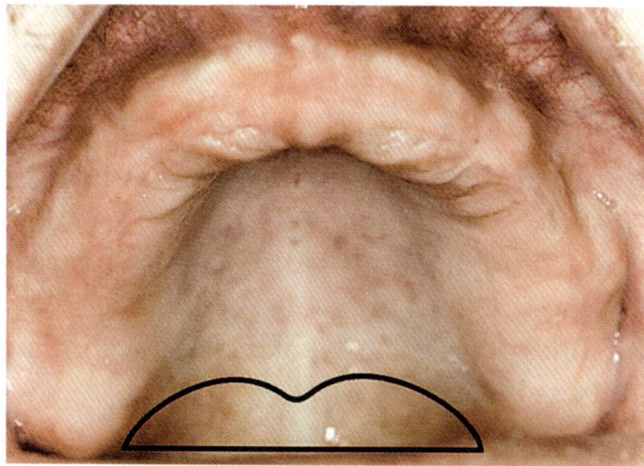

Fig. 4.16: Anterior and posterior vibrating lines.

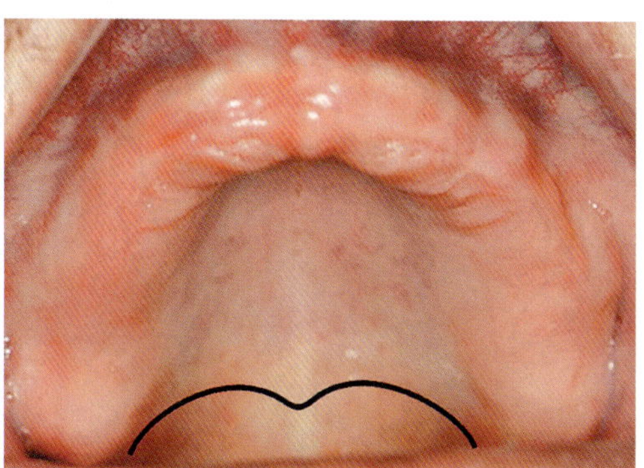

Fig. 4.15: Anterior vibrating line.

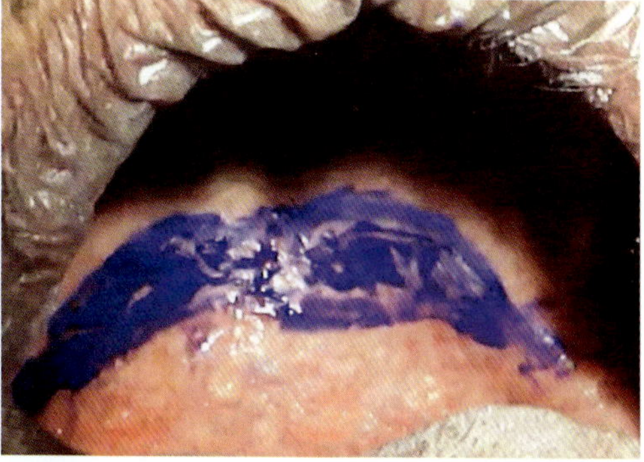

Fig. 4.17: Posterior palatal seal area—intraoral view.

Anatomical Landmarks: Edentulous Mandibular Arch

Paranjay Prajapati, Sneha Kulkarni

INTRODUCTION

Fabrication of complete denture for mandible is different than in maxilla due to presence of movable organs on both the sides, i.e., tongue and cheeks. This chapter deals with various anatomical landmarks of edentulous mandible.

Supporting Areas (Stress Bearing Areas)

- Buccal shelf area (primary stress bearing area)
- Retromolar pad (primary stress bearing area)
- Slopes of residual alveolar ridge (secondary stress bearing area).

Relief Areas

- Crest of residual alveolar ridge
- Mental foramen
- Genial tubercles
- Torus mandibularis
- Sharp mylohyoid ridge.

Valve Forming Structures (Limiting Areas)

- Labial vestibule
- Buccal frenum
- Buccal vestibule
- Alveololingual sulcus
- Pterygomandibular raphe.

SUPPORTING AREAS (STRESS BEARING AREAS)

Buccal Shelf Area (Figs. 5.1A and B)

It is at right angle to masticatory load making it appropriate for primary supporting area. It is made up of cortical bone and firmly attached

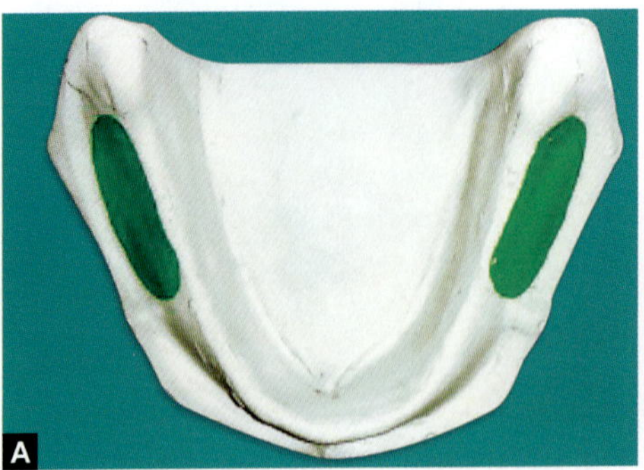

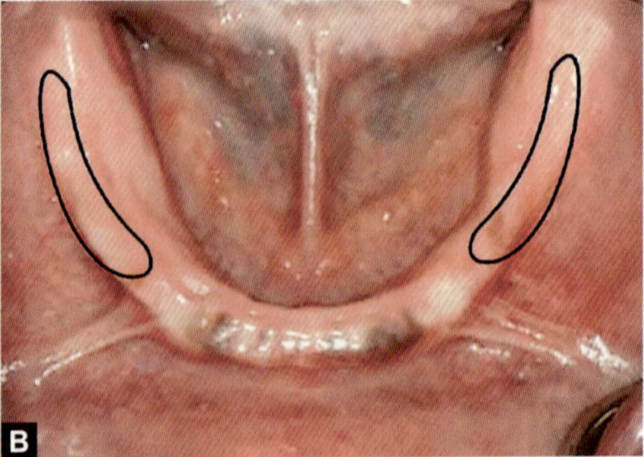

Figs. 5.1A and B: Buccal shelf area.

Box 5.1: Boundary of buccal shelf area.

- Anteriorly—Buccal frenum, posteriorly—retromolar pad
- Medially—Crest of residual alveolar ridge, laterally—external oblique ridge

mucosa with muscle fibers running parallel to the buccal shelf region **(Box 5.1)**.

Retromolar Pad (Figs. 5.2A and B)

It is triangular soft pad of tissue at posterior most end of mandibular edentulous ridge. The mandibular denture should cover the retromolar pad. The underlying bone is dense cortical bone and has muscle attachment to it **(Box 5.2)**. The bone is resistance to resorption in this area makes it stress bearing area. The denture should cover it to get good support.

Box 5.2: Contents of retromolar pad.

- Loose areolar tissue
- Glandular tissue
- Buccally fibers of buccinator muscle
- Lingually fibers of superior constrictor muscle
- Superoposteriorly pterygomandibular raphae
- Tendon of temporalis

Slopes of Residual Alveolar Ridge (Figs. 5.3A and B)

Slopes of residual alveolar ridge provide more support than crest. Both buccal and lingual slopes of mandibular residual ridge are secondary supporting areas. These slopes are made up of thin plate of cortical bone and are at acute angle to masticatory load.

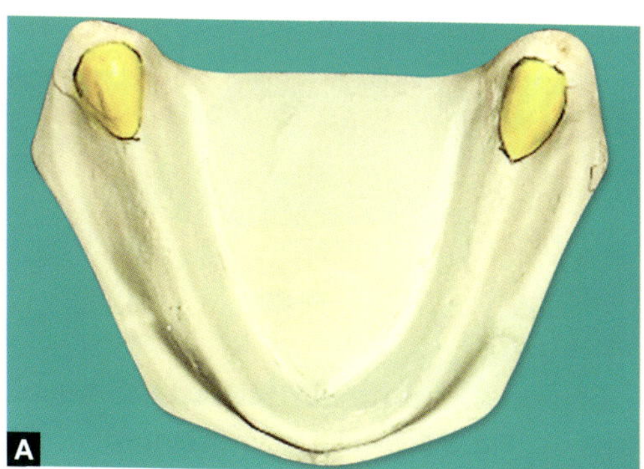

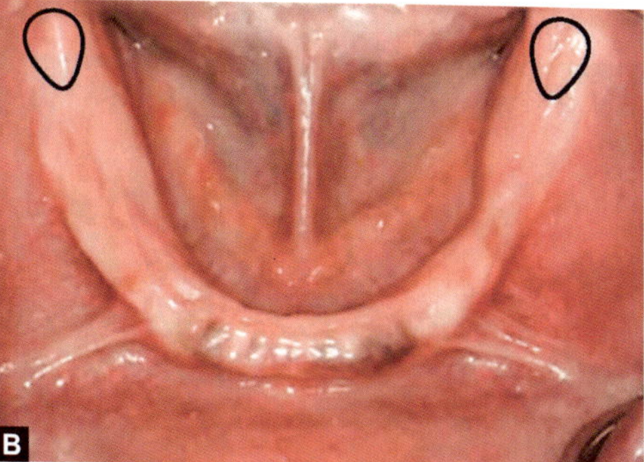

Figs. 5.2A and B: Retromolar pad.

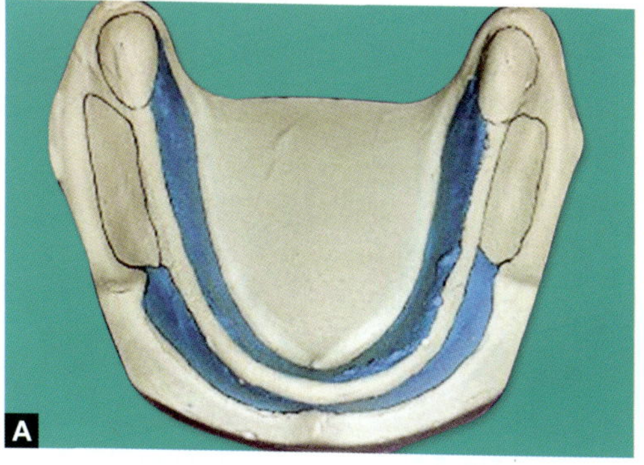

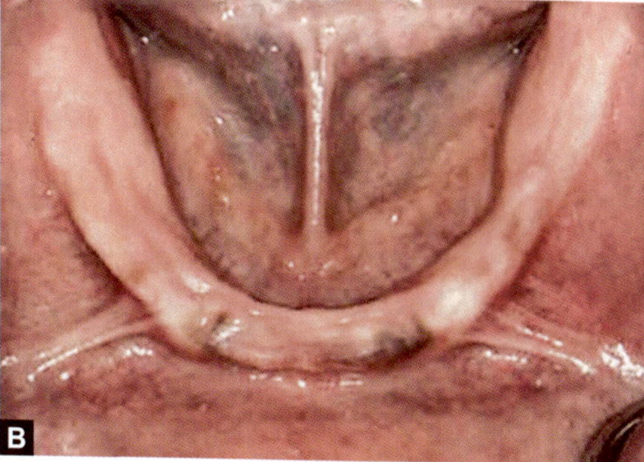

Figs. 5.3A and B: Slopes of residual alveolar ridge.

RELIEF AREAS

Crest of Residual Alveolar Ridge (Figs. 5.4A and B)

This area is relieved because of type of bone present on the crest of mandibular residual alveolar ridge. The bone in this area is cancellous. In spite of submucosa having fibrous connective tissue at the crest, this area cannot bear the masticatory load directly hence considered as relief area. It should be relieved when it is sharp and spiny or knife edge.

Mental Foramen (Fig. 5.5)

It is located between first and second premolars regions (see arrow in figure). Due to excessive ridge resorption it may lies close to crest of residual alveolar ridge. In such cases it should be relieved as pressure over the mental nerve coming out through foramen produces paresthesia in lower lip area see arrow in figure.

Genial Tubercle (Fig. 5.6)

They are small bony protuberance two to three in number. Located lingually near midline area near inferior border of mandible, and serve as attachment for genioglossus and geniohyoid muscles (See arrow in figure). They become prominent in severely resorbed ridge cases, so in such cases relief should be provided to prevent discomfort. However, the denture needs to be extended beyond them to complete the sublingual seal.

Torus Mandibularis (Figs. 5.7A and B)

It is bony prominence located bilaterally lingually near premolar region. Surgical removal is usually indicated. Torus mandibularis is covered with thin mucosa so

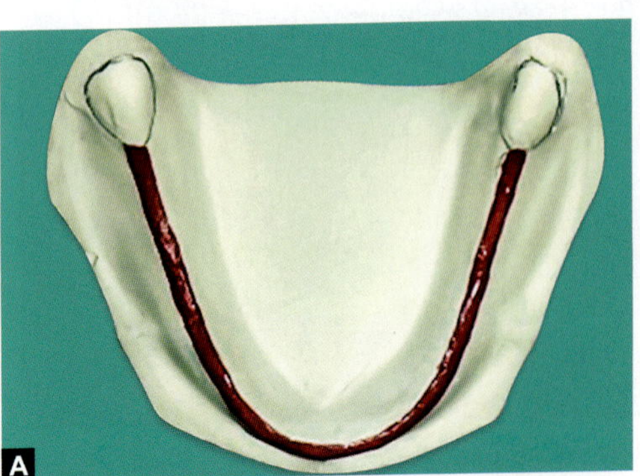

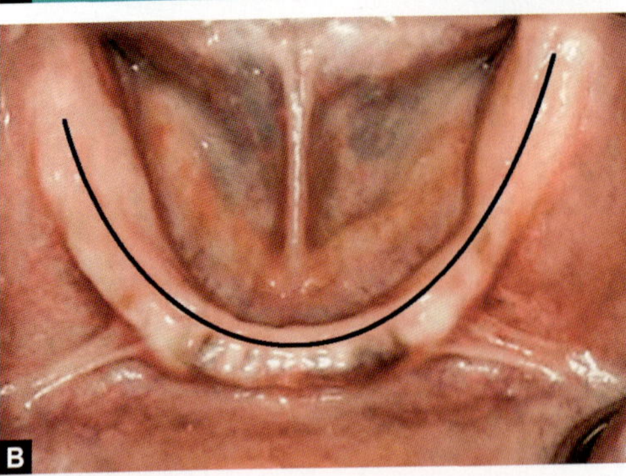

Figs. 5.4A and B: Crest of residual alveolar ridge.

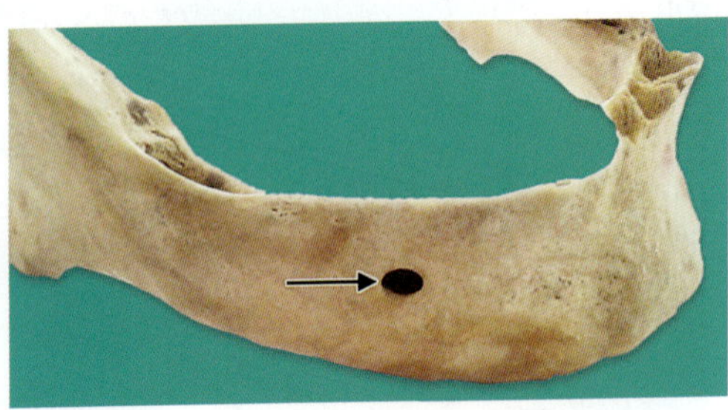

Fig. 5.5: Mental foramen (arrow).

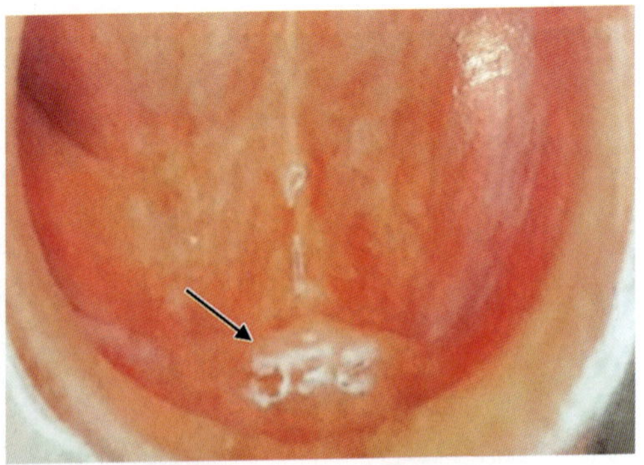

Fig. 5.6: Genial tubercle (arrow).

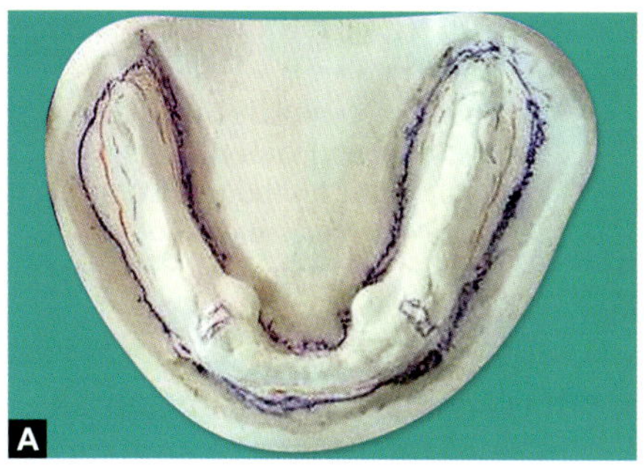
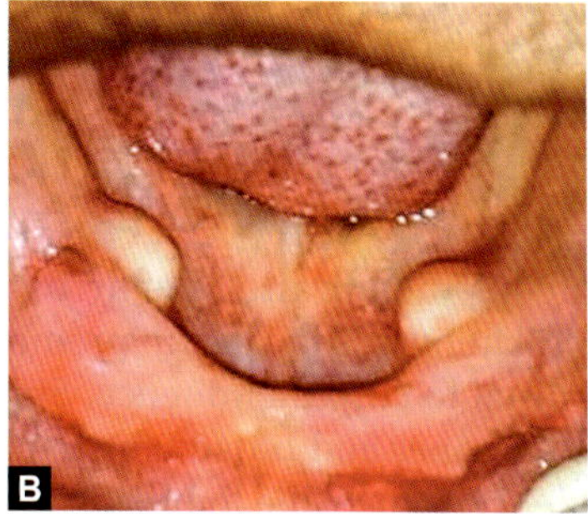

Figs. 5.7A and B: Torus mandibularis.

relief should be provided to prevent soreness in that area. Present only in 20% of population.

VALVE FORMING STRUCTURES (LIMITING AREAS)

Labial Frenum (Figs. 5.8A and B)

It is fold of fibrous band covered by mucous membrane at midline. It has attachment with orbicularis oris. Consider as active frenum. It should be properly housed in denture for enough clearance without compromising the seal.

Labial Vestibule (Figs. 5.9A and B)

It extends from labial frenum to buccal frenum. Overextension of denture in this region causes instability of denture or soreness of mucosa in this region. Muscle attachment in this area is near to the crest of the ridge which limits the extension of denture flange in this area. Recording of proper depth-width and proper

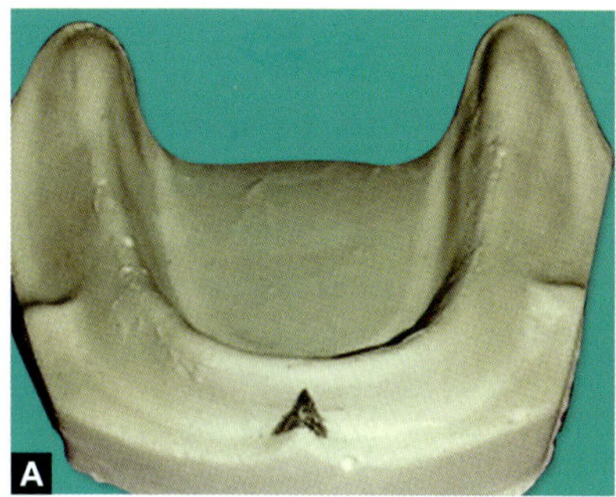
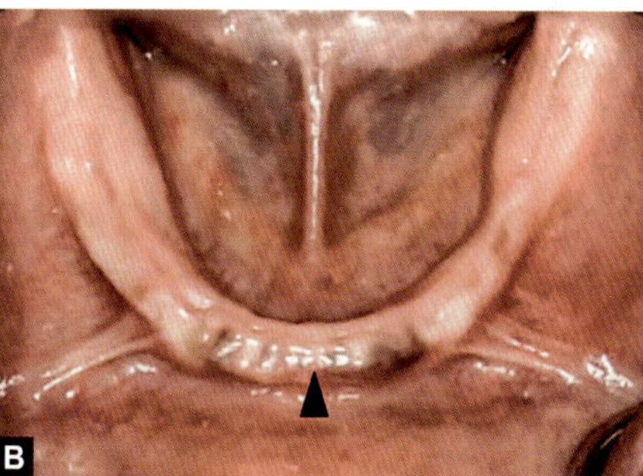

Figs. 5.8A and B: Labial frenum.

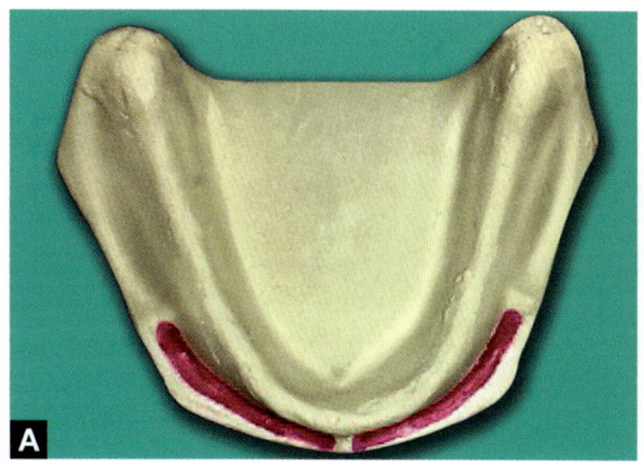
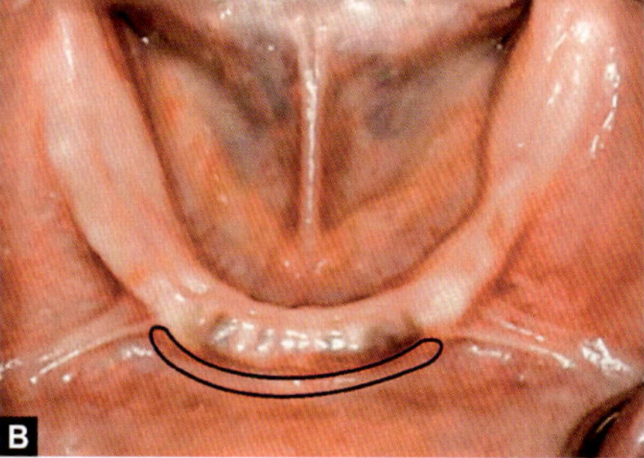

Figs. 5.9A and B: Labial vestibule.

contouring gives best esthetics to patient. Muscles in this region are incisivus, mentalis, and orbicularis oris (Im O).

Buccal Frenum (Figs. 5.10A and B)

Fold of mucous membrane (see arrow in figure). Buccal frenum is located in premolar region just distal to cuspid eminence. Single or double in number and broad fan shaped. It needs wider clearance due to broad shape. Located over depressor anguli oris muscle.

Buccal Vestibule (Figs. 5.11A and B)

It extends posteriorly from buccal frenum to the retromolar pad region bounded by residual alveolar ridge on one side and buccinator on the other side. This space is influenced by action of masseter muscle in the distobuccal border to produce a notch in the denture called as masseteric notch **(Box 5.3)**.

Box 5.3: Masseteric notch.

When masseter muscle contracts it pushes inward against the buccinator muscle producing a bulge into the mouth. It produces a notch in the denture flange called as masseteric notch

Lingual Frenum (Fig. 5.12)

It is a fold of mucous membrane. It attaches base of the tongue to supragenial tubercle (See arrow in figure). It should be registered in function. It usually occurs as a narrow and single band. It is a highly resistant and active frenum. It produces lingual notch in impression. It overlies the genioglossus muscle.

Alveololingual Sulcus (Fig. 5.13)

It is space between tongue and residual alveolar ridge. It extends from lingual frenum

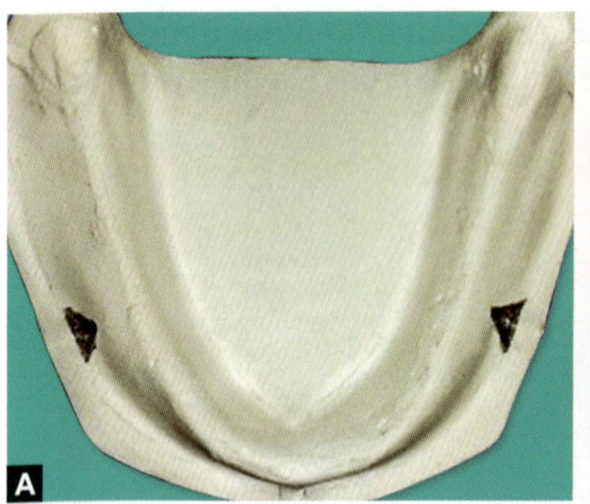

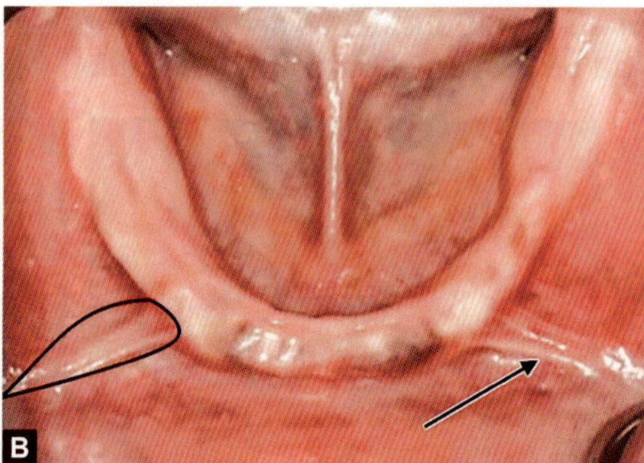

Figs. 5.10A and B: Buccal frenum (arrow).

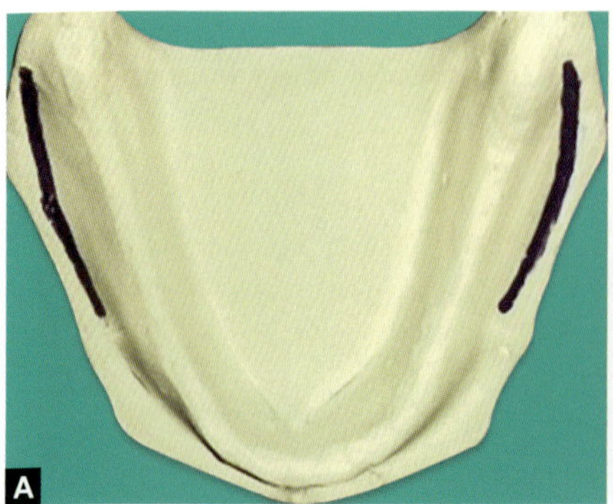

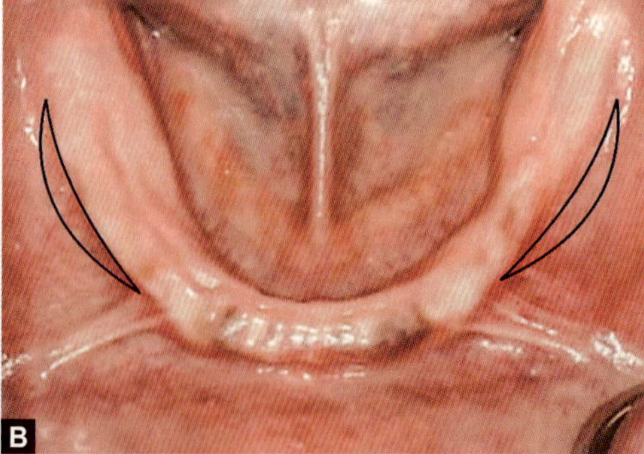

Figs. 5.11A and B: Buccal vestibule.

to retromylohyoid curtain. While making impression, borders of impression should be in contact with the floor of mouth when tongue touches the upper incisor region. Overextension of denture in this region causes soreness or instability.

The alveololingual sulcus can be divided in three parts as shown in **Table 5.1**.

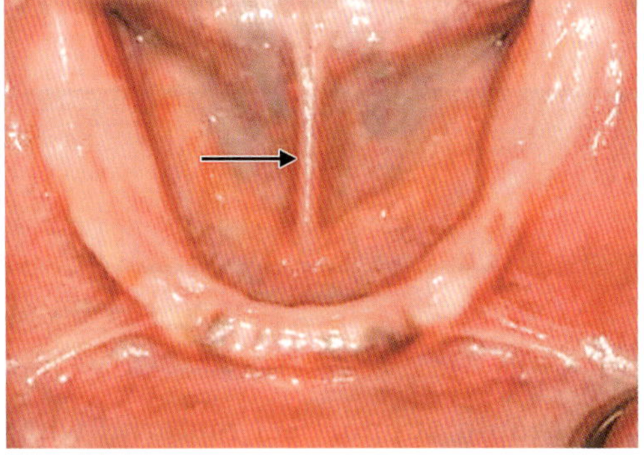

Fig. 5.12: Lingual frenum.

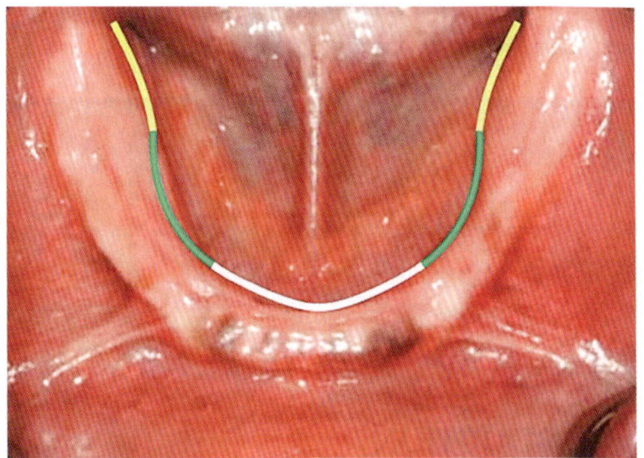

Fig. 5.13: Alveololingual sulcus.

Table 5.1: Three parts of alveololingual sulcus.

Name	*Anterior region*	*Middle region*	*Posterior region*
Synonym	Sublingual crescent area or sublingual fold	Mylohyoid area	Retromylohyoid area
Extension	From lingual frenum to premylohyoid eminence	From premylohyoid fossa to the distal end of mylohyoid ridge	Behind the end of mylohyoid ridge
Significance	❑ Lingual flange is short in this area anteriorly than posteriorly ❑ The lingual flange in this area should be in definite contact with mucosa of floor of the mouth to create peripheral seal	Lingual flange slopes medially toward tongue and extends below mylohyoid ridge to create peripheral seal	❑ Lingual flange passes in retromylohyoid fossa and turns lateral toward the ramus and forms typical "S" shape of lower denture ❑ This area is not influenced by mylohyoid muscle
Impression of area			
Denture base			

CHAPTER 6

Impression Trays

Paranjay Prajapati, Sneha Kulkarni

INTRODUCTION

Impression tray is device which used to carry impression material while making impressions. They are available in various designs and configurations. They are available in predetermined sizes and can be made individualized for particular patient. This chapter presents information on various types of impression trays and their indications.

DEFINITION

Impression Tray

A device used to carry, confine, and control the impression material while making the impression.

IDEAL REQUIREMENTS

- Impression trays must be rigid. Flexible trays cause distortion of the impression.
- It should be dimensionally stable.
- It should provide uniform space for impression material.
- It should be smooth to avoid injury to oral structure (borders and joint of handle and tray).
- It should not distort the tissue in vestibular area.
- It should support set material when removed from mouth so that a cast can be poured.
- If needed, it can be modified by dentist.

CLASSIFICATION

Impression trays can be classified according to their availability, use, and material used to fabricate it.

According to Use

- Stock/prefabricated
- Custom/special tray/individualized tray
- Sectional tray/quadrant tray
- Triple tray.

Stock/Prefabricated Impression Trays

These are available as readymade set of impression trays. They are available in different sizes. The size of stock tray is designated by a number. Stock trays are available for making edentulous and dentulous impressions. They are available as perforated and nonperforated trays. They are available in metal and plastic material. The metal trays can be used several times in different patients after sterilization. Plastic trays are usually of disposable variety. However, autoclavable plastic trays are also available. Stock trays are rigid and dimensionally stable (**Figs. 6.1 to 6.4**).

Custom/Special Tray/Individualized Tray

These trays are specially prepared to be used for a particular patient only and cannot be used for any other patient. It is fabricated on primary cast. It can be fabricated with self-cured polymethyl methacrylate acrylic resin, heat cure polymethyl methacrylate acrylic resin or light cured acrylic resin, thermoplastic resin, and shellac. Most commonly, modified self-cured acrylic resin known as "tray material" is used for fabrication of custom tray. "Tray material" is self-cures polymethyl methacrylate resin modified by adding filler particles. Most commonly added fillers are French chalk or pumice. Custom trays made up of "tray material" have *less polymerization shrinkage, better fit, and adaptation*. Custom trays should be 2 mm short of sulcus as they will be used for border molding procedure. Tray extension can be modified accordingly (**Fig. 6.5**).

Sectional Tray/Quadrant Tray

They are perforated trays made up of plastic or metal. They are available for anterior quadrant, right posterior quadrant, and left posterior quadrant. They are used to make

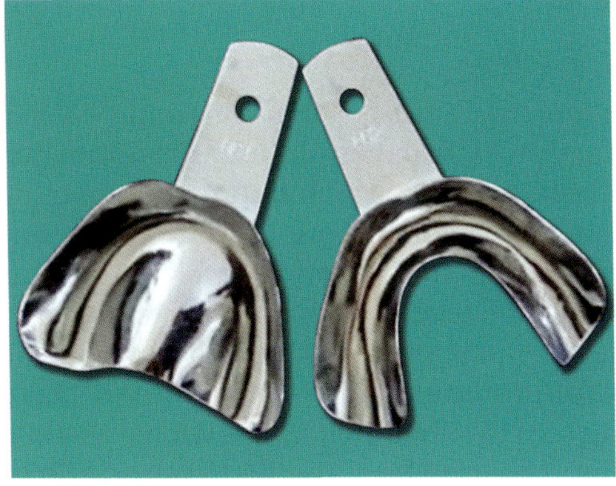

Fig. 6.1: Nonperforated stock tray for edentulous impression.

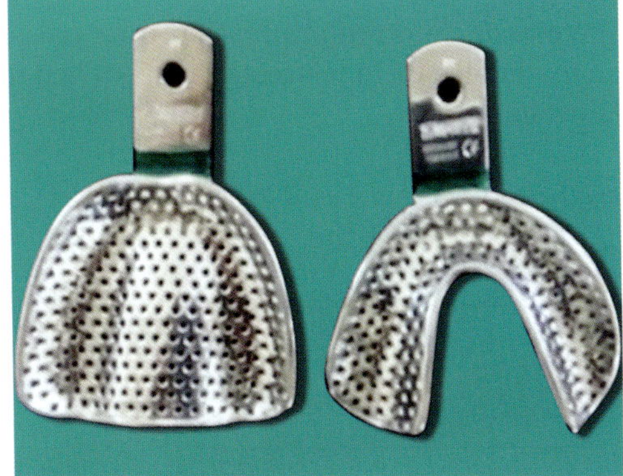

Fig. 6.2: Perforated stock tray for edentulous impression.

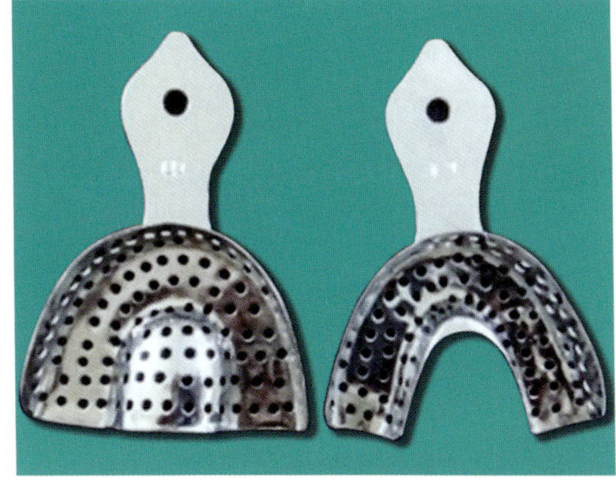

Fig. 6.3: Perforated metal stock tray for dentulous impression.

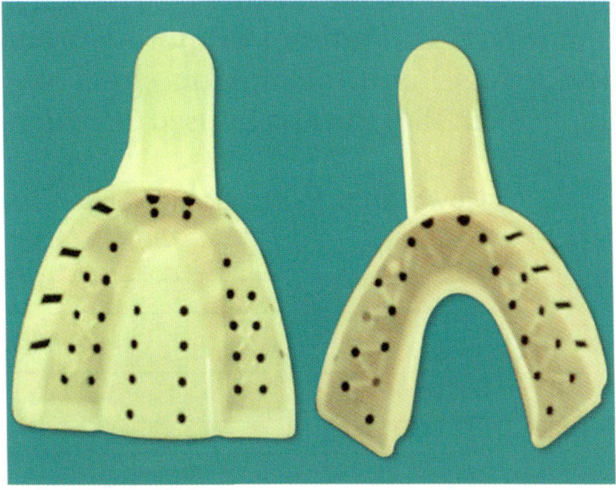

Fig. 6.4: Perforated plastic stock stray for dentulous impression.

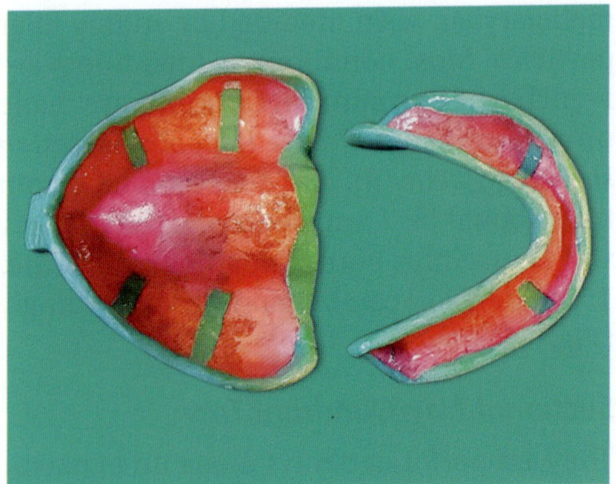

Fig. 6.5: Maxillary and mandibular custom trays.

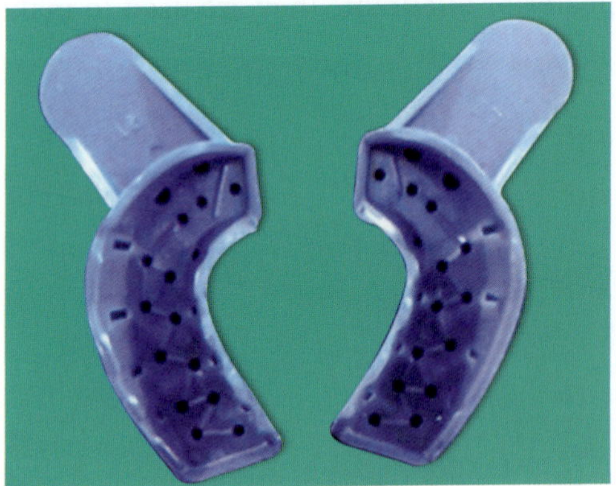

Fig. 6.6: Sectional trays.

sectional impression of a quadrant. They are usually used for making provisional or temporary restoration (temporary crown and bridge) and for making check cast impression. They can also be used for making

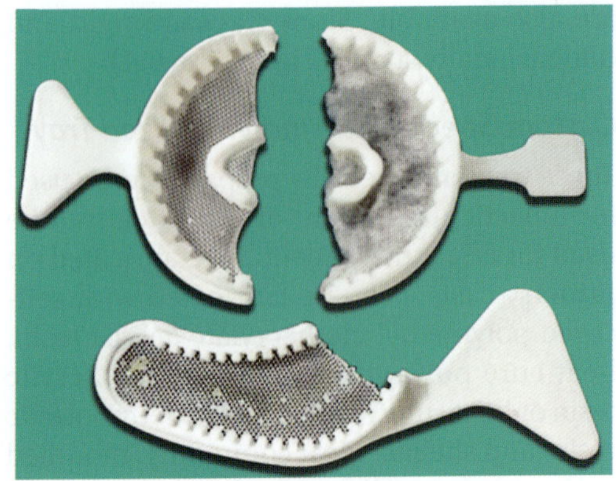

Fig. 6.7: Triple trays.

impression for single tooth restoration **(Fig. 6.6)**.

Triple Tray

These trays are used for making impression in fixed prosthodontics. These are trays with thin mesh or net on which impression material can be loaded on both the sides. With this tray, impression of teeth to receive prosthesis (prepared teeth), teeth opposite to prepared teeth, and interocclusal record can be made simultaneously. This way it gives three records together. Hence, it is known as triple tray. It is used for single tooth restoration or provisionalization **(Fig. 6.7)**.

Based on Tray Material

The classification of impression trays based on material used to fabricate them is given in **Flowchart 6.1**.

Flowchart 6.1: Classification of impression trays based on material used to fabricate.

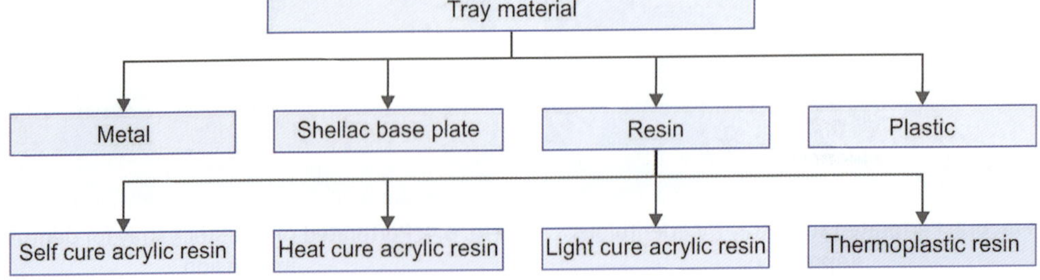

STOCK TRAYS

Classification of stock trays is given in **Flowchart 6.2**.

Perforated Stock Trays

Available for making impression of *edentulous* and *dentulous* arch **(Figs. 6.8A to C)**.

These trays have perforations all over. Perforations allow excess material to flow out **(Fig. 6.9)**. Excess material coming out from perforations gets entrapped and serves as mechanical locking of impression material with impression tray, thus preventing separation. These trays are used with elastic impression material which needs mechanical interlocking with tray.

Nonperforated Stock Trays

Available for making impression of *edentulous* and *dentulous* arch.

They are used for making edentulous primary impression **(Fig. 6.10)**. It is used with rigid impression material (impression compound). Nonperforated stock trays are also available for dentulous patient. It is used with agar impression material to make dentulous impression. However, special water-cooled rim locked trays are used with agar impression material.

Advantages and Disadvantages of Stock Trays

Advantages

- It is rigid and supports the impression material.
- Dimensionally stable.
- Tray is precisely fabricated and smooth so injury to oral tissue is avoided.
- **Multiple use:** It can be reused in several patients after sterilization.

Flowchart 6.2: Classification of stock trays.

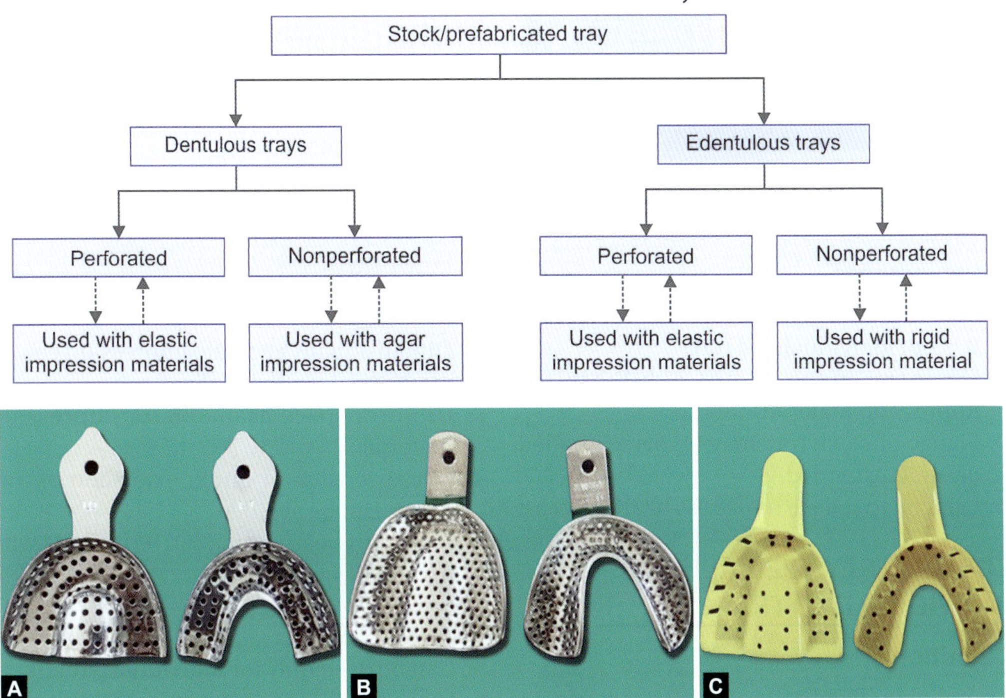

Figs. 6.8A to C: Perforated stock trays for dentulous and edentulous impressions.

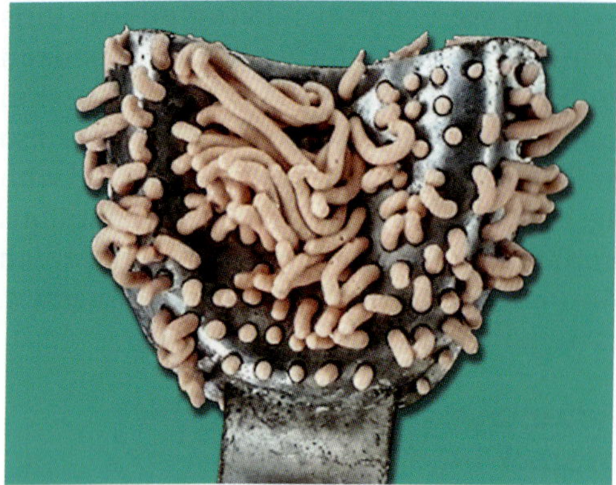

Fig. 6.9: Excess material entrapped in perforations.

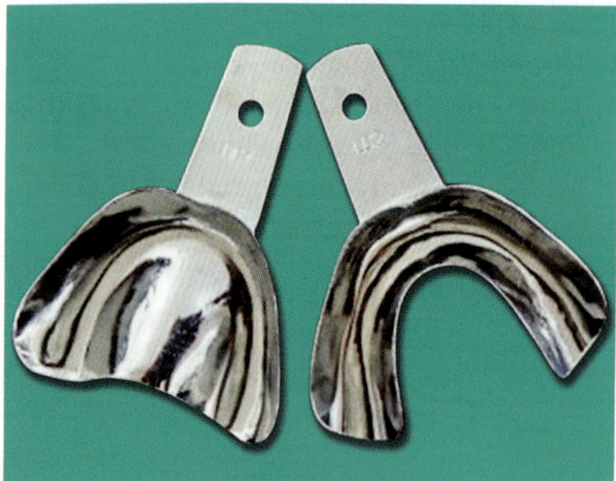

Fig. 6.10: Nonperforated stock trays for making edentulous primary impression.

Disadvantages

- Accurate impression is difficult to make as it is not individualized tray.
- Uniform space is not available for impression material.
- Flange of stock tray may be overextended or underextended.
- Difficult to relieve nonstress bearing areas.

CUSTOM TRAY/SPECIAL TRAY/ INDIVIDUALIZED TRAY

Definition

An individualized impression tray made on a cast recovered by pouring a preliminary impression (primary cast). It is used for making a final impression.

Stock trays are available in predetermined sizes which can be used for making primary impression. From this primary impression, a primary cast is made. On primary cast an impression tray is fabricated which is known as custom tray. Custom tray is an individualized tray and can be used for that particular patient only. Custom tray is used for making secondary or final impression.

Various Materials Used for Fabrication of Custom Trays

- Tray compound
- Tray acrylic (modified autopolymerizing acrylic resin)
- Shellac base plate **(Figs. 6.11A and B)**
- Vacuum formed thermoplastic resin sheets
- Old denture can also be used as custom tray
- Light cure acrylic resin
- Heat cure acrylic resin.

Parts of Custom Tray (Fig. 6. 12)

A. Tray body
B. Spacer
C. Tray handle
D. Tissue stops.

Advantages and Disadvantages of Custom Trays

Advantages

- Dimensionally accurate impression can be made as it is individualized tray.
- Uniform space available for impression material.
- Overextension or under extension of tray flange can be avoided.
- Nonstress bearing area can be relieved with the use of space.

Disadvantages

- Can be used only for individual patient.
- Fabrication is time consuming based on the material selected for it.

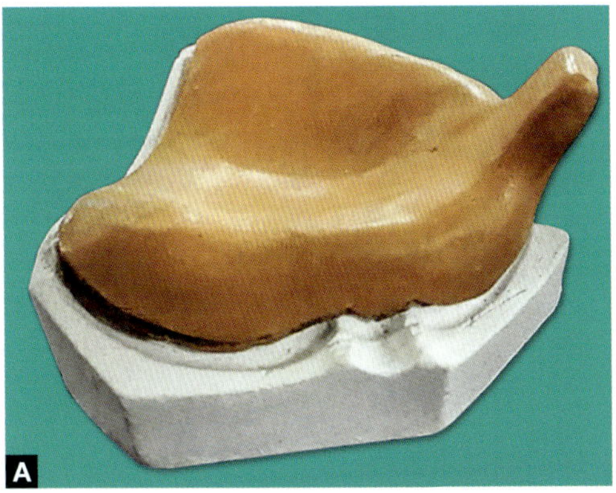

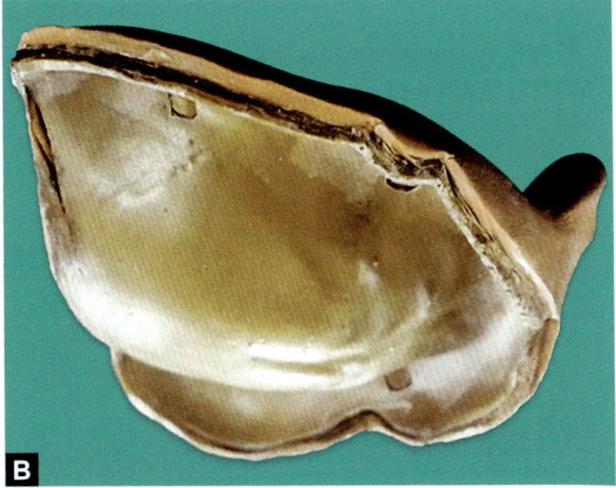

Figs. 6.11A and B: Maxillary custom tray fabricated with shellac and reinforced with impression compound.

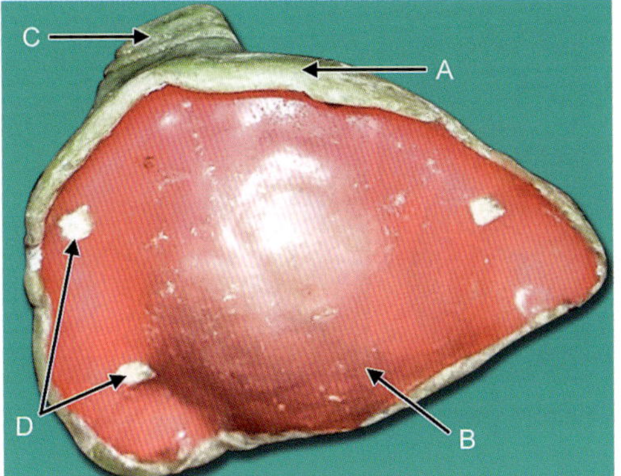

Fig. 6.12: Custom tray made of tray material.

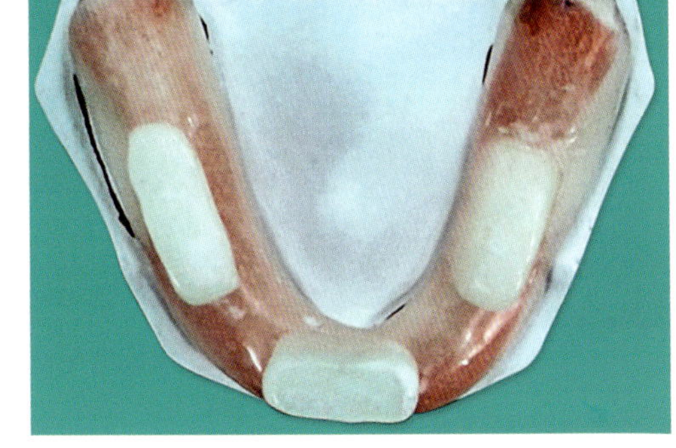

Fig. 6.13: Custom tray made with self-cure acrylic resin.

- Rigidity is less compared to a metallic stock tray.
- Dimensional stability is lesser compared to metallic stock tray.

Tray Handle

In stock tray, a horizontal tray handle is attached to anterior part of the tray body in both maxillary and mandibular trays. In custom trays, handles are of different dimensions and are placed at different angles than stock trays.

In maxillary custom tray, handle is placed on anterior region at midline at 45° angulation with the tray. This angulation is given to maxillary custom tray handle in accordance with angulation of residual alveolar ridge and anterior teeth in maxillary arch. The angulation also gives idea about the lip support and facilitate lip movement while doing border molding.

Mandibular custom tray handle is placed in anterior region at 90° angulation with tray. Sometime two extra finger rests are placed posteriorly in the molar region to equally distribute force while making impression **(Figs. 6.13 and 6.14)**.

Custom tray handle should be approximately 8 mm in length (Height), 8 mm in width, and 3–4 mm in thickness. The custom

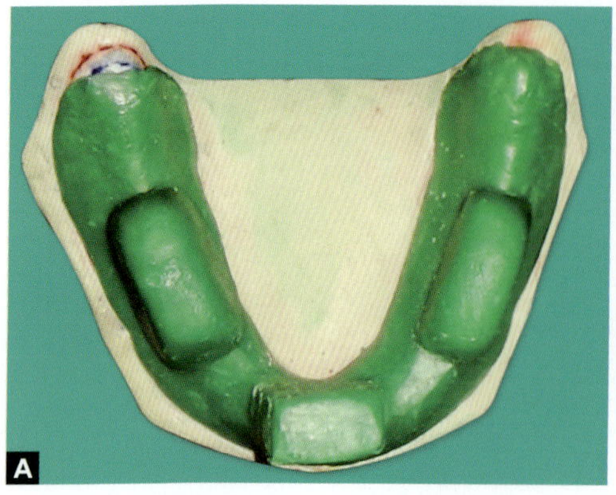

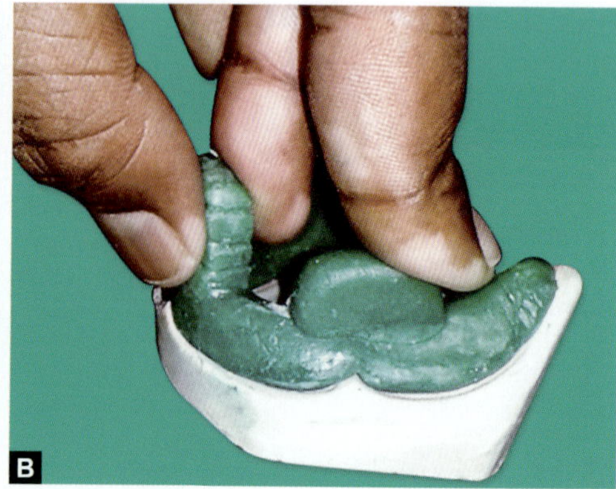

Figs. 6.14A and B: Mandibular custom tray with a handle and two finger rests.

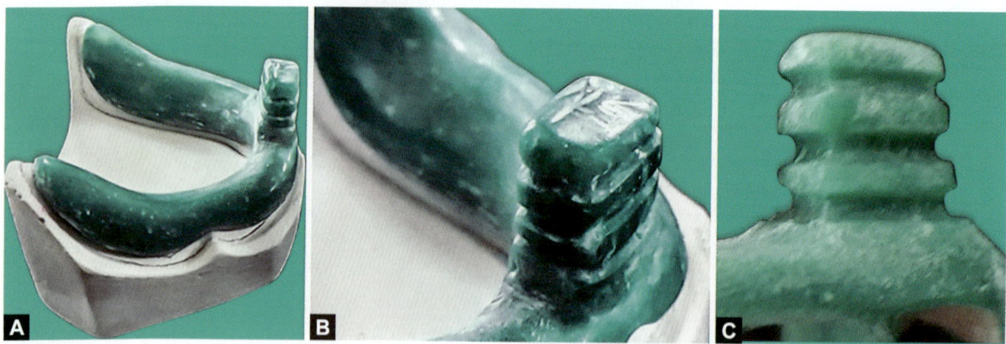

Figs. 6.15A to C: Grooved custom tray handle.

tray handle should be grooved to improve grip **(Figs. 6.15A to C)**.

Custom tray handle can be placed horizontally if needed. It should be placed such a way that it should not interfere during border molding **(Fig. 6.16)**.

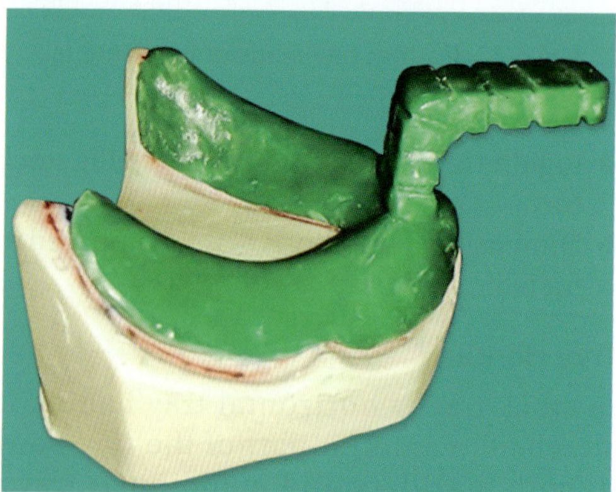

Fig. 6.16: Horizontal tray handle.

Perforations and Adhesives

It is essential that impression material firmly adhere to impression trays. This can be achieved either by perforations or by use of tray adhesive or by a combination of both. Perforations in tray provide mechanical interlocking between tray and impression material and tray adhesive provides chemical adhesion.

Excess impression material comes out from perforations and interlocks together to give mechanical retention between tray and impression material.

Adhesive solutions are used with alginate, polysulfide, polyether, and silicone impression materials. Tray adhesive is supplied as solution (apply with brush) or aerosol spray.

Tray adhesive for alginate is solution of resin in alcohol. Adhesive for elastomers is made up of silicone adhesive, alcohol, and colorant. Adhesive is supplied in umber glass bottle to protect it from sunlight. After application to tray, it is allowed to dry for 7–13 minutes before loading the impression material onto the tray.

CHAPTER 7

Complete Denture Impression

Paranjay Prajapati, Sneha Kulkarni

INTRODUCTION

For complete denture fabrication two impressions are made, i.e., primary impression and final impression. Different impression materials and impression trays are used for primary and final impressions. This chapter is about complete denture impressions.

DEFINITION

Impression

A negative likeness or copy in reverse of the surface of an objects.

OBJECTIVES OF COMPLETE DENTURE IMPRESSION MAKING

Preservation of Remaining Oral Tissue

It is always better to preserve what is remaining than to replace what is lost. The present health of oral tissue should be taken care while making impression or during prosthesis fabrication as it serves as foundation for prosthesis.

Be careful while making impression and avoid trauma to oral tissue. One should cover maximum foundation area in impression to divide masticatory force over wider area and minimize the resorption.

Provide Retention, Stability, Support, and Esthetics for the Denture

Retention

It is resistance of the prosthesis to the force acting in vertical direction away from the foundation.

Prosthesis should resist its removal when vertical force is applied against the path of insertion or path of placement of denture.

There are various factors which contribute for retention in complete denture. These factors are adhesion, cohesion, interfacial surface tension, and peripheral seal.

Stability

The property of prosthesis to be firm, steady, and resist the horizontal or rotational forces applied on it. If horizontal forces are applied to denture during various routine activities it should not become loose.

Factors affecting stability are thickness of denture border, contouring of polished surface, occlusal plane, neuromuscular control of patient, and adaptation of prosthesis with ridge slopes.

Support

The ability of denture to resist vertical forces directed toward the foundation (*Retention:*

Forces in vertical direction but away from foundation). Support depends on wide coverage of foundation area. Other factors affecting supports are amount of residual alveolar ridges, shape of palatal vault, buccal-self area, etc.

Achieve Esthetic

While making impression one should properly contour the borders and should get proper support for lips and cheeks. This will contribute in final outcome of denture esthetic.

IMPRESSION TECHNIQUES FOR MAKING EDENTULOUS IMPRESSION

Depending on Mouth Position While Making Impression

Closed Mouth Impression Technique

Occlusal rims are attached with impression trays and patient applies pressure on them. The tissue is recorded in displaced or functional position.

Open Mouth Impression Technique

Commonly used technique. Tissue is recorded in undisplaced condition. Mouth is partly opened and impression tray is held in position while making impression.

Depending on Pressure Applied on Oral Mucosa by the Impression Material While Making Impression

Mucocompressive/Pressure Technique (Green Brothers)

According to this technique tissue of oral cavity is recorded under pressure in their functional state. Pressure is applied on both stress bearing and nonstress bearing areas. Materials used for this technique are impression compound and impression waxes.

Mucostatic (Minimum Pressure Technique (Harry L Page)

According to this theory interfacial surface tension is the only factor responsible for denture retention. Pressure applied is very minimum and border molding is not done. Hence, the tissues are recorded in their rest position. Materials used for this technique are impression plaster and low viscosity material like light body.

Selective Pressure Technique (Boucher)

This theory combines advantages of both mucocompressive and mucostatic techniques. Mucocompressive concept is used while recording stress bearing areas and mucostatic concept used in recording relieving areas. Spacer is used to relieve relieving areas while making impression with custom impression tray. Border molding is done with custom tray. Material used for this technique is zinc oxide eugenol impression paste.

Modified/Special Impression Technique

- Flabby tissue
- Poor foundation
- Microstomia (sectional impressions).

TYPES OF EDENTULOUS IMPRESSION (FLOWCHART 7.1)

Primary/Preliminary/Diagnostic Impression

This impression is made for diagnosis and treatment planning of particular patient. The cast obtained by pouring this impression is used for fabrication of custom tray to make final impression.

Flowchart 7.1: Edentulous impression.

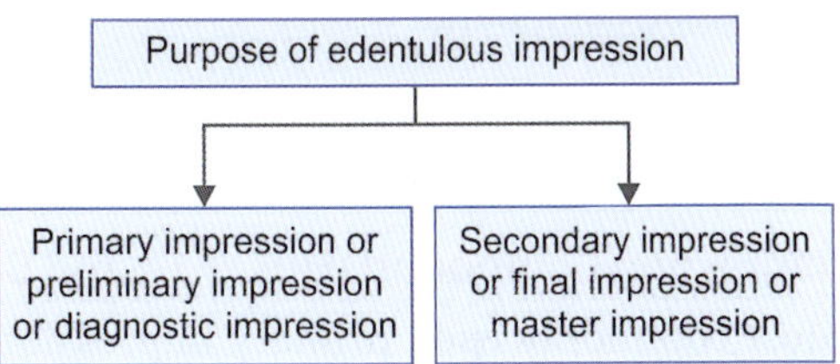

Secondary/Final/Master Impression

The final impression records fine details and proper border extensions. The cast retrieved after pouring final impression is used for fabrication of the complete denture and to achieve objectives of impression, i.e. retention, stability, support, preservation of tissue and esthetic.

WHAT SHOULD BE RECORDED IN AN IMPRESSION?

The maxillary impression should record labial and buccal frenums attachments, labial and buccal vestibule, residual alveolar ridge, palate, hamular notches, posterior palatal seal area, and coronomaxillary area.

The mandibular impression should record all frenum attachments, labial and buccal vestibule, buccal-self area, retromolar pads, sublingual area, mylohyoid ridge, retromylohyoid space, and sublingual crescent area.

PRIMARY IMPRESSION

Definition

A negative likeness made for the purpose of diagnosis, treatment planning or for the fabrication of a tray.

RATIONALE/NEED

Primary impression for complete denture should cover all landmarks and borders of denture foundation area. It should be accurate because it is used to pour primary cast on which custom tray is fabricated, which is used to make final impression. Mucocompressive technique is used for making primary impression with impression compound.

MATERIALS USED FOR MAKING PRIMARY IMPRESSION

Impression Compound (Figs. 7.1A and B)

Most commonly used primary impression material is impression compound. This material is rigid in nature; it becomes hard and inelastic after setting. It can be successfully used for making impression of denture foundation with no undercuts. If undercuts are presents then impression compound will not come out from undercuts, it may get distorted or may injure the mucosa and hence it is not advised for such undercut foundation.

Irreversible Hydrocolloid (Alginate) Impression Material

Sometime there are unilateral or bilateral undercuts present on the edentulous foundation area. In such cases impressions made with impression compound may not come out easily without distortion. In such

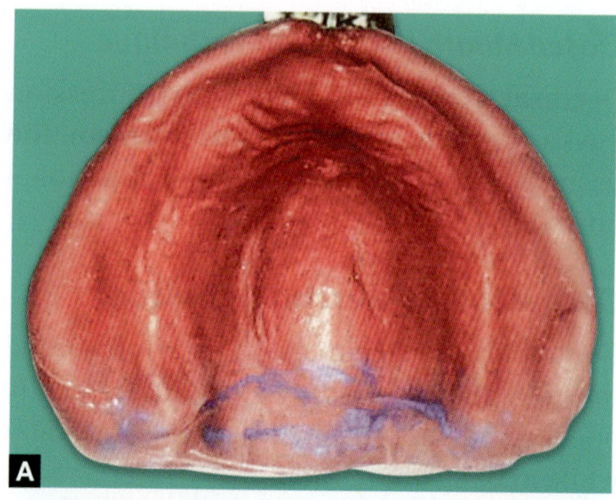

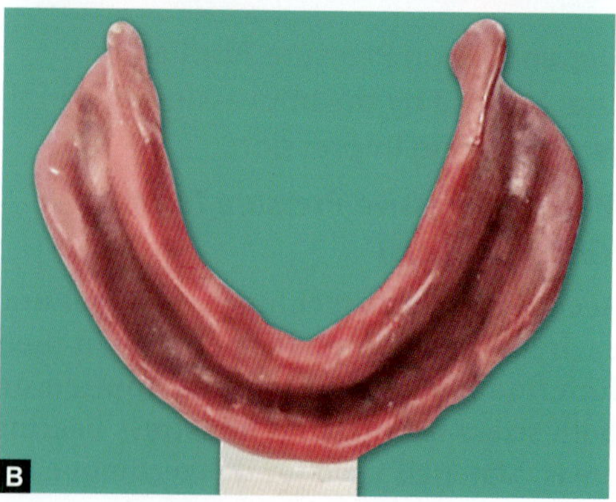

Figs. 7.1A and B: Maxillary and mandibular primary impressions made with impression compound.

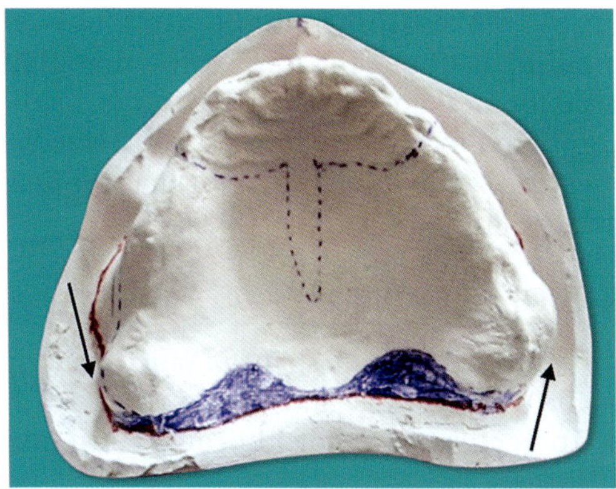

Fig. 7.2: Bilateral undercuts in maxillary cast-see arrows.

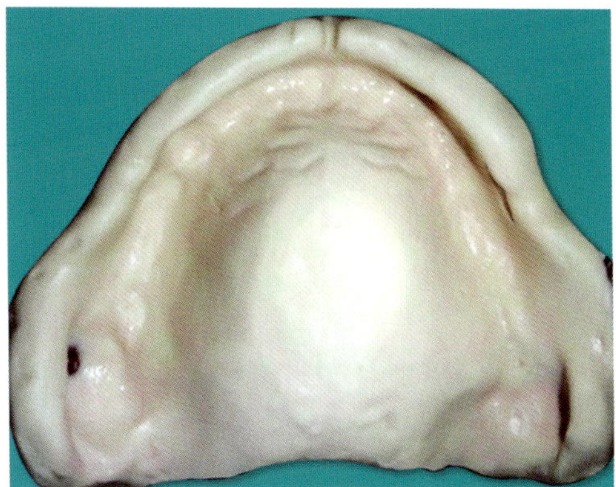

Fig. 7.3: Primary edentulous impression made with alginate.

patients, impression should be made with elastic material. Irreversible hydrocolloid is commonly used for this type of patients. As it is elastic in nature, it will allow easy removal of set impression without distortion of impression and without injury to patient. In some cases putty consistency of elastomeric impression material is also used **(Figs. 7.2 and 7.3)**.

IMPRESSION TRAYS FOR PRIMARY IMPRESSION

If impression material selected is impression compound then nonperforated edentulous stock trays are used.

If material of choice for primary impression is irreversible hydrocolloid then perforated edentulous stock trays are used.

FINAL IMPRESSION/SECONDARY IMPRESSION

Final impression of complete denture comprises of two different steps as follows:
1. Border molding
2. Impression of denture foundation.

Definition

Secondary impression: The impression that represents the completion of the registration of the surface or object.

Border molding: The shaping of the border areas of an impression tray by functional or manual manipulation of the tissue adjacent to the borders to duplicate the contour and size of the vestibule, OR

Determining the extension of the prosthesis by using tissue function or manual manipulation of the tissues to shape the border areas of an impression material.

Border Molding (Fig. 7.4)

In border molding, material is added over the borders of custom impression tray and inserted in patient's mouth. Various lip and cheek movements are performed by dentist and patient. These movements will shape added material and records the width and height of border (vestibule) and house the frenum attachments to prevent encroachment by denture. Border molding will help in achieving peripheral/border seal which is essential for denture retention and stability.

Two main objectives of border molding are as follows:
1. To shape the borders to allow muscle movements without interference with prosthesis.
2. To improve the border seal area to aid in retention of prosthesis.

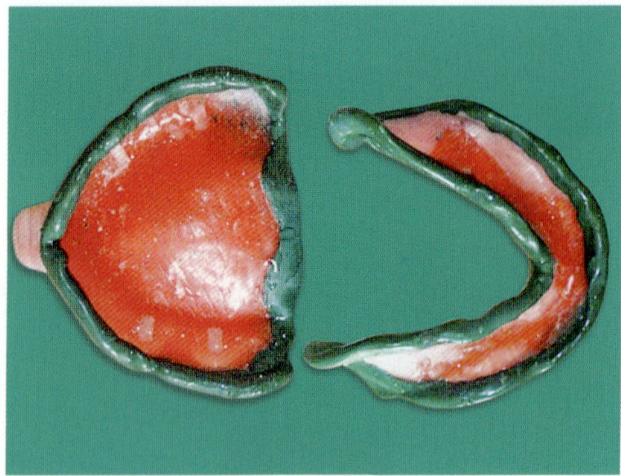

Fig. 7.4: Border molded custom trays.

Materials used for Border Molding

- Low fusing compound (greenstick compound)—most commonly used
- Polyether impression material
- Self-cure acrylic resin
- Impression waxes
- Tissue conditioner
- Pattern resin
- Wax (Adaptol)

Methods of Border Molding

- **Based on technique:**
  - Incremental or segmental technique
  - Single step or simultaneous technique
  - Closed mouth
  - Open mouth
- **Based on manipulation:**
  - Functional manipulation (movements provided by the patient)
  - Manual manipulation (movements done by dentist by manipulating cheek and lips)
  - Combination of functional and manual manipulation (some movements performed by patient and some done by dentist).

FINAL IMPRESSION MAKING

Final impression is made with custom tray which has better fit compared to the stock tray. Final impression is made after border molding is done. The impression materials used for final impression records fine details compared to primary impression. Selective pressure technique is used for making final impression.

RATIONALE/NEED

- To record accurate shape of mucosa lining the residual ridge and foundation area
- To accurately record border width and height
- To accurately record border configuration
- To produce master cast on which stable and retentive denture base can be fabricated.

Materials used for Making Final Impression

- Zinc oxide eugenol impression paste
- Noneugenol impression paste
- Addition/condensation silicone impression material
- Polyether impression material
- Polysulfide impression material.

> Addition/condensation silicone impression material, polyether impression material, polysulfide impression material are collectively known as *elastomers* or *elastomeric impression materials* or *rubber-based impression materials.*

Zinc Oxide Eugenol Impression Paste (Fig. 7.5)

Most commonly used material for making final impression is zinc oxide eugenol (ZOE) impression paste. Noneugenol impression paste is used when patient is suffering from smokers' palate, dry mouth, submucous fibrosis, burning sensation of mucosa, and if allergic to eugenol.

In severe undercut ZOE impression paste cannot be used as it become rigid after setting and cannot be removed without distortion,

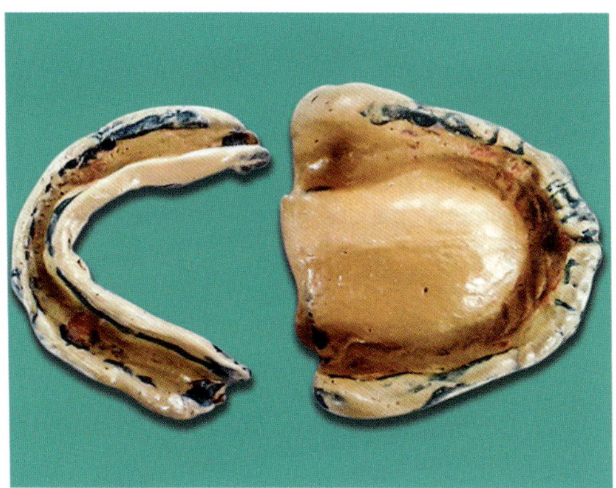

Fig. 7.5: Final impression of edentulous maxillary and mandibular arches made with zinc oxide eugenol impression material.

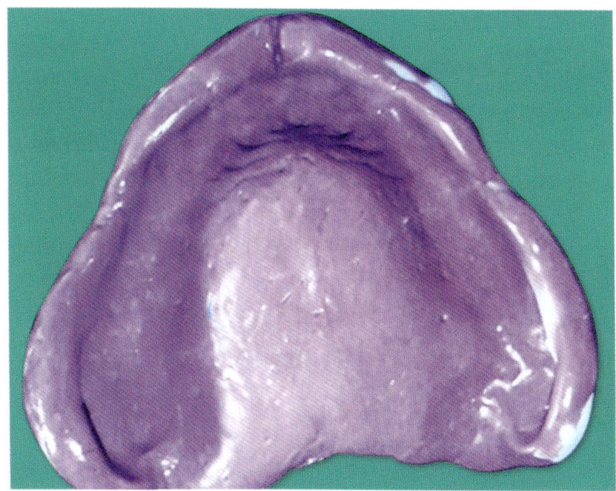

Fig. 7.6: Final impression of edentulous arch made with elastomeric impression material.

hence elastomeric impression materials (which are elastic after setting) are used in case of severe undercuts.

Elastomeric Impression Materials (Fig. 7.6)

Sometime, elastomeric impression materials, i.e., polyether, addition silicone, condensation silicone or polysulfide can also be used to make edentulous impressions. Light body or medium body consistency of elastomeric impression material is used to make final impression of complete denture. Elastomeric impression is made when there are severe undercuts located at different areas of edentulous arch.

VARIOUS IMPRESSION MATERIALS USED FOR EDENTULOUS IMPRESSION (TABLE 7.1)

Table 7.1: Advantages and disadvantages of various impression materials used for edentulous impression

Impression material	*Advantages*	*Disadvantages*
Impression plaster	❑ Accurate production of surface details ❑ Lesser tissue distortion ❑ Good flow ❑ No special equipment needed for manipulation	❑ Cannot be used when undercut present ❑ It may break due to brittleness ❑ Not suitable to record details due to saliva especially for mandibular arch
Impression compound	❑ It is self-supportive ❑ If not recorded properly can be re-soften and remade with same material ❑ Can be used as impression tray for impression	❑ Pressure applied on mucosa ❑ Not comfortable for heat sensitive patients ❑ Cannot be used for foundation with bony undercuts

Contd...

Contd...

Impression material	*Advantages*	*Disadvantages*
Irreversible hydrocolloid (alginate)	❑ Easy to manipulate ❑ Less pressure applied on tissue ❑ No need for hot water for manipulation ❑ Can be used for foundation with bony undercut	❑ Not self-supportive ❑ Cannot be corrected ❑ Cannot be reused ❑ Dimensional changes due to syneresis and imbibition
Reversible hydrocolloid (agar)	❑ Accurate impression ❑ Used in undercut	❑ Need expensive equipment for manipulation ❑ Manipulation is difficult ❑ Dimensional changes due to syneresis and imbibition
Zinc oxide eugenol impression paste	❑ Accurately records the details ❑ No displacement of tissue during impression making ❑ Beading-boxing can be done	❑ Taste is not good ❑ Messy to handle ❑ Distorts while removing from undercuts
Polysulfide	❑ Good working time ❑ High tear resistance	❑ Bad odor due to sulfur compound ❑ Messy in handling ❑ Stains clothes
Polyether	❑ Good dimensional stability ❑ Good tear strength ❑ Less distortion	❑ Very stiff after set ❑ Bad taste
Addition silicone	❑ Extremely high accuracy ❑ Dimensionally stable ❑ Repeated casts can be poured ❑ Less distortion on removal ❑ Easy manipulation	❑ Hydrogen gas as by product ❑ Expensive
Condensation silicone	❑ Adequate tear strength ❑ Less distortion on removal ❑ Good elastic properties	❑ Poor dimensional stability ❑ Less shelf life

CHAPTER 8

Dental Cast

Paranjay Prajapati, Sneha Kulkarni

INTRODUCTION

Dental cast represents denture foundation in absence of the patient. It is used for diagnosis and treatment planning. Denture is fabricated on cast made from impression of denture foundation. It is positive replica of the denture foundation and negative replica of the impression. It should be made properly for ease of handling and manipulation of material over it. This chapter deals with types of casts, methods of pouring of cast, its dimensions and characteristics.

DEFINITION

Cast

A life size likeness of some desired form.

Dental Cast

A replica of the tooth surfaces, residual ridge areas and/or other parts of the dental arch

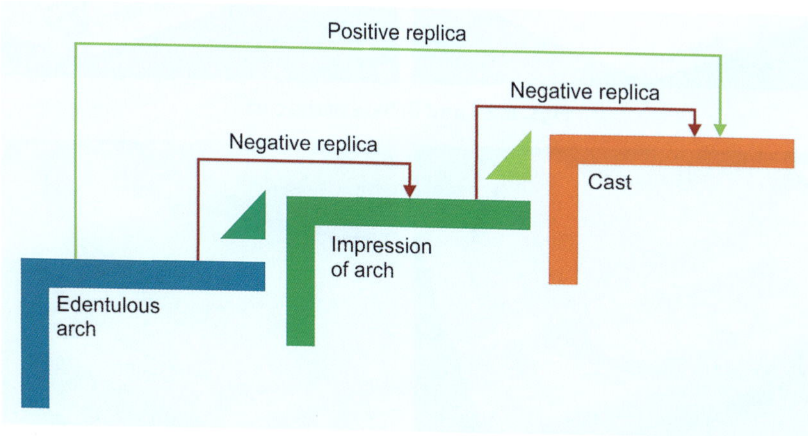

Fig. 8.1: Relation of positive and negative replica among arch, impression and cast.

and/or facial structures used to fabricate a dental restoration or prosthesis **(Fig. 8.1)**.

TYPES OF DENTAL CAST

Diagnostic Cast

It is made to diagnose the present condition of diseases or oral condition. Sometime mock surgical procedures are performed on diagnostic cast to estimate outcome. It is made up of dental plaster (type II gypsum).

Primary Cast

It is made from primary impression. Custom tray is fabricated on primary cast. It is poured in dental plaster (type II gypsum). It is made by inversion method.

Master Cast/Final Cast

This cast is obtained by pouring final/master impression. Usually prosthesis is fabricated on this cast. It is more accurate than primary cast and has more fine details. It is made with dental stone (type III gypsum). It is made by beading-boxing method.

IDEAL REQUIREMENTS OF THE CAST

- Cast should be neat, clean, and free of voids and blebs.
- The base should be of 15 mm in thickness **(Figs. 8.2A and B)**.
- Land area should be of 2–3 mm in height and width and slopped at 45° angulation **(Figs. 8.3A and B)**.

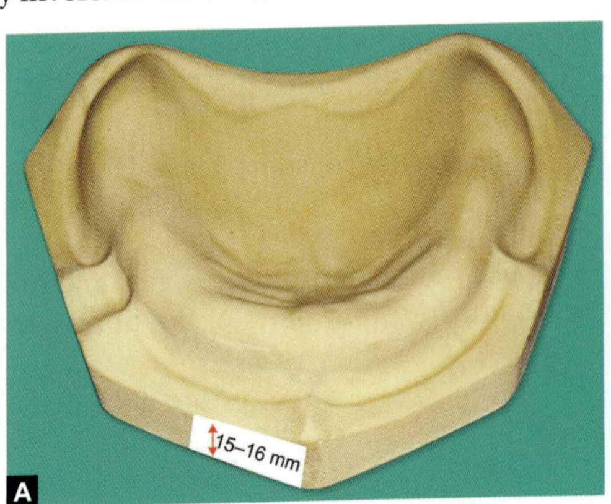

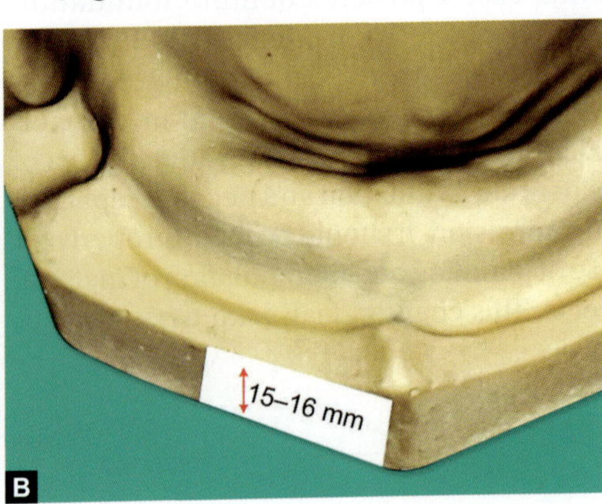

Figs. 8.2A and B: Base of the cast.

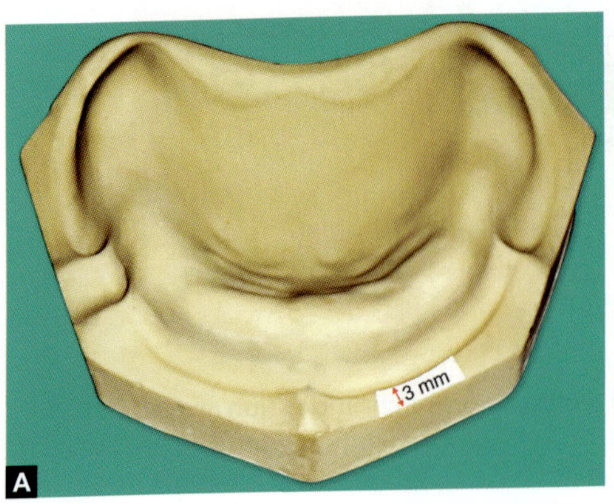

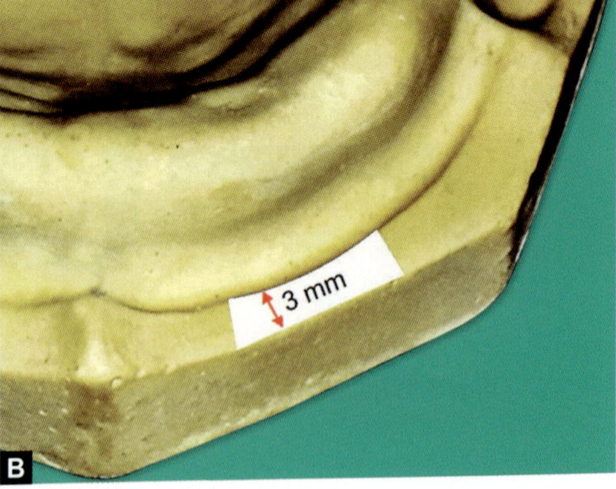

Figs. 8.3A and B: Land area of the cast.

- Denture foundation area should not be altered or represented as recorded in impression.
- Denture foundation area should be parallel to base of the cast.
- Land area should follow depth of vestibule.
- Cast should be labeled with patient name and OPD number.

PARTS OF DENTAL CAST

Dental cast has two parts namely:
1. Anatomic portion
2. Art portion.

Anatomic Portion (Fig. 8.4)

This part of dental cast is made by pouring impression of oral tissue. It represents anatomical landmarks or denture foundation area.

Art Portion

This portion is added to anatomic portion of cast to provide better strength and handling characteristic. It includes base of the cast, heel of the cast and land area of the cast.

The base and land area of cast are important as they imparts strength to the cast, preserve the depth and width of the sulcus, and protect anatomical landmarks/area of the cast **(Figs. 8.5A and B)**.

Base of the cast should have 15 mm thickness at the deepest part of the cast.

Land area should have 3-4 mm in height from sulcus and 3-4 mm width. Land area should be sloped outward at 45° angulation.

Refractory Cast (Fig. 8.6)

This cast is made from type IV gypsum. The material has characteristic of high strength and high expansion. This cast is used to fabricate wax pattern of cast partial framework. This cast can withstand high temperature.

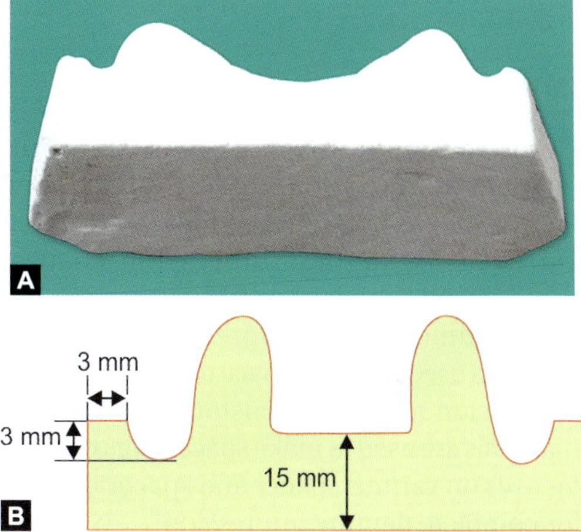

Figs. 8.5A and B: Section of the cast showing dimension of land area and base.

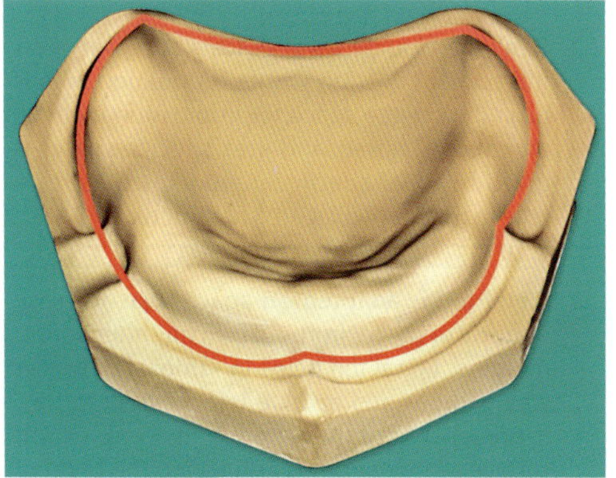

Fig. 8.4: Anatomical portion of the cast.

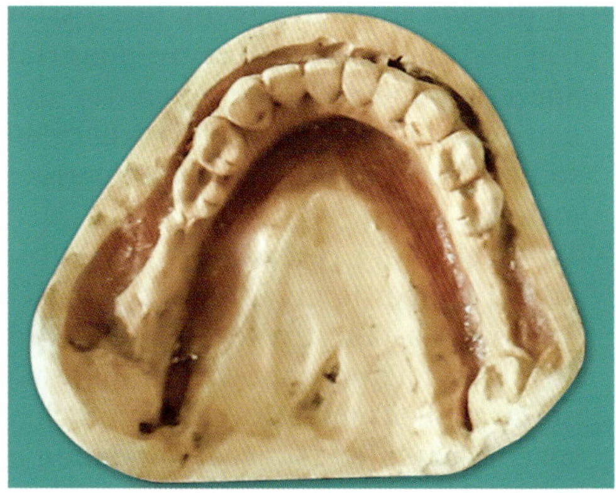

Fig. 8.6: Refractory cast.

CHAPTER 9

Spacer and Spacer Designs

JR Patel, Paranjay Prajapati

INTRODUCTION

Denture foundation area is made up of different type of anatomical structures among them some can bear the load and some cannot. During making final impression custom tray is used which should have provision to accommodate the impression materials. Spacer is used to create space to accommodate impression material in custom tray. Various materials are used to make spacer. This chapter focuses on various spacer and spacer designs for complete denture impression.

USES

- **To provide space in custom impression tray for the final impression material:** Spacer is removed from custom tray after border molding **(Fig. 9.1)**. This will create space in the custom tray for final impression material.
- **To selectively relieve the relieving areas:** Spacer is given in areas which cannot withstand the masticatory load. So while making impression, load will not be applied on those areas as sufficient space is provided for accommodation of material.

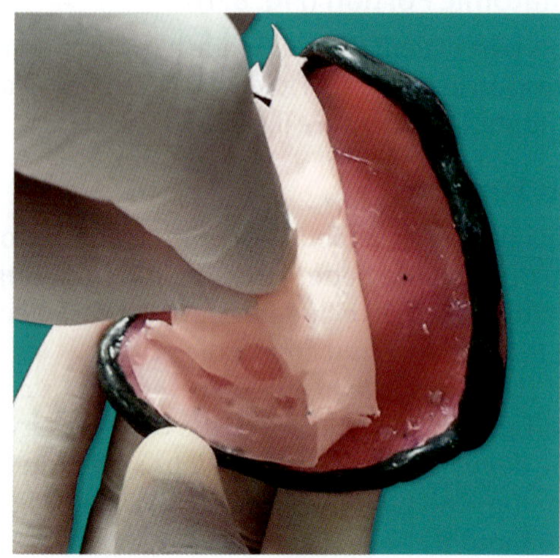

Fig. 9.1: Removal of spacer from custom tray.

- Generally double (two) spacers are given. First full spacer covering whole foundation area is placed to create space for impression material and above this second area specific spacer is given to cover specific anatomic structure to relieve that particular area or structure.

- Metal foil is adapted on spacer wax for easy removal of spacer from custom tray after border molding. Metal foil helps in removal of spacer wax without any residue left on custom tray. It prevents contamination of the impression surface of the tray thus enhancing the bond of impression material and adhesive to the tray.

MATERIALS USED FOR MAKING SPACER

- Base plate wax/modeling wax
- Casting wax
- Major connector wax
- Metal foil.

THICKNESS OF SPACER

The thickness of spacer should be kept such that it provides the sufficient impression material thickness without overloading the relieving areas. Neil recommended 0.9 mm thickness of casting wax as spacer. Boucher advocates for 1 mm thickness of base plate wax while Bernard and Frank suggest 2 mm thickness of base plate wax as spacer.

SPACER DESIGNS

Various designs proposed for spacer. Each design has its own significance. Operator can combine the spacer design according to the need of particular patient. Various spacer designs are as under.

Spacer Design by Roy MacGregor (Fig. 9.2)

He proposed to adapt metal foil in region of incisive papillae and midpalatine raphe.

Spacer Design by Neil (Fig. 9.3)

Neil recommends adaptation of 0.9 mm casting wax all over foundation area. Spacer is not adapted on posterior palatal seal (PPS) area.

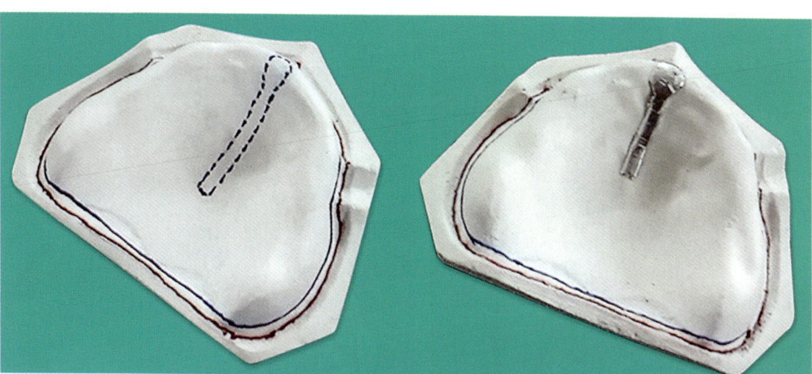

Fig. 9.2: Roy MacGregor's spacer design.

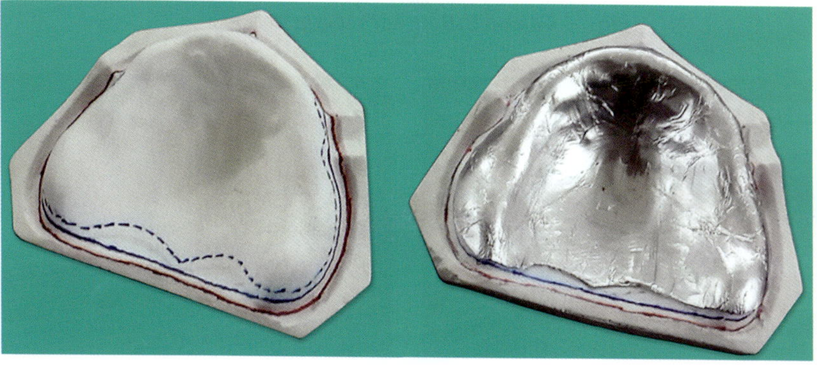

Fig. 9.3: Neil's spacer design.

Spacer Design by Boucher (Figs. 9.4A and B)

Boucher recommends placement of 1 mm base-plate wax on the cast except PPS area. For mandibular ridge, all the areas except buccal shelf are covered with wax.

Spacer Design by Morrow, Rudd, Rhoads (Fig. 9.5)

Full wax spacer 2-mm short of the resin special tray border is adapted all over. Placement of three tissue stops at equidistant from each other.

Spacer Design by Sharry (Fig. 9.6)

Adaptation of a layer of base-plate wax over the whole area outlined for tray. Placement of four tissue stops (2 mm in width located in molar and cuspid region which should extend from palatal aspect of the ridge to the mucobuccal fold).

Spacer Design by Bernard (Fig. 9.7)

Recommends a layer of pink base-plate wax (about 2 mm thick) attached to the areas of the cast that usually have the areas of the softer tissues.

According to the present concepts, stress bearing areas in the maxillary arch are crest of the alveolar ridge and horizontal plates of the palatine bone. Relieving areas are midpalatine raphe and incisive papilla.

Taking these into consideration Shetty et al. recommend following spacer design for the maxillary arch.

Sheet of wax (0.4 mm major connector wax) is placed in all the areas except the PPS area,

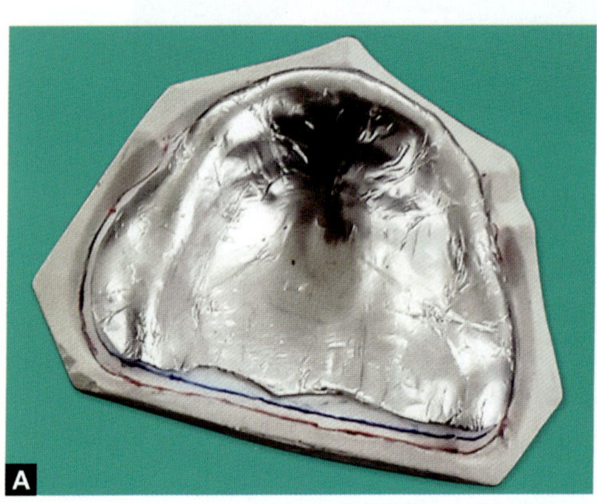

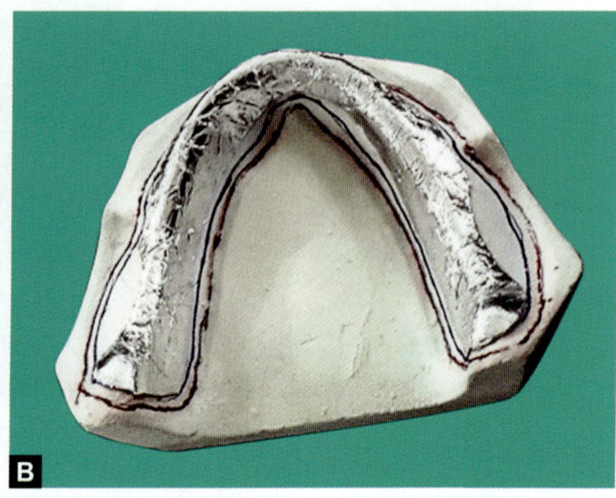

Figs. 9.4A and B: Boucher's spacer design.

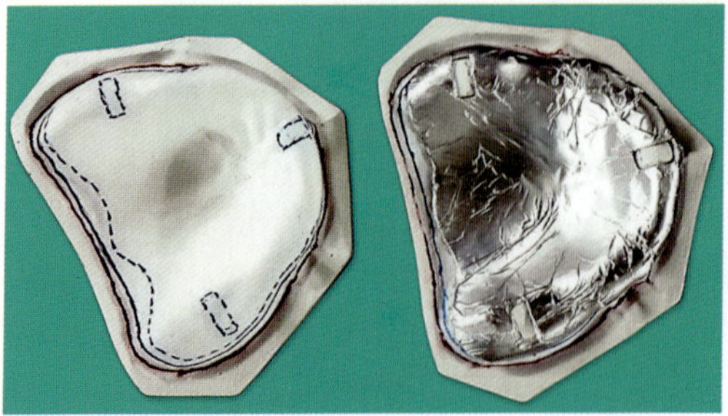

Fig. 9.5: Spacer design by Morrow, Rudd, Rhoads.

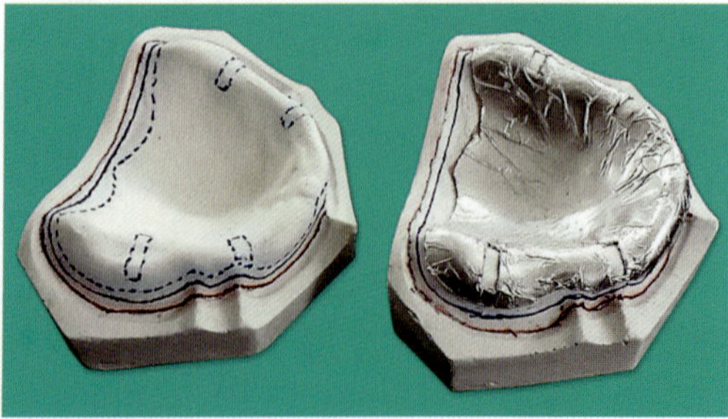

Fig. 9.6: Sharry's spacer design.

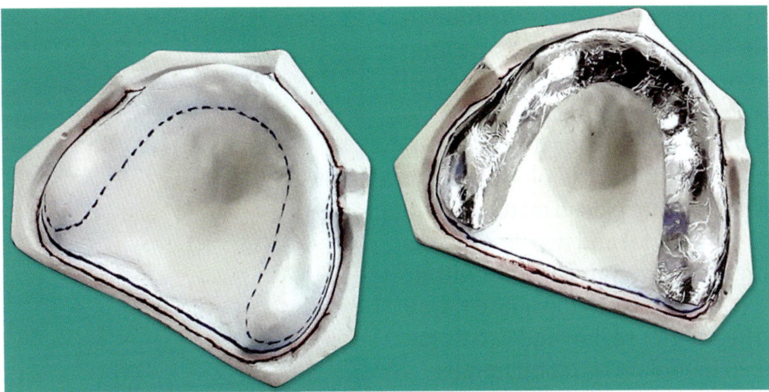

Fig. 9.7: Bernard's spacer design.

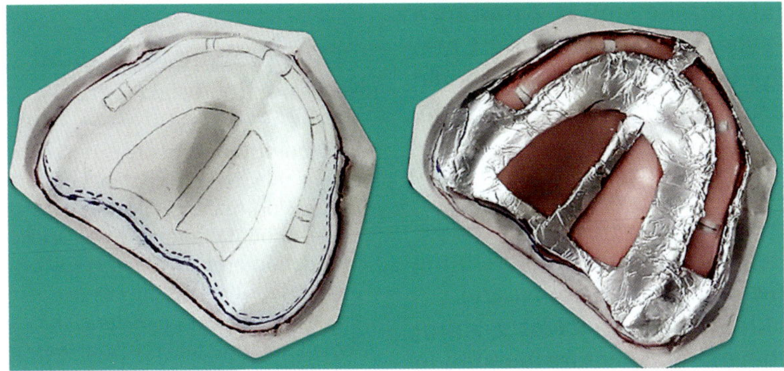

Fig. 9.8: Spacer design by Shetty et al.

as this area (PPS) requires to be compressed during the border molding procedures. A 1.5 mm modeling wax is adapted on top of the already adapted wax sheet.

After adapting the modeling wax tissue stops fabricated as shown in **Figure 9.8**.

SPACER THICKNESS FOR DIFFERENT IMPRESSION MATERIAL

Spacer thickness for different impression material shown in **Table 9.1**.

Table 9.1: Spacer thickness for different impression material.

S. No.	*Impression material*	*Spacer thickness*
1.	Impression plaster	1.5 mm
2.	Alginate	3.0 mm
3.	Zinc oxide eugenol	0.5 mm
4.	Elastomeric impression materials	0.5–1.5 mm (depends on viscosity of material)

TISSUE STOPS

A wax spacer is applied on primary cast before making custom impression tray. This spacer wax should be cut in 2–4 spaces to create window in spacer. When custom tray is fabricated over it, part of custom tray will be in direct contact with cast through the windows. This extended part of the custom tray is called as tissue stop.

Tissue stop is an extension (part) of custom tray. It is not a part of spacer.

The tissue stops can be three or four in numbers. Number and location of tissue stop is critical and they should be placed far from each other to cover more foundation area.

Usually, four tissue stops or minimum of three stops are placed. In case of four tissue stops, two tissue stops are placed on the canine region (one on either side) and two tissue stops are placed on molar region (one on either side). In case of three tissue stops, one tissue stop is placed in anterior region and two tissue stops are placed in molar region bilaterally.

It can be square or rectangular in shape. Square tissue stops can be 2 mm in size. The rectangular tissue stop is 2 mm by 4 mm in size (2 mm mesiodistally and 4 mm buccolingually). Rectangle tissue stops should cover the buccal and palatal slopes of the alveolar ridge.

USES

Tissue stops helps in stabilizing and orienting the custom tray while making impression.

They provide uniform space of 2-3 mm between custom tray and denture foundation and helps in free flow of material.

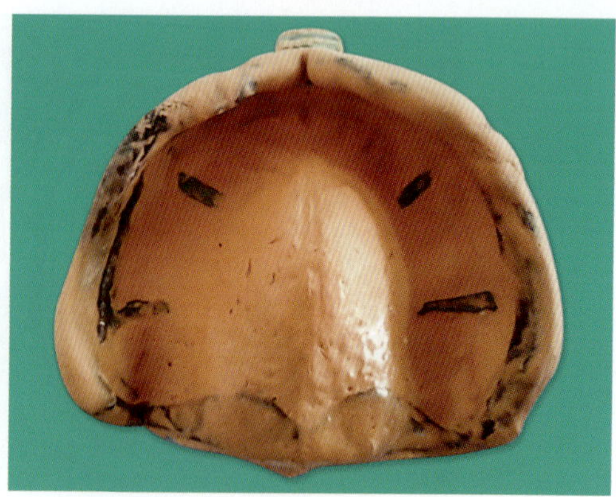

Fig. 9.9: Exposure of all four tissue stops.

They provide idea about thickness of impression material **(Fig. 9.9)**.

> If all four tissue stops are exposed in impression; it means they were in contact with oral tissue while impression making, the tray was stabilized and equal amount of pressure was applied all over the foundation area. If tissue stops on one side are unexposed, it means they were not in contact with tissue and impression material thickness is more in region and unequal pressure was applied by the material during impression making.

CHAPTER 10

Record Base

Paranjay Prajapati, Sneha Kulkarni

INTRODUCTION

Record base can be fabricated with various materials and methods. Wax occlusal rims are fabricated on records bases and jaw relation is recorded which is transferred on articulators. Artificial teeth are arranged on these records bases and trial is done. Record bases should be fabricated accurately to judge denture retention, stability, and esthetic.

DEFINITION

A material or device is representing the base of a denture. It is used for making maxillomandibular relation records and arranging teeth.

CLASSIFICATION

Based on Material

The record base can be classified based on material used to fabricate it as given in **Flowchart 10.1**.

Based on Use

The record base can be classified according to use as given in **Flowchart 10.2**.

> Permanent record bases are not discarded after dewaxing but it becomes part of finished complete denture.

Flowchart 10.1: Classification of record base according to material of fabrication.

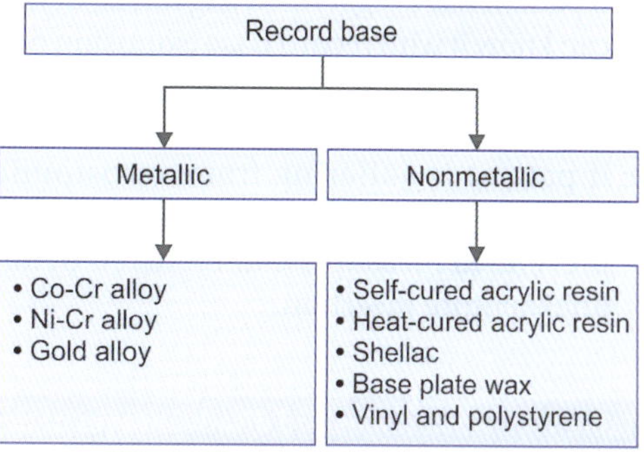

Flowchart 10.2: Classification of record base according to use.

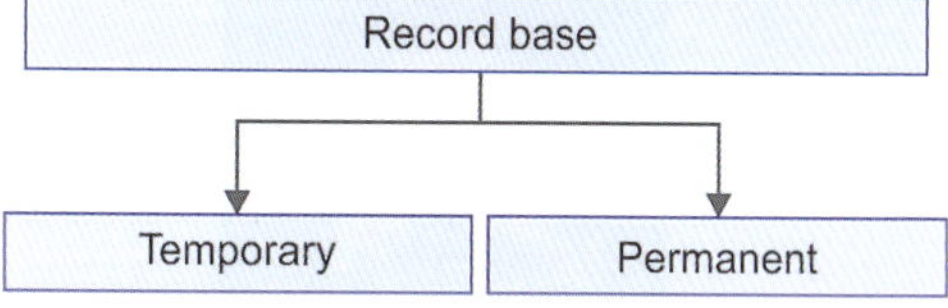

Denture base can be temporary and permanent. Temporary record base is made up of shellac, self-cured acrylic resin, vacuum formed vinyl and polystyrene, and base plate wax. This will be removed after dewaxing procedure and replaced by heat-cured acrylic resin to be a part of processed denture. All metallic denture bases and processed heat cure denture base are permanent denture bases. These will not be replaced after dewaxing but denture will be made and cured on these only.

Temporary record bases are discarded during dewaxing procedure (after jaw relation, teeth arrangement, and try in procedure is done) and replaced by denture base material.

DIAGNOSTIC USES

- It can give idea about overextension or underextension of border of first impression. Operator can get idea about the correctness of primary impression/primary cast as record base is made on primary cast.
- Patient and dentist both can get idea about acceptance and response to final denture. If patient has exaggerated gag reflex, dentist can know it with record base extension only and guide patient to manage with denture base and final denture.
- If patient is suffering from xerostomia, the final retention can be predicted and preventive measures can be taken before final denture insertion.
- Record base helps in establishing jaw relation record.
- It helps in recording of centric relationship.
- Allow setting of artificial teeth on it for wax trial.

IDEAL REQUIREMENTS

- It should be well adapted and accurately formed on final cast.
- It should be rigid and dimensionally steady.
- It should be stable on cast and on denture foundation in oral cavity.
- It should be free of voids on the surface that contact the oral mucosa.
- It should have smooth and rounded borders.
- It should be easily removable from cast.
- It must reproduce accurately the landmarks of final cast.

ADVANTAGES AND DISADVANTAGES OF DENTURE BASES

The advantages and disadvantages of denture bases are listed in **Table 10.1**.

Table 10.1: Advantages and disadvantages of denture bases.

S. No	*Types of denture base*	*Advantages*	*Disadvantages*
1.	Shellac denture base	❑ Easily fabricated ❑ Thickness is uniform ❑ Low cost ❑ Ease of availability ❑ Close adaptation ❑ Correction can be done	❑ Low strength ❑ Break at low force ❑ Distortion due to temperature change
2.	Self-cure acrylic record base	❑ Better strength ❑ Dimensionally stable ❑ No dimensional changes due to temperature change ❑ Close adaptation on cast	❑ Time consuming compared with shellac record base ❑ Maintenance of uniform thickness requires skills ❑ Unpolymerized monomer (residual) is serious hazard can cause allergic reaction

Contd...

Contd...

S. No	*Types of denture base*	*Advantages*	*Disadvantages*
3.	Light cure acrylic record base	❑ Easy manipulation and fabricate ❑ Available as readymade sheets ❑ Better adaptation and stable	❑ Requires special equipment for curing ❑ Brittle (low strength) compared to self and heat cure record base
4.	Processed heat cure acrylic resin record base	❑ Accurate, dimensionally stable ❑ This record base become part of denture ❑ Fabrication errors are less	❑ Time consuming ❑ Need separate cast for fabrication and articulation
5.	Metallic denture base	❑ Dimensionally most stable of all record bases ❑ It becomes part of denture ❑ Good conductor of heat ❑ For patient encountering frequent fracture of denture	❑ Fabrication is very time consuming ❑ Relining is difficult ❑ Some patient may evoke allergic reaction to metallic content
6.	Vinyl and polystyrene record base	❑ Easy fabrication ❑ Available as readymade sheets ❑ Close adaptation on cast	❑ Requires special equipment ❑ Low strength

CHAPTER 11

Mean Value Articulator

Paranjay Prajapati, Sneha Kulkarni

INTRODUCTION

The oral cavity is confined by maxilla and mandible with two temporomandibular joints (TMJs). During fabrication of prosthesis, some procedures are carried out in oral cavity and some are performed in dental laboratory in absence of patient. A mechanical device stimulating the two jaws and the TMJs is needed for ease of work. This device is "articulator".

DEFINITION

Articulator

Articulator is a mechanical device that represents the TMJs and the jaw members to which maxillary and mandibular casts may be attached to simulate some or all the mandibular movements.

CLASSIFICATION

Articulators are classified in several ways. The most common classification of articulator is based on their adjustability. Adjustability of articulator is judged based on their ability to accept face bow and various occlusal records which modifies condylar and incisal guidance accordingly.

Articulators can be classified according to:

- According to theories of occlusion
- Based on type of interocclusal records used
- Based on adjustability of the articulators
- Based on University of Michigan workshop.

Classification According to Theories of Occlusion

- **Bonwill theory articulator (Figs. 11.1A and B)**: This articulator was made by WGA Bonwill. This articulator is based on Bonwill's theory of equilateral triangle. According to this theory the teeth move in relation to each other as guided by the condylar and the incisor guidance. The equilateral triangle is formed between two condyles and condyles to midincisal point (of mandible). Theoretically the dimension of equilateral triangle is 4 inch.
- **Conical theory articulator (Figs. 11.2A and B)**: This theory was proposed by RE Hall. According to this theory the lower teeth move over the surface of upper teeth as over the surface of cone generating an angle of 45° with the central axis of cone tip 45° to the occlusal plane.
- **Spherical theory articulator (Figs. 11.3A and B)**: This articulator is based on Monson's theory of spherical occlusion.

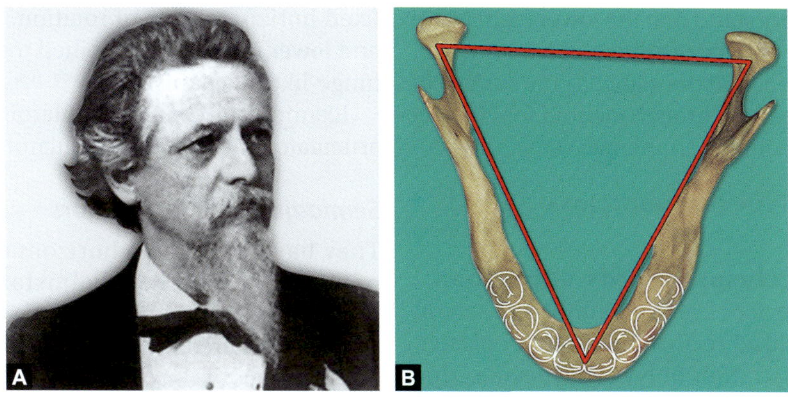

Figs. 11.1A and B: (A) WGA Bonwill; (B) Equilateral triangle.

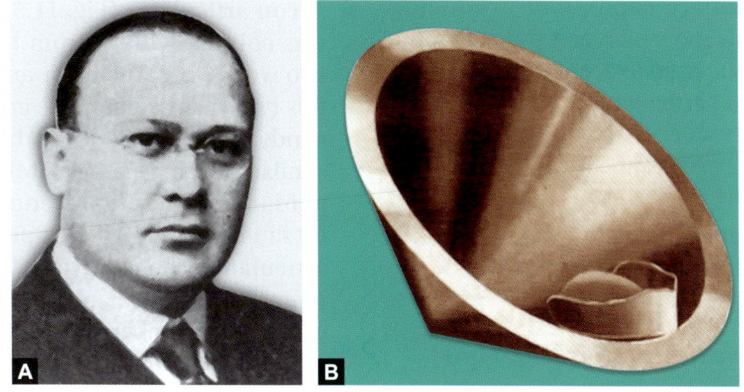

Figs. 11.2A and B: (A) Robert Hall; (B) Conical theory model.

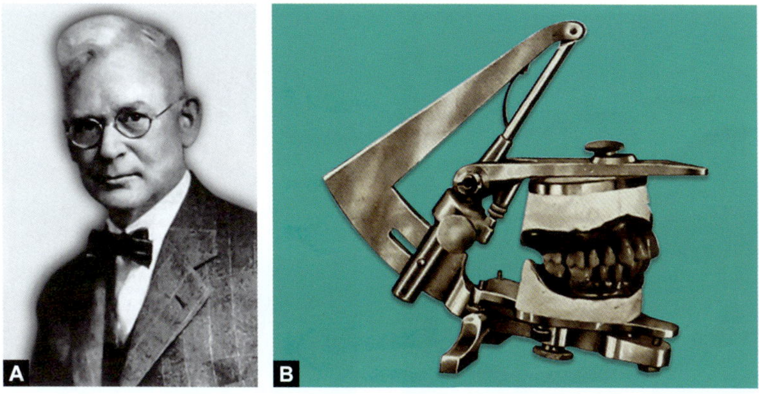

Figs. 11.3A and B: (A) Monson; (B) Monson articulator.

The theory states that the lower teeth move over the surface of sphere of 8 inch which has its center at the glabella. The surface of sphere passes through glenoid fossa along and articulating eminence.

Based on Type of Interocclusal Records Used

- **Interocclusal records adjustment:** These devices are programmed based on interocclusal records made up of plaster, bite registration polyvinyl siloxane, zinc oxide eugenol (ZOE) paste, and base plate wax.
- **Graphic records adjustment:** These articulators are capable of producing accurate jaw movements. A transographic record can be used to accurately locate the hinge axis on articulator.

Classification According to Adjustability of Articulators

- Nonadjustable articulators
- Semiadjustable articulators
- Fully adjustable articulators.

Nonadjustable Articulators (Fig. 11.4)

These are simple device to mount the casts. They are simple mechanical device which opens and close in one direction. They have fixed horizontal axis of rotation. The upper and lower members are joined together with hinge-like mechanism.

Examples are slab articulator and hinge articulator, mean value articulator.

Semiadjustable Articulators

They have adjustable horizontal condylar paths. They also have adjustable lateral condylar paths and incisal guide tables, and adjustable intercondylar distance. They accept face bow record.

These articulators are divided in two types based on arrangement of condylar guidance assembly.

1. **Arcon articulator (Fig. 11.5):** Term arcon was coined by Bergstrom by combining two words, i.e. articulator and condyle. In this type of articulator, the arrangement of condylar guidance and condylar element is similar to arrangement in TMJ. The condylar guidance which represents the glenoid fossa is attached with upper member of articulator. The condylar element which represents the human condyle is attached with lower member, e.g., Hanau wide-vue. *Advantages*: The face bow transfer, occlusal plane, and the relationship of opposing cast are preserved when articulator opened and closed.

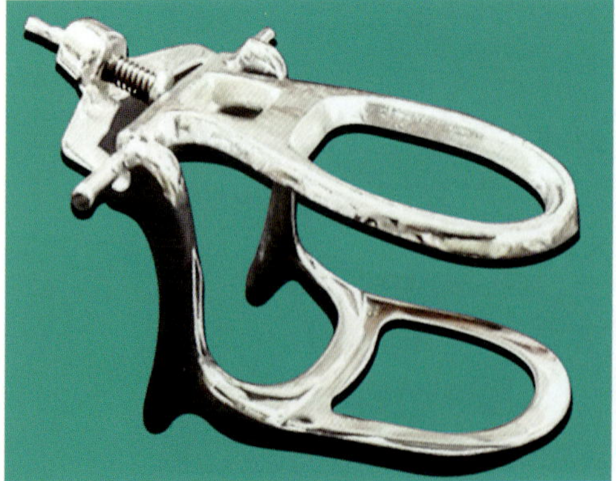

Fig. 11.4: Hinge articulator.

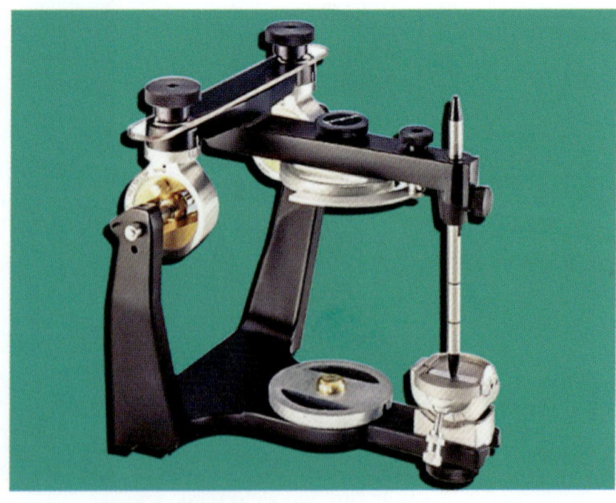

Fig. 11.5: Hanau wide-vue articulator—Arcon articulator.

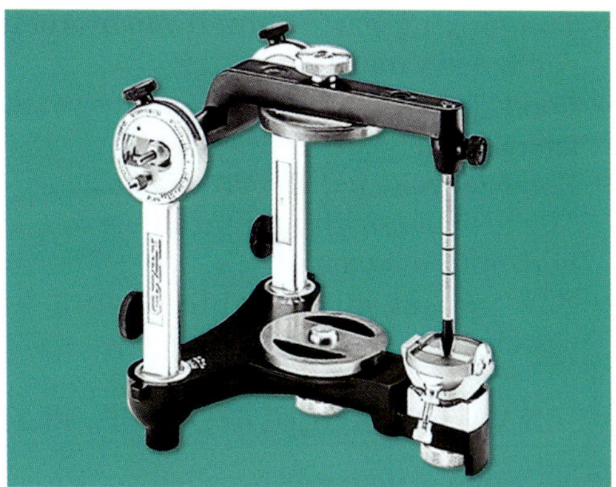

Fig. 11.6: Hanau H2 nonarcon articulator.

2. **Nonarcon articulators (Fig. 11.6):** In this type of articulators the position of condylar guidance and elements is reverse compared to human TMJ. The condylar guidance is attached with lower member and condylar element is attached with upper member, e.g., Hanau H2.

Fully Adjustable Articulators

They have ability to adjust according to patient's mandibular movements. They have provision to customize condylar guidance. They are highly precise in recording and understanding mandibular movements. Not widely used due to complexity. For example, is Stuart instrument gnathoscope.

Based on University of Michigan Workshop (Based on Ability to Simulate Jaw Movements)

Articulators may show single dimensional movement or they can show complex three-dimensional movements. The workshop on complete denture occlusion at the University of Michigan in 1972 classified articulators based on their ability to simulate jaw movements.

Class I

Simple device, capable of accepting single static record. Only vertical movement is possible.

Class II

These articulators perform horizontal and vertical movements but cannot orient the movement to TMJ with a face bow.

Class IIa

Limited eccentric motion is possible which is based on average value.

Class IIb

Limited eccentric motion is possible which is based on theories of arbitrary motion.

Class IIc

Limited eccentric motion is possible which is based on engraving records obtained from the patient.

Class III

They accept the face bow records but the facility is limited. They permit horizontal and vertical movements.

Class IIIa

They accept the face bow records. They accept static protrusive records.

Class IIIb

They accept static lateral, protrusive records.

Class IV

These articulators accept three-dimensional dynamic records. The point orientation of the cast can be achieved using face bow transfer.

Class IVa

Condylar path is determined by engraving records produced by the patient.

Class IVb

These articulators are similar to type IVa but they allow angulations in customization of condylar path.

Uses

- To diagnose the condition of occlusion in both natural and artificial dentition.
- To plan the treatment based on relationship of opposite natural or artificial teeth.
- To aid in the fabrication of restoration and prosthesis.
- To correct and modify complete restorations.
- To arrange artificial teeth.

Advantages

- Better visualization of cast and restorations in occlusion, especially from lingual side.
- Chair side and patient appointment time are reduced.
- No interference due to saliva, tongue, and cheek.
- Realeff effect eliminated (discrepancy due to resiliency of mucosa).
- Transfer of work from clinician to technician through articulators and vice versa.

Limitations

Since it is a mechanical instrument, it is subjected to error resulting from fatigue and wear.

It can simulate but not duplicate the jaw movements/relation.

Ideal Requirements

- It should hold casts in the correct horizontal and vertical relation.
- Provision to removal and reattachment of casts should be there.
- It should provide a positive anterior vertical stop.
- It should accept face bow transfer record using an anterior reference point.
- It should open and close in hinge movement.
- It should be made of noncorrosive and rigid material that resists wear and tear.
- It should not be bulky and heavy.
- There should be adequate space between the upper and lower member.
- The moving parts should move freely without any friction.
- Condylar guide should allow protrusive and lateral movements.
- Condylar guidance should be adjustable.
- The articulator should be adjustable in horizontal direction.
- The incisal guide table should be customizable (adjustable).

MEAN VALUE ARTICULATOR (FIG. 11.7)

Mean value articulator is called as "three-point articulator" or "free plane articulator". It is nonadjustable and nonarcon type of articulator. It is based on Bonwill theory of occlusion. According to this theory, an equilateral triangle of 4 inch formed between two condyles and from each condyle to midincisal point of mandibular incisors. It is capable of lateral and protruding movements based on the fixed average value in addition to hinge movements. Thus, these cannot be programmed to suit the individual requirement of a patient. The mean value of incisal guidance is fixed at 15°. Condylar guidance is fixed at 33° for mean value articulator.

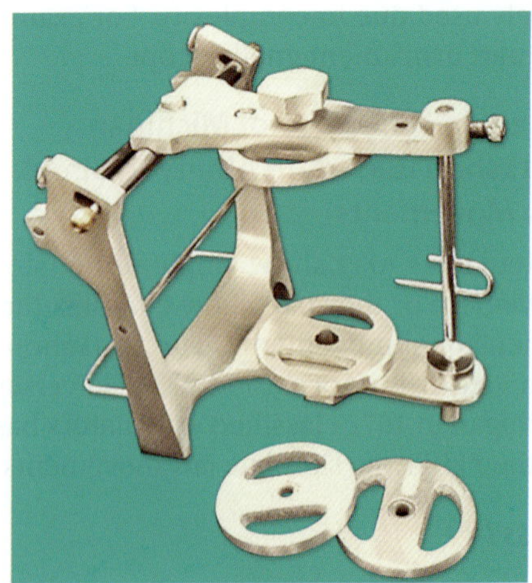

Fig. 11.7: Mean value articulator.

Various Models of Mean Value Articulator (Figs. 11.8A to D)

In mean value articulator, the intercondylar distance is 110 mm, condylar guidance is 30–33°, and incisal guidance is 15°. These are mean (average) values adopted for fabrication of articulator so known as mean value articulator.

Parts of Mean Value Articulators

Incisal Pin/Vertical Rod (Fig. 11.9)

It helps to keep a fixed distance between upper and lower member. It has a pointed tip resting on the center of incisal guide table. The upper flat surface should be flush with superior surface of upper member.

Condylar Shaft (Figs. 11.10A and B)

This is horizontal shaft attached with upper member of articulator. This attached in condylar slots. The length is 110 mm which represents intercondylar distance.

Midincisor Pin/Central Pin (Figs. 11.11A and B)

It is the anterior reference point. This is located at midpoint on incisal pin/rod. Relate to anterior occlusal plane. During mounting of wax occlusal rims this pin coincide with midline of occlusal rims. It helps during arrangement of maxillary central incisors according to midline and occlusal plane.

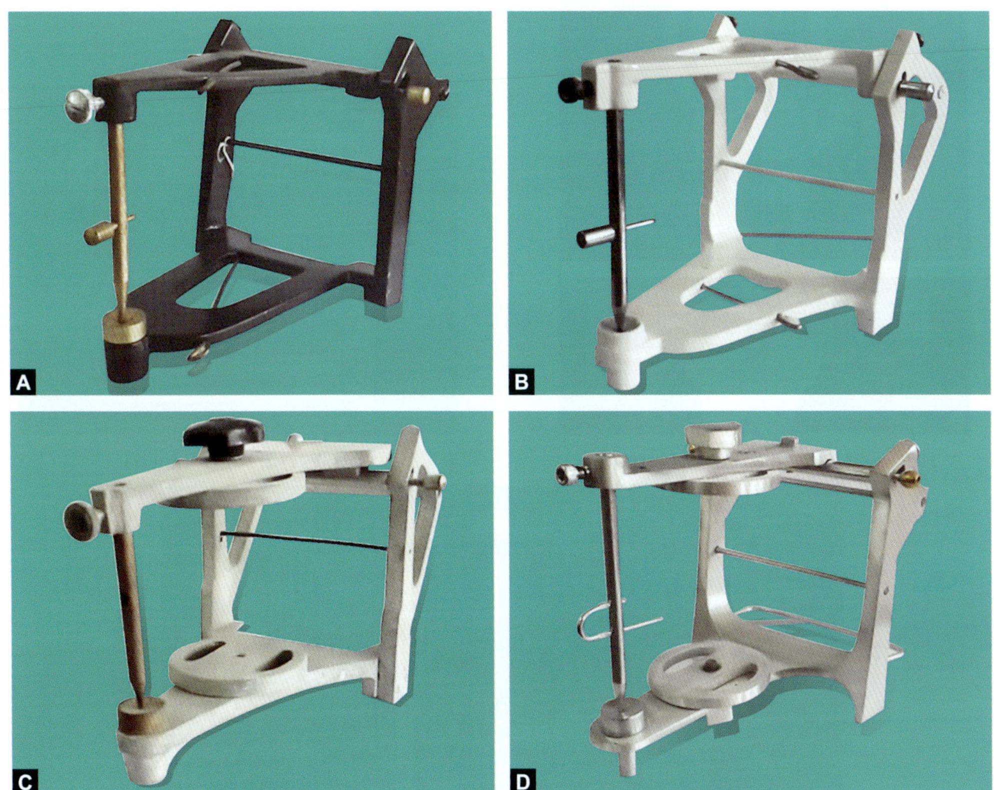

Figs. 11.8A to D: Various models of mean value articulator.

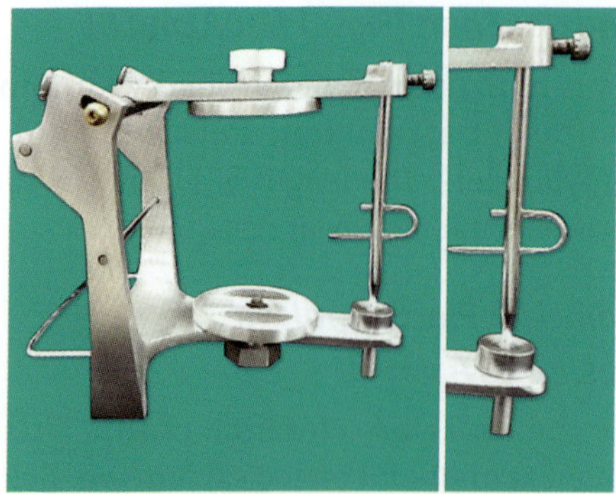

Fig. 11.9: Incisal pin/vertical rod.

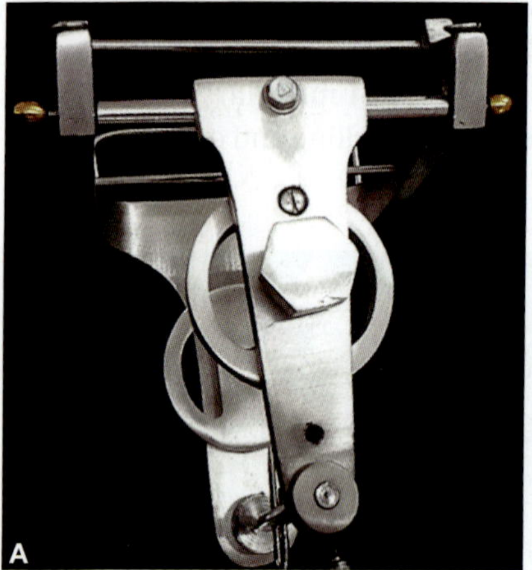

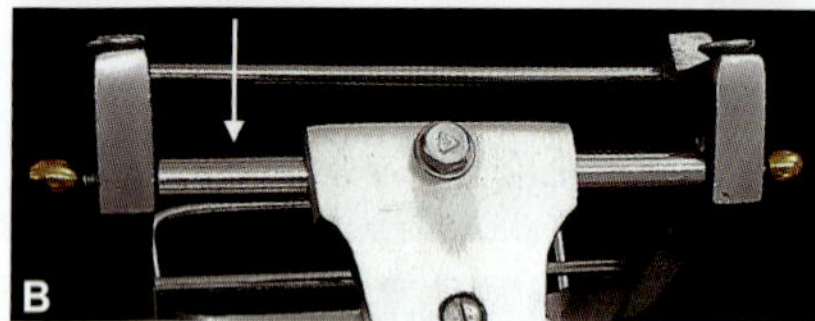

Figs. 11.10A and B: Condylar shaft.

Horizontal Bar (Fig. 11.12)

Two horizontal bars are attached in posterior region of articulator. Upper bar is supporting bar and the lower bar is known as horizontal orientation bar/rod. Orientation bar along with the midincisal pin form the plane of articulator. The plane of occlusion coincides with plane of articulator.

Upper Member (Fig. 11.13)

This represents maxilla on which maxillary cast may be attached (through mounting ring). It is triangular shaped. In anterior part incisal pin/vertical rod is attached and in posterior part two extensions corresponding to condyle elements are attached.

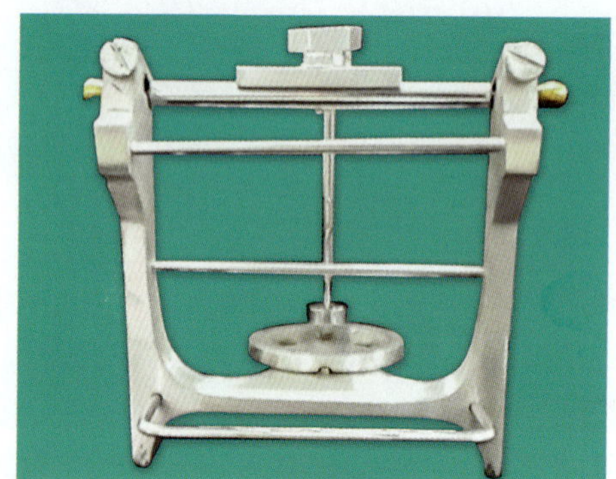

Fig. 11.12: Horizontal bar.

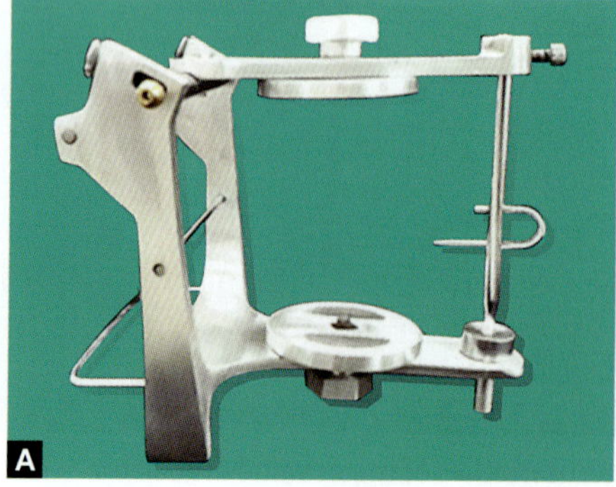

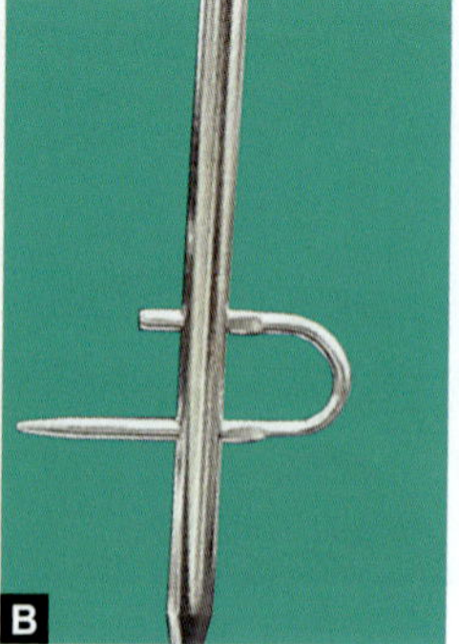

Figs. 11.11A and B: Incisor guide pin/central pin.

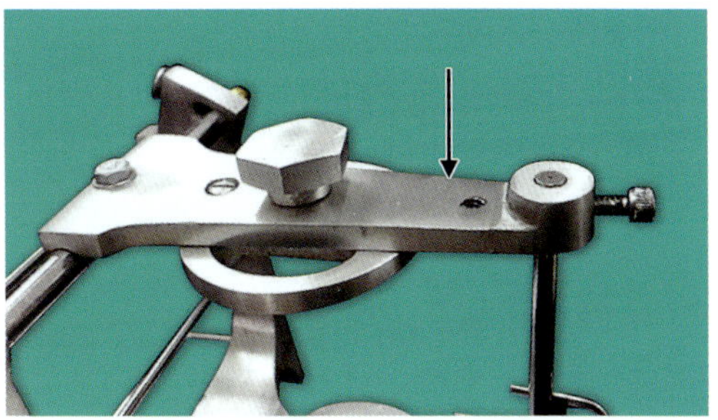

Fig. 11.13: Upper member of mean value articulator.

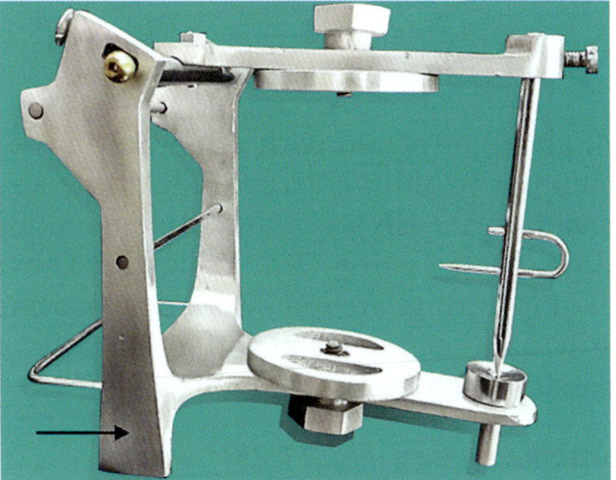

Fig. 11.14: Lower member of mean value articulator.

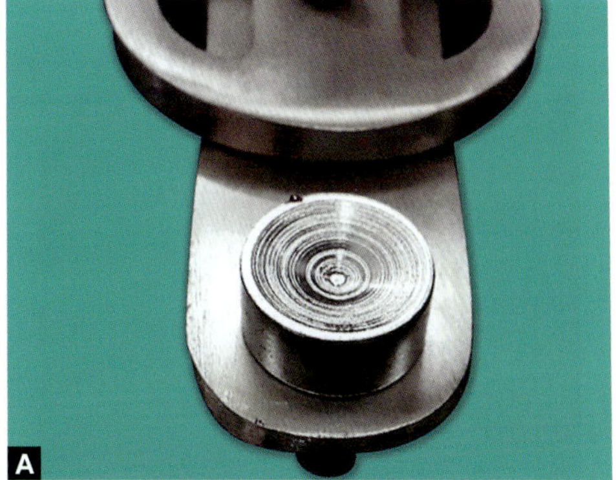

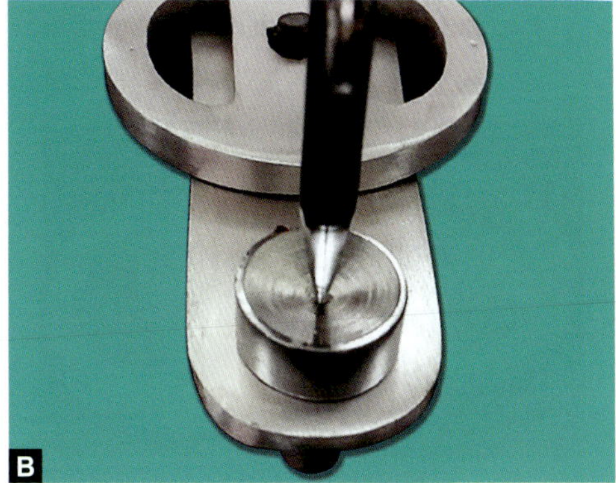

Figs. 11.15A and B: (A) Incisal guide table; (B) Vertical rod touching center of incisal guide table.

Lower Member (Fig. 11.14)

It is an "L"-shaped frame with vertical and horizontal arm.

Vertical part of "L" frame: Vertical arm of "L" frame is attached with upper member through condylar slots.

Horizontal bar is also attached on this part of lower member.

Horizontal part of "L" frame: In anterior region, anterior guide table is fixed.

In the center, mounting rim is attached on which mandibular cast is attached.

Incisal Guide Table/Anterior Guide Table (Figs. 11.15A and B)

It has a concave upper surface which gives the incisal guidance. The concavity is designed in such a way that it gives anterior guidance equal to 15°. Incisal pin/vertical rod is in contact with center of anterior guide table. The value of incisal guidance is fixed in mean value articulator.

Condylar Guidance (Fig. 11.16)

In mean value articulator condylar guidance is represented by a slot known as condylar slot/track. Condylar slot together with condylar elements make condylar guidance. Condylar elements are fixed in condylar slots. Spring assembly is attached in condylar slots/track to permit movements of condylar elements, when not in action it holds condylar elements in most posterior part of the slots. In mean value articulator condylar guidance is fixed at 33°.

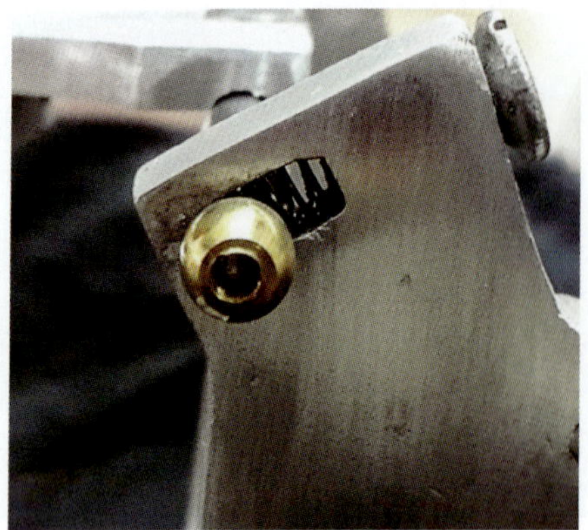

Fig. 11.16: Condylar guidance/slot of mean value articulator.

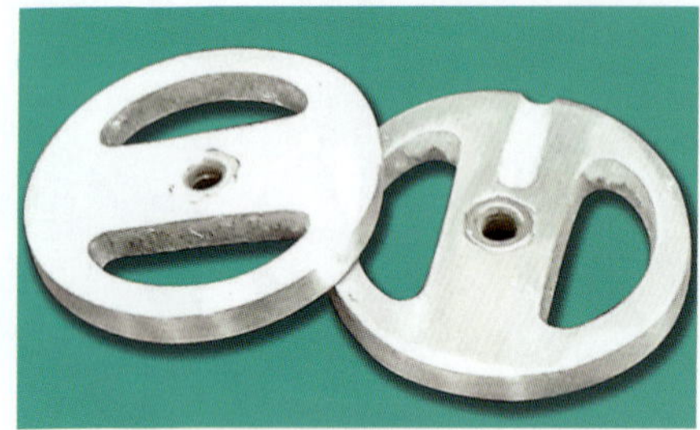

Fig. 11.17: Mounting rings/plates.

Mounting Rings/Plates (Fig. 11.17)

They are two in number, each attached with upper and lower member. Mounting plates/rings are attached with upper and lower member by thumb screws. Maxillary and mandibular casts are mounted on mounting rings/plates using dental plaster. These mounting rings are removable so that same articulator can be used with other case or patient with other set of mounting rings.

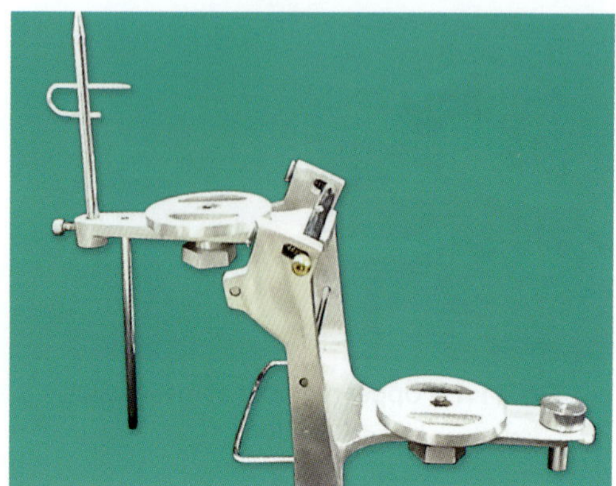

Fig. 11.18: Stabilizing rod stabilizes the upper member.

Stabilizing Rod (Fig. 11.18)

It is located in anterior part of upper member opposite to vertical rod. It prevents fall of upper member of articulator while working on it. It stabilizes the upper member.

CHAPTER 12

Indexing the Cast

Paranjay Prajapati, Sneha Kulkarni

INTRODUCTION

After recording jaw relation the same should be transferred to articulator for teeth arrangement and further laboratory procedures. Before mounting casts to the articulators, some modifications are done to the base of the casts for easy removal and accurate remounting. This chapter emphasizes on various indexing methods and briefs about mounting procedures.

INDEXING

Indexing is done on master cast. Indexing helps in remounting the casts in the same position on articulator after processing. Remounting is done to do selective grinding to eliminate processing errors.

REQUIREMENTS

- It should not weaken the cast
- Indexing should be free of undercuts
- Indexing procedure should be easy to perform
- It should permit easy removal and remounting
- It should be of use even if base of the cast is modified.

ARMAMENTARIUM

- Master casts
- Metallic scale
- Pencil
- BP blade No. 15 with handle/paper cutter.

TYPES

There are two types of indexing:

1. Groove indexing
2. Notch indexing.

Groove Indexing

In this method of indexing, "V"-shaped grooves are made across the base of the master cast.

For Maxillary Cast (Fig. 12.1)

Draw two lines that are perpendicular to each other through the center of the base of the cast.

For Mandibular Cast (Fig. 12.2)

Draw two lines that are on the thicker part of the cast. Draw these lines under the area of residual ridge as that is thicker area of the cast.

Make grooves along the lines. The grooves should be 3 mm in depth and 5 mm in width. The grooves can be made with 15 No. BP blade.

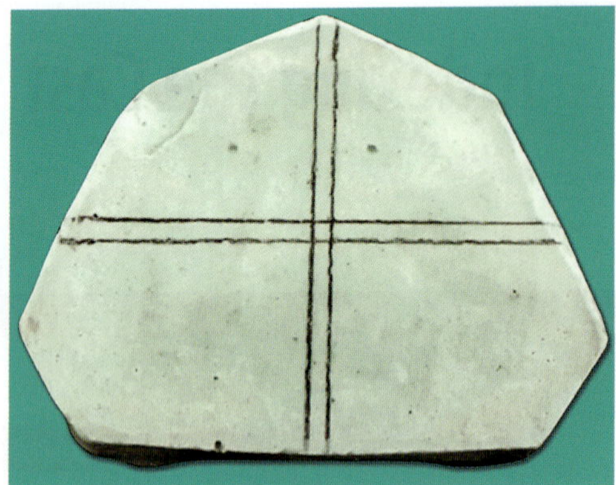

Fig. 12.1: Markings for groove indexing on maxillary cast.

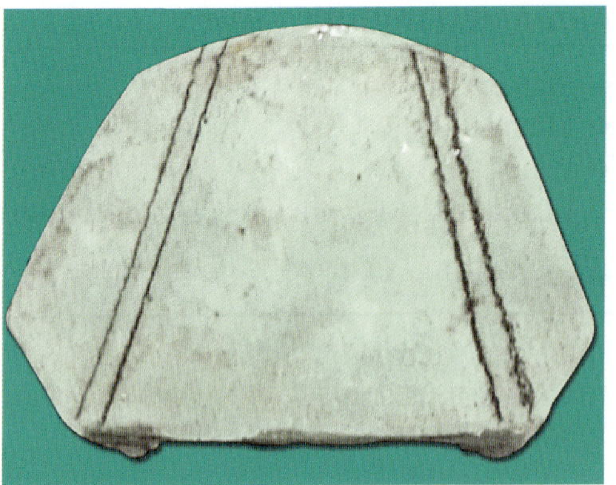

Fig. 12.2: Markings for groove indexing on mandibular cast.

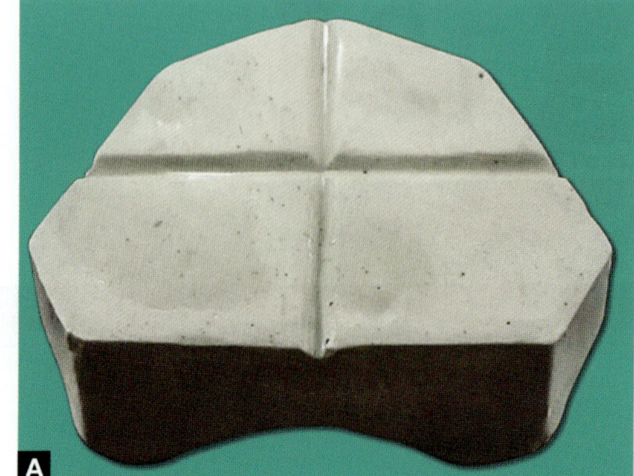

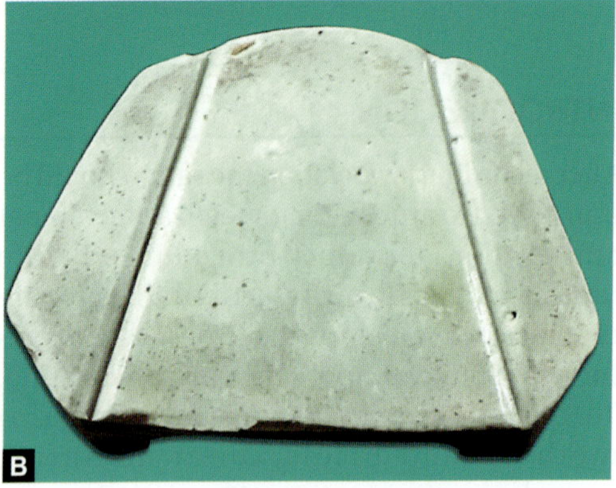

Figs. 12.3A and B: Groove indexing made on maxillary and mandibular casting.

Lathe mounted wheel which has been modified (sharpened) to make "V"-shaped groove can also be used for this purpose **(Figs. 12.3A and B)**.

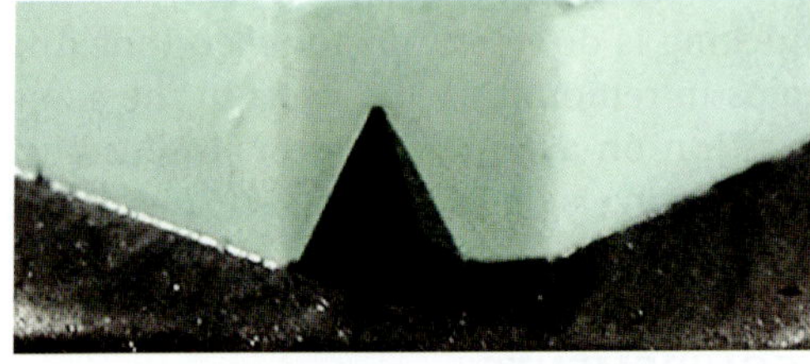

Fig. 12.4: Notch indexing.

Notch Indexing (Fig. 12.4)

In notch indexing "V"-shaped notches are created on the base of the cast. The notch should be 3 mm deep and 5 mm wide.

For Maxillary Cast (Figs. 12.5A to C)

Total four (04) notches are made for maxillary cast. Mark one notch in anterior, one in posterior and one on either side of the maxillary cast. Make notches using BP blade number 15.

For Mandibular Cast (Figs. 12.6A to C)

Total three (03) notches are made for mandibular cast. Mark one notch in anterior region and two in posterior region. Make notches using BP blade number 15.

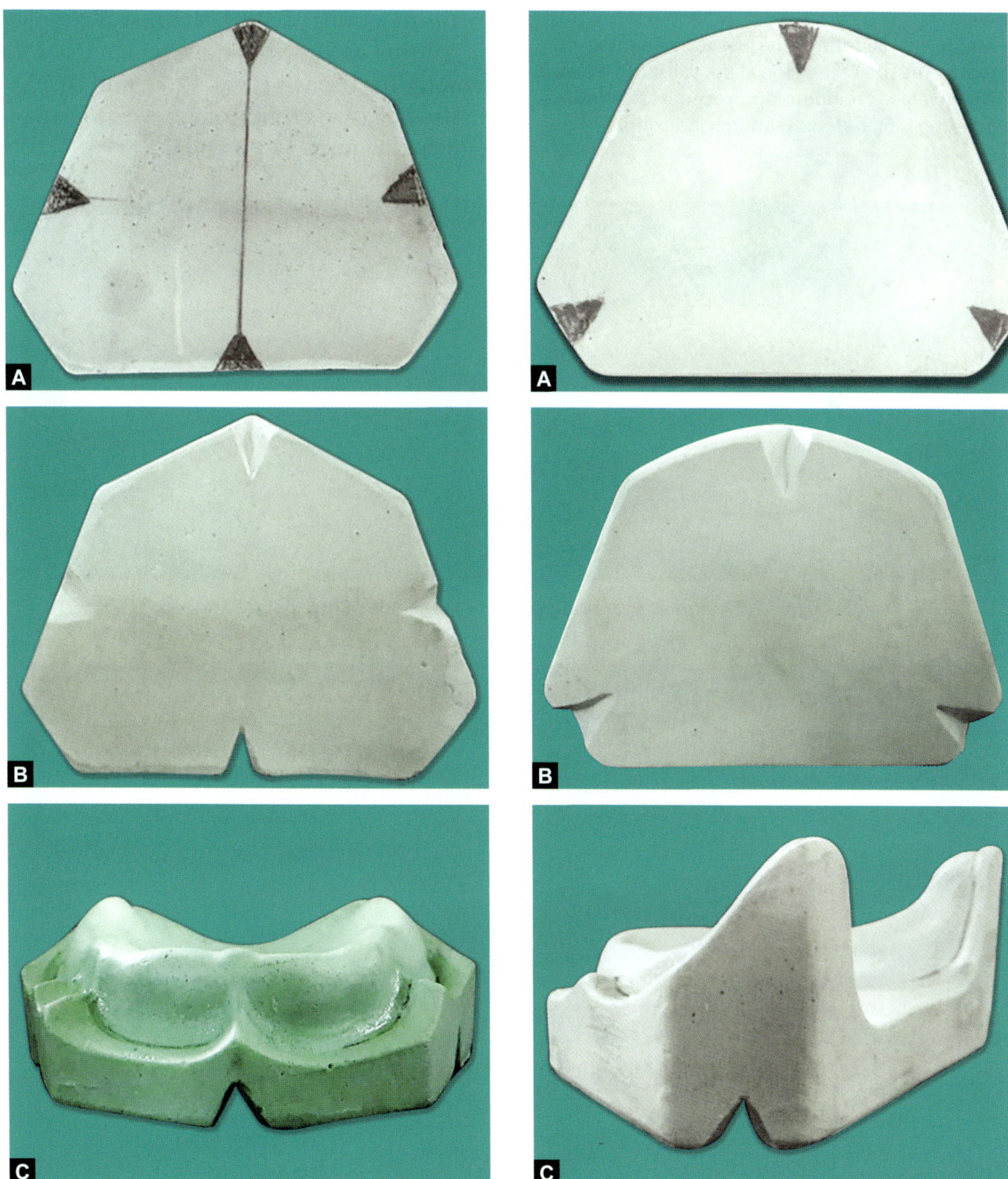

Figs. 12.5A to C: Notch indexing for maxillary cast.

Figs. 12.6A to C: Notch indexing for mandibular cast.

These indexing are made before mounting the casts on articulator. Sometimes it is necessary to reduce the size of base of the cast to fit in the flask during flasking procedure. During reduction of base thickness peripheral notch indexing will be trimmed and there will be loss of indexing.

If indexing is done with grooves, trimming may reduce the size of the groove but still it can be used effectively for remounting procedures so groove indexing is preferred over notch indexing.

The mounting plaster forms negative replica of grooves as shown below, which used for remounting of casts **(Figs. 12.7A and B)**.

The negative replica of groove indexing is shown in **Figures 12.8A and B**.

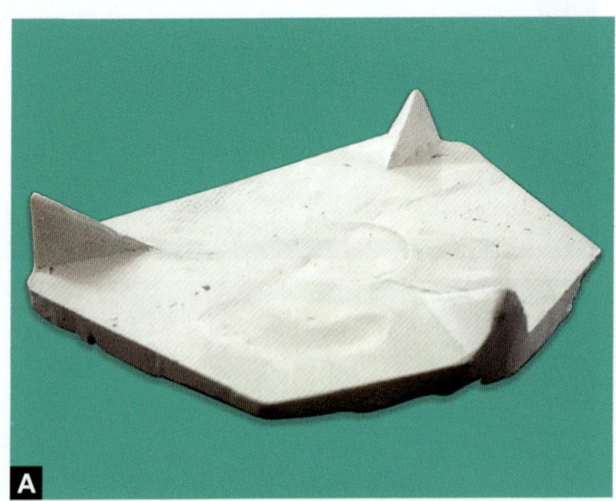

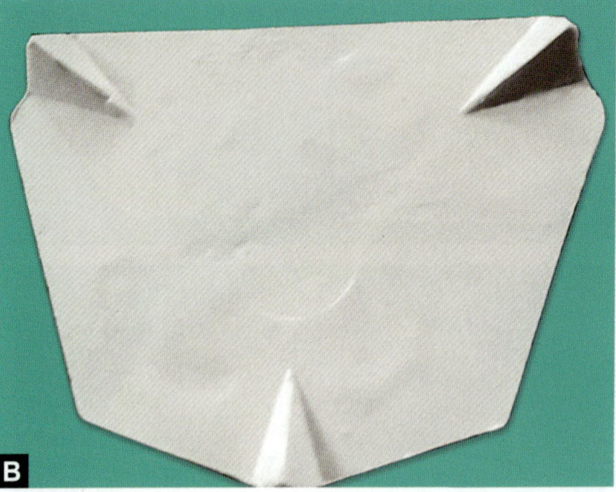

Figs. 12.7A and B: Mounting plaster extensions in notch indexing.

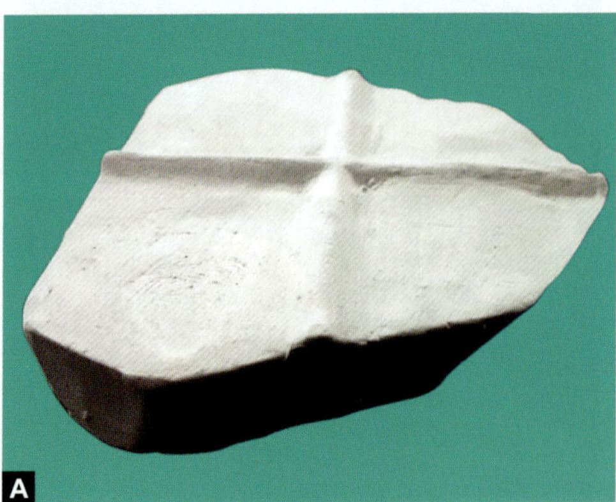

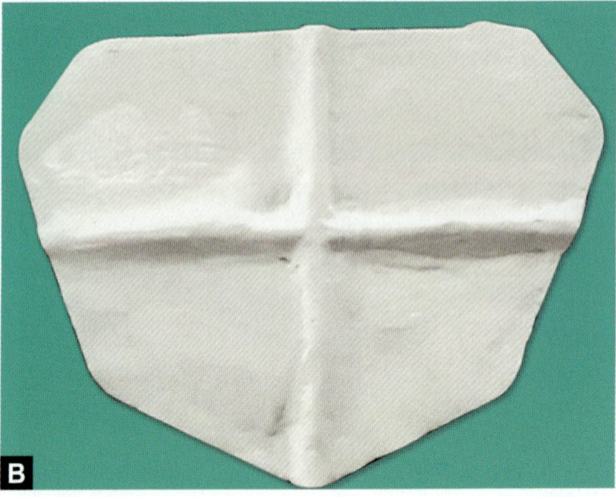

Figs. 12.8A and B: Mounting plaster extensions in groove indexing.

CHAPTER 13

Prosthetic Teeth

Rajesh Sethuraman, Paranjay Prajapati

INTRODUCTION

Artificial teeth or prosthetic teeth are considered as major factor determining the chewing efficiency of patient with prosthesis. Variety of artificial teeth in term of anatomy and materials are available in market. One should know how to select correct teeth which is most suitable for particular patient. This chapter focuses on important aspects of artificial teeth.

CLASSIFICATION OF PROSTHETIC TEETH

According to Material Used for Fabrication

- Acrylic teeth
- Porcelain teeth
- Composite teeth
- Acrylic teeth with amalgam inserts
- Acrylic teeth with metal occlusion.

According to Occlusal Anatomy of Teeth

- Anatomical teeth
- Semi-anatomical teeth
- Nonanatomical teeth.

ACRYLIC TEETH (FIG. 13.1)

Acrylic teeth are made up of acrylic, which bond chemically with denture base resin. They are available in various shapes and shades. They are most widely used denture teeth.

Indications

- When opposing teeth are acrylic teeth.
- When opposing teeth has metal occlusion.
- When less interarch space is available (in such case acrylic teeth can be trimmed easily to accommodate in available space).

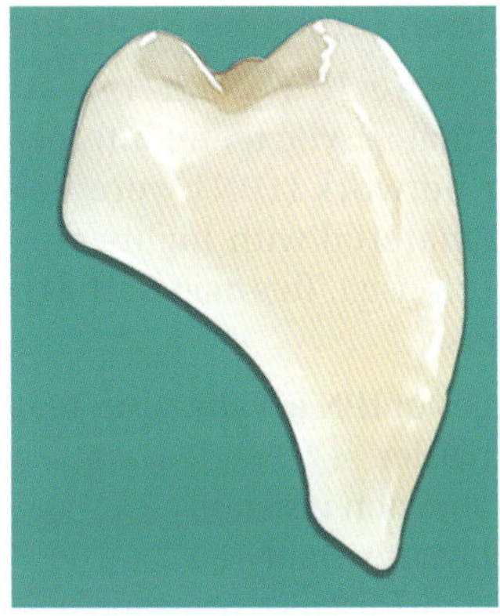

Fig. 13.1: Acrylic tooth.

Advantages

- They chemically bond with denture base material.
- They can be trimmed very thin to fit in available space.
- They do not abrade the opposing natural teeth.
- They can be easily polished.
- They can be easily modified to established occlusal contact with opposite teeth.
- They have less/softer impact sound (sound produced when opposite teeth come in contact).
- Less traumatic to denture foundation.

Disadvantages

- They wear with time.
- Subjected to abrasion if cleaning done with abrasive/rough substances.
- Due to wear, masticatory efficiency is reduced over a period of time.
- Stain and discolor easily.
- May need to be replaced due to excessive wear.
- Rebasing is difficult as acrylic teeth chemically attached with denture base.

Interpenetrating Polymer Network Acrylic Resin Teeth (IPN Resin Teeth)

To overcome low wear resistance of conventional acrylic teeth, interpenetrating polymer network (IPN) were developed. For IPN, material with highly cross-linked copolymer is used. This material has minimum or no fillers.

Advantages of IPN acrylic resin teeth are:

- More harder
- More abrasion resistant
- More heat resistant
- More stain/discolor resistant.

PORCELAIN TEETH (FIG. 13.2)

They are made up of porcelain (ceramic). There is no chemical bonding between porcelain teeth and acrylic resin. Porcelain teeth have metal pins or diatoric holes in ridge lap area, these features helps in mechanical bonding between porcelain teeth and denture base acrylic resin.

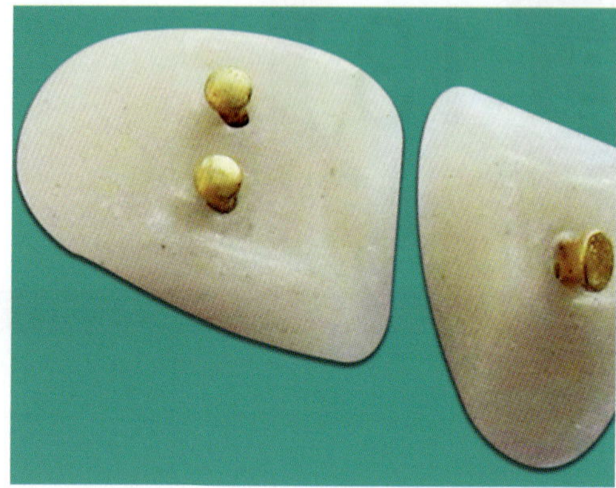

Fig. 13.2: Porcelain teeth with metal pins.

Indications

- Used where interarch space is sufficient and teeth placement can be done without trimming.
- Used with well-formed ridges.
- When patient demands high esthetic.
- When patient abrades acrylic teeth in short time, porcelain teeth are selected.

Advantages

- More resistant to wear compared to acrylic teeth.
- Good esthetic.
- Does not stain or discolor easily.
- Rebasing can be done easily as porcelain teeth are mechanically attached to denture base with the help of metal pins and channels within teeth.

Disadvantages

- No chemical bond with acrylic denture base.
- If used, opposite to the natural teeth they cause abrasion of natural teeth.

- As porcelain is brittle material, chipping and fracture is common with porcelain teeth.
- They have sharp impact sound (*clicking noise* comes when porcelain teeth contact with opposing arch porcelain teeth).
- Causes more trauma to denture foundation.

COMPOSITE TEETH

Composite teeth bond chemically to acrylic denture base material. Composite teeth have greater wear resistance compared to conventional acrylic resin teeth. They are more esthetic. They can be used opposing to natural dentition and opposing to acrylic teeth.

ACRYLIC TEETH WITH AMALGAM INSERTS/STOPS

In some clinical cases the acrylic resin teeth are placed opposite to porcelain teeth (when two opposite arches are not treated at same time). In such cases acrylic teeth abrade very quickly due to opposite porcelain teeth. To reduce this acrylic teeth wear, amalgam stops or inserts are prepared on acrylic teeth. To prepare these stops, cavities are prepares on occlusal surfaces of acrylic teeth and amalgam is placed in cavities. The contacts are established with opposite teeth before amalgam sets completely. This will establish the amalgam stops with proper occlusal contacts. Whenever patient chews, the amalgam stops come in contact with the porcelain teeth and prevent the direct contact of acrylic with porcelain teeth and reduce acrylic wear.

ACRYLIC TEETH WITH METAL OCCLUSION

To reduce the wear of acrylic teeth when opposing teeth are natural teeth or porcelain teeth or metal restorations, the acrylic teeth are modified with metal occlusion. The occlusal surface of acrylic teeth is prepared and wax pattern is made over it. Casting is done to convert the wax pattern in metal occlusion. The metal occlusion is then cemented to acrylic teeth to prepare acrylic teeth with metal occlusion **(Fig. 13.3)**.

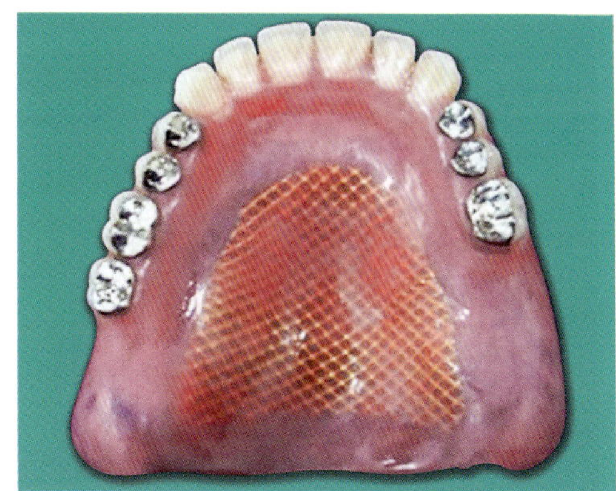

Fig. 13.3: Acrylic teeth with metal occlusion.

ANATOMICAL TEETH

Shape

Cuspal angulation: 33° or more (Figs. 13.4A and B).

Synonyms

Cusp teeth.

Indications

- Well-formed ridges.
- When teeth to be arranged in balanced occlusion (anterior and posterior simultaneous contacts of teeth in any centric or eccentric position).
- Patients with good neuromuscular control.

Advantages

- They have better chewing efficiency compared to semi-anatomic and non-anatomic teeth.
- They have more natural appearance.
- They penetrate food more easily.
- Act as a guide for proper jaw closure.

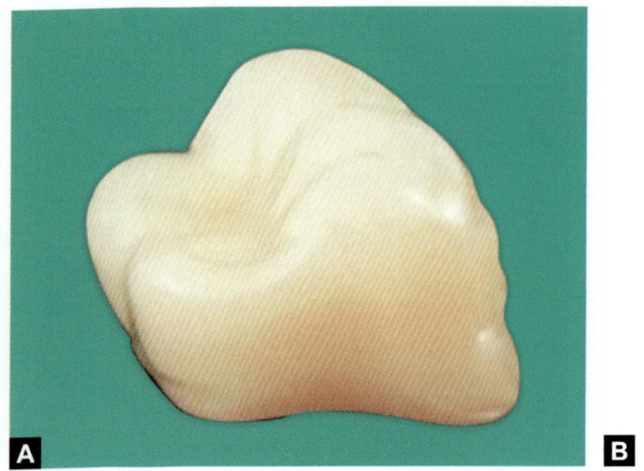

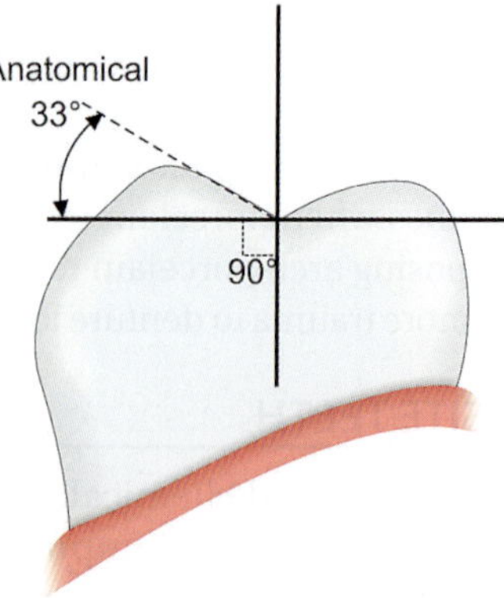

Figs. 13.4A and B: Anatomical tooth with 33° cuspal angulation.

- ❖ Resist rotation of the denture bases through cusp interdigitations.

Disadvantages

- ❖ More time-consuming procedure to arranged in balanced occlusion.
- ❖ Posterior teeth placement restricted by opposing fossa and cusps.
- ❖ Denture bases need frequent relining to keep occlusion stable and balanced.
- ❖ More occlusion disharmony during settling and difficult to correct by adjustment.
- ❖ Precise jaw closure and base stability required for interdigitation.
- ❖ Difficult to adapt to abnormal jaw relationship (class II and class III).
- ❖ Increased horizontal forces due to deep cuspal angulation.

SEMI-ANATOMICAL TEETH

Shape

Cuspal angulation: 20° **(Figs. 13.5A and B)**.

Synonyms

Low cusp teeth, modified cusp teeth.

Indications

- ❖ Well-formed ridges and fair ridges.
- ❖ When balanced occlusion to be achieved.
- ❖ In patient with mild jaw discrepancies.

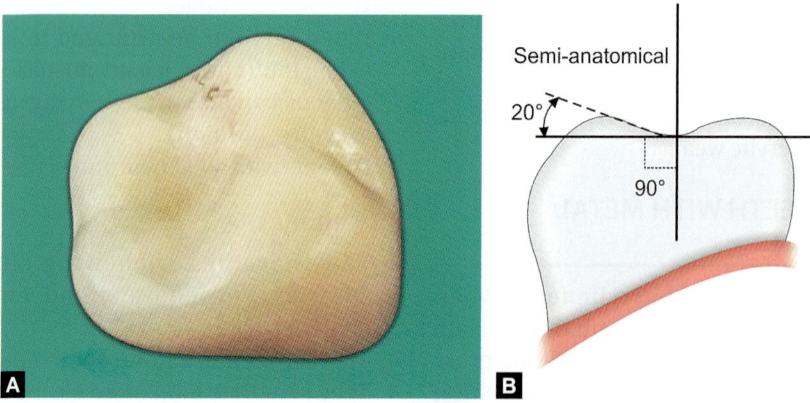

Figs. 13.5A and B: Semi-anatomical tooth with 20° cuspal angulation.

Advantages

- Balanced occlusion can be easily obtained.
- Good chewing efficiency compared to nonanatomic teeth.
- Better esthetic compared to nonanatomic teeth.
- Shallow cuspal inclination generates less horizontal forces compared to anatomic teeth.

Disadvantages

- *Poor esthetic* compared to anatomic teeth.
- *Lesser chewing efficiency* compared to anatomic teeth.

NONANATOMIC TEETH

Shape

Cuspal angulation: 0° **(Figs. 13.6A and B)**.

Synonyms

Cusp less teeth, monoplane teeth, monoline, and zero degree teeth.

Indications

- Patient with poor ridge (severely resorbed ridge).
- Patient with poor neuromuscular control.
- Patient with jaw discrepancies.
- When crossbite tooth relation is indicated.
- Indicated to use for patient with uncoordinated closure and poor neuromuscular control, i.e., patients suffering from parkinsonism, dyskinesia, and stroke.

Advantages

- Quick arrangement of teeth.
- Less force transferred to residual alveolar ridge.
- Prevent destruction of tissue.
- Freedom of occlusal movements (from centric to eccentric position).
- Does not lock the mandible in one position.
- Permits the use of less time-consuming technique.
- Adapt easily to class II and class III jaw relations.
- More easily adjusted after changes in vertical and horizontal relations.
- Easier to arrange in crossbite.

Disadvantages

- *Least chewing efficiency* compared to semi-anatomic and anatomic teeth.
- *Least esthetic* compared to semi-anatomic and anatomic teeth.
- Difficult to arrange in balanced occlusion.

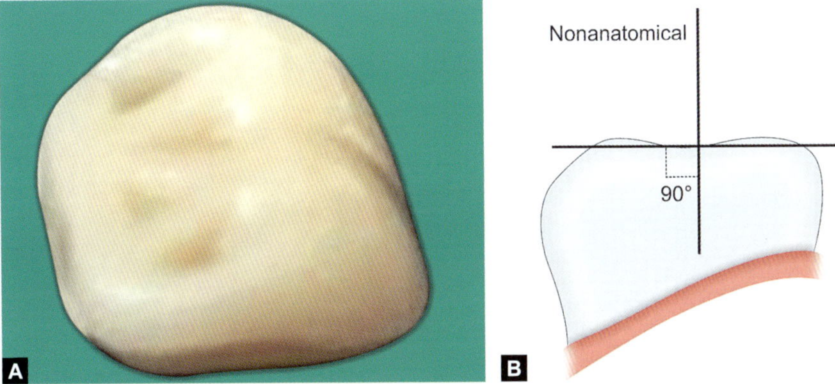

Figs. 13.6A and B: On anatomic tooth with 0° cuspal angulation or flat cusps.

THE PROSTHETIC TEETH SET (FIG. 13.7)

Prosthetic teeth are available as full set of 28 teeth including six anterior and eight posterior teeth (Total 14 teeth/arch) for each maxillary and mandibular arch. Some manufacturer provide anterior and posterior teeth separately also. Artificial teeth sets do not have third molars. They are attached on plastic card through wax. This plastic card is called as "tooth card" and wax used for this is "carding wax" **(Fig. 13.8)**.

Shape

Prosthetic anterior teeth are usually available in square, tapered, and ovoid shapes.

Shade

They are available in various shades like A1, A2, A3, A3.5, A4, B1, B2, B3, B4, C1, C2, C3, C4, D2, D3, D4, E1, F1, and F2.

Size

Artificial teeth are available in various sizes. The size of teeth is designated by a number. Number describes the combined width of anterior teeth and A2 is the shade **(Fig. 13.9)**.

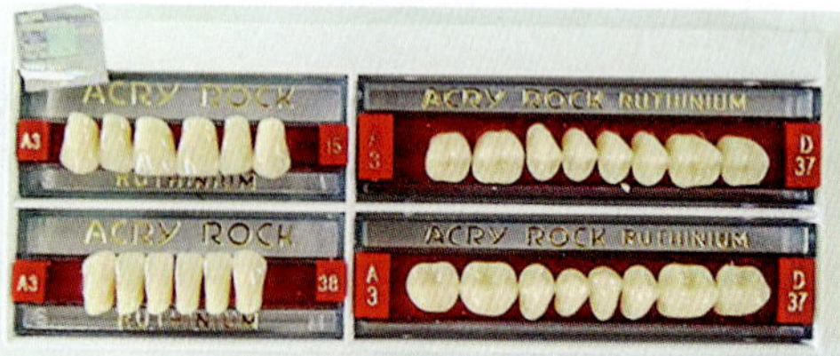

Fig. 13.7: Acrylic teeth set.

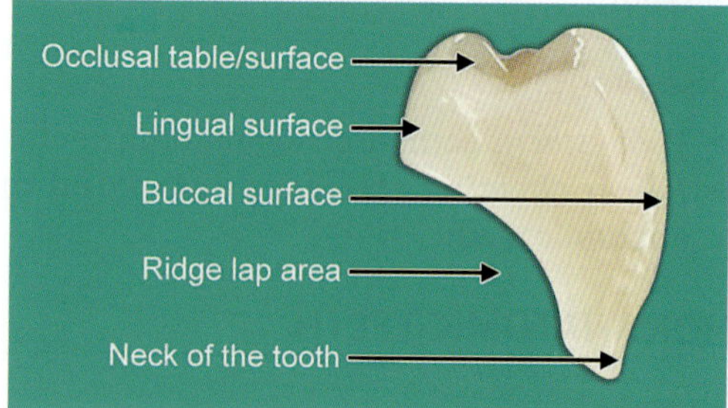

Fig. 13.8: Parts/surfaces of tooth.

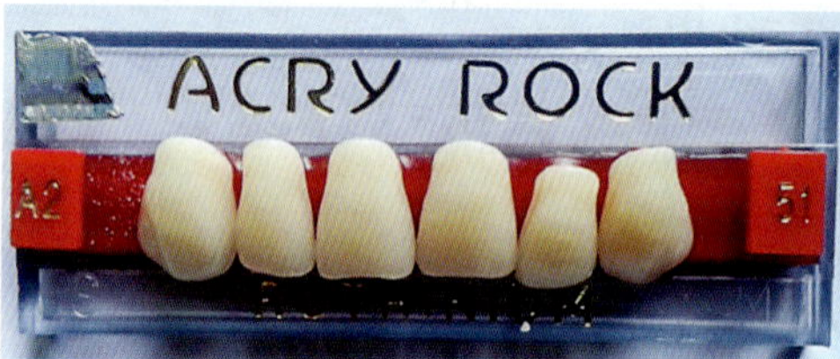

Fig. 13.9: Tooth card with anterior teeth.

Teeth Selection: Brief Overview

Rajesh Sethuraman, Paranjay Prajapati

INTRODUCTION

Teeth selection is important procedure which requires knowledge of denture foundation and patient's demand of esthetic. Various factors affect the selection of teeth like, available bone support, type of mucosa, the relationship of edentulous jaws with each other and patient demand. This chapter briefly explains about various available methods used to select artificial teeth.

DEFINITION

The selection of a tooth or teeth of a shape, size, and color to harmonize with the individual characteristics of a patient.

OBJECTIVES OF TEETH SELECTION

- The anterior teeth selected should be esthetically acceptable and should perform their function.
- Posterior teeth selected should aid in denture stability and should be efficient in mastication.
- They should not abuse the tissue over residual ridges.
- They should maintain correct vertical dimension.
- They should not impair the speech.

ANTERIOR TEETH SELECTION

Esthetic is the prime objective in selection of artificial anterior teeth. Before selection of teeth one should inform the patient and should approve it from patient. During anterior teeth selection various parameters are taken into considerations. They are as follow:

- Size of the teeth
- Shape of the teeth
- Color/shade of the teeth
- Material of teeth (acrylic, porcelain, etc.).

Selection of Teeth Size

Various factors are considered during selection of proper teeth size. Three main factors are: (1) Width—mesiodistal width; (2) Length—incisogingival length; (3) Thickness—labiolingual thickness. There are various subjective and objective methods available for selection of teeth size (**Tables 14.1 to 14.5**).

Selection of Teeth Shape

Shape of artificial teeth can be selected using preextracted and postextracted records of the patient. Commonly used method is based on classification proposed by *Leon and Williams*. According to them the *shape of teeth should be inverse of the shape of face*. The shape of

Table 14.1: Use of pre-extraction record of patient.	
Diagnostic cast	Casts with natural teeth can give idea about teeth size and shape. It is most reliable pre-extraction record
Photographs of patient	Information like size, shape and also color of patient's natural teeth can be achieved. Facial view of patient is important for teeth placement and lip support
Radiographs of patient	Dentist can get information regarding the size and shape of natural teeth of patient and based on that the artificial teeth can be selected. Radiographic errors like elongation and shortening may give false idea

Table 14.2: Use of postextraction record of patient.	
Extracted teeth	Preserved extracted teeth by patient is the best guide in selection of size and shape of artificial teeth. They may get discolored after extraction so not used for determination of color
Previous prosthesis	Old prosthesis is important to know about shape, size, and color of teeth previously used

Table 14.3: Use of anthropometric methods.	
Combined width of maxillary anteriors	Bizygomatic width/3.3
Width of maxillary central incisor	Bizygomatic width/16
Total width of mandibular anteriors	4/5* (total width of maxillary anteriors)
Width of maxillary lateral incisor is 2 mm less than central incisor	
Width of maxillary canine is 1 mm less than width of central incisor	
Cranial circumference is measured at forehead level and divided by 10 gives total width of maxillary anteriors	

the maxillary central incisor should resemble the facial form (shape of face) if it was placed upside down. The teeth selection based on facial form is also known as geometric theory.

Table 14.4: Use of anatomical landmarks.	
Using size of maxillary arch	Mark three points. One on crest of incisive papilla and one each on both hamular notches. Join them together to form a triangle. Measure each side and combine them. Total value obtained is equal to total width of maxillary anterior and posterior teeth
Using corners of the mouth	Make markings on maxillary occlusal rim matching to corners of the mouth. These markings indicates distal surface of canine. Hence distance between these two markings gives combined width of maxillary anterior teeth
Use of canine eminence	If canine eminences are clearly seen bilaterally, measure the distance between them following the ridge contour. This will give combined width of maxillary anterior teeth

Table 14.5: Selection of incisogingival length and labiolingual thickness.	
Using smile line as guide	During jaw relation ask patient to smile. Mark the lower border of upper lip. Generally, neck of teeth coincides with lower border of smiling upper lip (smile line). Select teeth slighter longer so that denture base will not be visible
Interarch space	If available interarch space is less, the teeth with less incisogingival length should be selected. With more interarch space longer teeth should be selected
Using length of face as guide	Length of maxillary central incisor = Distance between hairline and tip of chin/16
Thicker teeth are more esthetic as they can be placed rotated and spaced out	

The facial form is identified by connecting the following points on the face.

- The forehead
- Zygomatic arch
- Angle of mandible.

Table 14.6: Classification of facial form.

Square facial form	*Square tapering facial form*	*Tapering (tapered) facial form*	*Ovoid facial form*

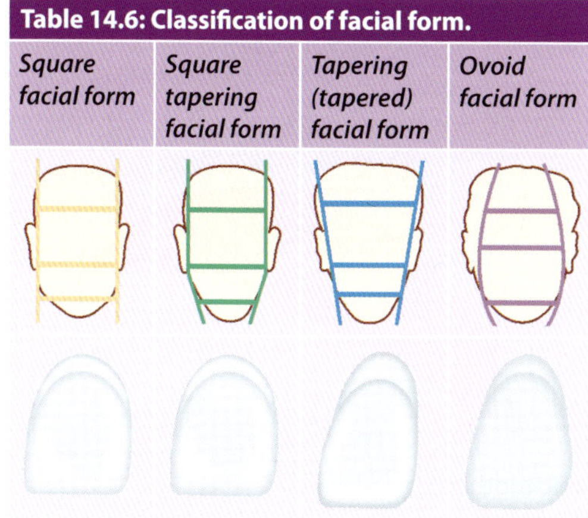

According to this the facial form can be classified as given in **Table 14.6**.

Selection of Teeth Color/Shade (Table 14.7)

In selection of tooth shade, components of color, i.e., hue, value, and croma play a major role. Apart from these opacity, translucency, transparency, metamerism, and fluorescence are also important factors.

Table 14.7: Selection of teeth color/shade.

Age	In young patient lighter shade is preferred. For old patients darker shade is selected as teeth become darker and yellower in old age
Color of face	The shade of teeth should be in harmony with skin color. For fair complexion patient, lighter color teeth with high value should be selected. For darker complexion dark color teeth with low value should be preferred
Color of eye and hair	There is relation between color of eye and hair to the skin color. Earlier this factor was also considered for teeth selection but nowadays eye and hair color can be changed with artificial lenses and hair dyes so not considered for selection of teeth shade

POSTERIOR TEETH SELECTION

Selection of Size of Posterior Teeth (Table 14.8)

If teeth are placed beyond maxillary tuberosity, it results in tipping of denture and cheek biting. If teeth are placed on retromolar pad (as it is displaceable tissue) results in tipping of denture during mastication.

Selection of Shape of Posterior Teeth

Posterior teeth are available in various shapes. Their selection for edentulous patient depends on ridge condition, jaw discrepancies, and systemic conditions (poor neuromuscular control, Parkinsonism).

- Anatomical teeth—when ridges are well formed **(Fig. 14.1)**.
- Semi-anatomic teeth—used when ridges are fair **(Fig. 14.2)**.
- Nonanatomic teeth—used when ridges are poor **(Fig. 14.3)**.

Table 14.8: Selection of size of posterior teeth.

Mesiodistal width	Maxillary teeth should be selected such that they occupy space between distal of canine to maxillary tuberosity and mandibular teeth should occupy space between distal of mandibular canine and beginning of retromolar pad
Buccolingual width	Narrow occlusal table is selected. It reduces amount of forces transferred on foundation area. It allows sloping of flanges and adaptation of cheek and tongue to flanges and maintains denture stability. Narrow occlusal table facilitate escapement of food during mastication
Occlusogingival length	Selected based on available interarch space. Long teeth selected in more interarch space and shorter teeth selected in case of less interarch space

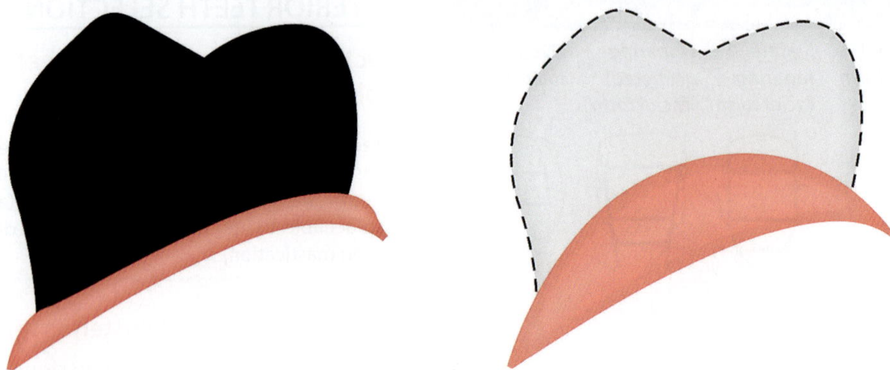

Fig. 14.1: Anatomic tooth.

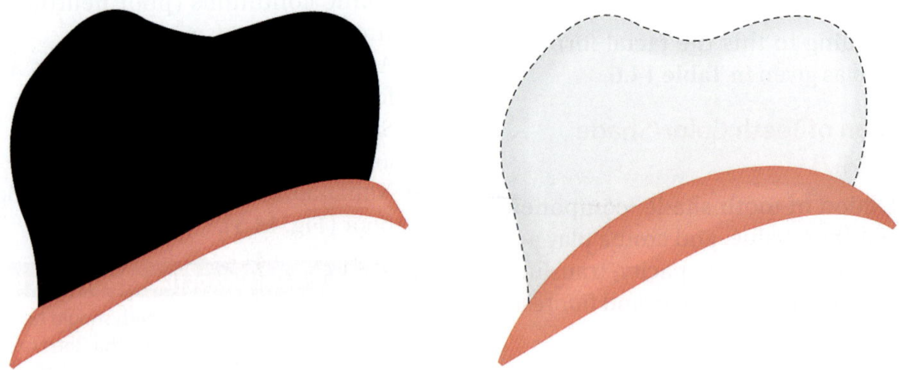

Fig. 14.2: Semi-anatomic tooth.

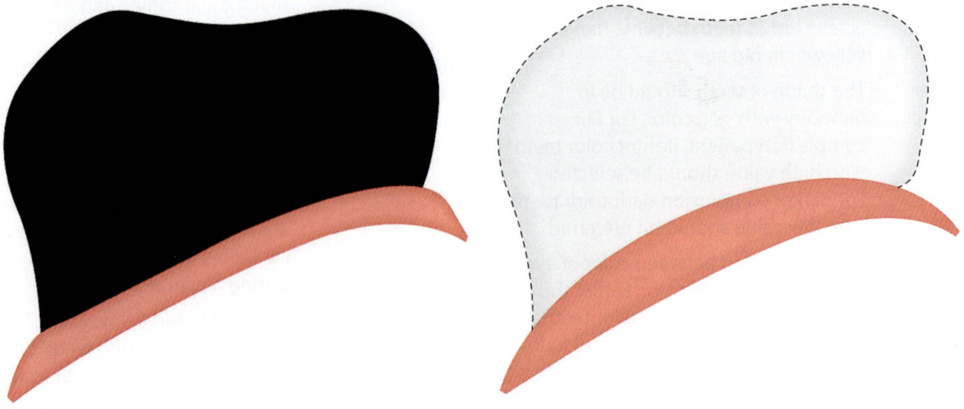

Fig. 14.3: Nonanatomic tooth.

DENTOGENIC CONCEPT (SPA GUIDELINES)

This concept was proposed by Frush and Fisher. They suggested guidelines for selection and arrangement of teeth based on three factors, i.e., (1) Sex (2) Personality, and (3) Age.

Sex

The characteristic difference in teeth of male and female is listed in **Table 14.9**.

Personality

Flush and Fisher used personality spectrum consisting in see **Table 14.10**.

Age

According to dentogenic concept the visibility of maxillary and mandibular teeth varies according to age of the patient. In young age patient, there is considerable exposure of maxillary central incisors but in old aged patient there is no exposure. The opposite occurs for mandibular teeth, less exposure of mandibular teeth for young patient and more exposure of mandibular incisors for old aged patients.

Natural teeth wear with increasing age in most of the patients; this can be duplicated in denture by grinding the incisal edges of anterior teeth.

Gingival papillae in old age become blunted and shortened; this should be duplicated in denture wax up.

Table 14.9: Character of male and female patients.

Character	*Male patients*	*Female patients*
Tooth form	Square or cuboidal	Spherical
Color	Darker shade	Lighter shade
Labial surface	Flat mesiodistally and incisogingivally	Curved mesiodistally and incisogingivally
Incisal angles	Sharper incisal angles	Rounded incisal angles
Width	Broader lateral incisor and other teeth	Narrow lateral incisor and other teeth
Cervical area	More prominent	Less prominent
Canine arrangements	More prominent and turned out at incisal edge	Less prominent and turned in at incisal edge

Table 14.10: Personality spectrum (Flush and Fisher).

Delicate personality	It is fragile and frail. Light colored, round feminine looking teeth are selected for this kind of patients
Medium personality	This is moderate and most common personality type. Majority patients have medium personality. Teeth which have blend of both delicate and vigorous characteristics are selected
Vigorous personality	This type is hard and aggressive. Broad teeth with sharp angles and dark color is suitable for this personality

Lines, Planes, and Curves in Prosthodontics

YG Naveen, Jignesh Chaudhari

INTRODUCTION

Some lines and planes are used as reference and guides for various prosthodontic procedures. This chapter describes various lines, planes, and curves related to prosthodontic specialty.

LINES IN PROSTHODONTICS

These guidelines are used as reference during fabrication of occlusal rims on maxillary and mandibular casts.

Maxillary Guidelines (Fig. 15.1)

M line: Midline between center of incisive papilla and fovea palatine. It divides cast into right and left halves.

R line: Crest line from distal of canine to the crest of maxillary tuberosity.

B line: Line between right and left second premolars.

C line: Line between distal of canine and point X.

Mandibular Guidelines (Fig. 15.2)

M line: Midline between labial frenum and midpoint between both retromolar pads.

R line: Line between distal part of canine and anterior part of retromolar pad.

B line: Line joining right and left second premolars.

C line: Line between distal of canine and point X.

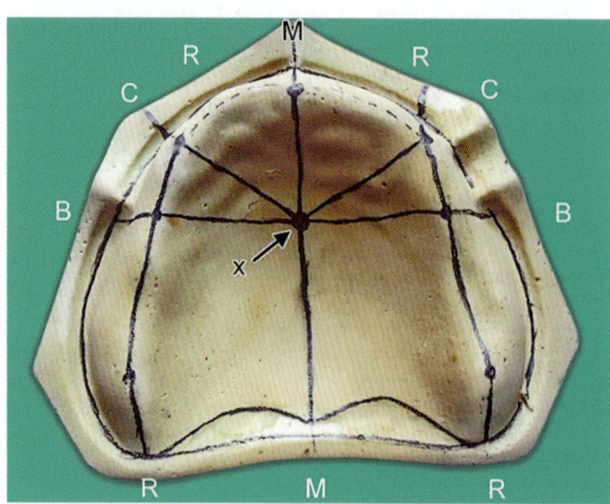

Fig. 15.1: Maxillary guidelines.

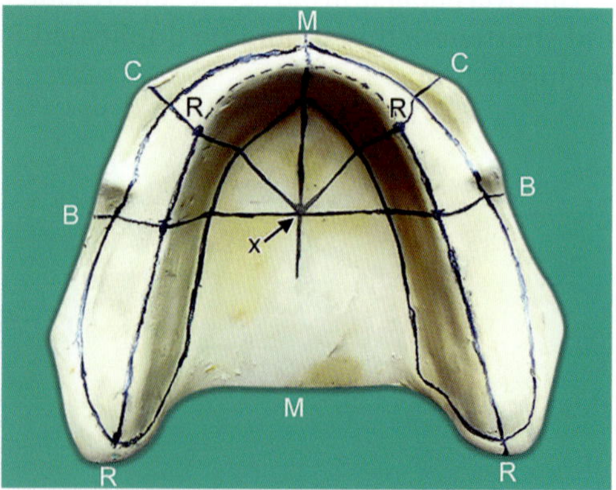

Fig. 15.2: Mandibular guidelines.

PLANES IN PROSTHODONTICS

Camper's Plane: (Ala-tragus Plane/ Bromell's Plane) (Fig. 15.3)

A plane established by the inferior border of the ala of the nose and the superior border of the tragus of both ears. This is also known as ala-tragus plane or line. This plane is used to establish occlusal plane during jaw relation.

Occlusal Plane (Fig. 15.4)

Occlusal plane is one where maxillary and mandibular teeth occlude with each other. In instance of occlusal rims plane of occlusal is established at level of interface when maxillary and mandibular rims are in contact with each other (the plane between maxillary and mandibular occlusal rims).

Plane of Articulator (Fig. 15.5)

For mean value articulator plane of articulator is established by midincisal pin and posterior reference bar/rod.

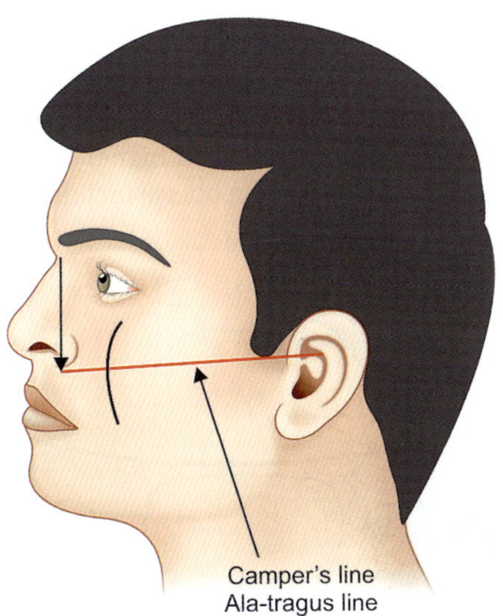

Fig. 15.3: Campers plane: (ala-tragus plane/ Bromell's plane.

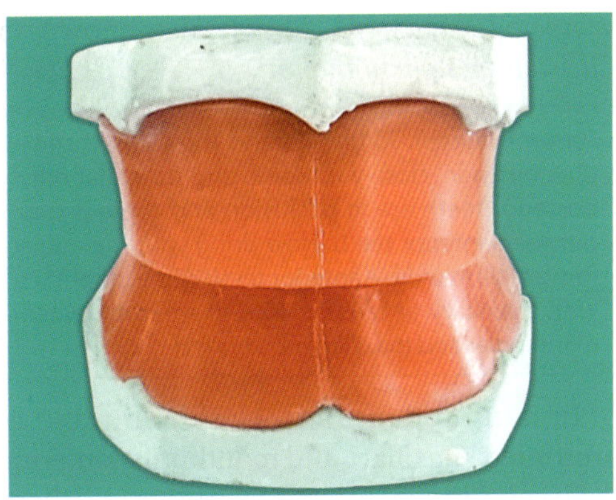

Fig. 15.4: Occlusal plane.

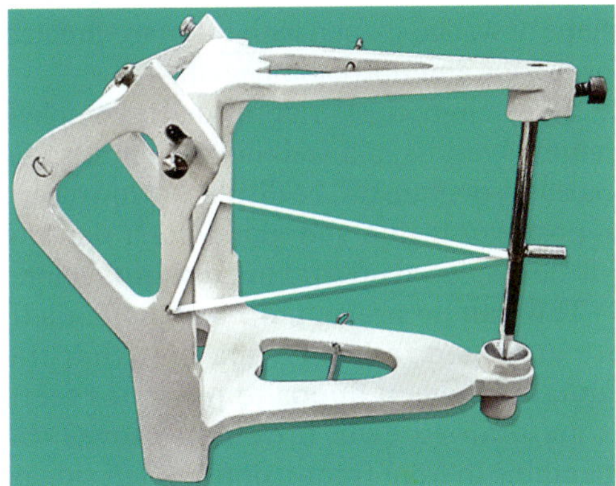

Fig. 15.5: Plane of articulator.

CURVES IN PROSTHODONTICS

Various imaginary curves exist in natural dentition. These curves are due to anteroposterior and lateral inclination of individual tooth. During teeth arrangement these curves should be reproduces by aligning the artificial teeth.

When posterior teeth are in occlusion, there is disocclusion (gap formation) between maxillary and mandibular anterior teeth. When protrusive movement is performed (bring the mandible forward), mandibular anterior teeth come in contact with maxillary anterior teeth, resulting in disocclusion of posterior teeth. This is called as *"mutually protected occlusion"*. This is also known as *Christensen's phenomenon.*

> *Perform yourself*: To understand the Christensen's phenomenon, close your teeth and note that only posterior teeth are in occlusion and there is gap between anterior teeth. Now bring your mandible forward till mandible anterior teeth come in contact with maxillary anteriors. Note the gap between mandibular and maxillary posteriors.

In natural dentition when mandible is protruded, maxillary and mandibular anterior teeth come in contact with each other and there will be disocclusion (space) between upper and lower posterior teeth. This space is triangular in shape or wedge shaped with the apex directed toward the anterior/canine teeth.

If the same occlusion is provided in complete dentures results in instability of denture, i.e., maxillary denture will be displaced downward in posterior region and mandibular denture will be displaced upward in posterior region.

This can be prevented; if artificial teeth are arranged in such a manner that the contact between opposite posterior teeth is maintained even if patient moves the mandible in front (protrusion), or left side or right side (left and right lateral movements).

In any position or movement there is constant contacts maintained in anterior teeth and posterior teeth. This concept of maintaining bilateral, simultaneous, anterior and posterior occlusal contact of teeth in centric and eccentric position is called as "*balanced occlusion*". Balanced occlusion gives stability to complete denture.

CURVES IN NATURAL DENTITION

Anteroposterior Curve

Curve of Spee (Fig. 15.6)

This curve was described by German anatomist Ferdinand Graf Spee in 1890.

It is defined as the anatomic curve established by the occlusal alignment of the teeth, as projected onto the mesial plane, beginning with the cusp tip of mandibular canine and following the buccal cusp tips of the premolar and molar teeth, continuing through the anterior border of the mandibular ramus, ending with the anterior most portion of the mandibular condyle.

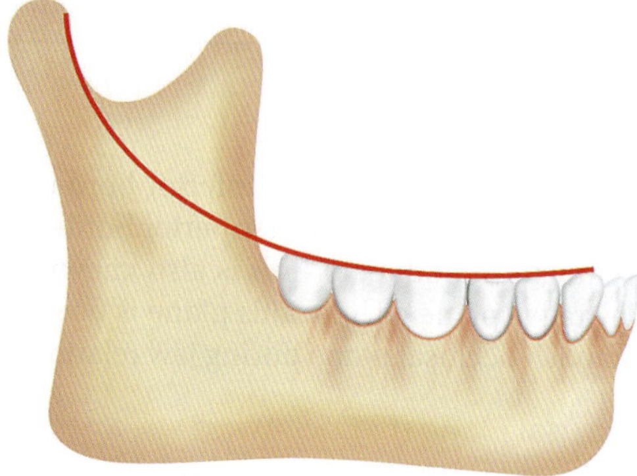

Fig. 15.6: Curve of Spee.

Mediolateral Curves

Curve of Wilson (Fig. 15.7)

It is mediolateral curve that contacts the buccal and lingual cusp tips on each side of the arch. It results from lingual inclination of mandibular molar, making the lingual cusps lower than the buccal cusps. Accordingly, the buccal cusps of maxillary molars are placed higher than the palatal cusps resulting in buccal inclination of

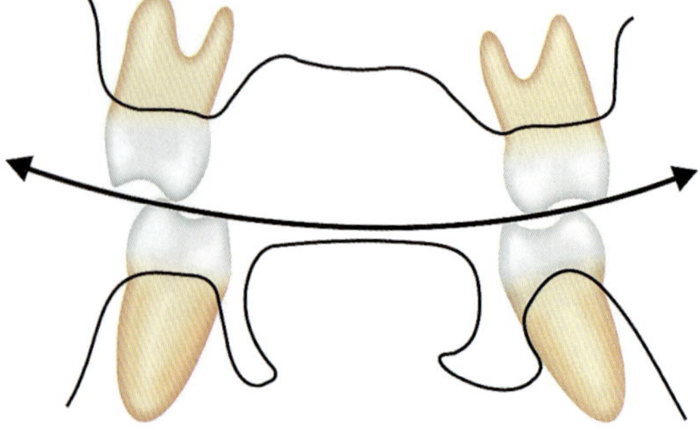

Fig. 15.7: Curve of Wilson.

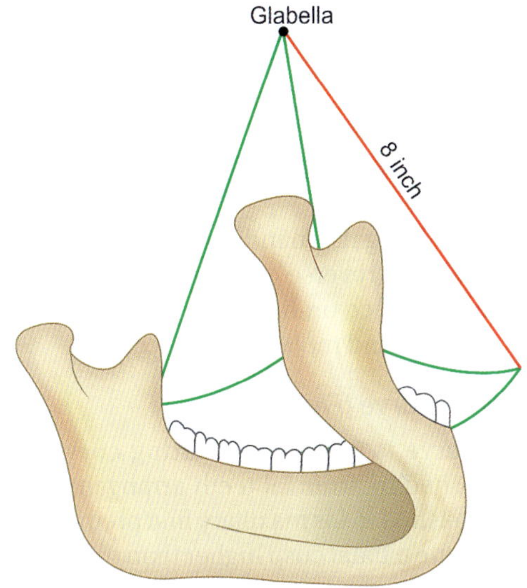

Fig. 15.8: Curve of Monson.

maxillary molar teeth. This arrangement results in concave curve for maxillary arch and convex curvature in mandibular arch.

Curve of Monson (Fig. 15.8)

It is defined as the curve of occlusion in which each cusp and incisal edge touches or conforms to a segment of a sphere of 8 inches in diameter with its center in the region of glabella.

This curve is based on spherical theory of occlusion proposed by Monson.

COMPENSATING CURVE

Compensating curves are artificial counterpart of natural curves. They are established during arrangement of complete denture teeth.

Definition

It is defined as the anteroposterior curvature (in the median plane) and the mediolateral curvature in the frontal plane in alignment of the occluding surfaces and incisal edges of the artificial teeth that are used to develop balanced occlusion.

They are called as compensating curved because they compensate for the space formed between the maxillary and mandibular posterior teeth during protruding and lateral mandibular movements. These curves compensate for Christensen's phenomenon occurring in natural dentition, so that maxillary and mandibular posterior teeth occlude with each other and there will not be any space between them during any eccentric movement of mandible. They hence help in achieving balanced occlusion in complete denture and provide stability to complete denture.

Curves in Artificial Dentition

- **Anteroposterior compensating curve:** Compensating curve for curve of Spee.
- **Mediolateral compensating curves:**
  - Compensating curve for curve of Wilson
  - Compensating curve for curve of Monson
- Pleasure curve
- Reverse curve.

Compensating Curve for Curve of Spee

This compensating curve can be established at the distal marginal ridge of the first posterior replacement tooth and continue through the second molar. It is incorporated into artificial occlusion by raising distal portion of the first and second molars to conform to the curve. This is usually done to maintain posterior balancing contact and to compensate for the spacing that occurs between maxillary and mandibular posterior teeth during protrusive movements of mandible.

Mediolateral Compensating Curves

- **Compensating curve for curve of Wilson:** This compensating curve can be achieved by tilting maxillary molars such that the buccal cusps are higher than the palatal cusps and mandibular molars are tilted lingually to make lingual cusps lower than buccal cusps. This compensating curve is important for lateral balance of occlusion.

- **Compensating curve for curve of Monson:** This curve runs across the buccal and palatal cusps of maxillary molars. This is important to achieve lateral balance of occlusion.

> Wilson curve runs opposite to the direction of Monson curve and hence called as "anti-Monson curve".

Pleasure Curve

It is defined as helicoidal curve of occlusion that when viewed in the frontal plane conforms to a curve that is convex superiorly except for the last molars which reverse the pattern.

This was proposed by Maximum Pleasure to provide balanced occlusion and better stability. Maximum Pleasure proposed to modify the mandibular teeth occlusal surfaces to a reverse curve by tilting the mandibular teeth buccally. He proposed reverse curve in premolars, flat occlusal surface on first molars and Monson curve on second molar for balance.

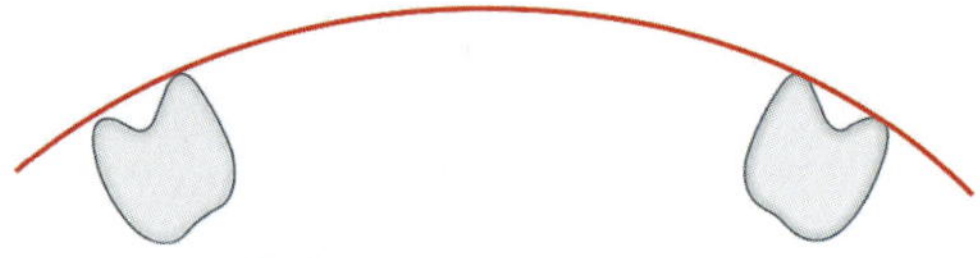

Fig. 15.9: Reverse curve.

Reverse Curve (Fig. 15.9)

This curve is not compensating curve but established in artificial teeth arrangement. It is established in for maxillary first premolar by raising the palatal cusp higher than the buccal cusp (reverse than usual arrangement pattern, i.e., buccal cusp higher than palatal).

CHAPTER 16

Complete Denture Occlusion: An Overview

Rajesh Sethuraman, JR Patel

INTRODUCTION

Occlusion means "contact". Occlusion in prosthesis is required to achieve esthetic, stability, and chewing ability. This chapter focuses on different concepts and types of complete denture occlusion.

DEFINITION

Occlusion: The relationship between the occlusal surfaces of the maxillary and mandibular teeth when they are in contact.

OBJECTIVES

- It should provide maximum intercuspation of the maxillary and mandibular teeth in centric relation
- Should minimize harmful lateral forces
- Should be designed to provide stability to complete denture
- Should maintain comfort and well-being of the patient
- Should be designed such a way that it can guide jaw closure
- Occlusion should not cause any trauma to underlying soft and hard tissue.

DIFFERENCES BETWEEN NATURAL AND ARTIFICIAL OCCLUSION

The teeth in natural dentitions are retained by periodontal tissues. In complete denture all the teeth are on denture bases seated on denture foundation.

In natural dentitions the teeth receive individual occlusal load and can move independently to adjust to occlusal load. The artificial teeth move as a whole unit on denture foundation.

Malocclusion of natural teeth may not be harmful for years. Malocclusion of artificial teeth induces an instant response and involves all of the teeth and the denture base.

Horizontal or rotational forces on natural teeth during function affect only the teeth involved and are usually well tolerated, whereas in artificial occlusion, the effect involves all of the teeth on the denture bases and is traumatic.

In natural teeth, the second molar is the favored area for masticating hard foods. Heavy pressures of mastication in the second molar region with artificial dentition will tilt the prosthesis.

In natural teeth, prematurities are avoided due to neuromuscular system control. In artificial occlusion any prematurely causes instability due to lack of feedback.

CLASSIFICATION

Angle classified occlusion in three classes based on relationship of opposing posterior teeth **(Table 16.1)**.

THEORIES OF OCCLUSION

Bonwill's Theory of Occlusion

According to this theory of occlusion, the teeth move in relation with each other as guided by the *condylar and incisal guidance*. This theory is also known as "Theory of equilateral triangle". According to this, distance between two condyles is equal to distance between condyle and midincisor point of mandible. Each side of this triangle measures 4 inch (all sides measure equal distance of 4 inch, so called as equilateral triangle).

Conical Theory of Occlusion

This theory was proposed by RE Hall. According to this theory mandibular teeth move over the surface of the maxillary teeth as if they are moving over the surface of a cone, generating an angle of 45° with the central axis of the cone tipped at 45° to the occlusal plane.

Table 16.1: Angle classification.

Class I	The mesiobuccal cusp of the maxillary first molar occludes in the buccal groove of the mandibular first molar
Class II	The distobuccal cusp of the maxillary first molar occludes in the buccal groove of the mandibular first molar
Class III	The mesiobuccal cusp of the maxillary first molar occludes in the embrasure between the mandibular first and second molars

Spherical Theory of Occlusion

This theory was proposed by Monson. According to this theory, mandibular teeth move over the surface of the maxillary teeth as over a surface of sphere with a diameter of 8 inch. The center of the sphere located in the region of glabella. The surface of sphere passes through the glenoid fossa and articulating eminences.

TYPES/CONCEPTS OF THE COMPLETE DENTURE OCCLUSION

Balanced Occlusion

Definition

The bilateral, simultaneous, anterior, and posterior occlusal contact of teeth in centric and eccentric positions.

In this type of occlusion there is bilateral, simultaneous, anterior, and posterior occlusal contact of teeth in centric and eccentric positions. This type of occlusion provides good stability of denture due to simultaneous contacts. In most cases anatomical teeth are used for arrangement. Difficult and time consuming to get balanced occlusion. It enhances retention and stability of complete denture. Balanced occlusion distributes forces equally all over the denture-bearing area resulting in reduced resorption of alveolar bone.

Factors Influencing Balanced Occlusion

Condylar guidance: It is angle generated by condyle and the articular disk traversing the contour of glenoid fossa.

Incisal guidance: The influence of contacting surfaces of maxillary and mandibular anterior teeth.

Plane of occlusion: It is average plane established by the incisal and occlusal surfaces of teeth.

Cuspal inclination: Cuspal inclination is slope of a cusp with the occlusal plane.

Compensating curve: Anteroposterior and mediolateral curves in alignment of artificial teeth are used to develop balanced occlusion.

Lingualized Occlusion

Definition

This form of denture occlusion articulated the maxillary lingual cusps with the mandibular occlusal surfaces in centric, working, and nonworking mandibular positions (the term is attributed to Earl Pound and was first describes by S Howard Payne, in 1941).

This form of denture occlusion articulates the maxillary lingual cusps with the mandibular occlusal surfaces in centric, working, and nonworking mandibular positions. Carry advantages of both anatomical and non-anatomical teeth.

Monoplane Occlusion

Definition

An occlusal arrangement wherein the posterior teeth have masticatory surfaces that lack any cuspal height.

This type of occlusion arrangement is achieved using nonanatomic or monoplane teeth. Philosophy behind this type of arrangement is to elimination of cusps and so minimizing the lateral forces which ultimately enhance the denture stability. Anterior teeth are arranged with 2 mm overjet and zero overbite. Easy to arrange teeth according to this scheme but chewing efficiency is less due to monoplane/nonanatomic teeth.

NEUTROCENTRIC CONCEPT OF OCCLUSION

This concept was proposed by Devan. It expresses the centralization of occlusion forces that act on the basal seal when mandible is in centric relation with maxilla. Teeth are arranged flat with no medial or lateral inclination. No compensating curves are incorporated.

CHAPTER 17

Making Primary Impression of Maxillary and Mandibular Edentulous Foundations

Paranjay Prajapati, Sneha Kulkarni

INTRODUCTION

Correctly made primary impression is base for fabrication of good quality, well-fitting complete denture. Primary impression should be made with great care as it is important to fabricate custom tray which is needed for making final impression. Various materials can be used for making primary impression depending upon condition of denture foundation area. In present chapter we will learn to make impression of edentulous maxillary and mandibular arches with impression compound and alginate impression material.

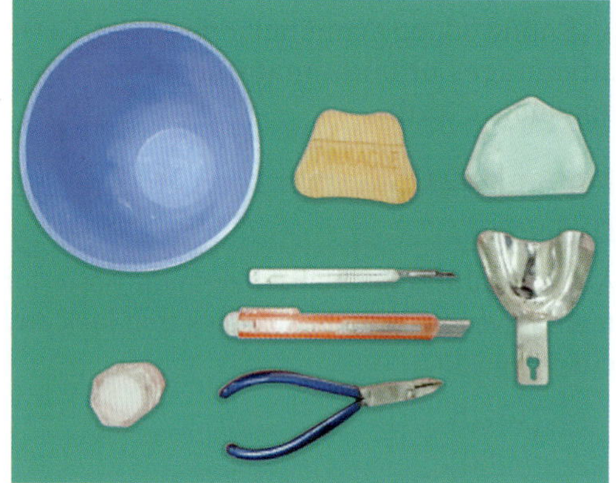

Fig. 17.1: Instruments and materials.

INSTRUMENTS AND MATERIALS (FIG. 17.1)

- Maxillary edentulous cast
- Large clean rubber bowl
- Maxillary and mandibular edentulous nonperforated stock metal trays
- BP blade and handle
- Pliers
- Vaseline
- Impression compound.

MAKING PRIMARY IMPRESSION

Step 1

Take edentulous casts of maxillary and mandibular arch. Select proper edentulous nonperforated maxillary and mandibular trays such that they cover denture bearing area and limiting area. Ensure that there is space of 5–6 mm between tray and cast to load impression material. Posteriorly it should cover hamular notch and posterior palatal seal area. Mandibular tray should cover retromolar pads posteriorly. Sometime you may need to modify tray flanges with pliers **(Figs. 17.2A to C)**.

Step 2

Lightly grease model/cast with Vaseline to prevent adherence of impression material with it or wet the cast in slurry water for few minutes.

Step 3

Take water at temperature of 55–60°C in a clean rubber bowl. Break the impression compound into pieces and place into hot water in bowl and allow it to soften **(Figs. 17.3A and B)**.

Put cloth or small handkerchief at the bottom of rubber bowl containing hot water. This will prevent adhesion of impression compound with rubber bowl.

Step 4

After softening it should be kneaded for uniform mixing **(Figs. 17.4A to C)**.

Step 5

Kneaded soften compound is loaded on the impression tray in form of pellet and roughly shape it like arch **(Figs. 17.5A to C)**.

For mandibular arch impression, the impression compound is rolled in rope shape

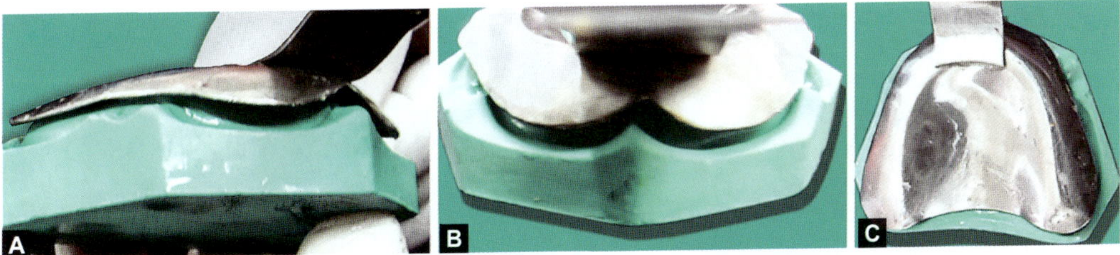

Figs. 17.2A to C: Checking tray extension.

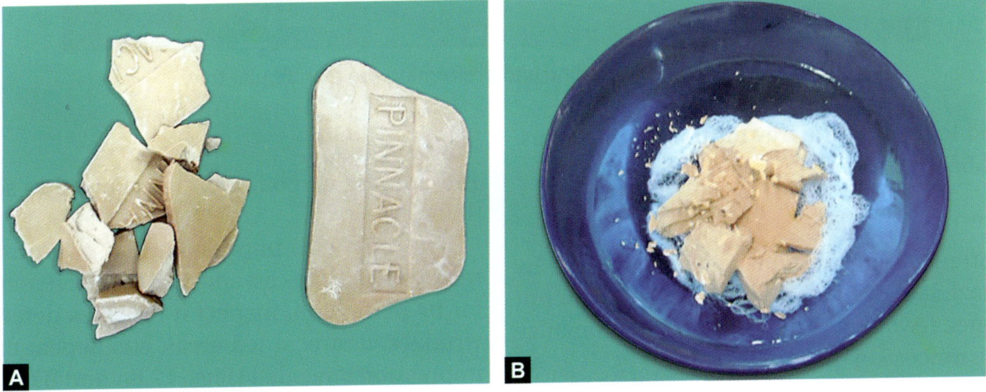

Figs. 17.3A and B: Break impression compound in small pieces and put them into hot water to soften.

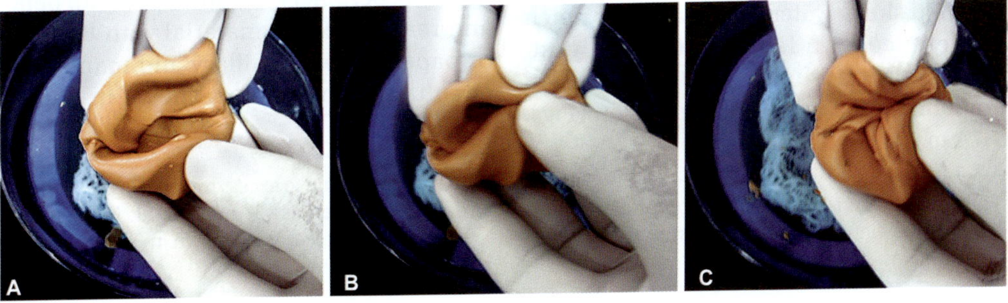

Figs. 17.4A to C: Kneading of impression compound for uniform mixing.

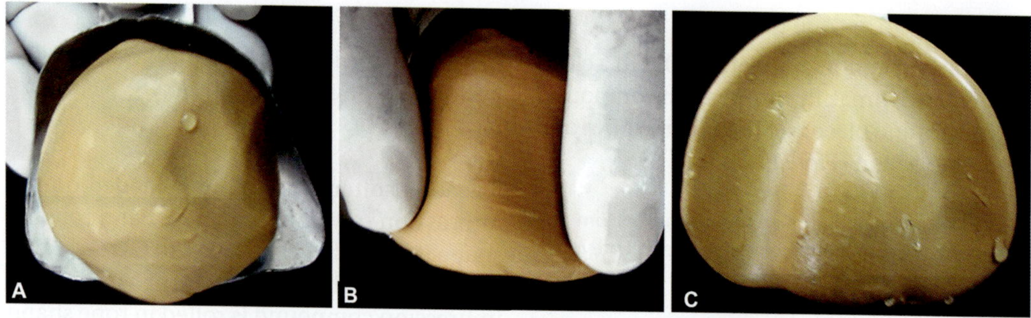

Figs. 17.5A to C: Loading the maxillary tray and preforming.

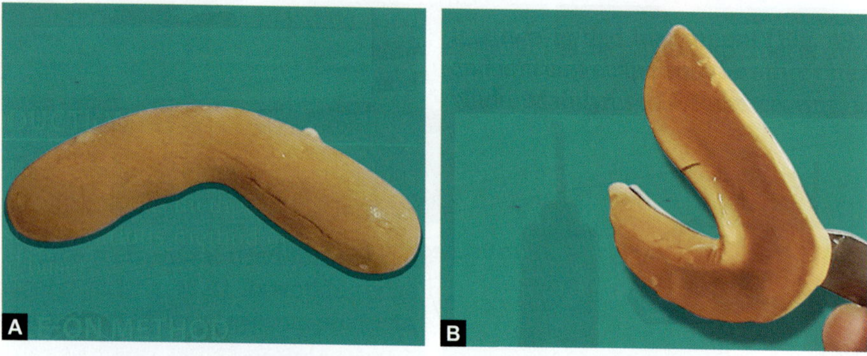

Figs. 17.6A and B: Loading and preforming the mandibular tray.

and loaded on the tray for preforming (**Figs. 17.6A and B**).

Step 6

Soften the impression material surface by Glazing and do tempering by dipping in hot water. (Avoid over glazing, it may traumatize the mucosa in oral cavity).

Step 7

Now, loaded tray is placed over the cast soaked in slurry water, taking anterior notch as reference with labial frenum on cast. Apply proper pressure to flow the impression compound and record the impression (**Figs. 17.7A to C**).

> Fold excess material on back side of impression tray, this will prevent dislodgement of impression from the tray (Figs. 17.7A to C).

Step 8

The impression compound is allowed to set (harden).

The tray with impression compound is removed from the cast and read the impression for its perfection. Inspect it for gross defect, wrinkles, nonrecorded areas, etc. Repeat the impression if needed (**Figs. 17.8A and B**).

Step 9

Mark the periphery of impression with pencil and remove excess material with BP blade or paper cutter. Maxillary and mandibular edentulous impressions shown in **Figures 17.9A and B**.

> Do not try to remove excess material in bulk, slowly remove it otherwise it may break impression. Peeling it in small area as shown in Figures 17.10A and B is correct method.

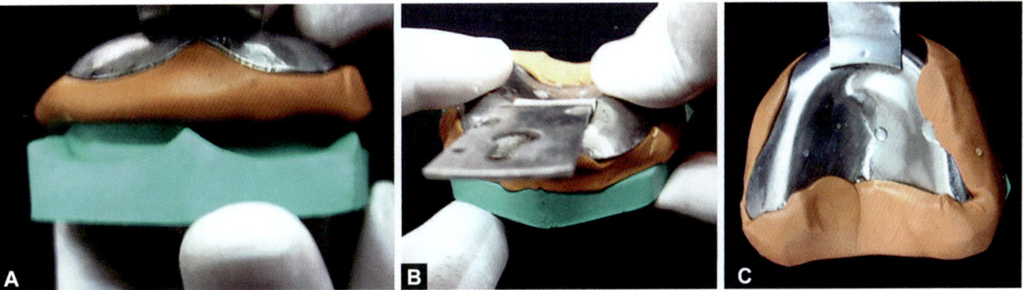

Figs. 17.7A to C: Making impression of maxillary foundation on cast.

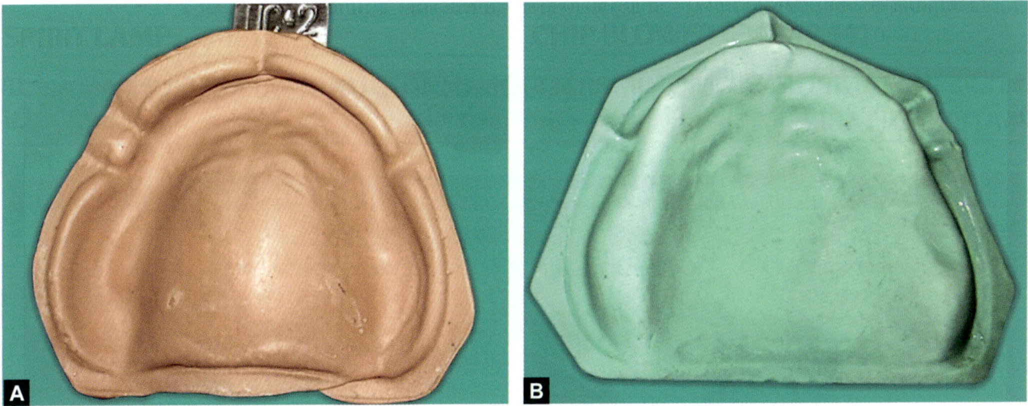

Figs. 17.8A and B: Maxillary primary impression and cast.

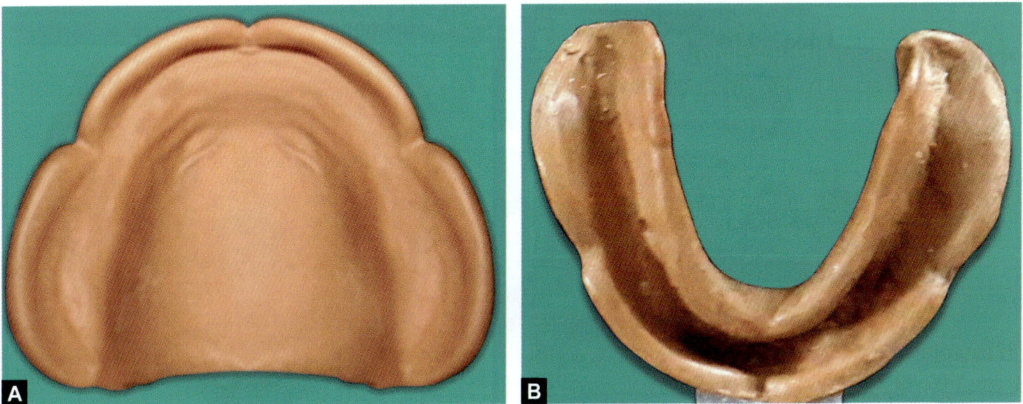

Figs. 17.9A and B: Maxillary and mandibular primary impressions.

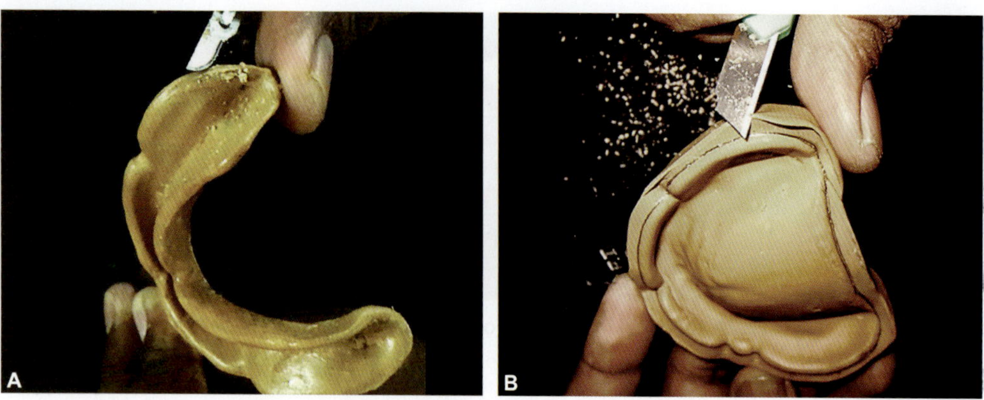

Figs. 17.10A and B: Trimming of excess material using BP blade or paper cutter.

STEPS IN MANIPULATION OF IMPRESSION COMPOUND/IMPRESSION MATERIAL (TABLE 17.1)

Table 17.1: Steps in manipulation of impression compound impression material.

Steps	*Purposes*
Breaking of impression material into pieces	Increases surface area, fast softening.
Softening	For proper consistency and manipulation.
Kneading	For uniform mixing of material.

Contd...

Contd...

Steps	Purposes
Loading	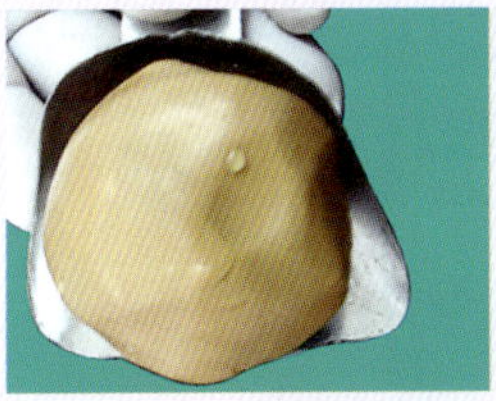 To carry the material on impression tray.
Preforming	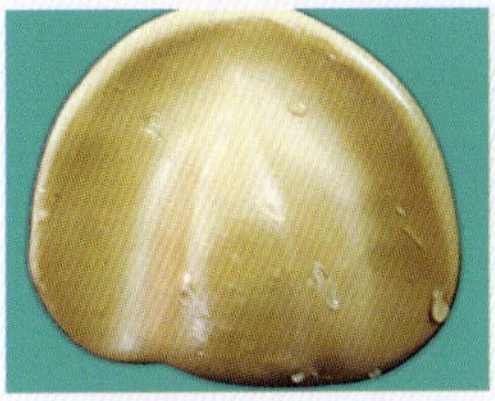 Giving the shape of edentulous area/arch to allow easy flow of material.
Glazing	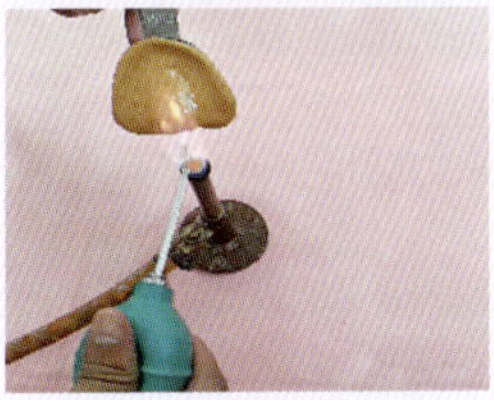 Heating the surface of compound over the flame to record the minute surface details with minimum distortion of whole bulk of loaded material.
Tempering	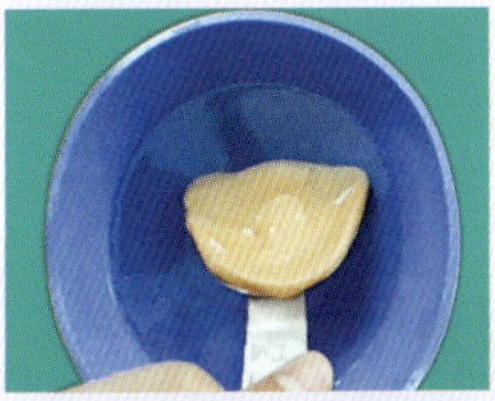 To reduce the temperature of loaded material around 45°C this is tolerated by oral tissues.
Placing tray in patient's mouth	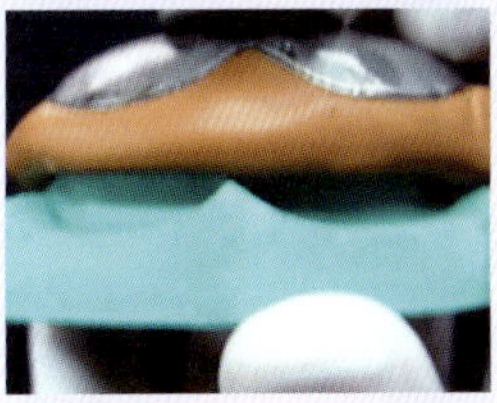 To make impression. (Take reference of labial frenum while placing the tray and making impression)
Removal of impression from mouth/cast	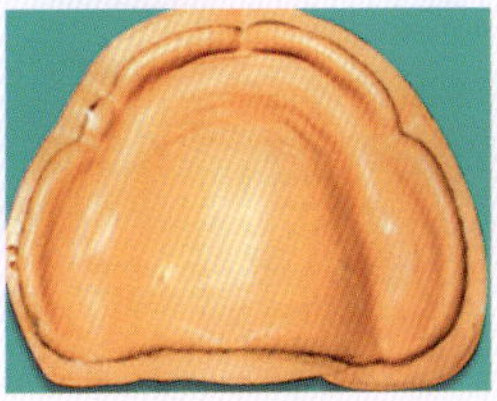 To read correctness and completeness of impression.

Contd...

Contd...

Steps	Purposes
Coding the impression	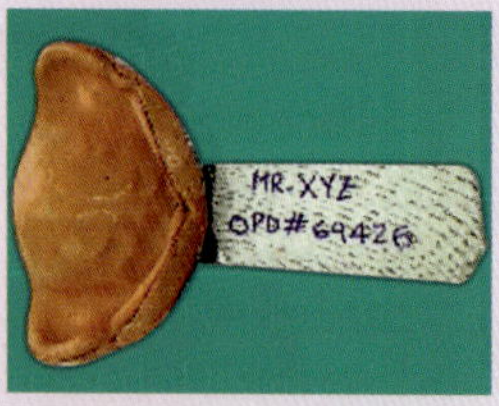 To identify
Disinfection	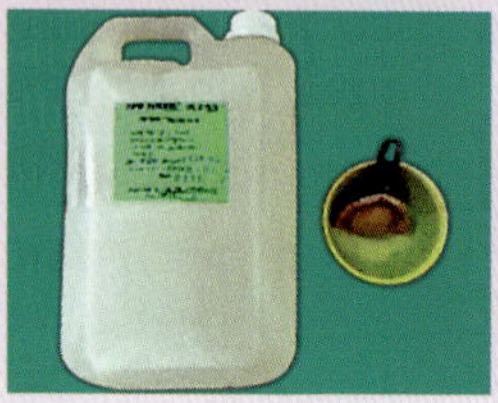 To prevent cross infection.

CHAPTER 18

Pouring/Making of Dental Cast

Paranjay Prajapati, Sneha Kulkarni

INTRODUCTION

Dental cast serve as replica of denture foundation in absence of patient. Dental cast is made by pouring suitable gypsum product in impression. The present chapter inform about available methods for making dental casts.

METHODS OF MAKING CAST

- Inversion method
- Beading-boxing method
- Plaster pumice method.

Here, most widely used two methods, i.e., inversion method for pouring primary impression and beading-boxing method for pouring final impressions are discussed in detail.

Making Primary Cast by Inversion Method

This method is mainly used for making diagnostic and primary cast. This method involves three phases namely: (1) Pouring the impression; (2) Retrieval of the cast; and (3) Finishing of the cast. This method is also known as *"two stage pouring method".*

Armamentarium used for this procedure are **(Fig. 18.1)**:

- Primary impression
- Large rubber bowl
- Dental plaster
- Plaster spatula
- Porcelain tile
- Plaster knife
- Warm water (55–60°C temperature)
- Sandpaper.

Pouring of Impression

Step 1: Impression made of edentulous cast is rinsed with water and disinfectant. Measured quantity of water is taken in rubber bowl. Weighed quantity of dental plaster (according to recommended water powder ratio by the manufacturer) is sifted in water. This is spatulated to form a creamy mix **(Fig. 18.2)**.

Step 2 (Figs. 18.3 and 18.4): Put some quantity of this mix in one corner of impression

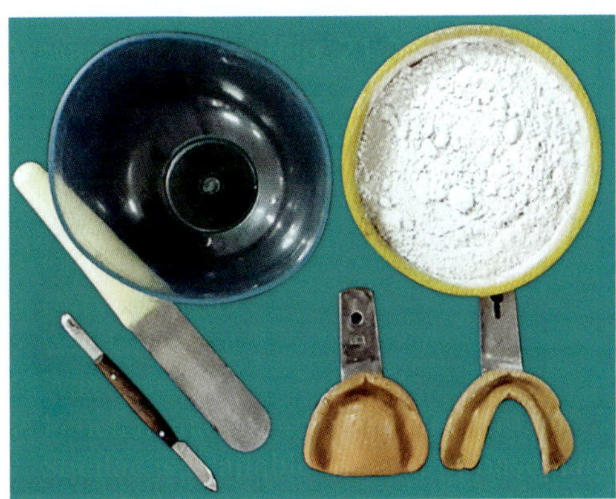

Fig. 18.1: Armamentarium for pouring cast.

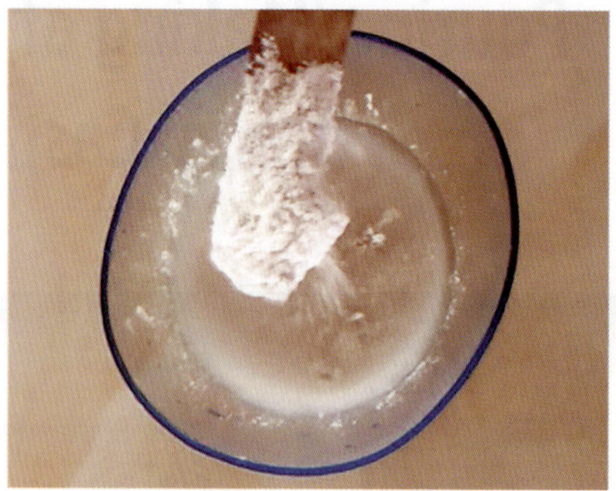

Fig. 18.2: Manipulation of dental plaster.

and allow it to flow till the other corner by vibrating/tapping the impression. This will avoid incorporation of air bubble while pouring. Cover the impression completely.

Step 3: Make some serrations as shown in **Figures 18.5A and B** to create undercuts or place some plaster blebs. This helps in mechanical union between first pour and second pour. The base of the cast is made after the initial set of the first pour.

Step 4 (Figs. 18.6A to C): Rest of creamy mix is placed on the porcelain tile and roughly given the shape of base of the cast and impression is inverted over it.

Step 5 (Figs. 18.7A and B): Allow initial set to take place. Plaster is shaped according to desired form of cast base using plaster knife. Excess material is removed beyond the borders of impression. Allow the material to set completely. In case of mandibular impression, remove plaster from tongue space till the stock tray borders.

Impression borders should not be covered more than 2–3 mm. Covering tray border in excess results in fracture of land area while retrieval of the cast **(Figs. 18.8A to C)**.

Retrieval of Cast

Step 1 (Fig. 18.9): After the plaster is set completely, the poured impression with base

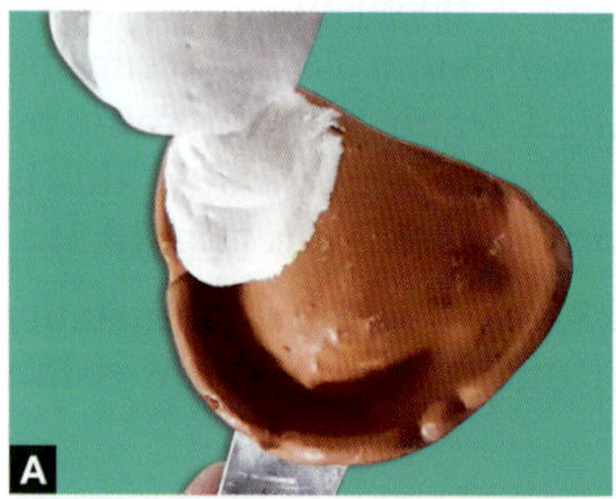

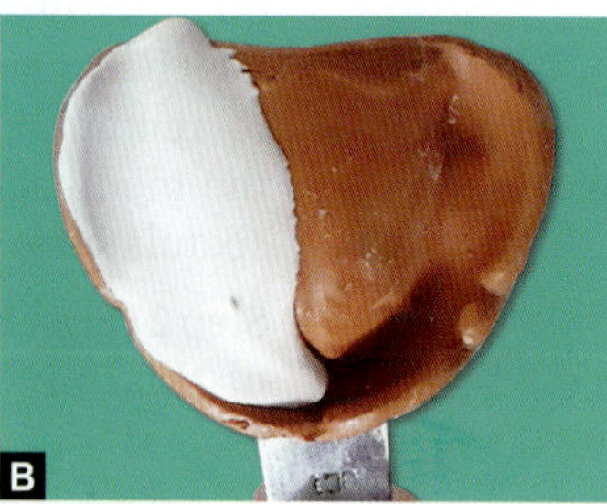

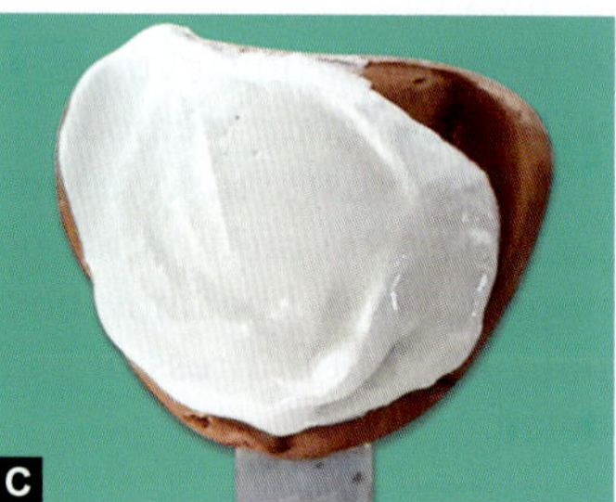

Figs. 18.3A to C: Pouring of maxillary primary impression.

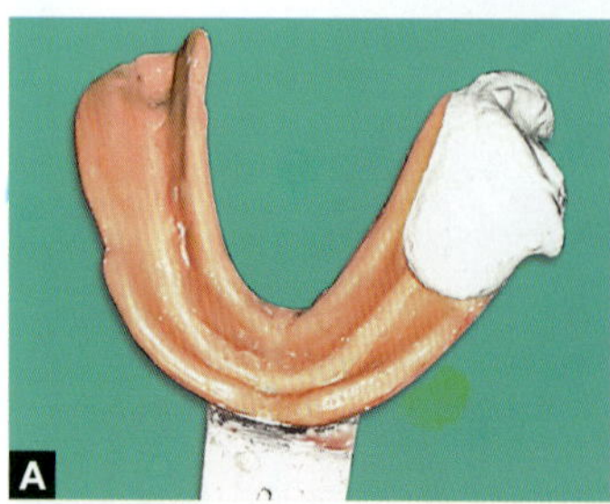

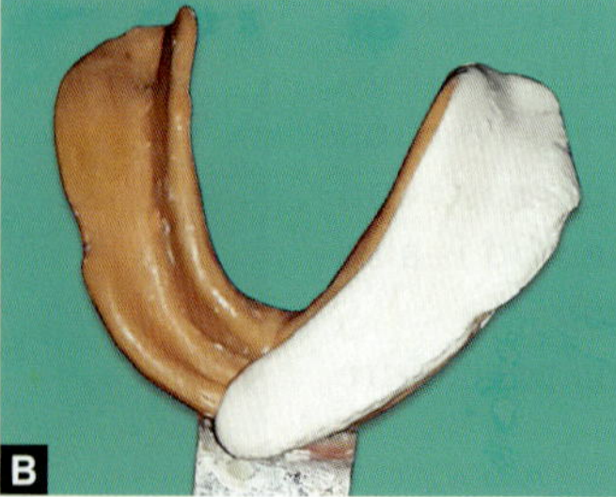

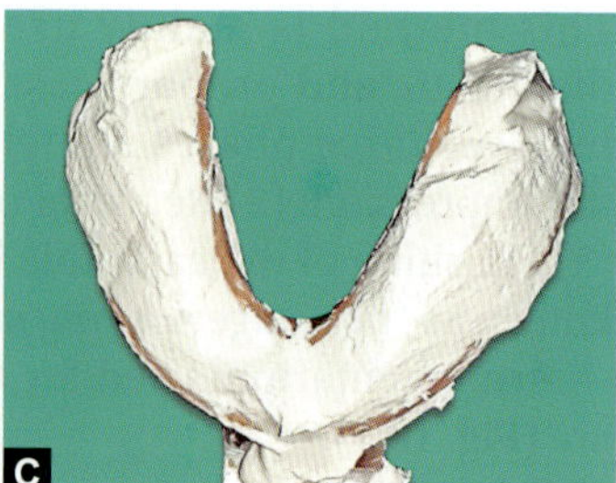

Figs. 18.4A to C: Pouring of mandibular primary impression.

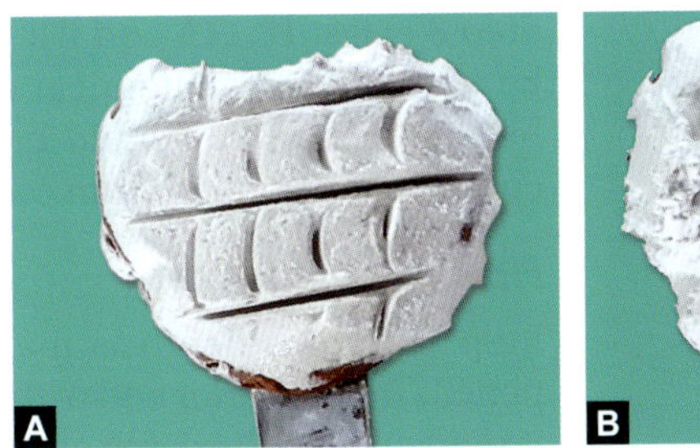
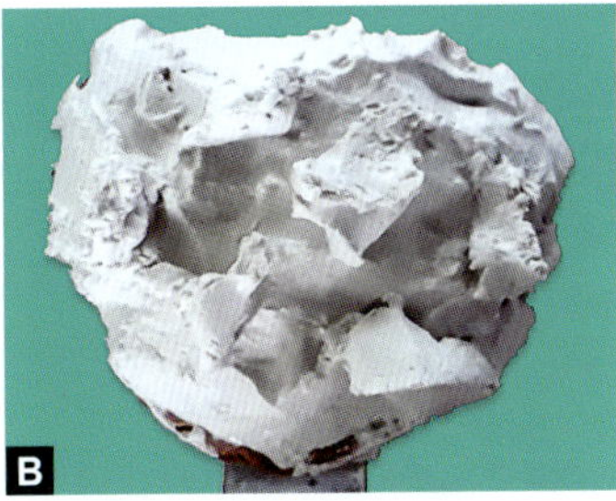

Figs. 18.5A and B: Making retentive grooves on first pour.

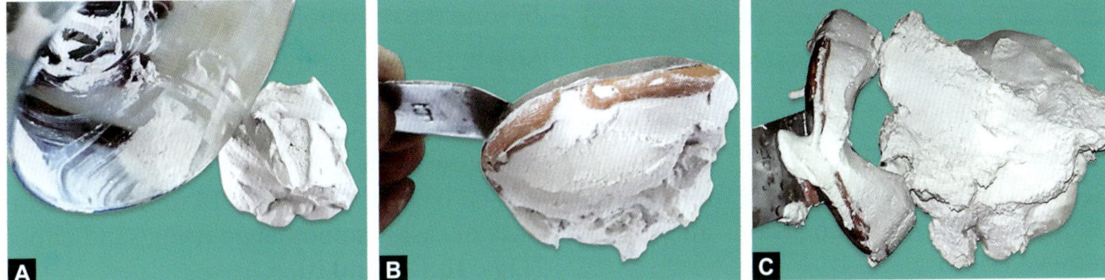

Figs. 18.6A to C: Placing maxillary and mandibular impressions on second mix.

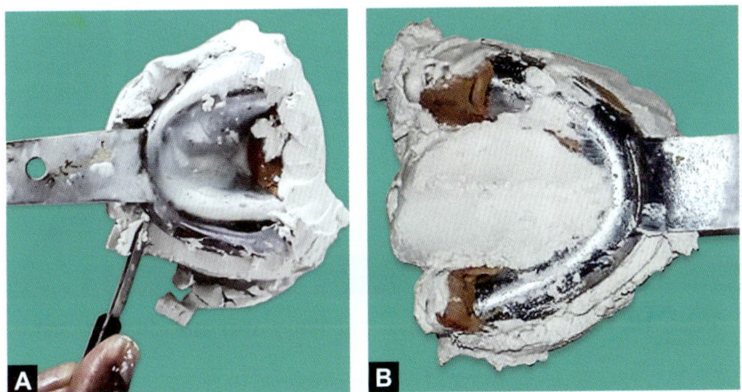

Figs. 18.7A and B: Shape the base of maxillary and mandibular casts after pouring impressions.

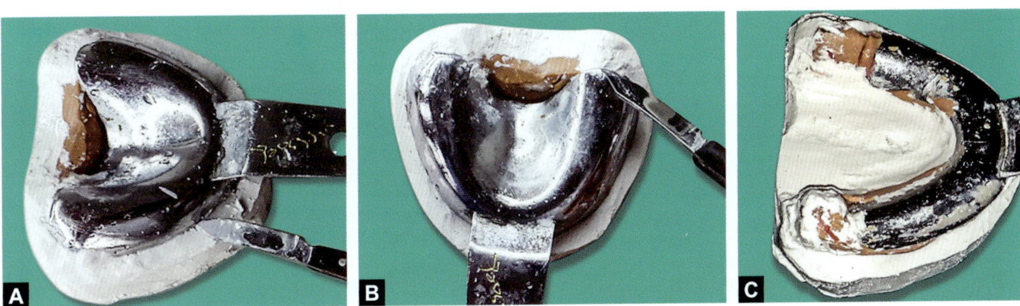

Figs. 18.8A to C: Do not cover impression borders excessively.

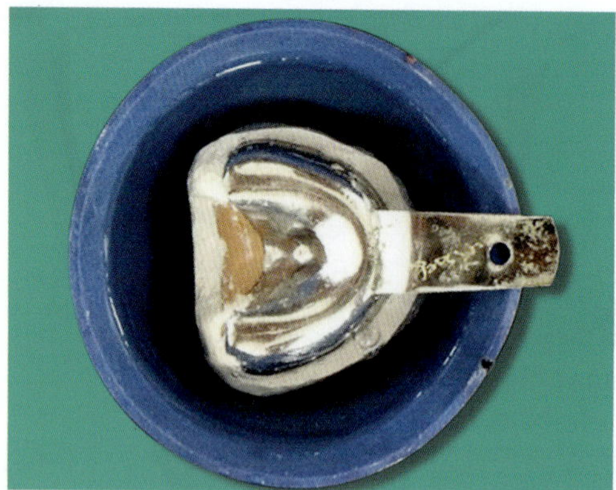

Fig. 18.9: Place cast with impression in hot water.

is placed in large rubber bowl with hot water having temperature of 55–60°C.

Step 2 (Figs. 18.10A to C): Compound is allowed to soften in hot water and cast is retrieved slowly.

Step 3 (Figs. 18.11A and B): The cast should be checked for anatomical details. Any air bubble or nodule should be eliminated or corrected to obtain a clean cast.

Finishing of the Cast

Step 1: Sulcus depth is marked using red pencil. The posterior end of the maxillary cast is marked from the depth of hamular notch on one side to hamular notch on other side. The posterior end of mandibular cast is marked beyond the retromolar pad of both the sides.

Step 2: The cast is trimmed using a plaster knife in such a way that the land area of the cast is 3 mm high and 3 mm wide. It slopes downward and outward by 45° or should be straight.

The base of the cast is 15 mm thick. The base of cast is smoothened using sand paper **(Figs. 18.12A and B)**.

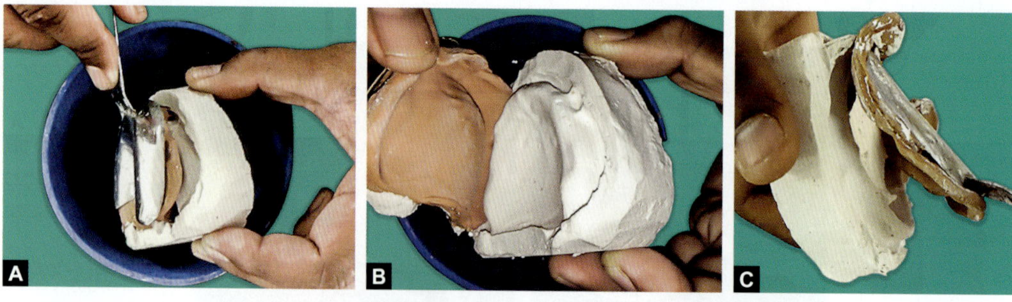

Figs. 18.10A to C: Retrieval of maxillary and mandibular cast.

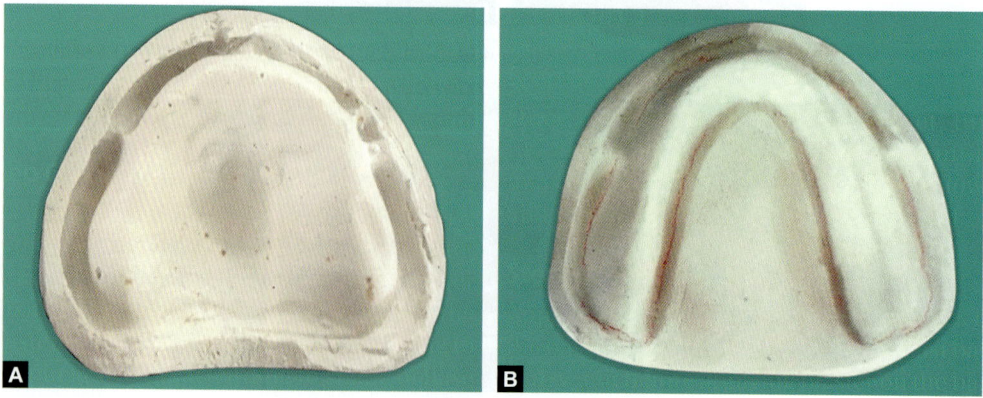

Figs. 18.11A and B: Observe cast for any defect.

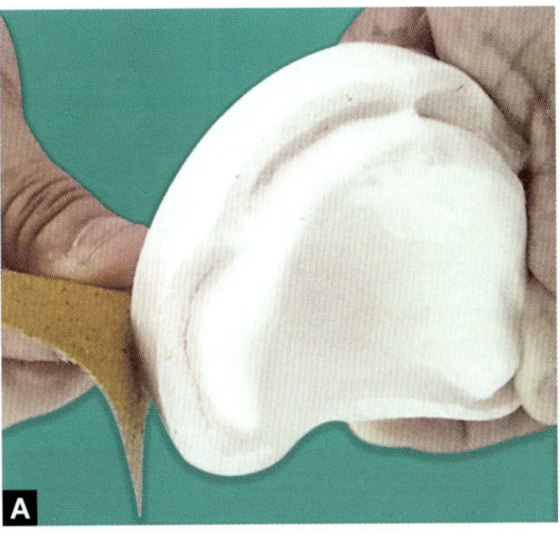

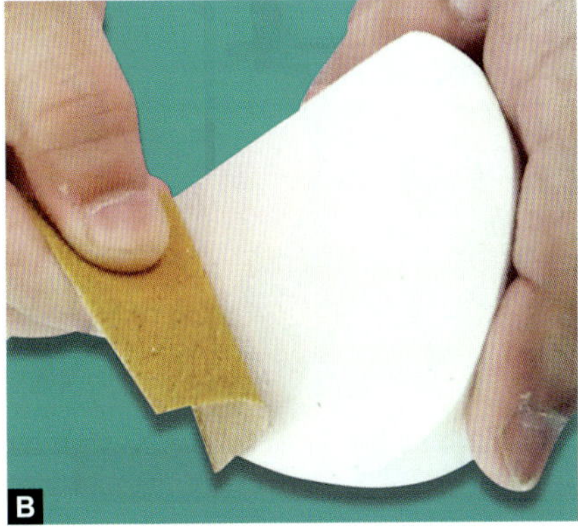

Figs. 18.12A and B: Smoothening of base of the cast with sand paper.

Do not alter the anatomical area of the cast with sand paper or by any means.

Step 3 (Fig. 18.13): Label the cast with your name and registration or roll number on its side.

(On patients' cast OPD number and patient name is written).

Pouring Cast by Beading-Boxing Method

The final impression is made for recording of fine details with precision. The final cast is made with beading-boxing method. This method gives more precise cast that needs no or minimum corrections after retrieval. In this method, one can control or predetermine the thickness of base by adjusting the height of boxing wax.

Instruments and Material (Figs. 18.14A and B)

- Maxillary and mandibular impressions
- Rubber bowl
- Plaster spatula
- Beading wax
- Boxing wax
- Dental stone
- Sand paper.

Beading wax is available in square or round shapes and in various colors. Boxing wax is available in various colors and lengths **(Figs. 18.15 and 18.16)**.

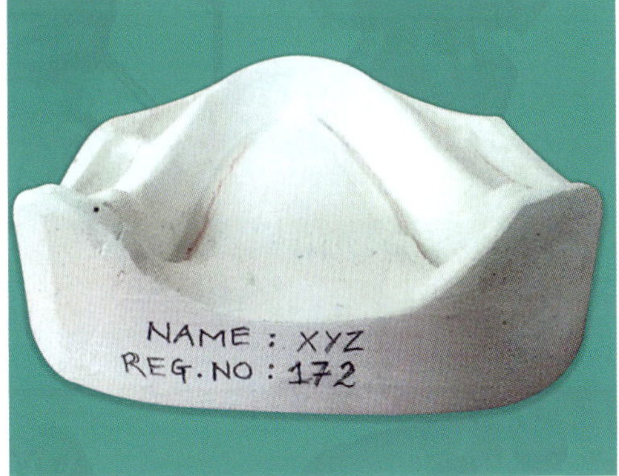

Fig. 18.13: Labeling the cast.

Procedure

Step 1: Wash final impression and disinfect it. Place markings 2–3 mm away from the impression borders as shown in **Figure 18.17**.

Step 2: Beading wax is placed 3 mm below the sulcus extension (borders) of impression. It is sealed with hot wax spatula to bead the impression. Placement of beading wax 2–3 mm below the impression borders forms height of land area on cast. The thickness of beading wax ensures thickness of land area on the cast. It should be 3 mm **(Figs. 18.18A to C)**.

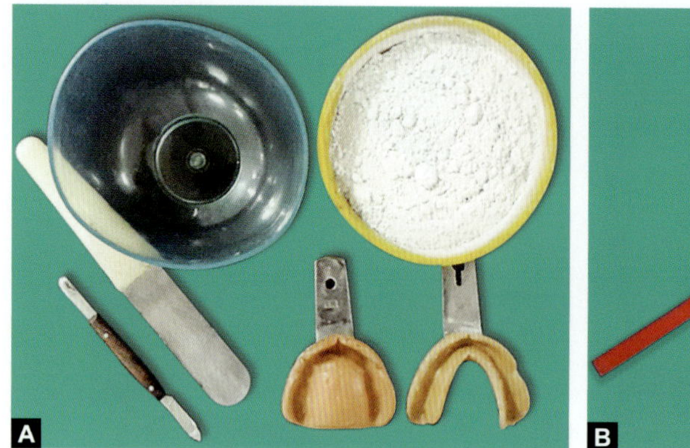

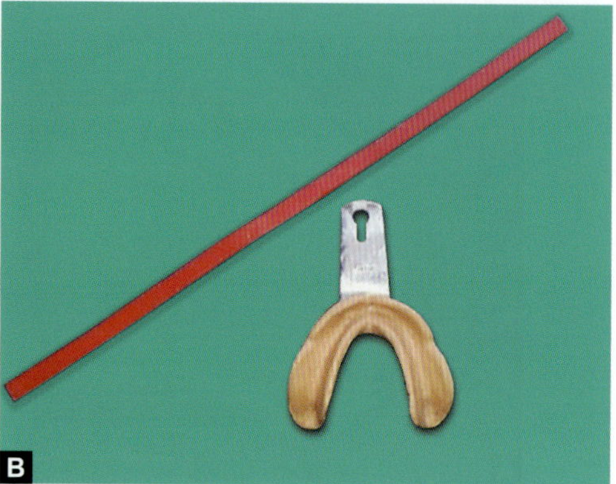

Figs. 18.14A and B: Instruments and material required in beading-boxing method.

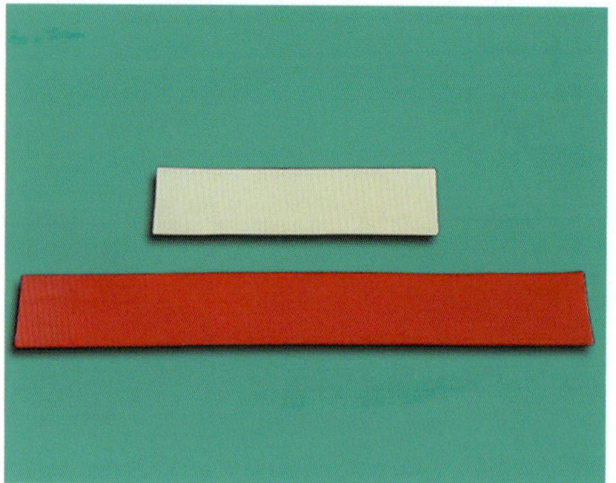

Fig. 18.15: Boxing wax available in various color and length.

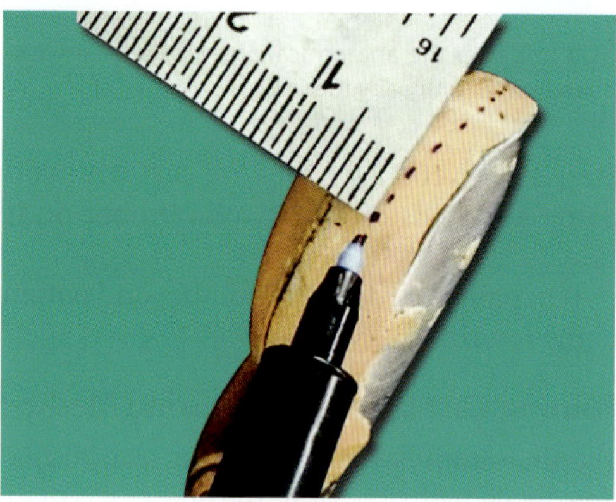

Fig. 18.17: Placing markings 2–3 mm from tray borders.

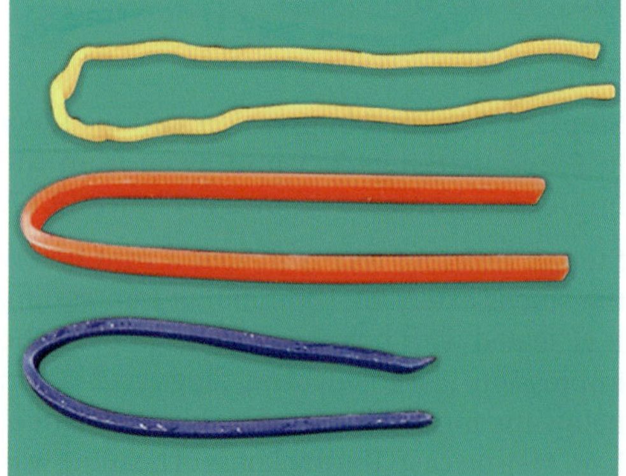

Fig. 18.16: Beading wax available in various shapes and color.

Step 3: Boxing wax is sealed to the beading wax such that the impression is boxed in. Height of boxing wax provides thickness of base of the cast **(Figs. 18.19A to C)**.

> In case of mandibular impression, a tongue-shaped modeling wax is placed in tongue space after beading to create tongue space in cast.

Step 4 (Figs. 18.20 and 18.21): Pour some water in boxed in impression to ensure that it is sealed perfectly. This ensures perfect sealing of beading and boxing wax and there is no seepage from where plaster can flow out. Dental stone or plaster is mixed in bowl

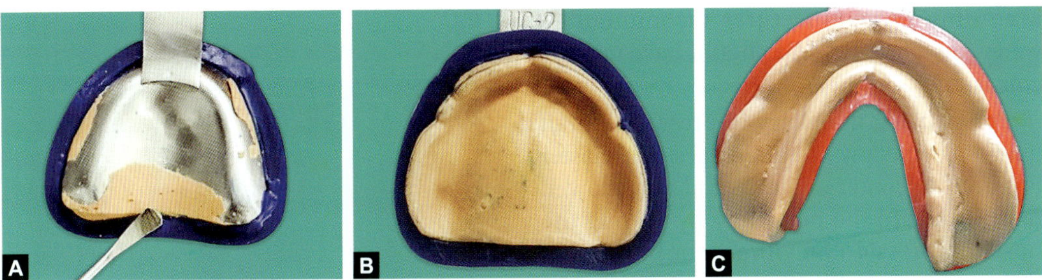

Figs. 18.18A to C: Beading the maxillary and mandibular impressions.

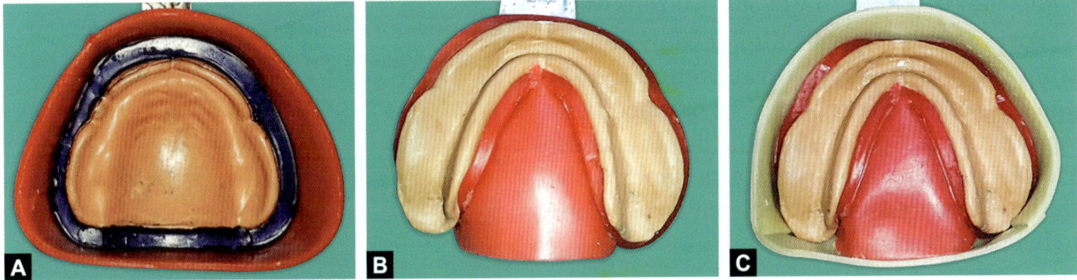

Figs. 18.19A to C: Boxing maxillary and mandibular impressions.

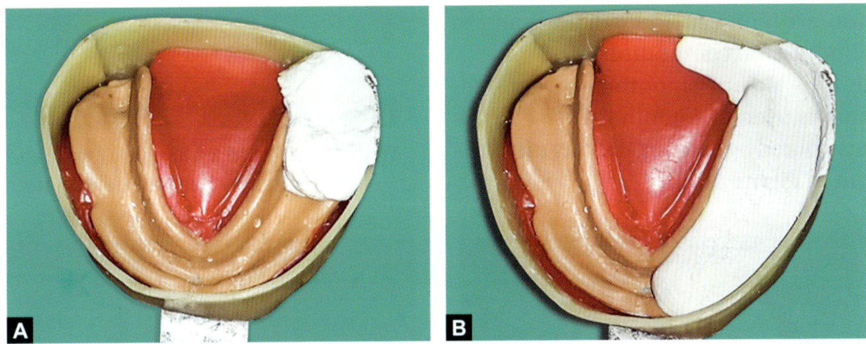

Figs. 18.20A and B: Pouring the impressions.

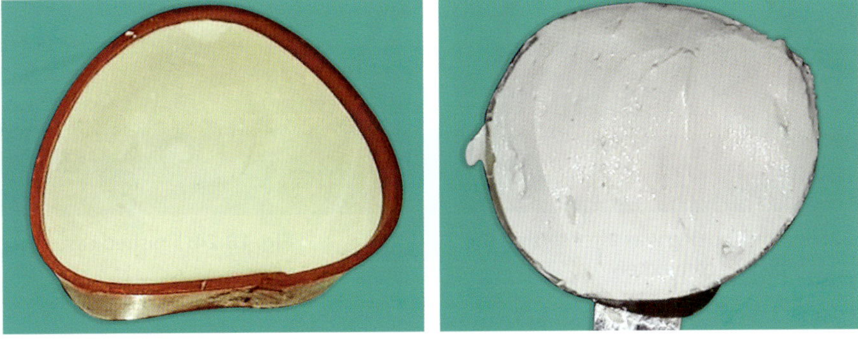

Fig. 18.21: Pouring the boxed impression till the height of boxing wax.

according to manufacturer recommended water-powder ratio. Mix should have creamy consistency.

For pouring maxillary impression, small quantity of creamy mix of dental stone/plaster is placed in center of palate and it is allowed to flow toward the periphery by putting the boxed impression on vibrator or by tapping the impression. Plaster/stone is added in small increments till the boxed impression is completely covered till the height of boxing wax.

For pouring mandibular impression, dental stone/plaster is placed on retromolar area and impression is either tapped or placed on vibrator to make plaster flow till the other end. Plaster/stone is added in small increments till the boxed impression is completely covered up to height of boxing wax.

Step 5 (Figs. 18.22 and 18.23): Once dental stone/plaster sets completely, beading and boxing wax are removed. Put it in hot water to remove impression compound.

Cast is finished and smoothen as required. Sand paper is used to smooth the base of the cast. Casts poured by beading–boxing methods are shown in **Figure 18.24**.

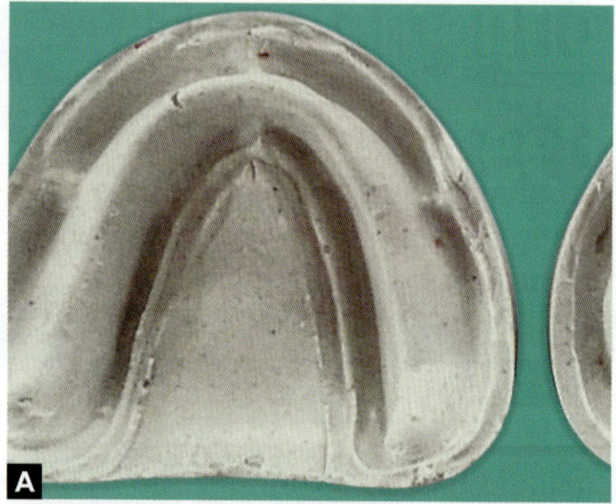

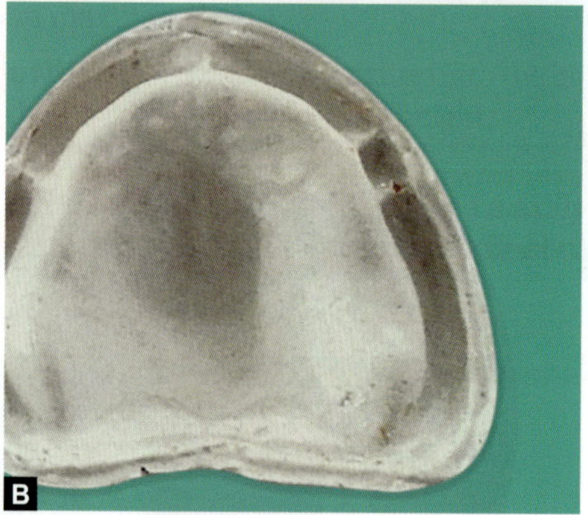

Figs. 18.23A and B: Maxillary and mandibular casts poured by beading-boxing method.

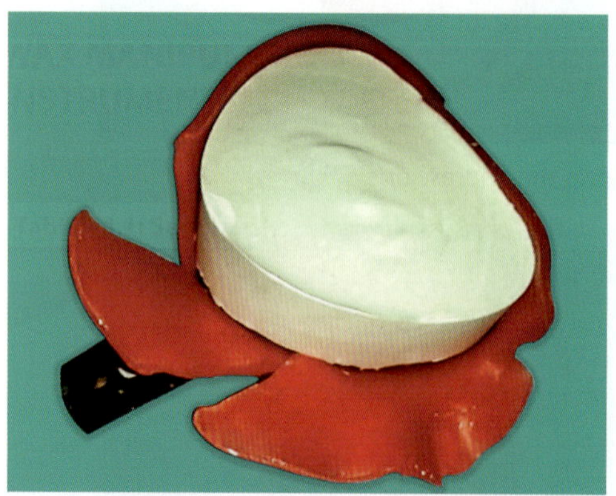

Fig. 18.22: Remove boxing wax after setting the plaster completely.

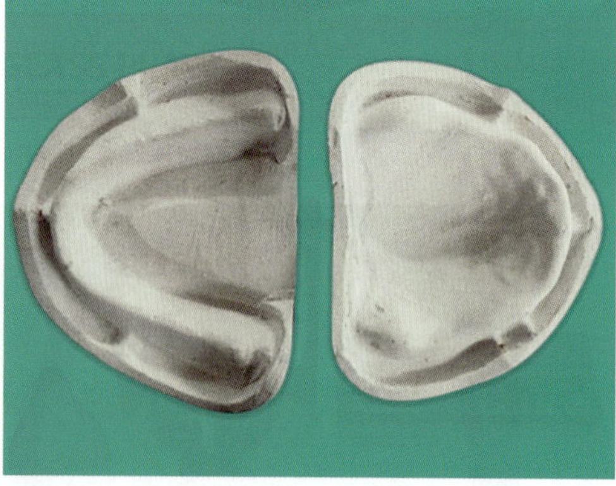

Fig. 18.24: Finished casts.

CHAPTER 19

Adaptation of Spacer on Primary Cast

Paranjay Prajapati, Sneha Kulkarni

ARMAMENTARIUM

- Maxillary and mandibular primary casts
- Spacer wax or modeling wax
- Red and blue pencils
- Rubber bowl with hot water
- BP Blade No. 15 with handle.

Guiding Lines

Step 1 (Fig. 19.1)

Mark midline using the frenum as the reference point. Mark outline of sulcus on primary cast. Sulcus line is marked in deepest part of sulcus. A red color pencil can be used for marking sulcus line. Sulcus line is continuous line. In posterior aspect of maxillary cast, red line is drawn 1 mm beyond posterior vibrating line.

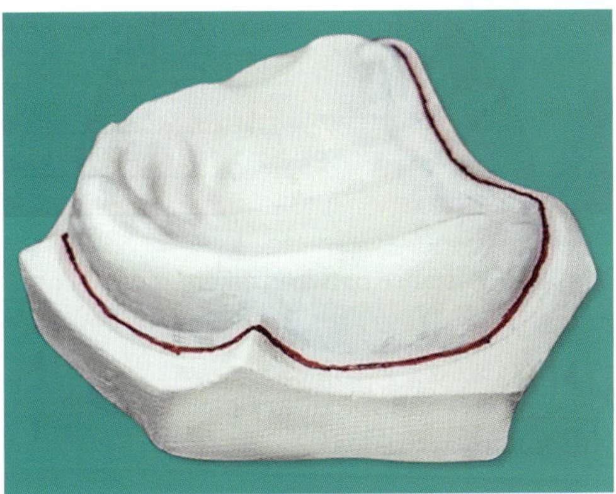

Fig. 19.1: Marking the sulcus outline on the cast.

Step 2 (Figs. 19.2A and B)

Place scale in the sulcus and mark several points 2 mm away from sulcus line at different areas. Join these points as a bold line 2 mm away from the sulcus on labial and buccal side of the cast. Use blue color pencil for this line.

This line (continuous blue line) is 2 mm short of sulcus line. It indicates extension of custom tray border. The blue line is not marked 2 mm short in posterior aspect of casts.

Step 3 (Figs. 19.3 to 19.5)

Draw spacer outline. This line is drawn as dotted line. Draw it at a level 2 mm short of the tray outline. In posterior part of maxillary cast, this line is limited till the anterior vibrating line of posterior palatal seal area.

Step 4 (Fig. 19.6)

Outline of tissue stops: Four tissue stops are marked on maxillary cast, two anteriorly (canine region) and two posteriorly (molar region). On mandibular cast, two tissue stops are marked in canine region.

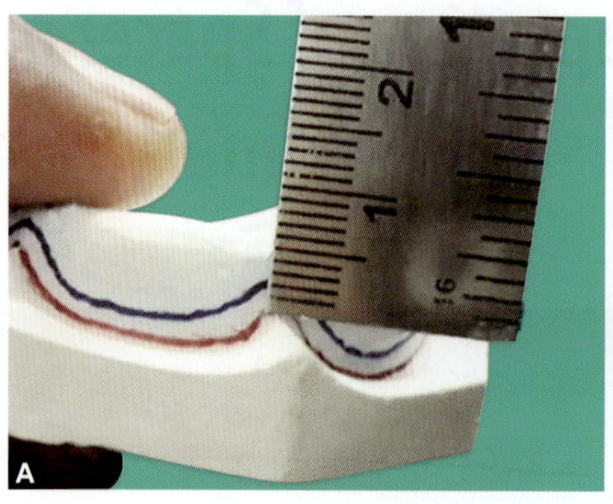

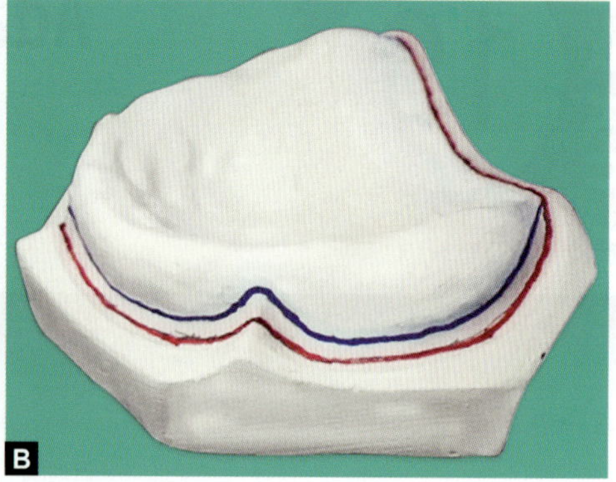

Figs. 19.2A and B: Marking tray outline 2 mm short of sulcus line.
Note: See the posterior extension of line.

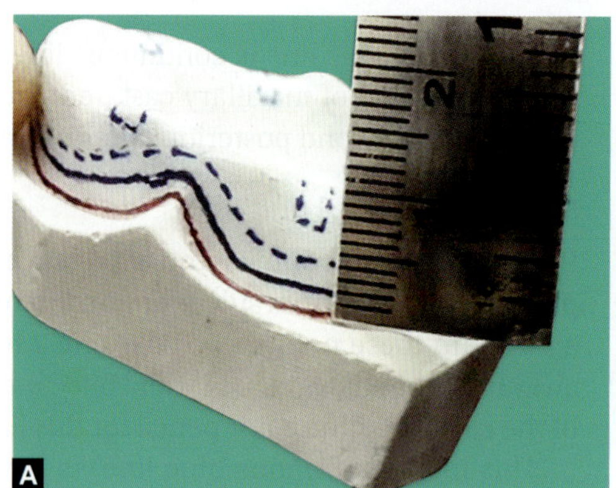

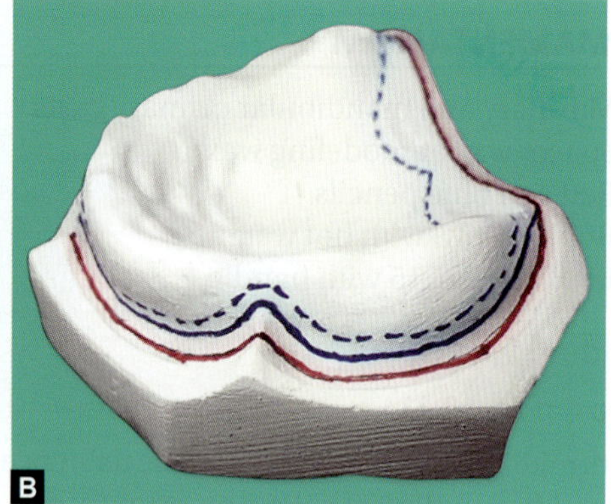

Figs. 19.3A and B: Draw spacer line 2 mm short of tray extension line.

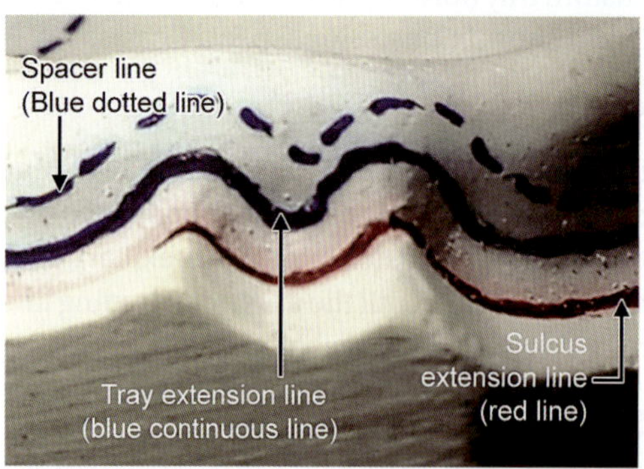

Fig. 19.4: Showing guidelines on casts.

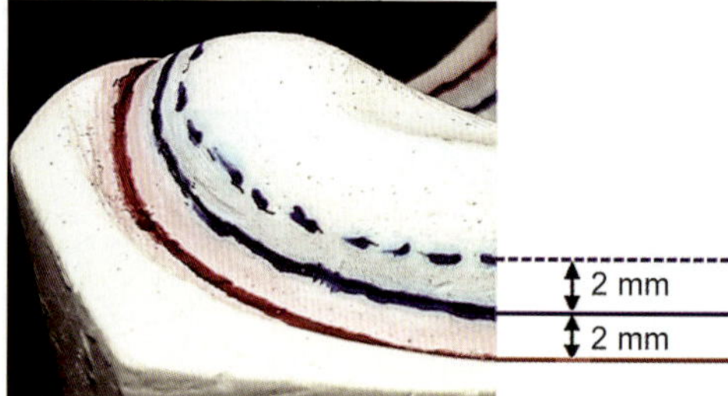

Fig. 19.5: Distance between different guidelines.

Adaptation of Spacer

Step 1 (Figs. 19.7A and B)

Take half sheet of modeling wax (or spacer wax) and soften it over the Bunsen burner. Place it over the maxillary cast and adapt it without any wrinkles.

Step 2 (Figs. 19.8A to C)

Put a cut on wax at the level of spacer line (dotted line) with No. 15 BP blade. Take care

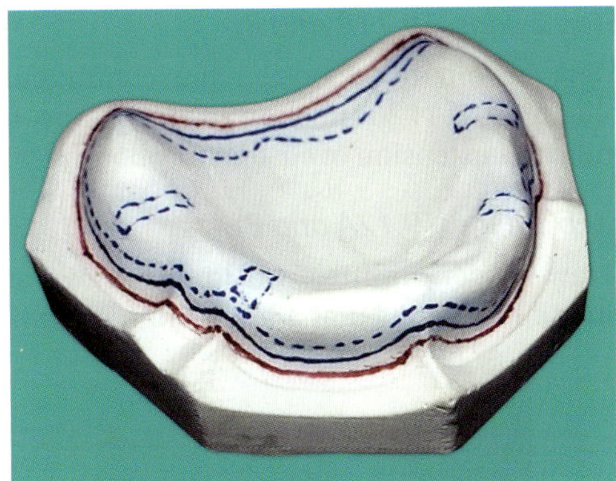

Fig. 19.6: Guidelines with tissue stops.

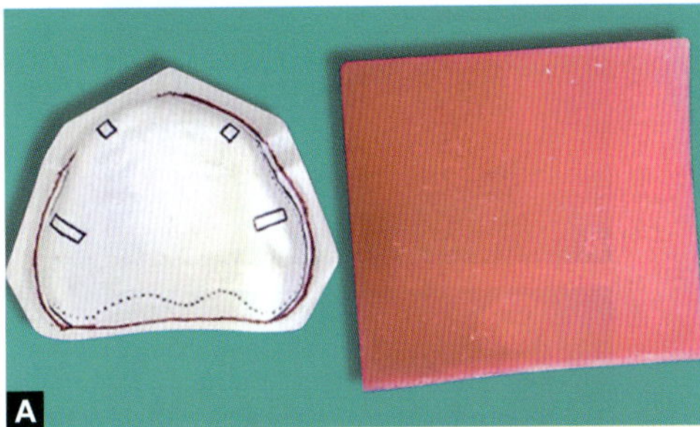

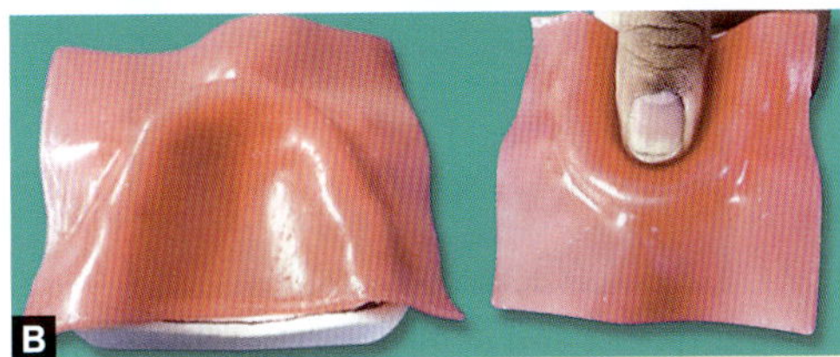

Figs. 19.7A and B: Adaptation of modeling wax on cast.

not to scratch cast with blade. Remove excess wax beyond the dotted line.

Step 3 (Figs. 19.9A and B)

Cut the tissue stops area according to outline to make window in spacer wax. The spacer is

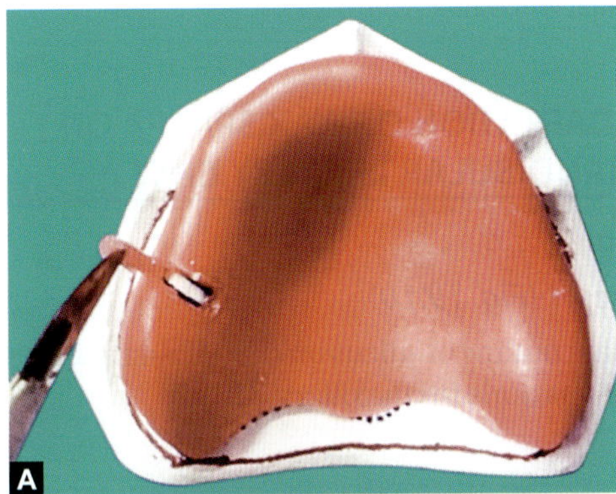

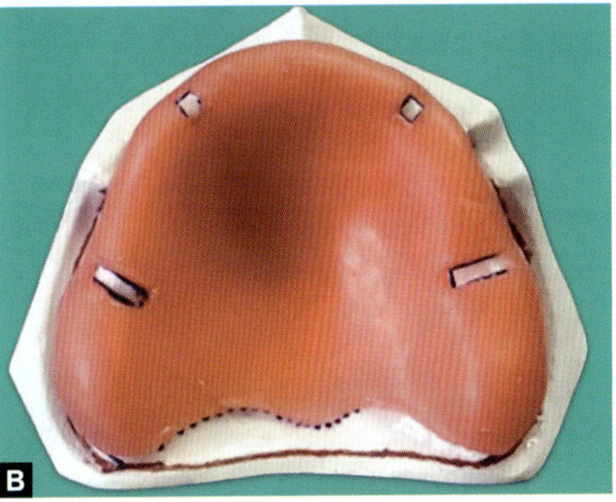

Figs. 19.9A and B: Creating window for fabrication of tissue stops.

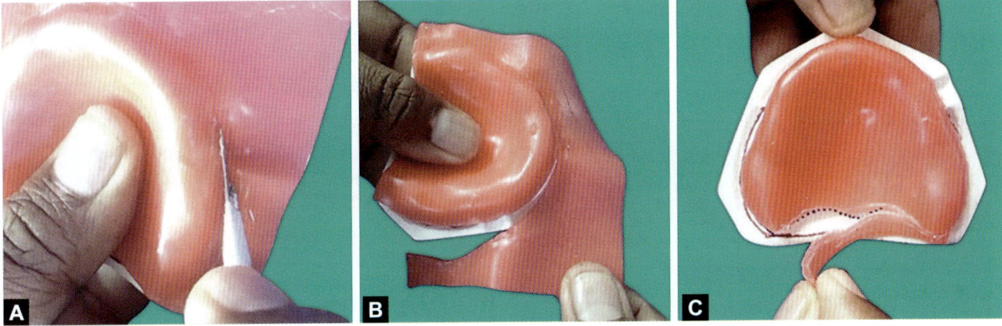

Figs. 19.8A to C: Cut the modeling wax along the spacer line.

4 mm short of sulcus and limited till the anterior vibrating line in posterior palatal seal area.

Wax is cut and removed from spacer according to tissue stop outline. This will create window in the spacer wax. This is not the tissue stop. Tissue stop is the extension of custom tray (through this window) that is in contact with cast.

ADAPTATION OF WAX SPACER ON MANDIBULAR PRIMARY CAST

Guiding Lines

Step 1 (Fig. 19.10)

Mark outline of sulcus on mandibular primary cast as done for maxillary cast.

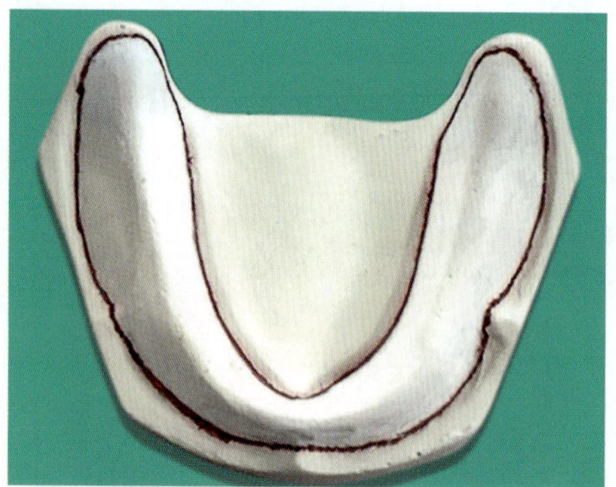

Fig. 19.10: Drawing the sulcus line.

Step 2 (Figs. 19.11A and B)

Mark custom tray extension line (continuous blue line). It is 2 mm short of sulcus line. It indicates extension of custom tray border.

Step 3 (Figs. 19.12A and B)

Draw spacer outline. This line is drawn as dotted line. Draw it at a level 2 mm short of

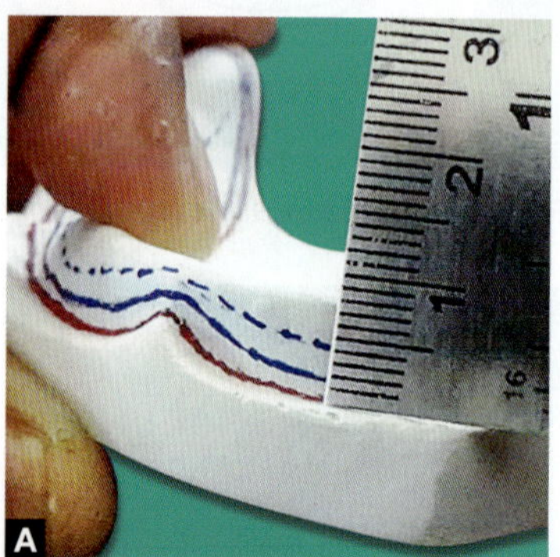

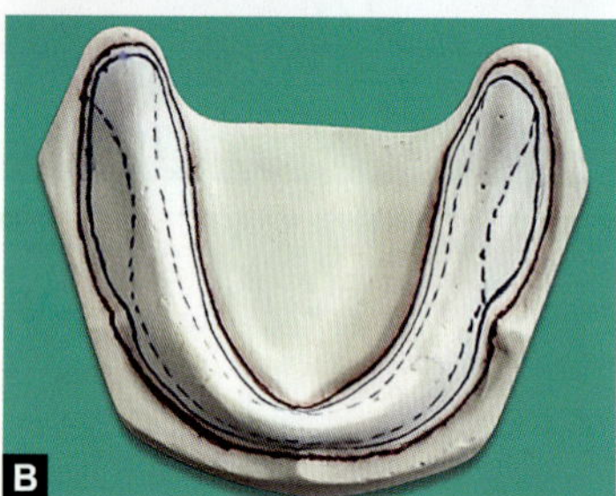

Figs. 19.12A and B: All guidelines drawn on mandibular cast.

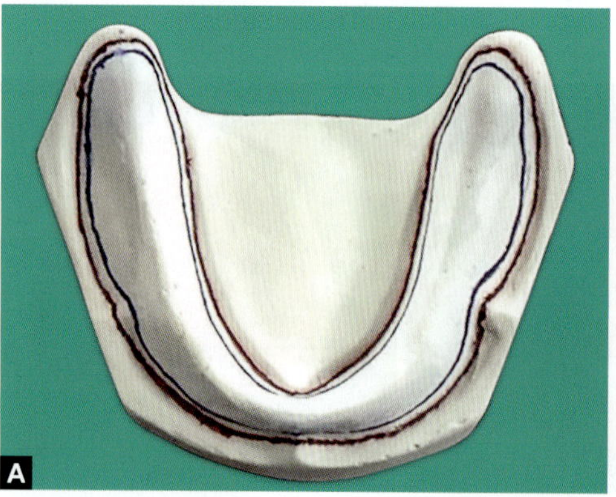

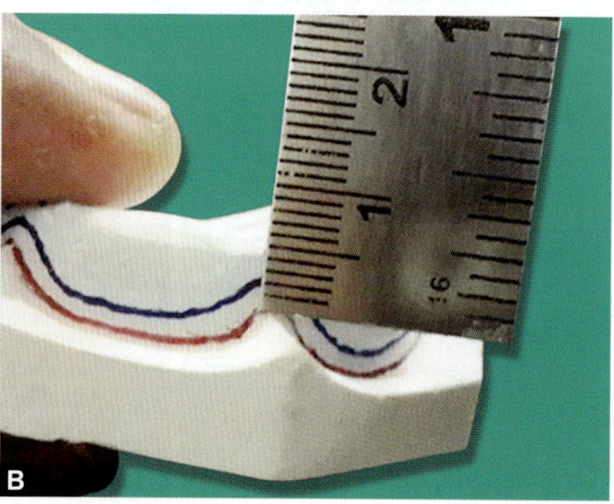

Figs. 19.11A and B: Marking tray extension line 2 mm short of sulcus line.

the tray outline. In case of mandibular cast the buccal-shelf area is not covered with spacer as it is primary stress bearing area. Mark outline for two tissue stops (2 × 2 mm) on mandibular cast at canine region.

> Buccal-shelf area itself acts as tissue stop. So no separate tissue stops are made in posterior region of mandibular cast.

Adaptation of Spacer

Step 1 (Figs. 19.13A and B)

Take half sheet of modeling wax and roughly shape it according to arch shape, soften it over the Bunsen burner. Place it over the mandibular cast and adapt it without any wrinkles.

Step 2 (Figs. 19.14A to C)

Put a cut on wax at the level of spacer line (dotted line) with No. 15 BP blade. Take care not to scratch cast with blade. Remove excess wax beyond the dotted line. Remove spacer wax from buccal-shelf area.

Step 3 (Fig. 19.15)

Cut the tissue stops area according to outline to make window in spacer wax. The spacer is 4 mm short of sulcus. Make sure that there is no spacer on buccal-shelf area.

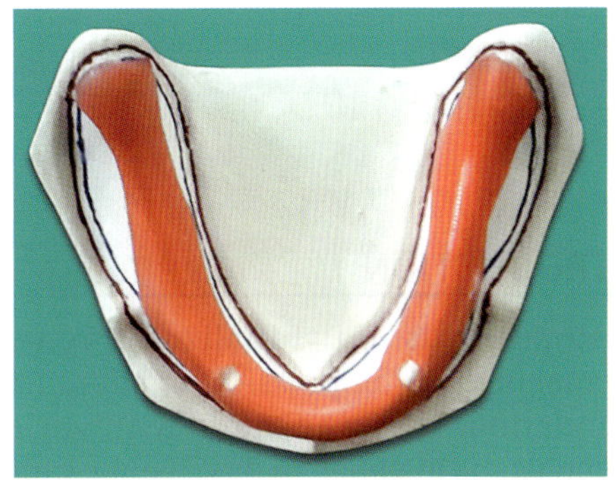

Fig. 19.15: Spacer adapted on mandibular cast.

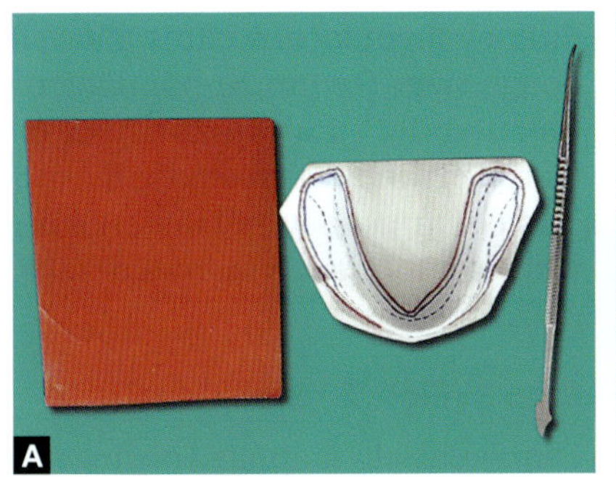
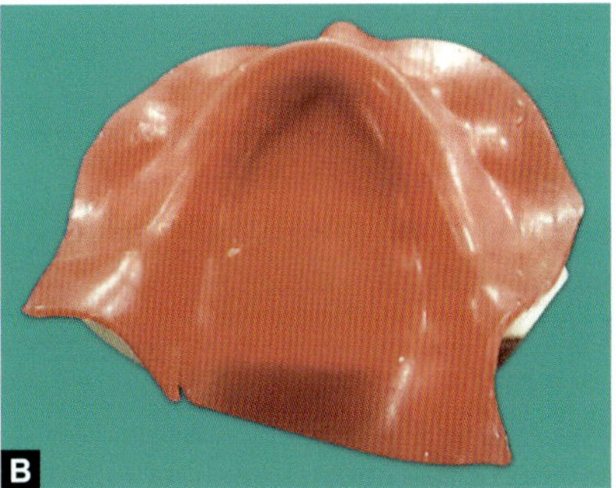

Fig. 19.13A and B: Adaptation of modeling wax to create spacer.

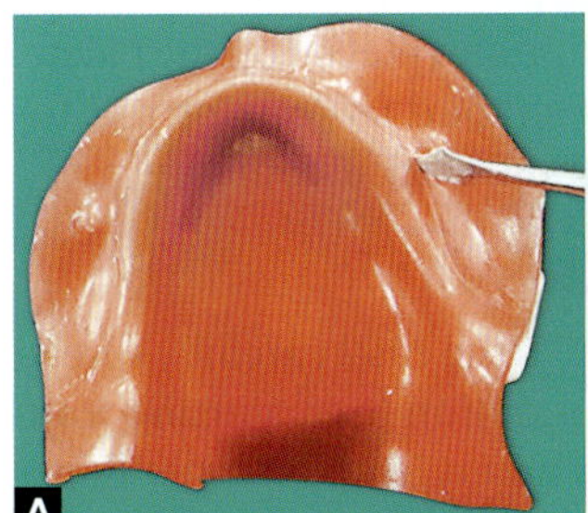
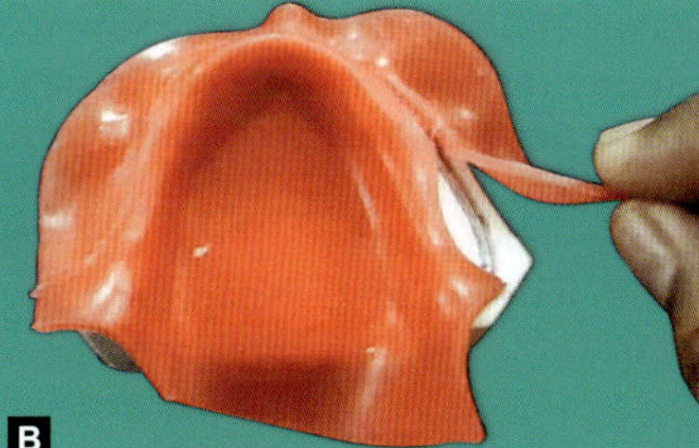
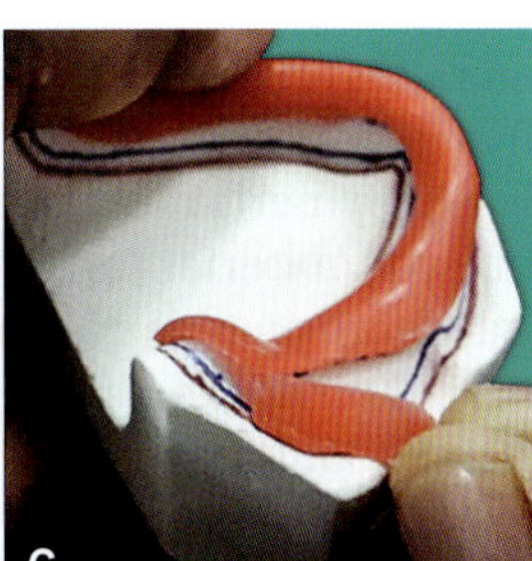

Figs. 19.14A to C: Cut modeling wax at the level of spacer line.

Fabrication of Custom Tray on Maxillary and Mandibular Primary Casts

Paranjay Prajapati, YG Naveen

INTRODUCTION

Custom tray is individualized tray used for making final impression of edentulous foundation. It can be made with various materials and methods. In this chapter, various materials and methods are demonstrated to make custom trays on maxillary and mandibular primary casts.

ARMAMENTARIUM

- Primary casts with adapted spacer.
- Tray material (or self-cure acrylic resin).
- Porcelain jar with lid.
- Mixing spatula.
- Petroleum jelly.
- Lathe and acrylic trimmer.

In present demonstration, maxillary custom tray is fabricated using tray material. Tray material is self-cure acrylic resin with more amounts of filler particles added. This material has good dimensional stability (fit) due to less polymerization shrinkage but requires bulk of material for strength. The custom tray fabricated of tray material should have minimum thickness of 2–3 mm for providing stability and strength to custom tray.

Step 1 (Figs. 20.1A and B)

Cold mould seal is applied on cast using fine bristle brush. Application of cold mould seal is done in one direction only. No need to apply cold mould seal on wax spacer. Small brush is used to apply separating medium on windows created for tissue stops.

Step 2 (Figs. 20.2A to C)

Tray material is mixed with monomer in porcelain jar according to recommended ratio by manufacturer. It is allowed to attain dough stage for proper handling of material. Meanwhile, small quantity of material is placed in windows created to make tissue stop. This confirms that tray material is in contact with cast through windows to take up shape of tissue stops.

Step 3 (Figs. 20.3 and 20.4)

Petroleum jelly is applied on fingers to prevent material adhesion. Material in dough stage is taken out from the porcelain jar and kneaded to give desired shape and placed on the palate. Acrylic dough is shaped as rope or roll for fabrication of mandibular custom tray.

Step 4 (Figs. 20.5A to C)

Adapt the material to the casts carefully spread it all over the foundation area starting from palatal area to periphery. Apply proper finger pressure while adapting the resin over cast. Avoid excessive pressure while adaptation otherwise it will over thin the resin. Minimum

2–3 mm thickness of tray material should be maintained all over. Tray material should cover all of the denture foundation area till the sulcus. Avoid excessive thickness on palatal part.

For mandibular custom tray, take out material from porcelain cup and shape it like a roll and put it on residual ridge. Start spreading the material all over the edentulous ridge. Cover retromolar pad bilaterally. Do not apply

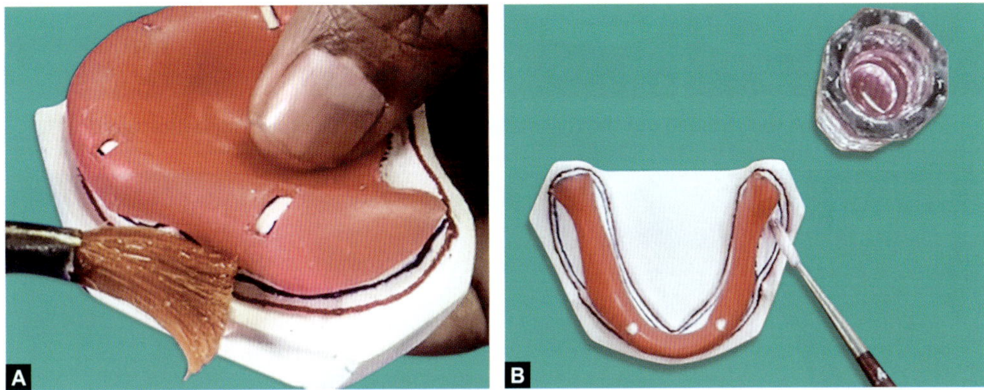

Figs. 20.1A and B: Application of cold mould seal on cast and on windows made for tissue stops.

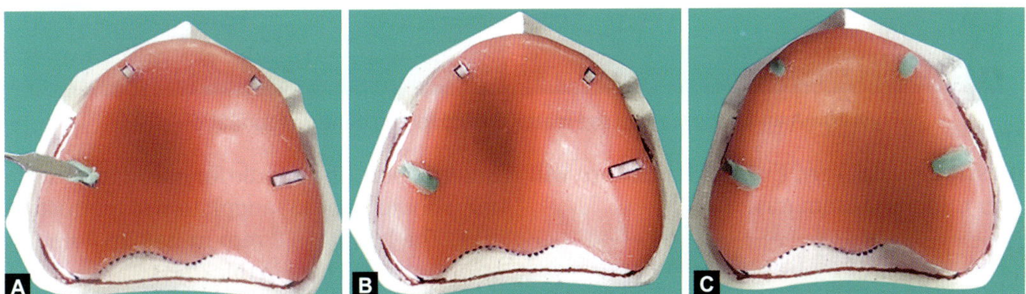

Figs. 20.2A to C: Creating tissue stops by putting tray material in windows for tissue stops.

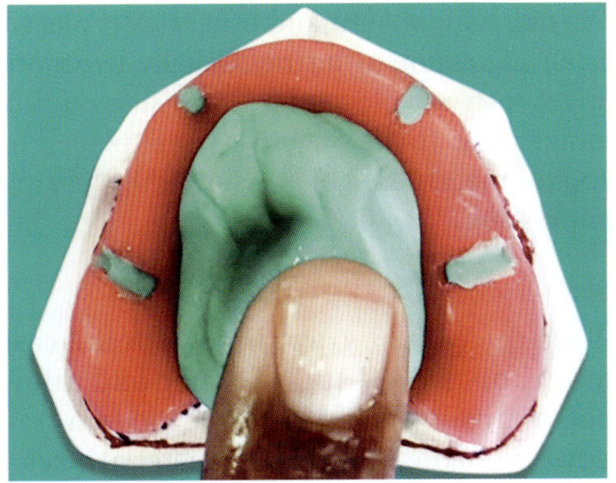

Fig. 20.3: Tray material is placed on palate.

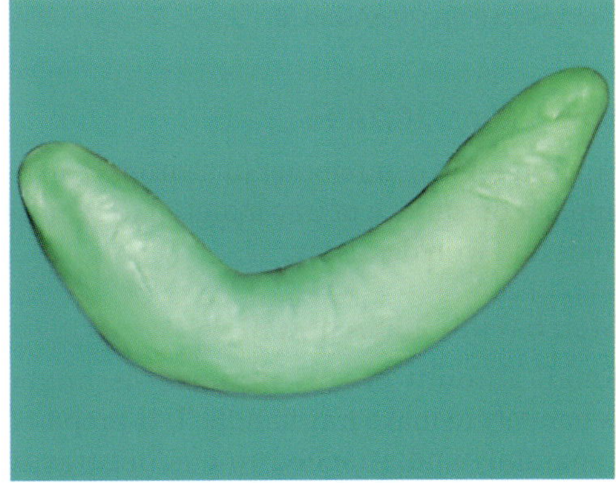

Fig. 20.4: Shape the acrylic dough as roll.

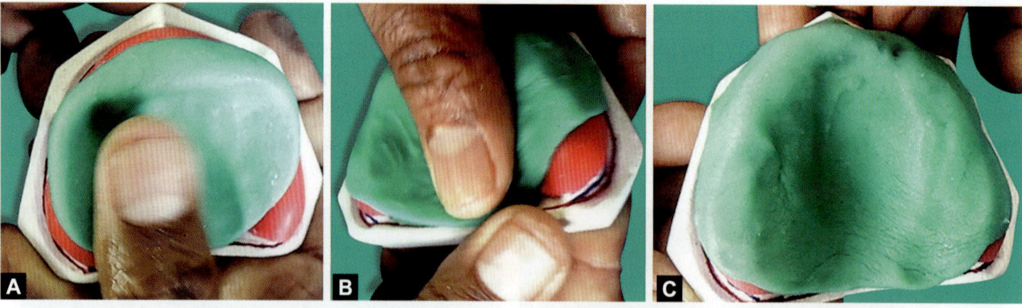

Figs. 20.5A to C: Spread out the tray material to cover the denture foundation area.

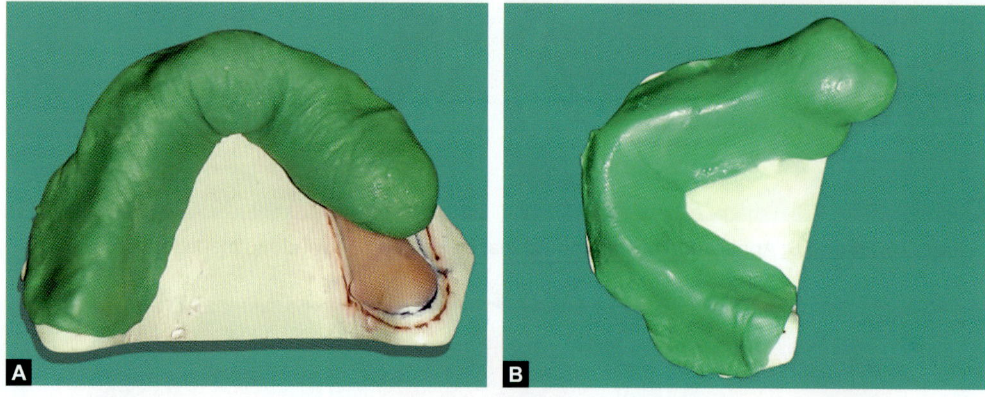

Figs. 20.6A and B: Spreading the material to cover the denture foundation area.

pressure excessively. Excessive pressure will over thin the custom tray.

Remove excess tray material from the borders with Le Cron carver so that the borders extend only up to the tray line. However, if the material has passed late dough stage, do not attempt to cut excess. This will drag tray borders and make it uneven and distorted **(Figs. 20.6A and B)**.

Step 5 (Figs. 20.7A to C)

Small amount of monomer (2–3 drops) can be applied on surface of tray material to remove folds and wrinkles if any.

Step 6 (Figs. 20.8A and B)

Small amount of tray material is mixed separately to make tray handle. It is prepared separately and attached to custom tray in anterior part. The handle for maxillary custom tray should be at 45° angulation to the custom tray. The handle is 8 mm in height, 8 mm in width, and 3–4 mm in thickness.

For Mandibular Custom Tray (Figs. 20.9A and B)

The tray handle for mandibular tray is placed at 90° angulation to the tray. Usually, two more finger rests are placed on either side on first molar area. These finger rests are placed to apply equal amount of pressure while making impression.

Step 7 (Figs. 20.10A and B)

Place the custom tray along with the cast into rubber bowl full of water and allow polymerization. Separate the custom tray slowly from the cast once the material is set.

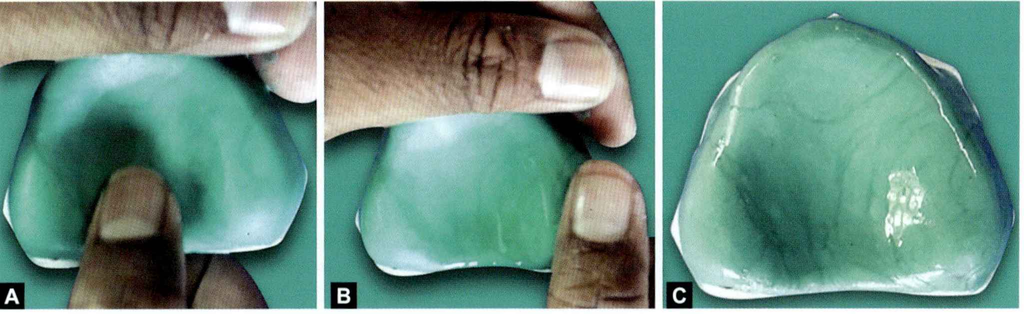

Figs. 20.7A to C: Remove folds and wrinkles.

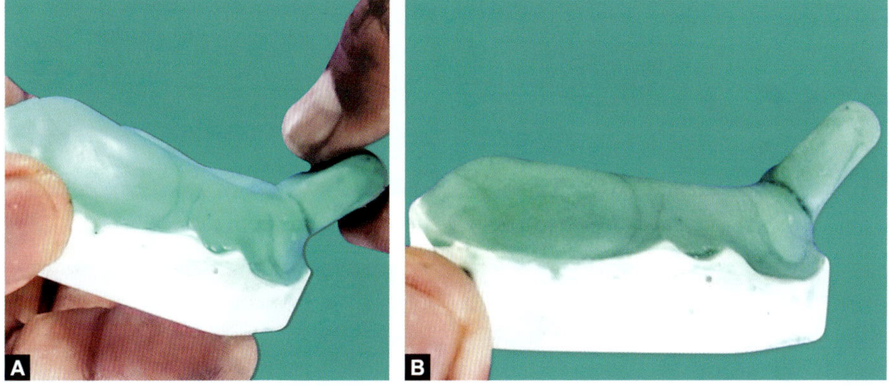

Figs. 20.8A and B: Handle is attached at 45° angulation in anterior part of maxillary custom tray.

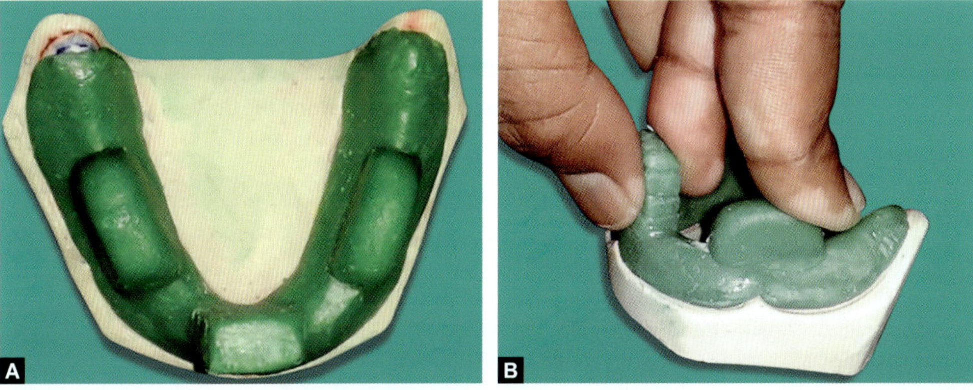

Figs. 20.9A and B: Mandibular custom tray with a handle and two finger rests.

Inspect the custom tray. The tissue stops and spacer should be at same level. All tissue stops should be well formed and should be in contact with cast.

Step 8 (Figs. 20.11A to C)

Trim the excess material beyond the land area on the lathe machine. Use the acrylic trimmer to shorten the tray borders 2–3 mm from the sulcus line.

Step 9 (Figs. 20.12A and B)

Maintain the thickness of the tray borders up to 2–3 mm. Make wide notches for all frenum with straight fissure metal or acrylic laboratory bur. Make the tray borders rounded. There should be no sharp projections, otherwise it may traumatize the oral tissue while border molding procedure.

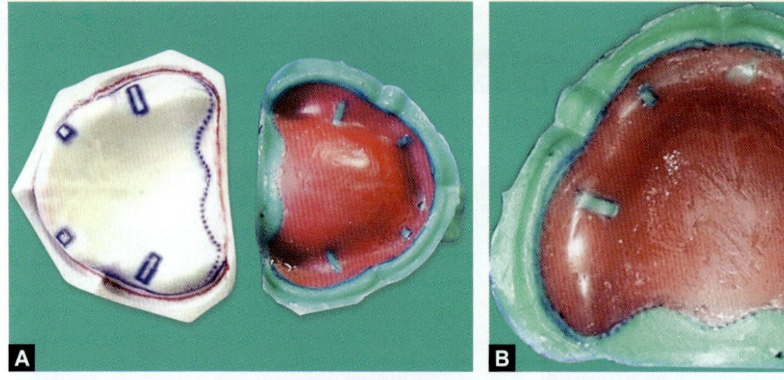

Figs. 20.10A and B: Retrieve the custom tray from cast.

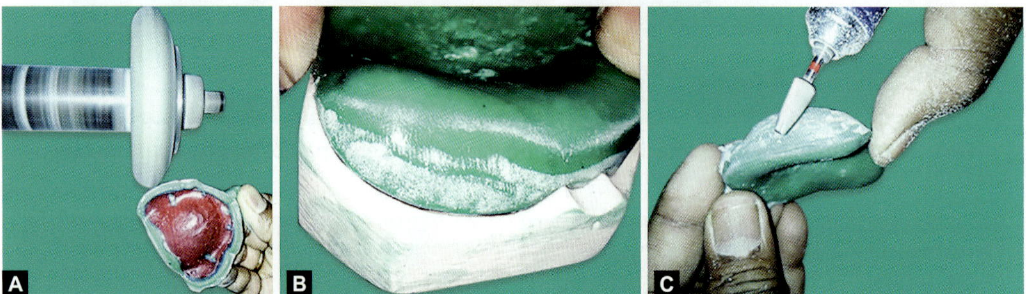

Figs. 20.11A to C: Trimming the excess material beyond the borders.

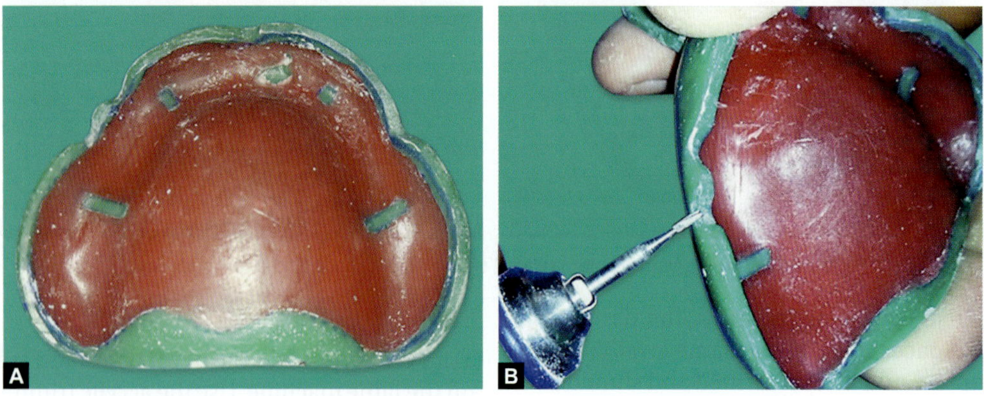

Figs. 20.12A and B: Create notches for frenum using straight fissure laboratory bur.

Step 10 (Figs. 20.13 to 20.15)

Some grooves are prepared on the tray handle. This will improve the grip in tray handling by the dentist. Make sure that the custom tray is 2–3 mm short of the sulcus line drawn on the primary cast. Enough space is created in the form of notch for frenum.

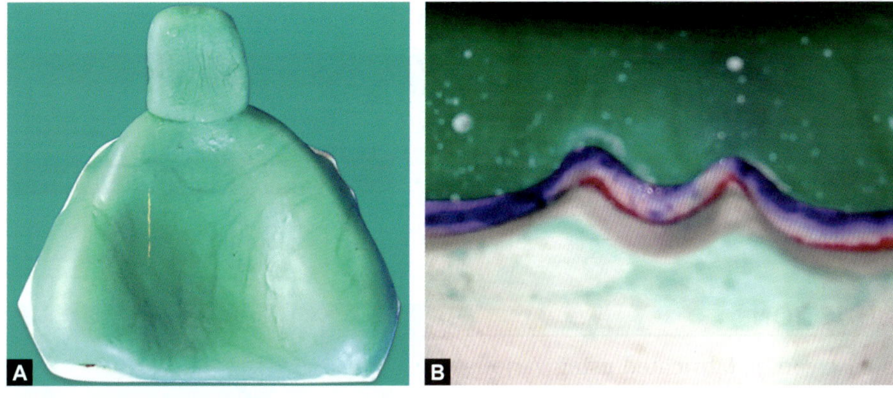

Figs. 20.13A and B: Custom tray is 2 mm short of sulcus and clearance is provided for frenums.

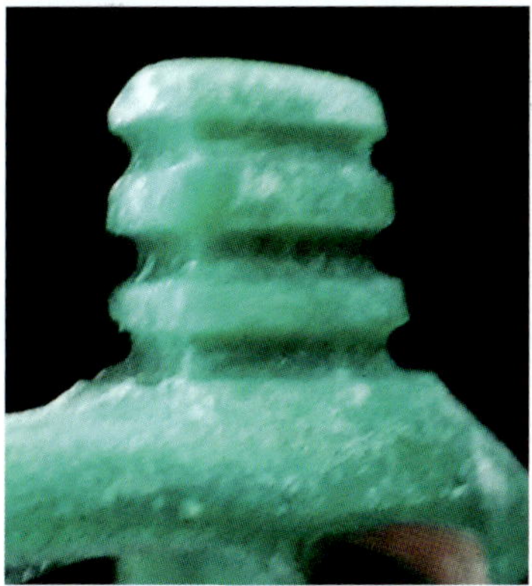

Fig. 20.14: Make grooves on tray handle to improve grip.

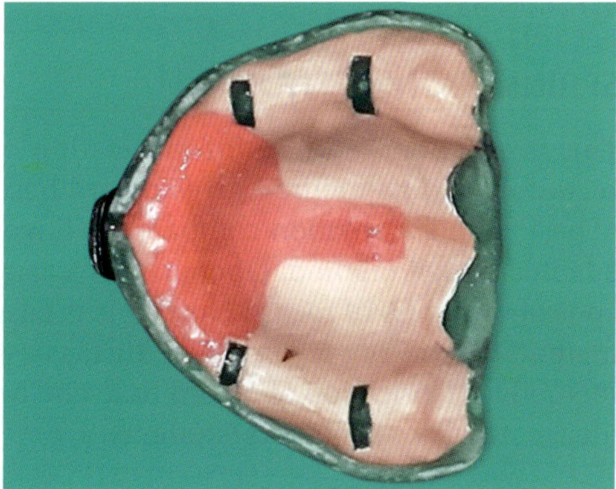

Fig. 20.15: Tissue surface of maxillary impression tray with spacer.

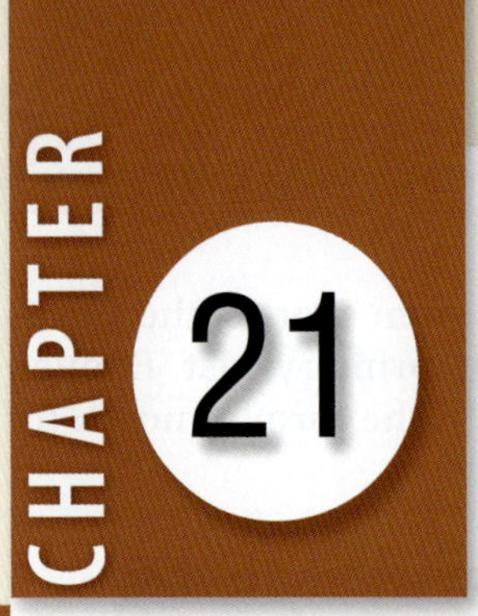

CHAPTER 21 Fabrication of Denture Base/Record Base

Paranjay Prajapati, Sneha Kulkarni

INTRODUCTION

Record base can be fabricated using various materials with various methods. This chapter demonstrates various method of fabrication of record base.

SPRINKLE-ON METHOD

This is excellent method for fabrication of record base. This method gives record base of best fit and adaptation compared to finger adapted dough method. Operator can easily control thickness of record base. This is easy method to fabricate record base. This is easy method for fabrication of record base and an ideal method for beginners/students.

Armamentarium (Fig. 21.1)

- Maxillary final cast
- Self-cure acrylic resin in dispenser
- Self-cure monomer
- Syringe
- Cold mold seal
- Painting brush
- Dappen dish.

Step 1 (Figs. 21.2A and B)

Mark denture borders with indelible pencil in the sulcus depth. Apply cold mold seal (separating medium) on maxillary cast with painting brush. Repeat application 2–3 times to achieve even coating of it.

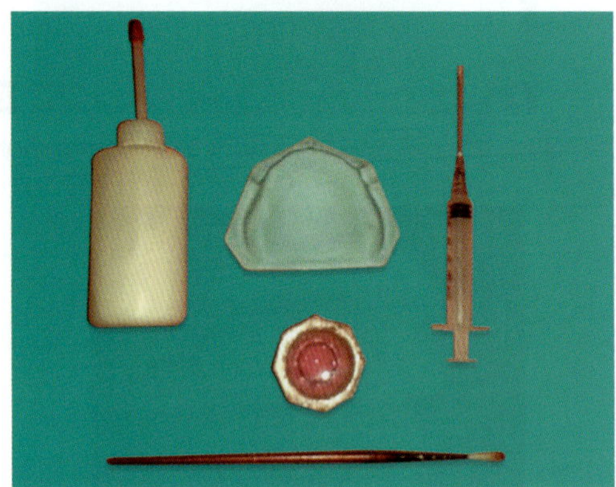

Fig. 21.1: Armamentarium required for fabrication of record base.

Step 2 (Figs. 21.3A and B)

Apply desired quantity of self-cure polymer on smaller area of cast and saturate it with monomer liquid. Repeat the procedure as needed. A syringe can be used for dropping the monomer on polymer.

Step 3 (Fig. 21.4)

Apply material in sulcus in such a way that it fills sulcus evenly. This will record proper width and depth of sulcus. Proper recording

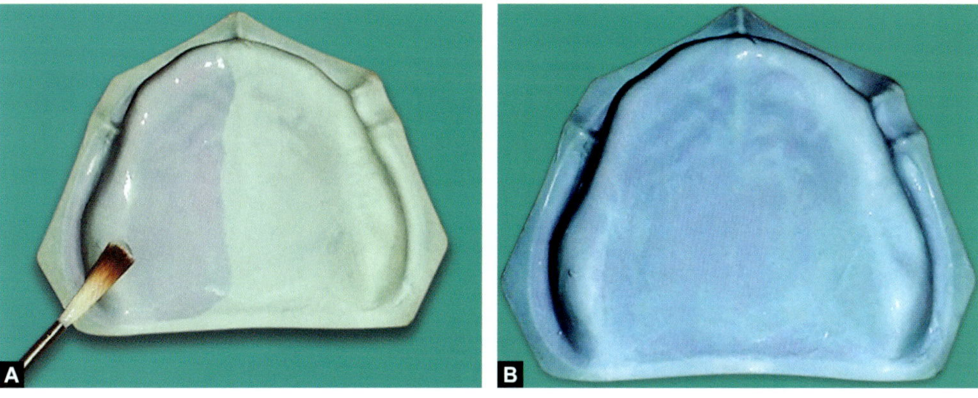

Figs. 21.2A and B: Application of cold mold seal with brush.

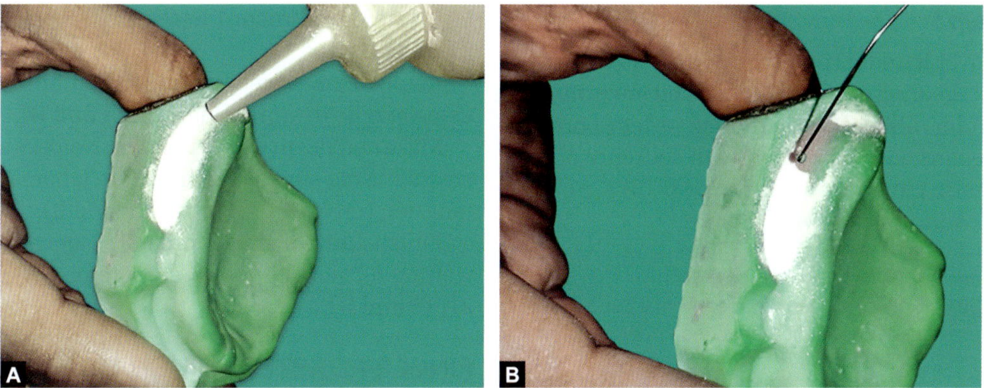

Figs. 21.3A and B: Application of polymer and saturating it with monomer.

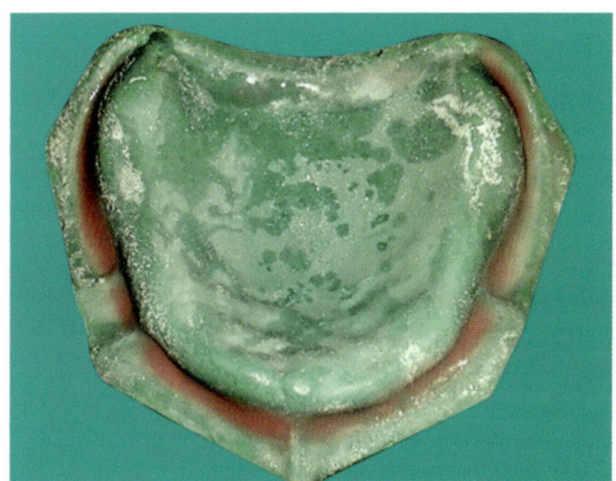

Fig. 21.4: Making record base and recording sulcus depth and width.

of width and height of sulcus is essential to achieve retention of record base.

> Use small plastic bottle with nozzle to dispense polymer powder and syringe with needle to dispense monomer liquid drop by drop. Bend needle as shown in picture for easy use and visualization.

Step 4 (Figs. 21.5A and B)

Repeat the procedure until even thickness of denture base of around 2–3 mm is achieved. Extend the procedure all over the cast to cover entire denture foundation area with the acrylic resin.

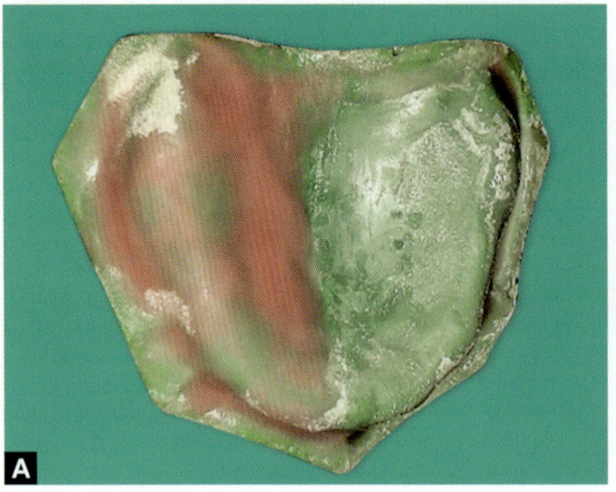
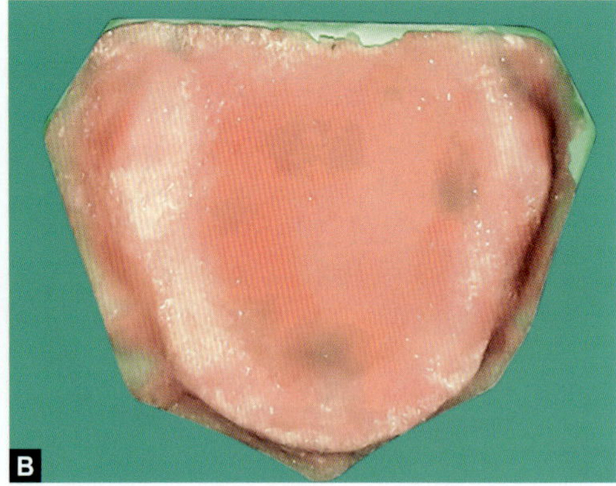

Figs. 21.5A and B: Continue making record base on other area till it covers whole denture foundation area.

Step 5

Cover it under rubber bowl for 10–20 minutes for creating monomer saturated environment under rubber bowl to reduce surface porosity. Record base fabricated with self-cure acrylic resin can be cured in pressure pot for 20 minutes at 20 psi pressure.

> Record bases cured under pressure have less porosity. Record base cured at normal atmospheric pressure has better fit than cured under pressure.

Step 6

Remove it carefully with sharp instrument without damaging the cast or record base. Examine cured record base carefully **(Figs. 21.6A and B)**.

Remove any excess material from borders using acrylic trimmer **(Figs. 21.7A and B)**.

Make notches to relieve frenums. Notches are created using small straight fissure laboratory tungsten carbide bur **(Figs. 21.8A and B)**.

Finish and polish it. Store it in water while waiting for next appointment/exercise **(Figs. 21.9A and B)**.

FINGER ADAPTED DOUGH METHOD

An alternate method of making record base is finger adapted dough method. Instead of sprinkling on polymer and saturating it with

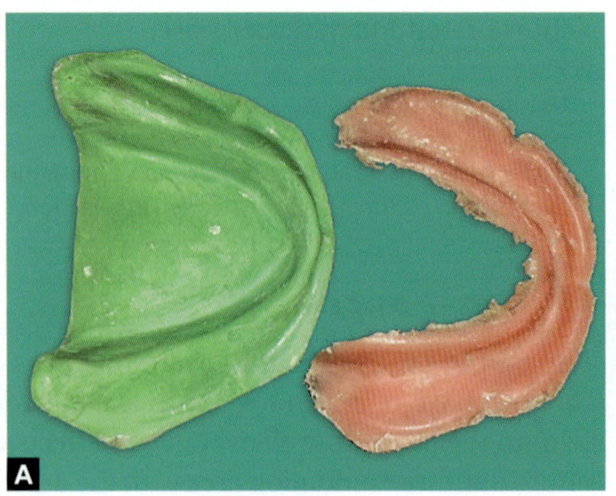
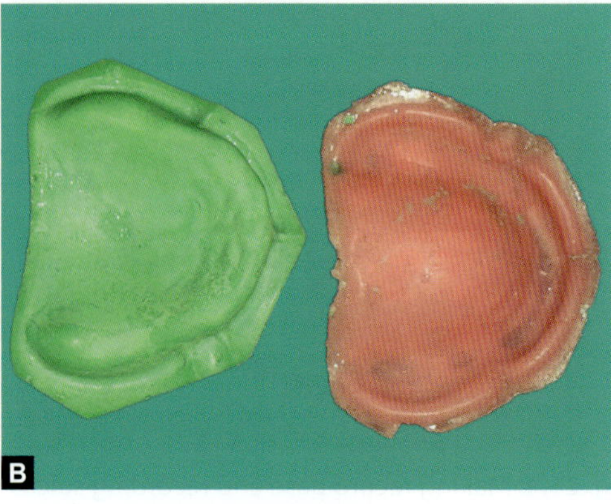

Figs. 21.6A and B: Retrieve the record base after polymerization.

monomer, mix the polymer and monomer together until the mixture attains dough consistency.

When the polymer-monomer mixture attains dough consistency, it is removed from the porcelain jar and adapted on cast in such

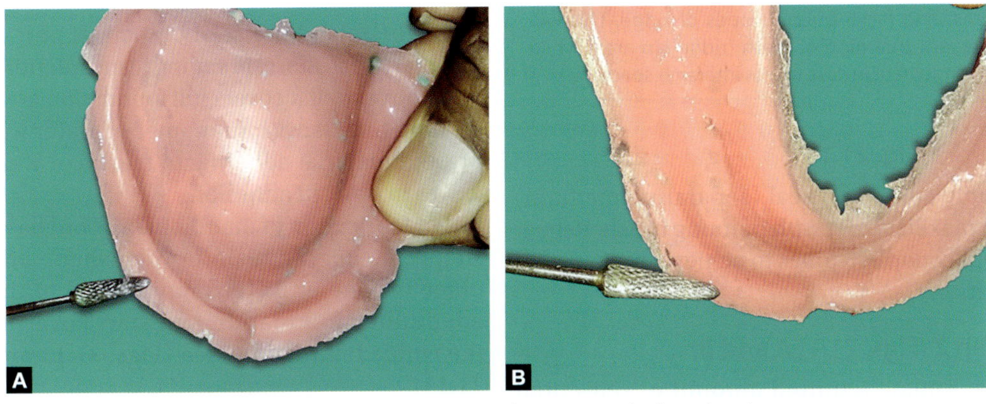

Figs. 21.7A and B: Trimming of excess acrylic from borders.

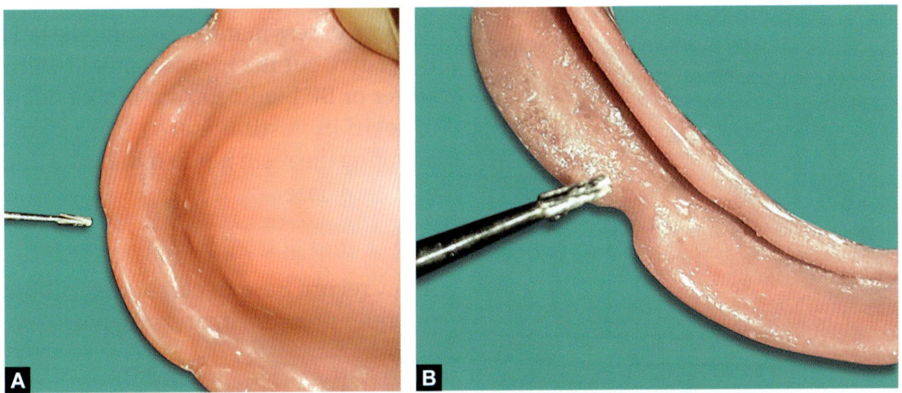

Figs. 21.8A and B: Creating notches to relieve frenums.

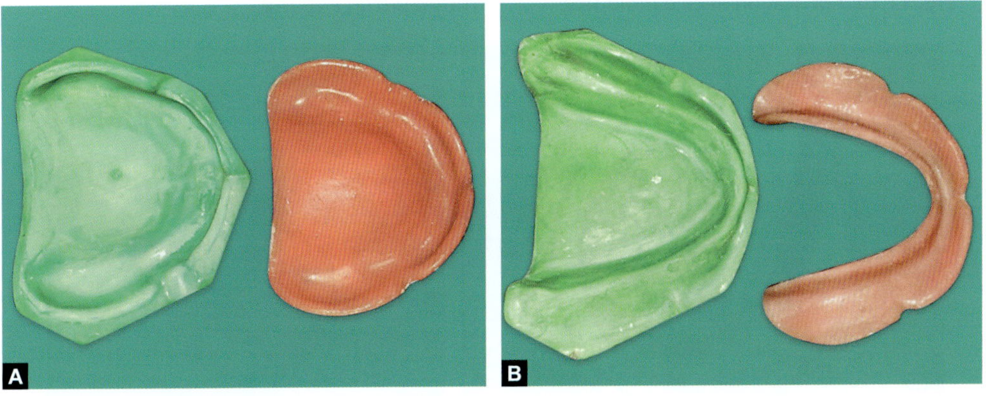

Figs. 21.9A and B: Finished maxillary and mandibular record bases.

a way that the record base of even thickness of 2–3 mm is fabricated.

Thickness of record base is kept 1–1.5 mm over crest and facial/buccal slopes of ridge. This will prevent trimming of teeth (ridge lap area) while arrangement in case of less interarch space.

Step 1 (Fig. 21.10)

Apply cold mold seal (separating medium) on maxillary cast with painting brush. Repeat application 2–3 times to achieve even coating of it.

Step 2 (Figs. 21.11A and B)

Manipulate required amount of self-cured polymer and monomer in porcelain jar and wait till it attains dough consistency. Apply Vaseline on palm and collect material from porcelain jar, mix it well using finger.

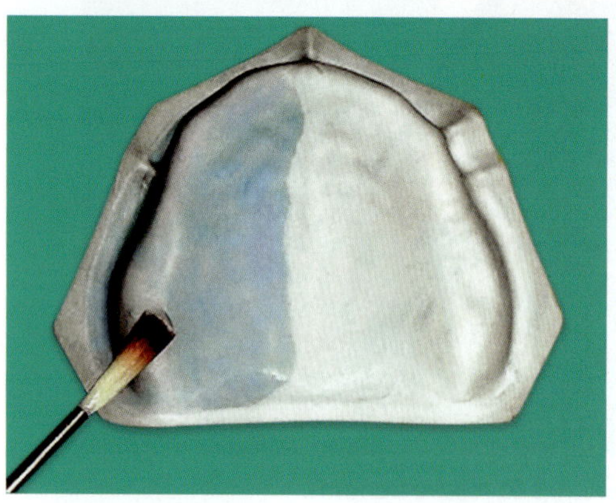

Fig. 21.10: Application of cold mold seal.

Step 3 (Figs. 21.12A to C)

Place the mixed material on palatal part of maxillary cast. Start spreading it and adapting it on the cast till it covers full foundation area. Wetting fingers with monomer or water will prevent material adhering to fingers or wear gloves to prevent adhesion.

For fabrication of mandibular record base, shape the acrylic resin in rope shape and place on one end (retromolar pad) of the edentulous foundation and start covering the whole foundation area **(Figs. 21.13 and 21.14)**.

Step 4 (Figs. 21.15A and B)

Remove excess material beyond the land area. If needed, cut the excess material with paper cutter or BP blade. Ensure proper adaptation of resin in vestibule area. Take care while adapting the resin not to reduce the thickness of record base.

Step 5 (Fig. 21.16)

Allow record base to cure under rubber bowl or under pressure in pressure pot.

Step 6 (Figs. 21.17A and B)

Make notches to relieve all the frenum. Smooth rough surface if any.

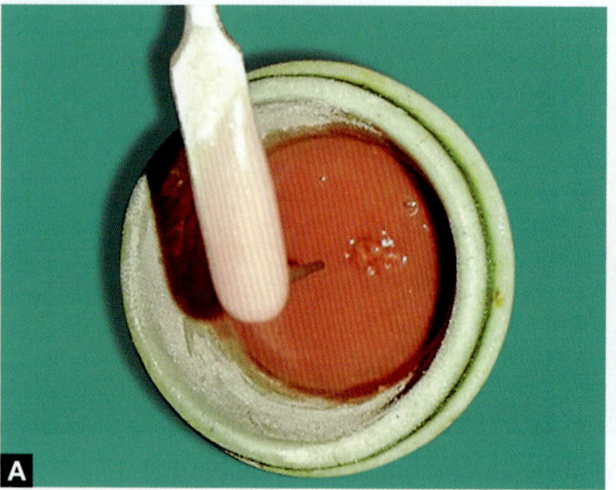

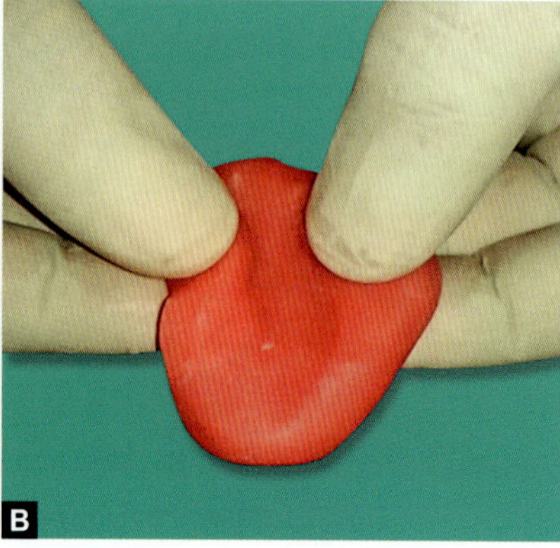

Figs. 21.11A and B: Manipulation of self-cure acrylic resin.

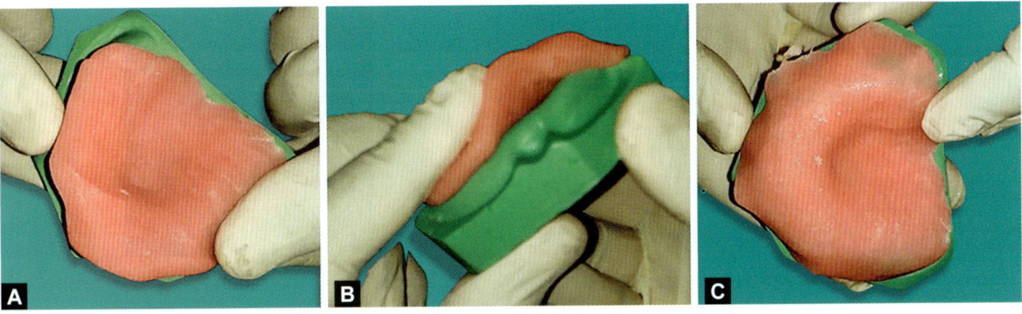

Figs. 21.12A to C: Finger adaptation of acrylic resin in dough stage.

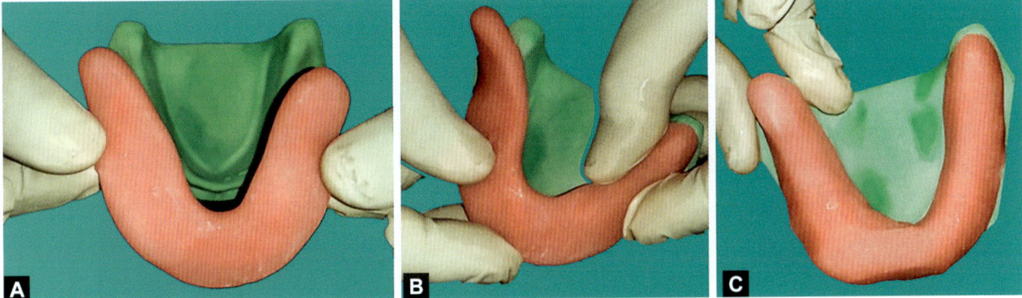

Figs. 21.13A to C: Start adapting acrylic from one end and cover whole foundation area.

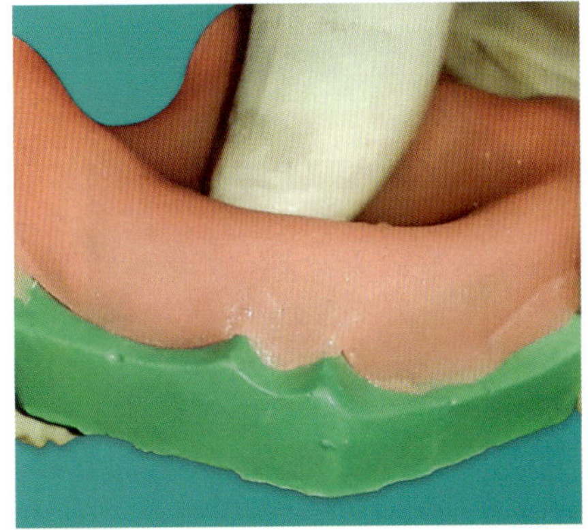

Fig. 21.14: Take care to cover sulcus properly. The thickness should be maintained.

FORMING RESIN SHEET TO FABRICATE RECORD BASE (FIGS. 21.18 TO 21.23)

A modification to finger adapted dough method is to roll the acrylic dough in a sheet of desired thickness and adapting it on cast to fabricate record base.

Acrylic dough can be rolled in sheets by pressing it between two lubricated glass slabs or by using the stone mold.

Resin sheets can also be fabricated by pressing the resin dough between two lubricated glass slabs.

FABRICATION OF RECORD BASE BY SHELLAC BASEPLATE

Armamentarium (Fig. 21.24)

- Final cast
- Shellac baseplate
- Slurry water
- Cotton
- Chip blower
- Curved scissors
- Wax knife
- Wax spatula
- Pencil to mark borders and frenum.

Shellac is available in form of baseplates **(Fig. 21.24)** in different shapes for maxillary

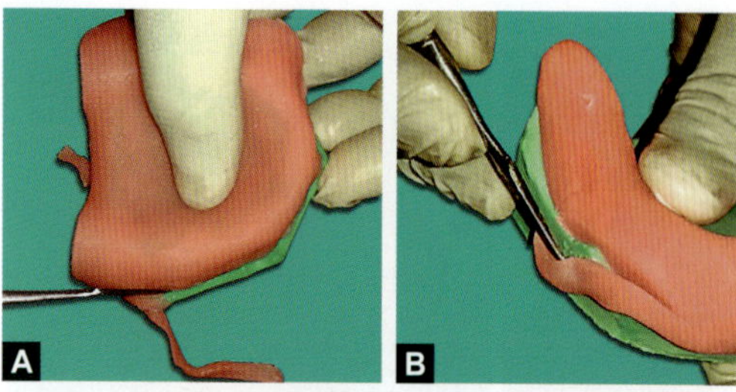

Figs. 21.15A and B: Removal of excess material beyond land area.

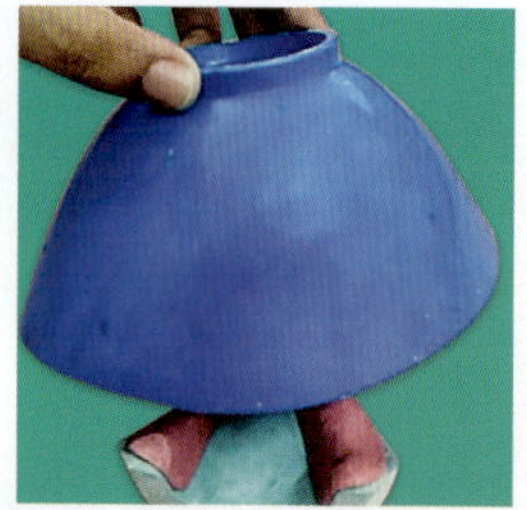

Fig. 21.16: Cover the record base under rubber bowl till it set completely.

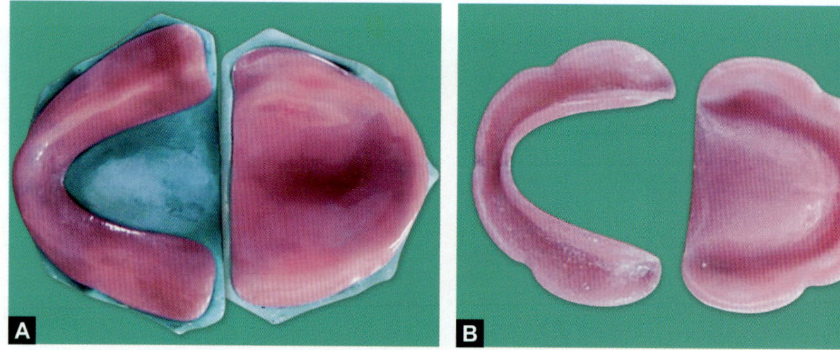

Figs. 21.17A and B: Polished surface and tissue surface of record base.

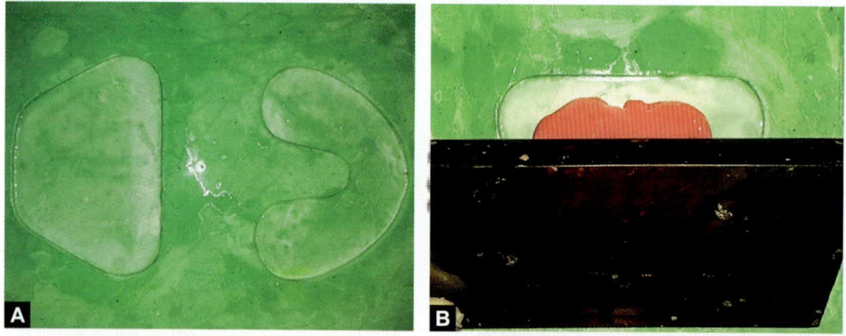

Figs. 21.18A and B: Stone mold to make acrylic resin sheet, press resin dough in stone mold by glass slab.

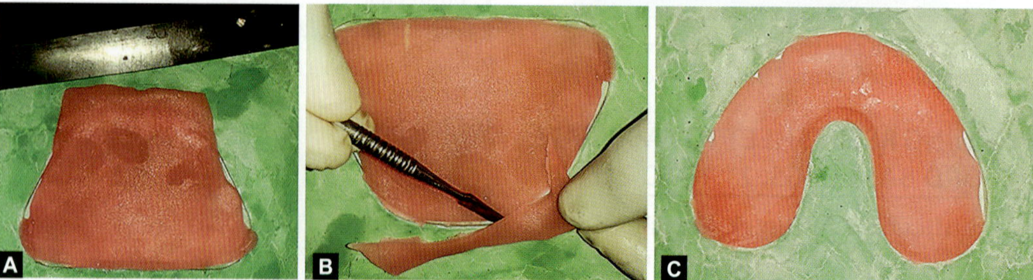

Figs. 21.19A to C: Cut the excess material extending out from the boundary.

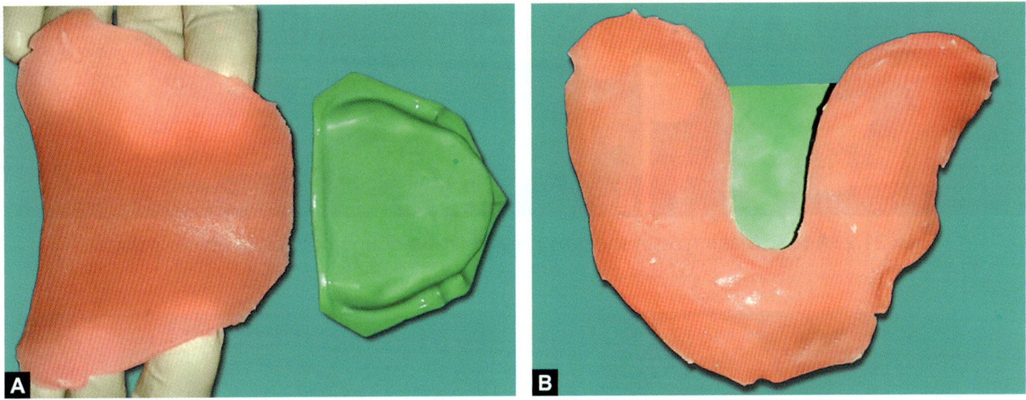

Figs. 21.20A and B: Adapt resin sheets on casts to fabricate record base.

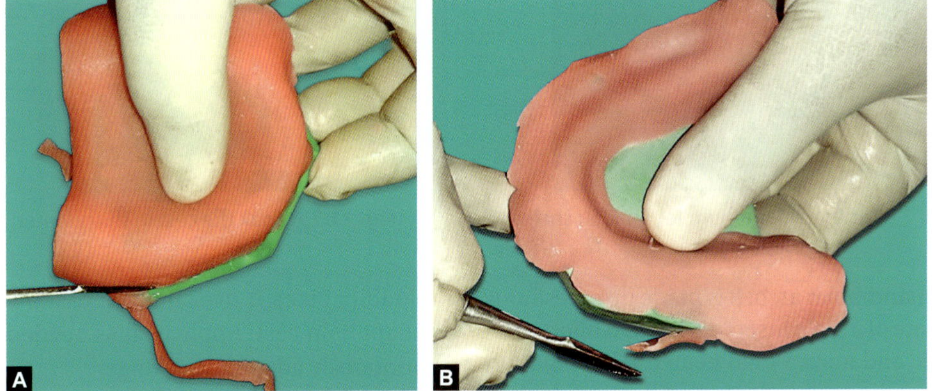

Figs. 21.21A and B: Trim excess material with BP blade.

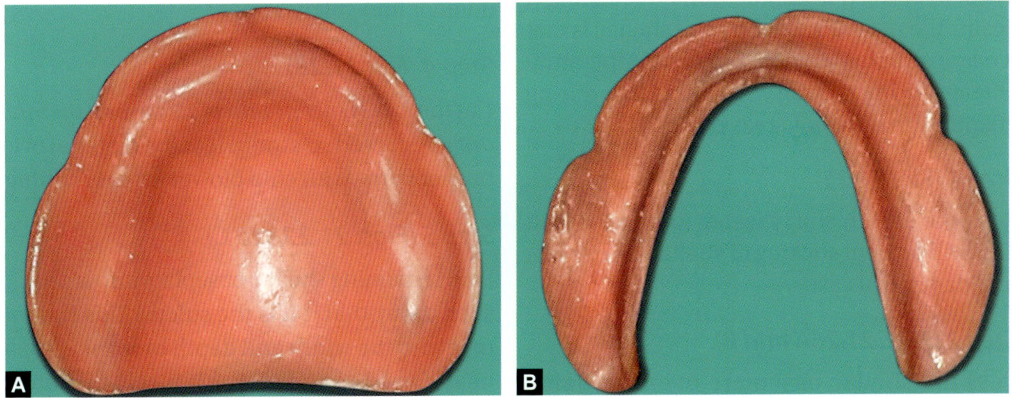

Figs. 21.22A and B: Maxillary and mandibular record bases after polymerization.

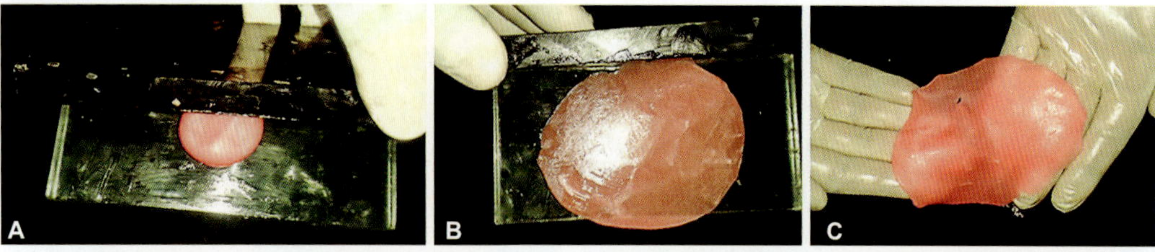

Figs. 21.23A to C: Making resin sheet by pressing resin dough between two glass slabs.

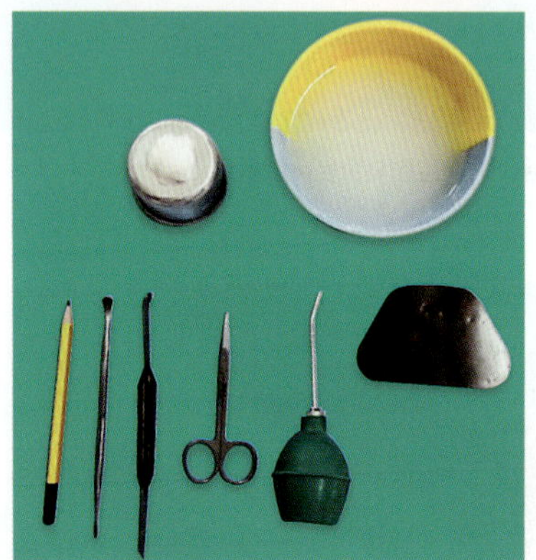

Fig. 21.24: Armamentarium for making shellac record base.

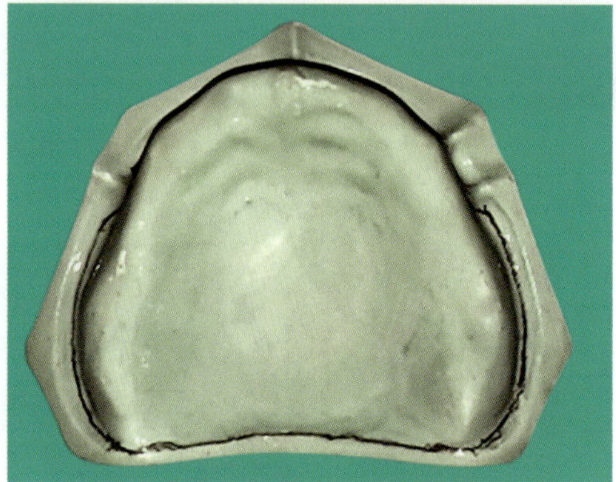

Fig. 21.25: Soak the cast in slurry water.

and mandibular arch. It is made up of resinous exudate of a scale insect and added fillers such as talc and mica. When heated it become soft and can be easily adapted on cast, on cooling become rigid and dimensionally stable. It is easy to manipulate and adapt shellac. If needed, correction can be done by heating it again. The main disadvantage of shellac is that it may lose its initial adaptation by temperature change during making wax rim on it or during adapting on different areas on cast.

Step 1 (Fig. 21.25)

Soak the cast in slurry water to make it wet. This will prevent sticking of shellac on the cast and damage of cast.

Step 2 (Figs. 21.26A and B)

Pass the shellac baseplate over the flame of Bunsen burner till it become soft and moldable. Place it over the wet cast and try to adapt it on cast. Apply heat as needed and continuously adapt it with finger.

Step 3 (Fig. 21.27)

Use curved end of wax knife or wax spatula to adapt it into sulcus.

Step 4 (Fig. 21.28)

Cut the *excess shellac baseplate beyond the land area* by curved scissors. Heat the material over burner flame with chip blower for easy cutting.

Step 5 (Figs. 21.29A to C)

Fold remaining shellac baseplate into sulcus in such a way that it fills the sulcus. This is done to record the width and depth of sulcus. Apply heat if needed and merge it nicely to remove rough area.

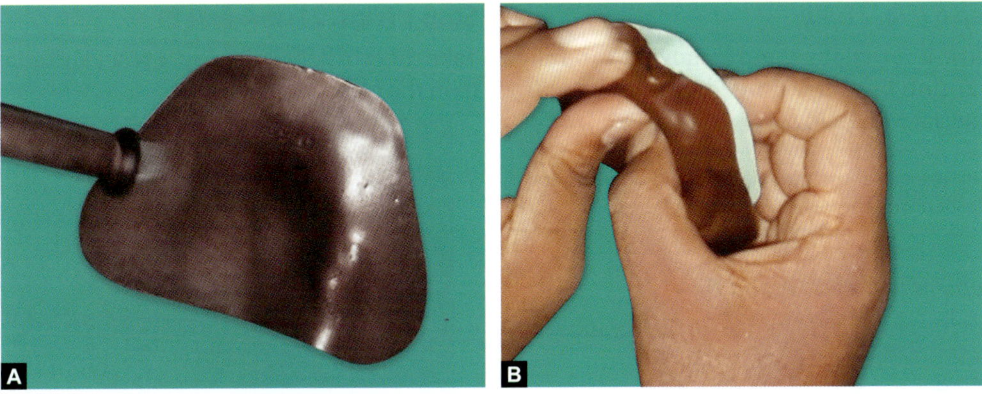

Figs. 21.26A and B: Soften the baseplate before adapting on cast.

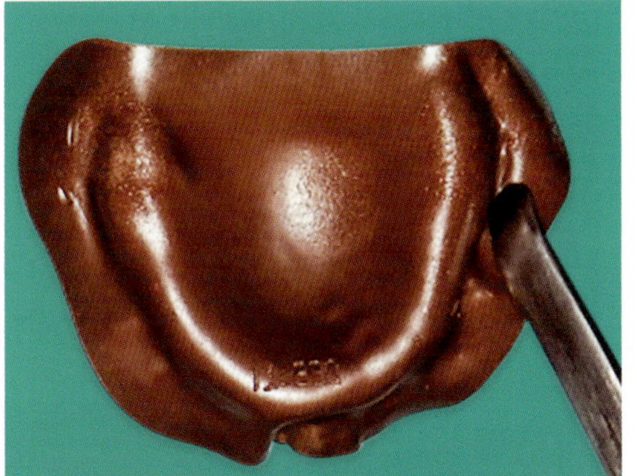

Fig. 21.27: Adapt the baseplate in the sulcus area with blunt end instrument like wax knife.

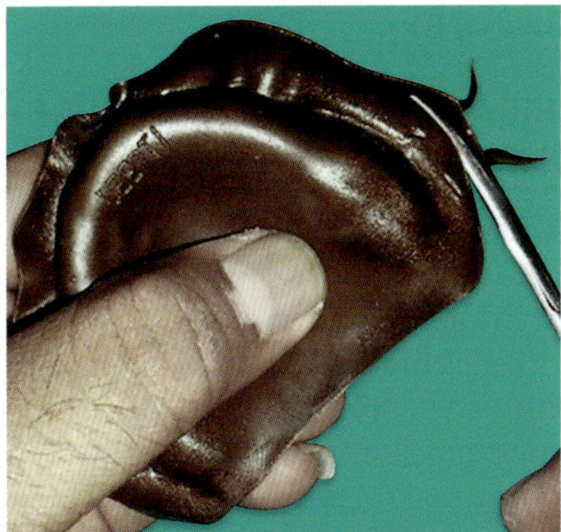

Fig. 21.28: Cut the excess material beyond the land area.

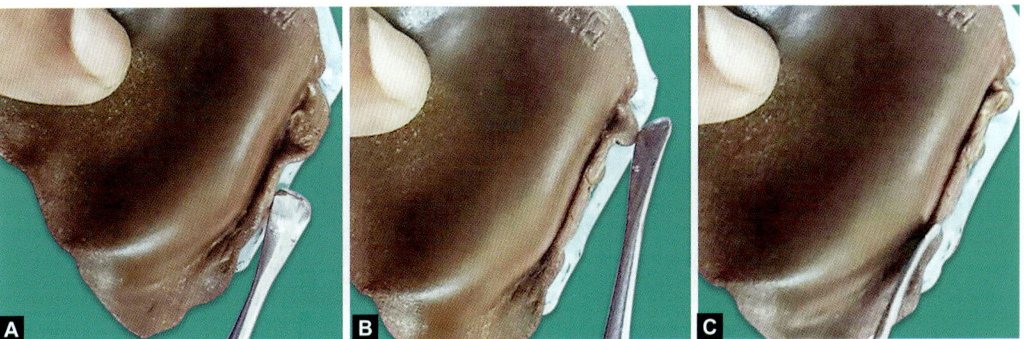

Figs. 21.29A to C: Adapting the remaining material into sulcus to record width and depth of sulcus.

Step 6 (Fig. 21.30)

Allow it for cooling and remove it carefully. Examine borders, if needed remove extra material with filling.

> The margin of the baseplate should be filled and flushed with the vestibular depth of the cast.

Step 7 (Figs. 21.31A and B)

Provide enough clearance for all frenum.

Step 8

Inspect the borders and smooth them with sandpaper wherever needed **(Fig. 21.32)**.

Shellac record base is ready for use **(Figs. 21.33A and B)**.

FABRICATION OF RECORD BASE BY LIGHT CURE ACRYLIC RESIN

Light cure resin is available in sheets in light protected box. It is easy to adapt, shape, and adjust the light cure resin sheet on the cast. It is very quick method for fabrication of record base but costly compared to other material and methods. It requires special equipment for polymerization of light cure resin. Sheets are available in uniform thickness **(Fig. 21.34)**.

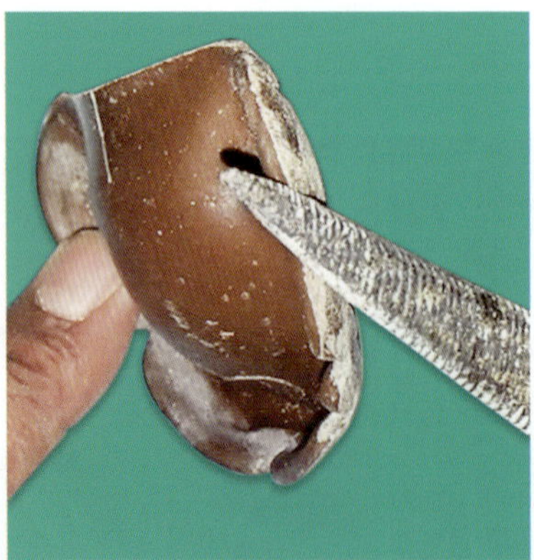

Fig. 21.30: Filling is done to smoothen the rough areas.

Step 1 (Figs. 21.35A and B)

Take sheet of light cure acrylic resin and adapt it on the cast.

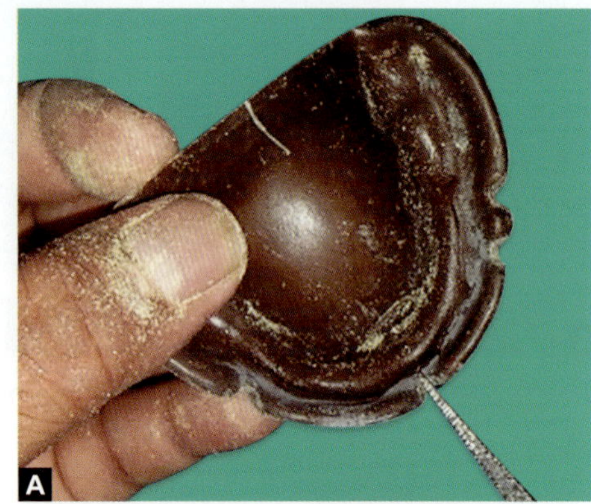

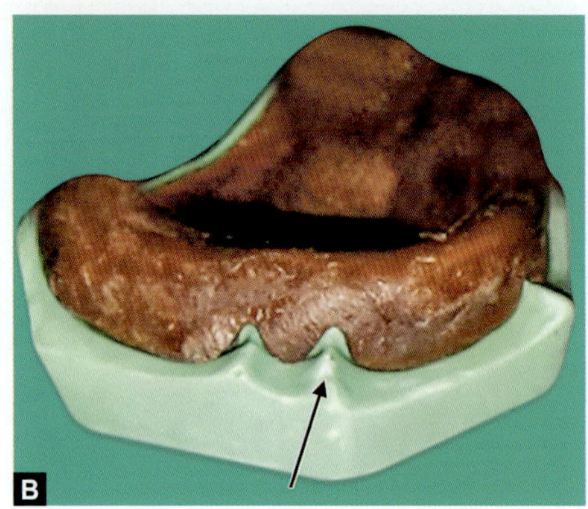

Figs. 21.31A and B: Provide clearance for frenum.

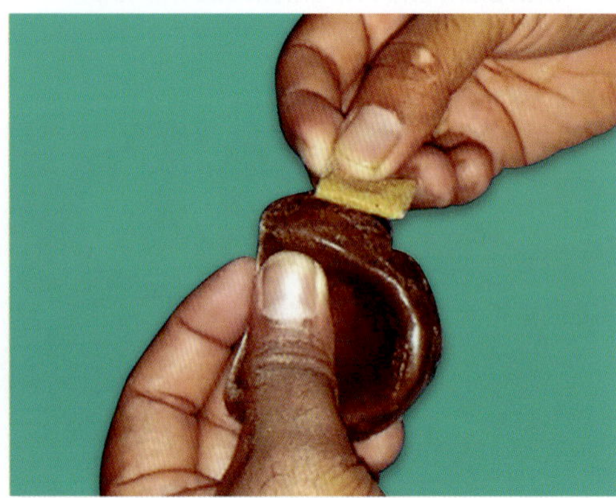

Fig. 21.32: Do sandpapering to remove roughness wherever needed.

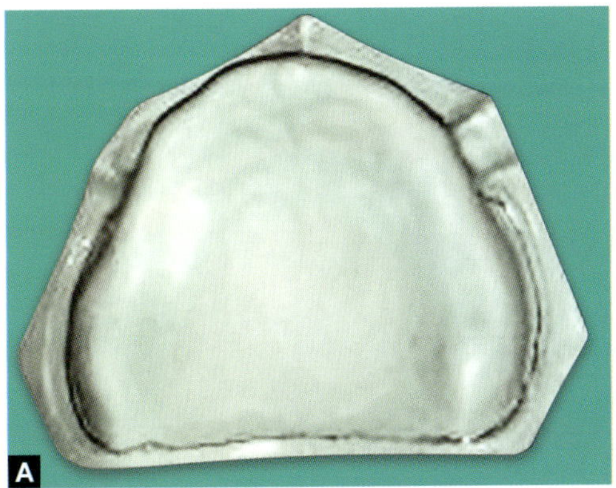

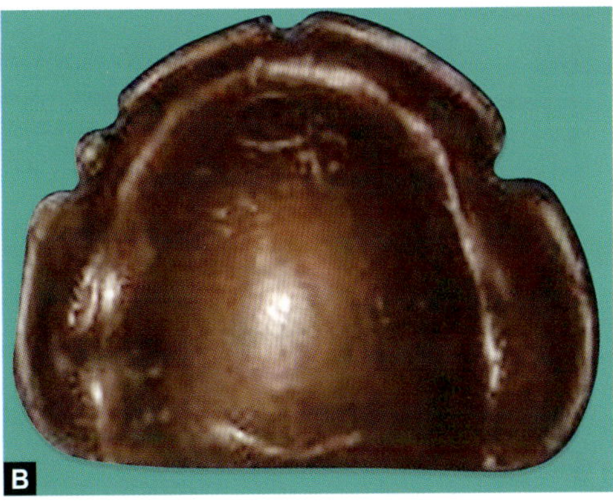

Figs. 21.33A and B: Shellac record base.

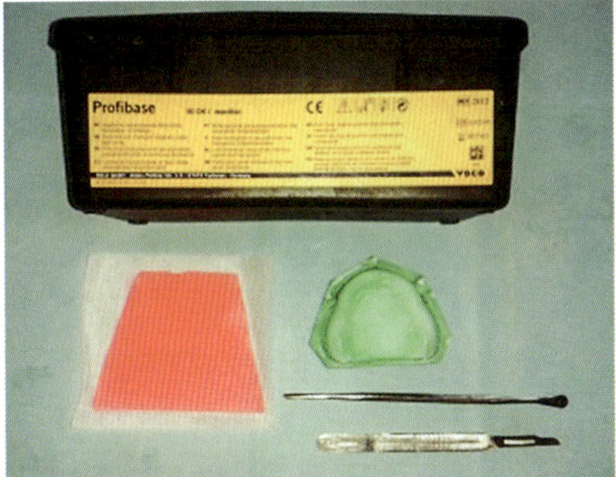

Fig. 21.34: Light cure resin sheet with box and other armamentarium

Step 2 (Figs. 21.36A and B)

Cut extra material beyond the land area with BP blade.

Step 3 (Fig. 21.37)

Adapt material in sulcus area with wax spatula.

Step 4 (Figs. 21.38A and B)

Cure it in curing chamber for 10 minutes.

Step 5

Inspect the borders. Trim and smoothen if needed **(Figs. 21.39A and B)**.

Light cure denture base is ready for use.

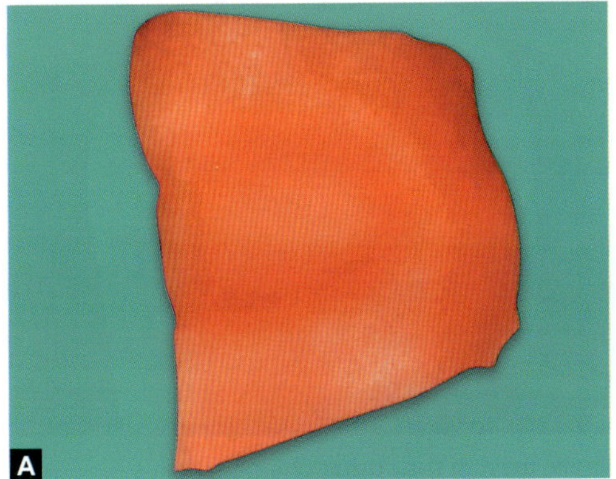

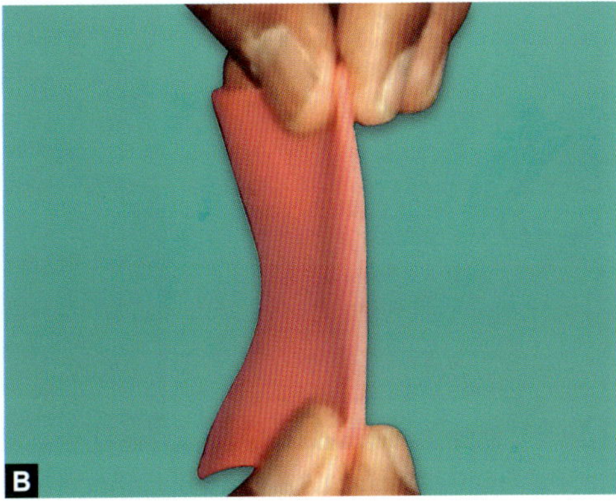

Figs. 21.35A and B: Adapt light cure resin sheet on the cast.

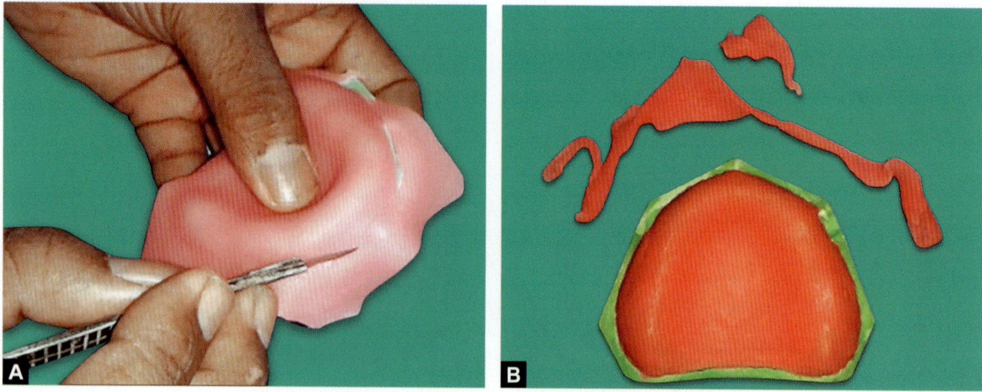

Figs. 21.36A and B: Cut the excess material beyond the land area.

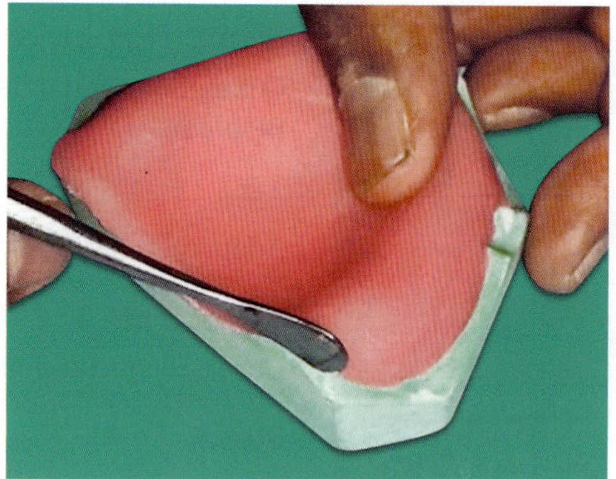

Fig. 21.37: Adapt the material in the sulcus.

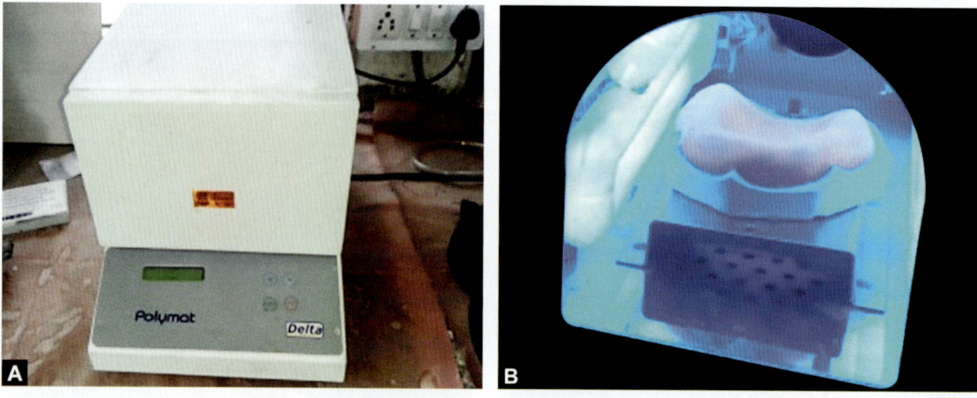

Figs. 21.38A and B: Light curing of acrylic resin in the curing chamber.

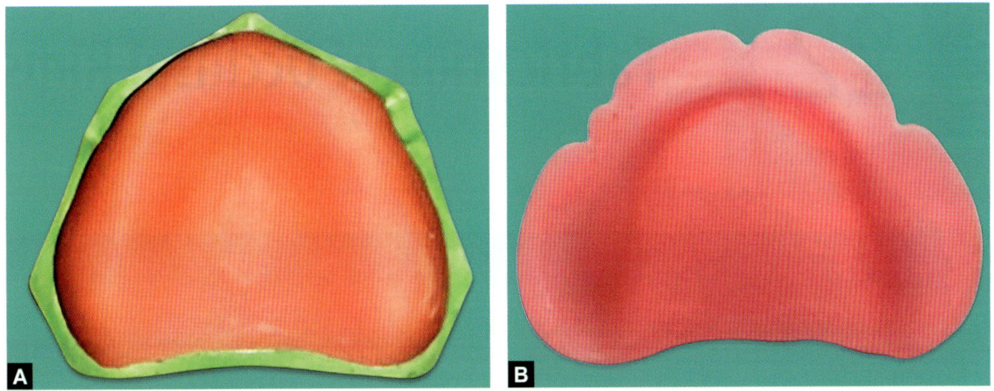

Figs. 21.39A and B: Light cured record base—external surface and tissue surface.

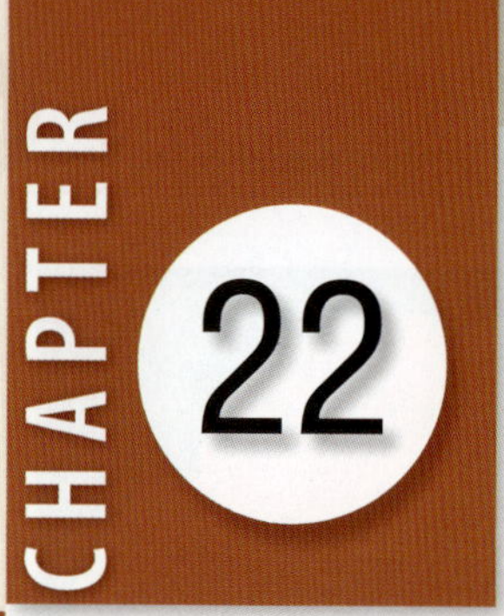

CHAPTER 22 Fabrication of Occlusal Rims

Paranjay Prajapati, Sneha Kulkarni

INTRODUCTION

This chapter explains fabrication of wax occlusal rims using rolled wax technique. This is the most commonly used method for fabrication of occlusal rims. Follow the procedure step by step for accurate fabrication of occlusal rims.

ARMAMENTARIUM (FIG. 22.1)

Maxillary and mandibular master casts with record base.

- Modeling wax
- Pencil or marker pen

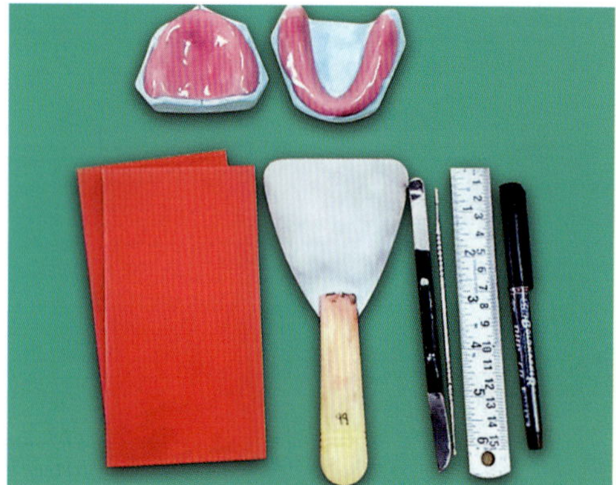

Fig. 22.1: Armamentarium of maxillary and mandibular master casts.

- Bunsen burner
- Wax knife
- Wax carver
- Wax spatula
- Hot plate
- Metallic scale.

FABRICATION OF MAXILLARY OCCLUSAL RIM

Step 1 (Figs. 22.2A and B)

Take a sheet of modeling wax. Heat it over the flame of Bunsen burner to soften it. Fold it from one end (approximately 0.5 cm). Take care not to melt it. Continuously soften it and roll it to prevent air bubble entrapment during rolling.

Step 2 (Fig. 22.3)

Roll the full wax sheet to get wax roll of diameter of around 2–3 cm. Place one end of the rolled wax on posterior aspect of record base (maxillary tuberosity) and follow the arch contour till the other posterior end.

Step 3

Apply downward pressure on wax roll by holding it in between index finger and the

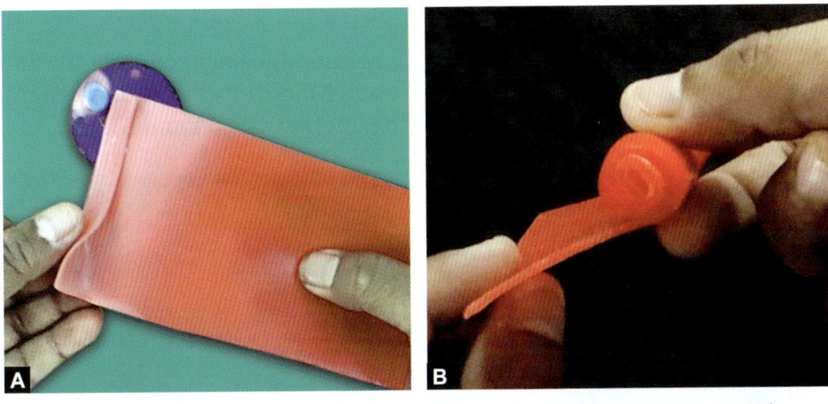

Figs. 22.2A and B: Softening the wax sheet over Bunsen burner and rolling it to make wax roll.

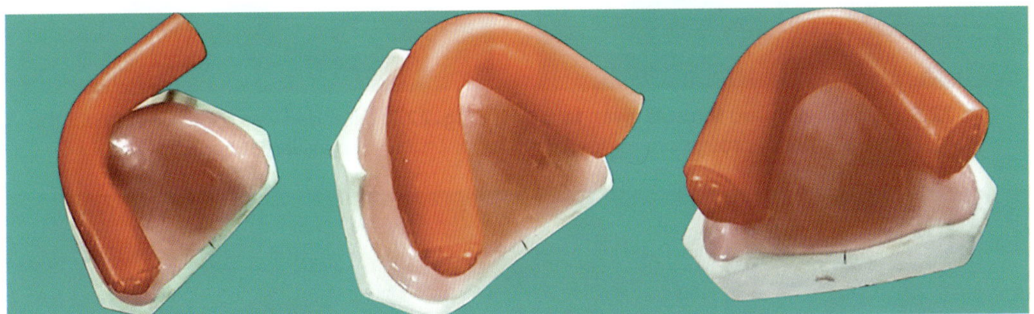

Fig. 22.3: Placement of wax roll following the arch shape.

thumb to extend it along the borders. Follow the arch contour while doing this to maintain the arch form **(Fig. 22.4)**.

Step 4

Give inside to outward push (thrust) in anterior region. This is done to give inclination to anterior rim. The inclination (protrusion) should be 12–15°. Due to inclination, maxillary rim becomes thinner anteriorly compared to posteriorly **(Fig. 22.5)**.

Step 5

Seal the adapted wax on buccal and lingual peripheries using hot wax spatula or wax knife. Add or remove wax to fill up voids, spaces, and irregularities. Smooth the buccal surface maintaining the arch form **(Figs. 22.6A to C)**.

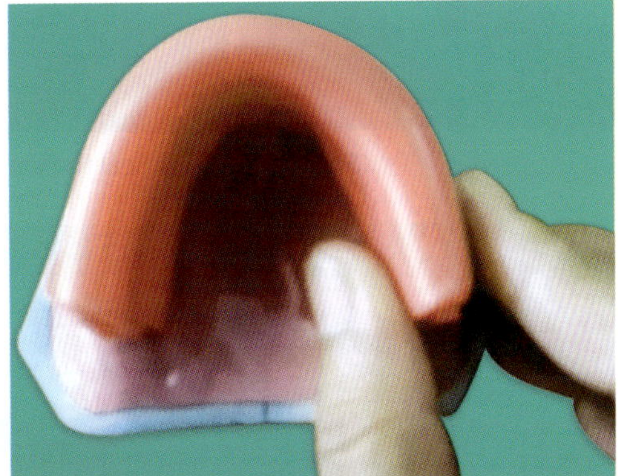

Fig. 22.4: Extend the wax till the borders of record base using index finger and thumb.

Step 6 (Fig. 22.7)

Cut the wax roll if extended over the maxillary tuberosity.

Step 7

Measure the height of occlusal rim in canine area. Mark it 2–3 mm more than required height **(Figs. 22.8A and B)**.

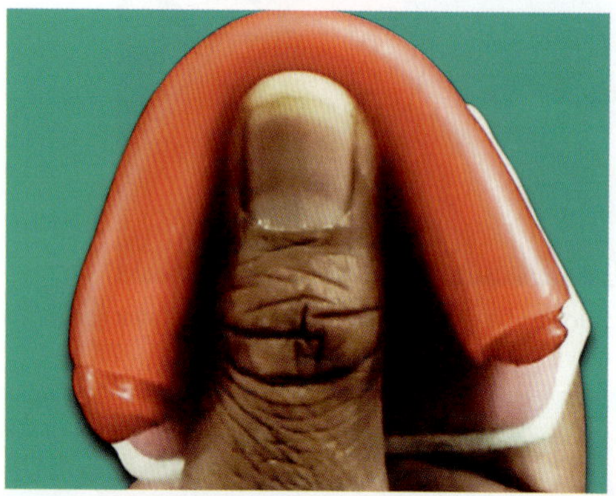

Fig. 22.5: Inside to outward thrust is given to achieve anterior protrusion.

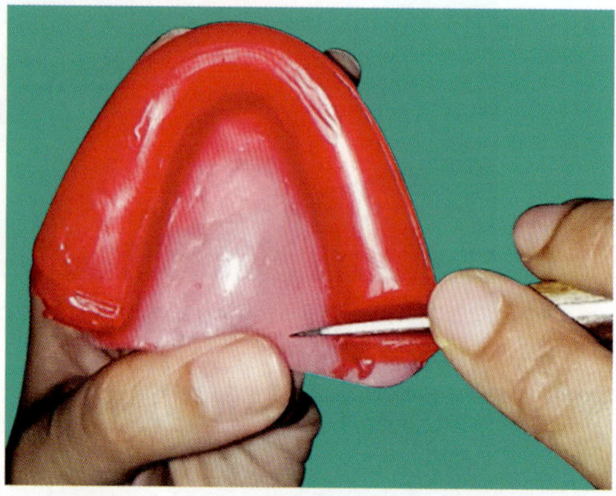

Fig. 22.7: Extended was roll to be cut over the maxillary tuberosity.

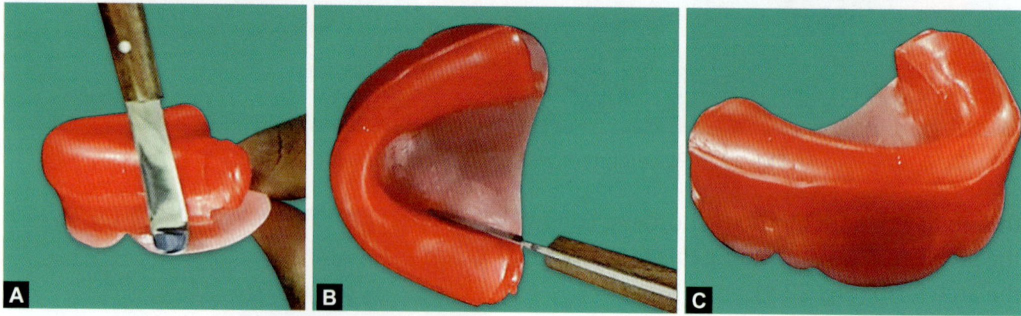

Figs. 22.6A to C: Seal the wax on all peripheries of record base.

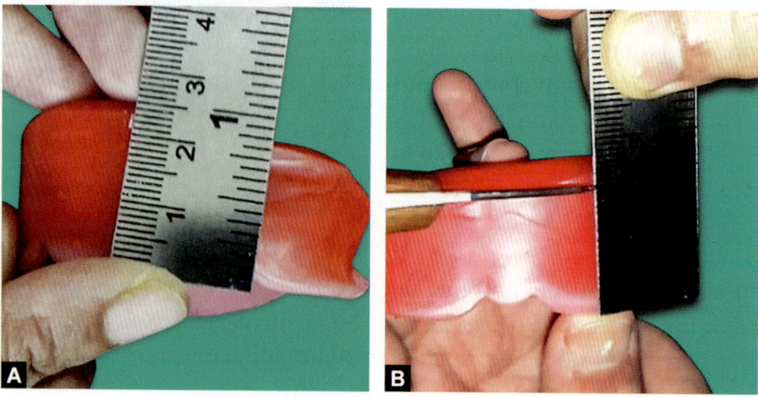

Figs. 22.8A and B: Measure and mark the height of oculars rim in canine area.

Step 8

Reduce the excess height by using hot plate. Perform this procedure very slowly and frequently check the plane during the reduction. The hot plate is used for reduction of height and to make plane of occlusion **(Figs. 22.9A and B)**.

Step 9

Make anterior height 20-22 mm in canine region and posterior height 18 mm in molar region from border of record base. Adjust the anterior width 5-6 mm and posterior width 8-10 mm **(Figs. 22.10A to D)**.

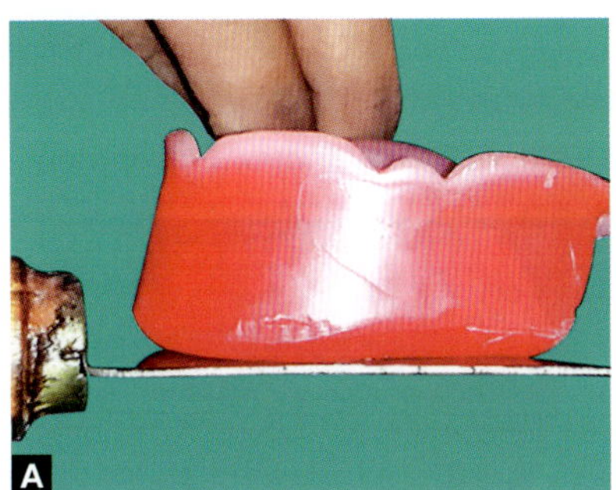

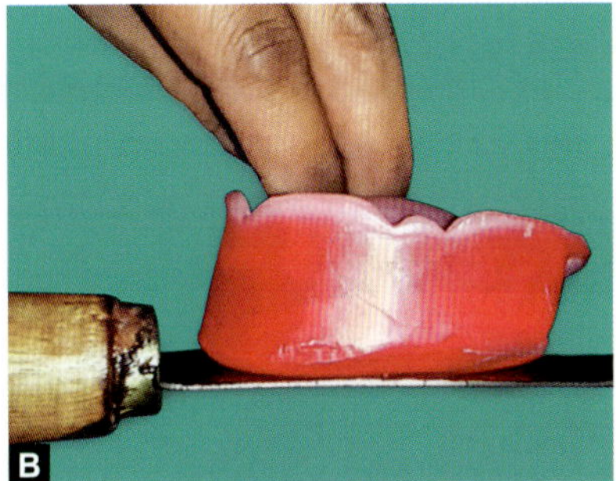

Figs. 22.9A and B: Reduction of height of occlusal rim and establishing the occlusion plane.

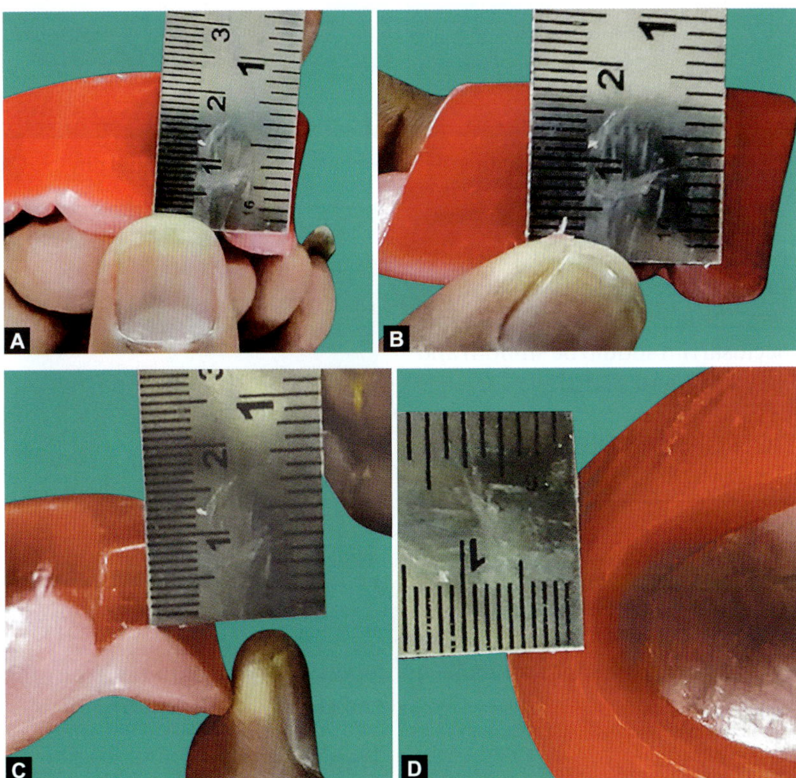

Figs. 22.10A to D: Anterior height 20–22 mm in canine region and posterior height 18 mm in molar region from border of record base.

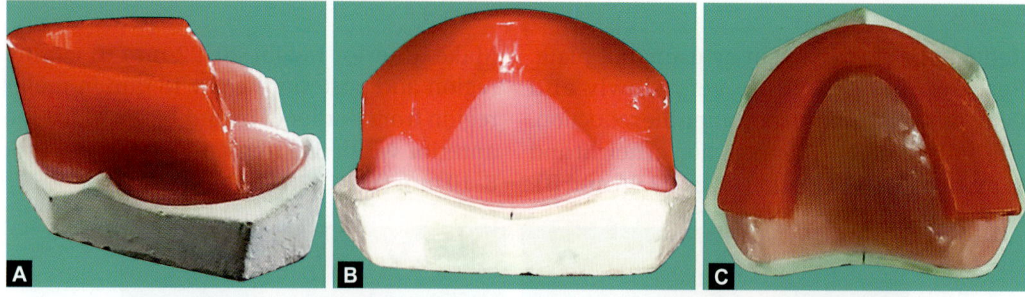

Figs. 22.11A to C: Maxillary occlusal rim—side view, palatal view, and top view.

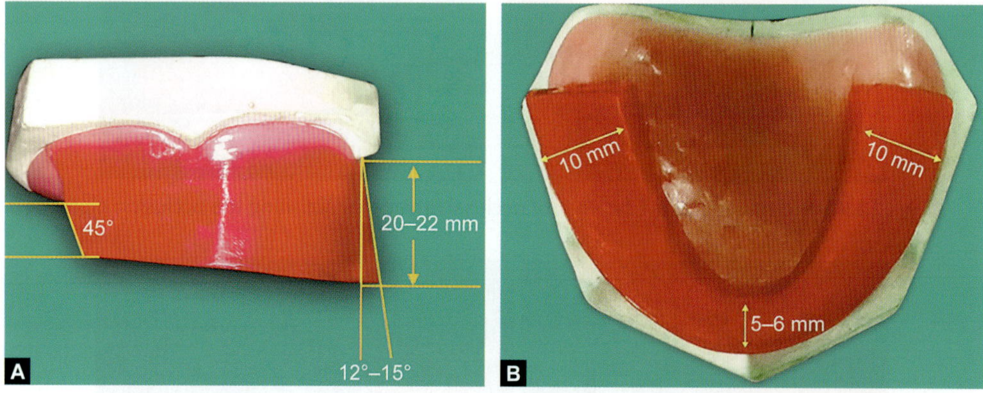

Figs. 22.12A and B: Various measurements of maxillary occlusal rim.

Step 10

Remove excess wax from the borders. Check the tissue surface of record base, it should be free of any wax. The labial, buccal, and lingual surfaces of occlusal rim should be smooth and polished **(Figs. 22.11 and 22.12)**.

FABRICATION OF MANDIBULAR OCCLUSAL RIM

Step 1

Take a sheet of modeling wax. Heat it over the flame of Bunsen burner to soften it. Fold it from one end (approximately 0.5 cm). Take care not to melt it. Continuously soften it and make a wax roll **(Fig. 22.13)**.

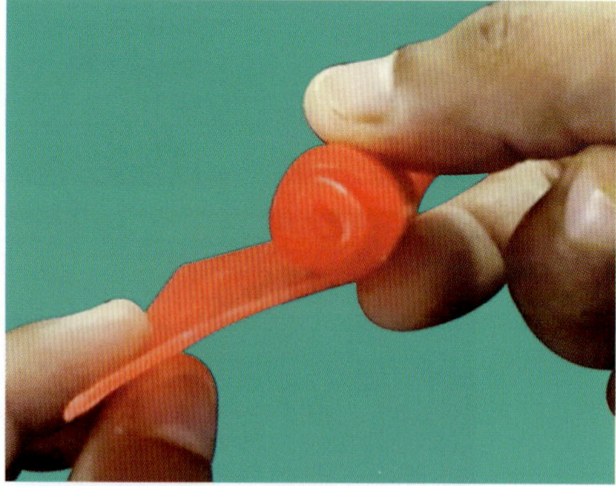

Fig. 22.13: Rolling the wax sheet.

Step 2

Place one end of the rolled wax on posterior aspect of record base (retromolar pad) and follow the arch contour till the other posterior end **(Figs. 22.14A and B)**.

Step 3

Apply downward pressure on wax roll by holding it in between index finger and the

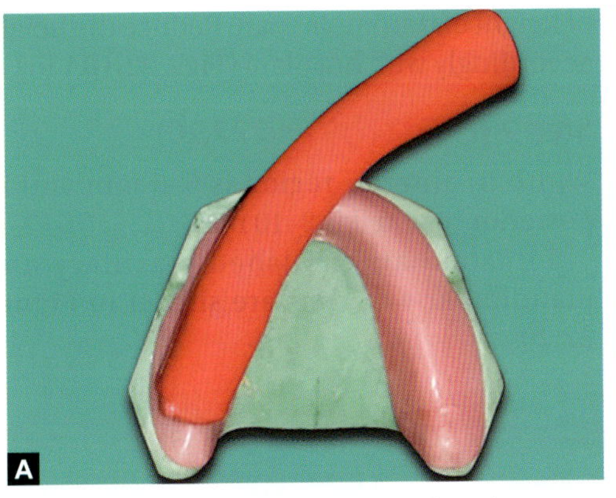

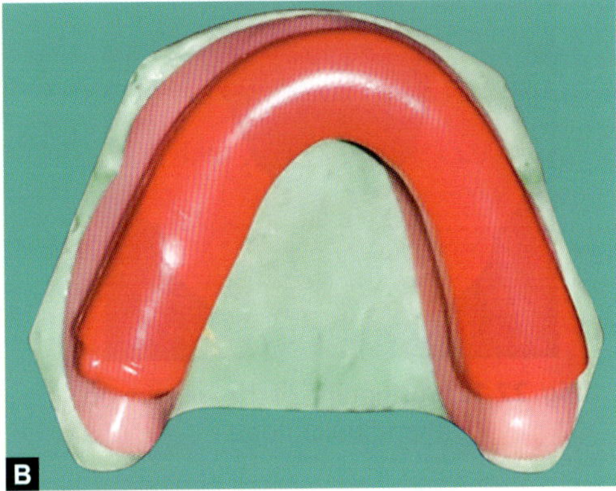

Figs. 22.14A and B: Placing wax rolls following the arch contour.

thumb to extend it along the borders. Follow the arch contour while doing this to maintain the arch form **(Fig. 22.15)**.

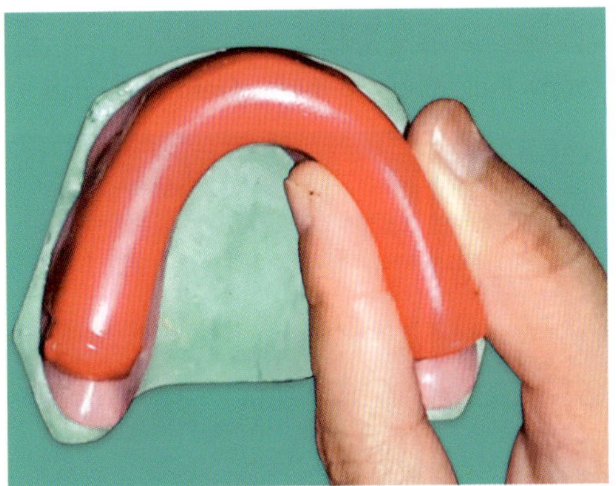

Fig. 22.15: Extend the wax till the borders of record base using index finger and thumb.

Step 4 (Figs. 22.16A to C)

Seal the adapted wax on buccal and lingual peripheries using hot wax spatula or wax knife. Add or remove wax to fill up voids, spaces, and irregularities. Smoothen the buccal surface maintaining the arch form.

Step 5 (Fig. 22.17)

Position the wax rim on mandibular ridge according to guiding lines. The rim should be extended till anterior aspect of retromolar pad. Position the wax rim equally on the buccal and lingual aspect of the crest of the ridge.

Step 6

Mark the height of 16 mm in canine region. Posteriorly height of wax rim is till two-thirds

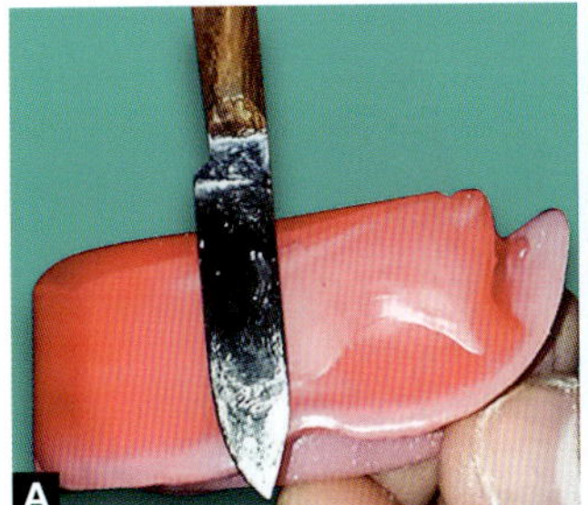

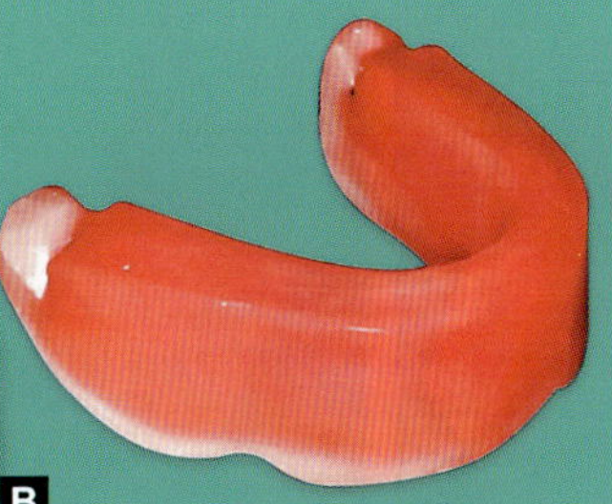

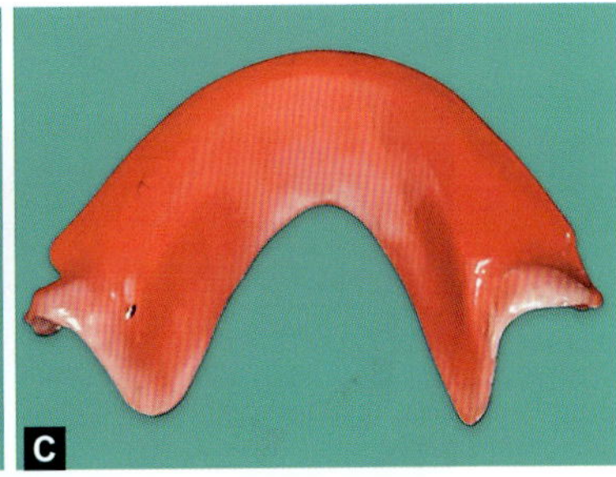

Figs. 22.16A to C: Sealing the wax on denture base.

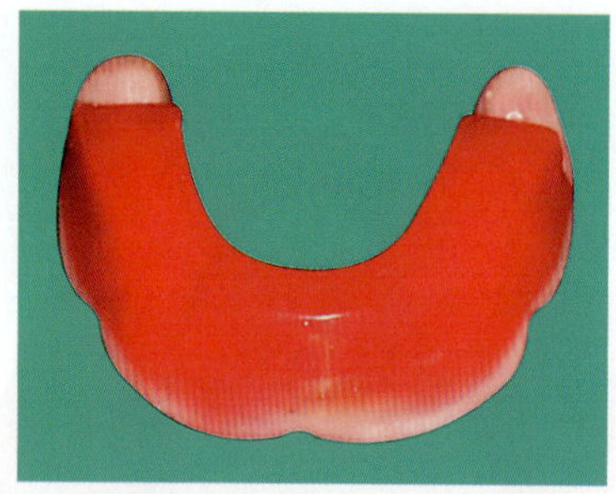
Fig. 22.17: Positioning of the wax rim on mandibular ridge.

of height of retromolar pad. Reduce the height accordingly with hot plate **(Figs. 22.18A to C)**.

Step 7 (Figs. 22.19 and 22.20)

Width in anterior region is 5-6 mm and in posterior region it is 8-10 mm.

Finished and polished maxillary and mandibular wax rims are shown in **Figure 22.20**.

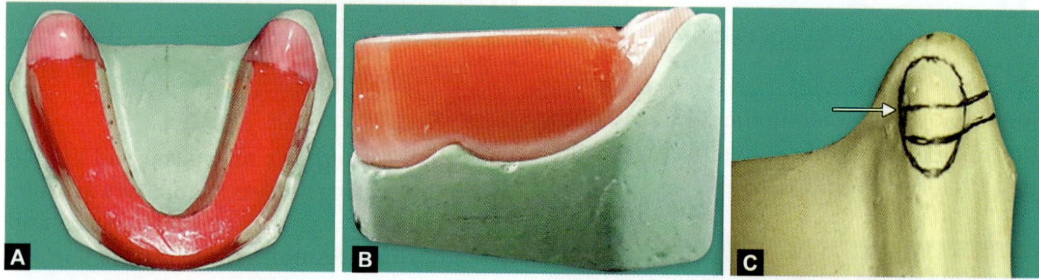
Figs. 22.18A to C: Adjust the height of occlusal rim—arrow indicating two-thirds of retromolar pad.

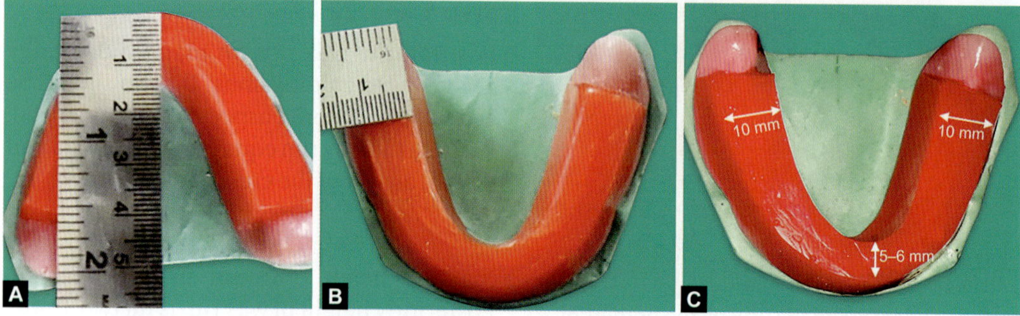

Figs. 22.19A to C: Adjust the width of occlusal rim.

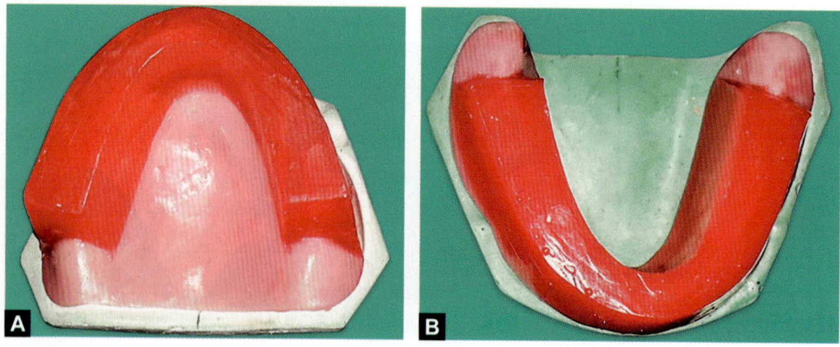
Figs. 22.20A and B: Finished and polished maxillary and mandibular wax rims.

CHAPTER 23

Mounting Occlusal Rims on Articulator

Paranjay Prajapati, Sneha Kulkarni

INTRODUCTION

Mounting is done to position wax occlusal rims and casts on articulator and fix them in particular position. This chapter demonstrates simple method to mount casts on mean value articulator.

ARMAMENTARIUM

Maxillary and mandibular occlusion rims with casts **(Fig. 23.1)**.

- Mean value articulator
- Dental plaster
- Rubber bowl and plaster mixing spatula

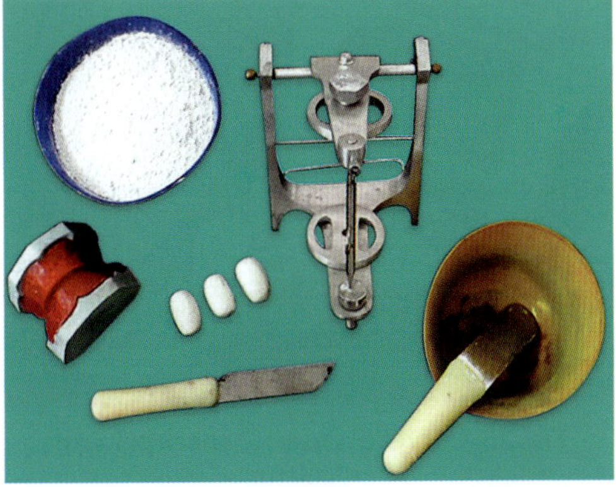

Fig. 23.1: Armamentarium of maxillary and mandibular occlusion rims with casts.

- Wax knife
- Modeling clay
- Thread
- Petroleum jelly.

Step 1

Indexing should be done on the base of the master cast using any of the indexing method (groove indexing or notch indexing). Midline is marked on both the occlusal rims taking labial frenum (on the cast) as reference. Maxillary and mandibular rims are placed together in such a way that maxillary rim overlaps the mandibular rim labially by 2 mm. Midline of maxillary and mandibular rims should coincide with each other **(Figs. 23.2A and B)**.

> Horizontal overlapping of mandibular rim by maxillary rim is essential to achieve overjet in teeth arrangement.

Step 2

The rims are sealed together to maintain the horizontal overlapping. Sealing is done in molar area by marking cross by hot wax knife. This sealing will prevent movement of hot wax rims during mounting procedures and maintains them in specific position **(Figs. 23.3A to C)**.

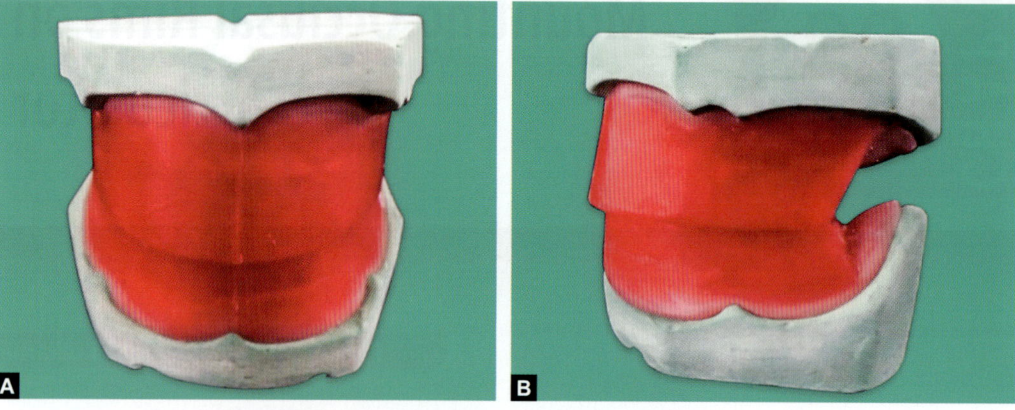

Figs. 23.2A and B: Midline of maxillary and mandibular rims coincides with each other.

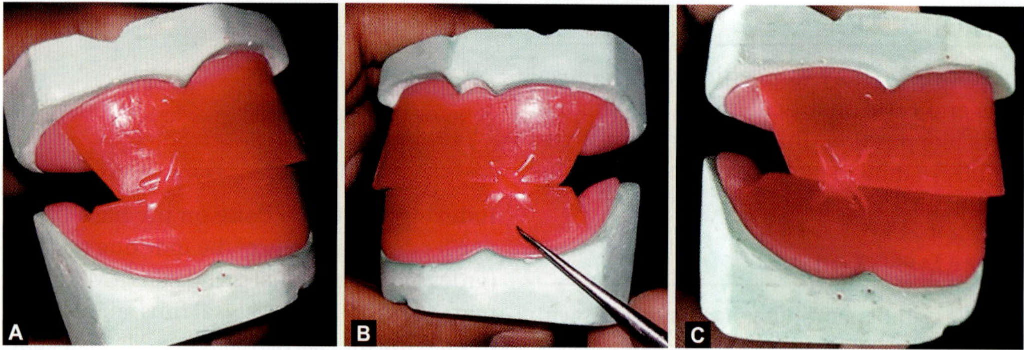

Figs. 23.3A to C: Sealing the wax rims at molar area.

The rims are sealed at specific position. The interface of two rims is occlusal plane. In the articulator, anterior reference point is central pin and posterior reference is provided by posterior reference rod. Central pin and posterior reference rod form the plane of articulator (or plane of orientation).

While mounting, the occlusal plane should coincide with articulator plane (or plane of orientation).

A thread tied on posterior reference rod can be used to verify position of occlusion rim **(Fig. 23.4)**.

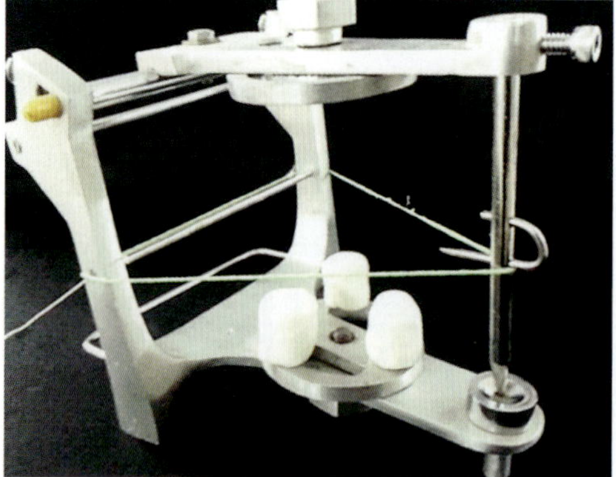
Fig. 23.4: Thread is used to check plane of articulator.

Modeling clay is placed on mounting ring of lower member of articulator. The sealed rims are placed on the clay accordingly that the central pin is in midline and it is at the level of occlusal plane (between maxillary and mandibular rims).

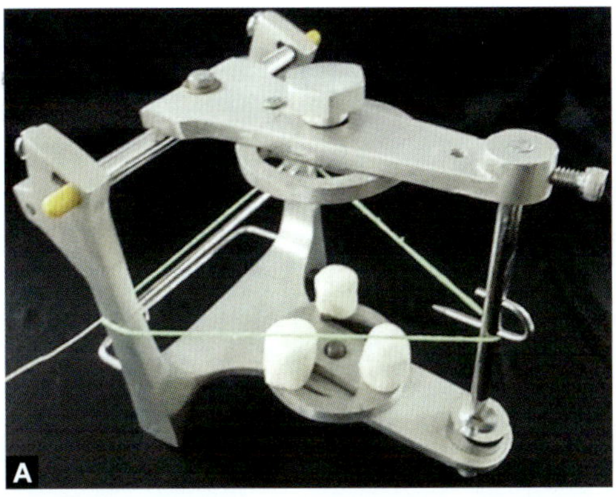

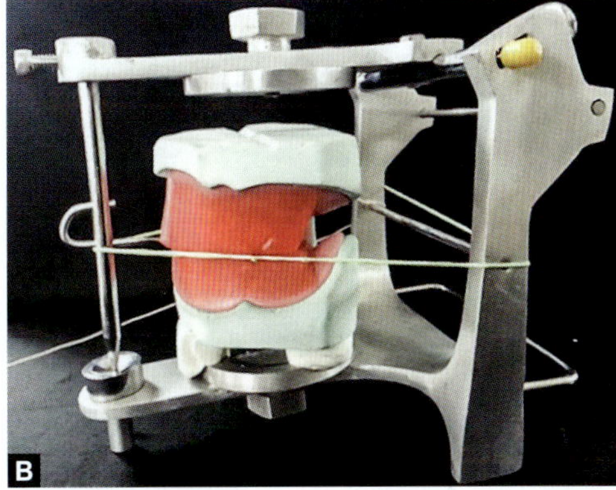

Figs. 23.5A and B: Occlusal plane should coincide with plane of articulator.

The position of rims is adjusted in such a way that the occlusal plane (on wax rim) matches with the articulator plane. The thread can be used for checking the match of two planes **(Figs. 23.5A and B)**.

> Before adjusting the rims on articulator, make sure that the central pin is fully seated in its position.

Check the matching of two planes at eye level as shown in **Figure 23.6**.

Step 3

Apply thin coat of petroleum jelly in index (grooves or Vshaped notches) **(Fig. 23.7)**.

Step 4

Mix dental plaster in homogeneous and creamy consistency using rubber bowl and spatula. Pour mixed plaster in grooves or notches made on base of the maxillary cast using wax knife **(Figs. 23.8A and B)**.

Step 5

Pour remaining mixed plaster on the whole base of the maxillary cast. Apply plaster on mounting ring also. Close upper member of articulator. Allow plaster to fill the spaces provided in mounting ring. Remove excess plaster coming out from mounting ring and

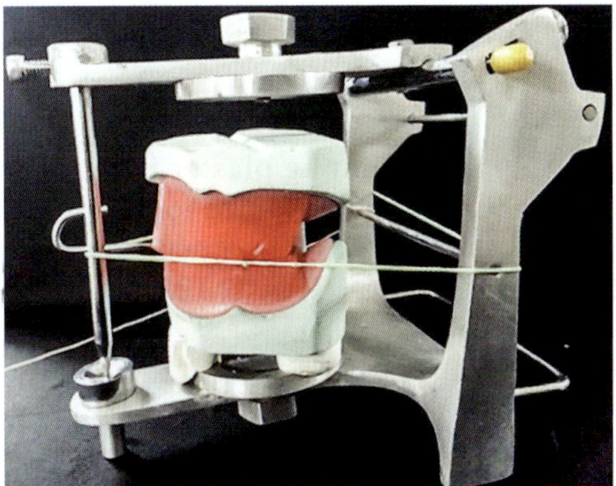

Fig. 23.6: Matching of two planes at eye level.

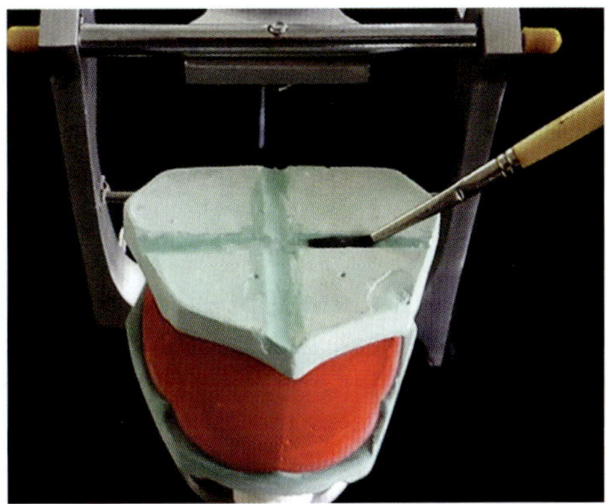

Fig. 23.7: Application of petroleum jelly in index.

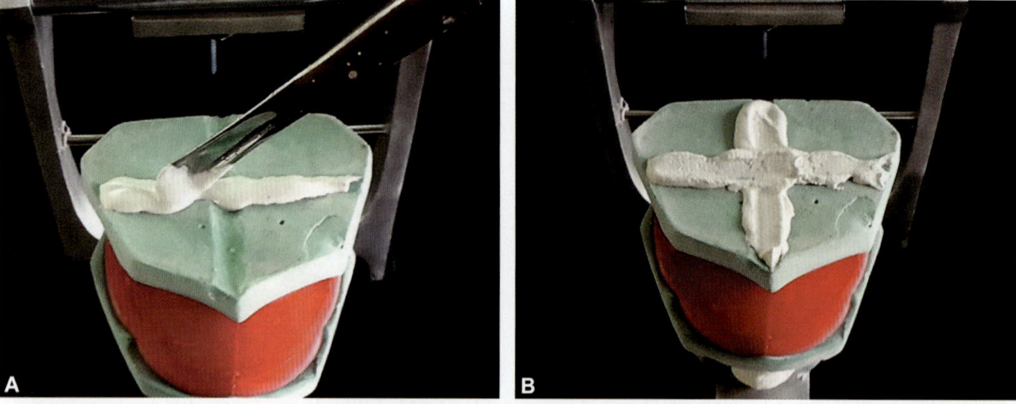
Figs. 23.8A and B: Pouring the plaster in index.

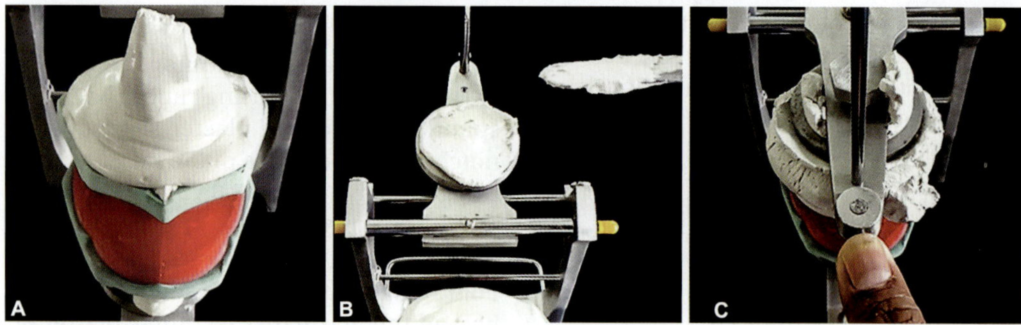
Figs. 23.9A to C: Place mounting plaster on base of the cast, on mounting ring, and close the upper member.

make it parallel to upper surface of mounting ring (**Figs. 23.9A to C**).

> Plaster used for mounting should be creamy in consistence. If it is not creamy and free flowing then during closing the upper member, pressure will be exerted on casts and this may change position of rims which leads to discrepancy of planes.

Step 6 (Figs. 23.10A to C)

Try to shape mounting plaster according to the shape of cast. Add or remove plaster as needed. Use flat metal strip like plaster mixing spatula or wax knife for shaping the plaster. Shape mounting plaster according to periphery of cast (according to shape of base of the cast).

Step 7

Use wet cotton or finger to smooth the mounting plaster and allow it to set (**Figs. 23.11A to C**).

Step 8

Once upper mounting plaster is set, turn the articulator upside down for mounting mandibular cast. Open the articulator slowly and remove the clay (**Figs. 23.12A and B**).

Step 9

Apply thin coat of petroleum jelly on index on the base of mandibular cast. Wet the cast base with water before applying plaster on the base (**Figs. 23.13A and B**).

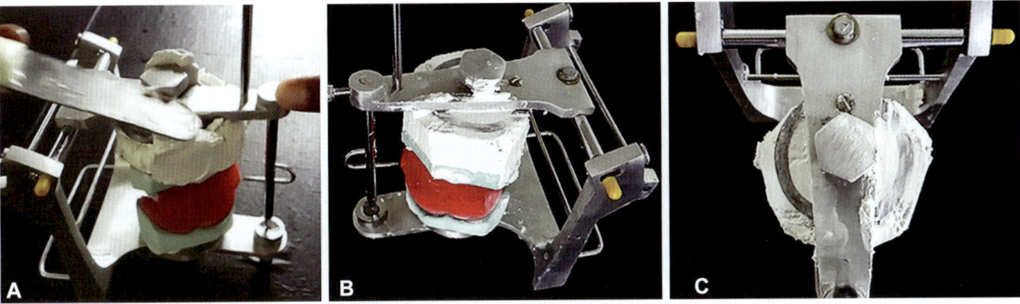

Figs. 23.10A to C: Shaping the mounting plaster on articulator.

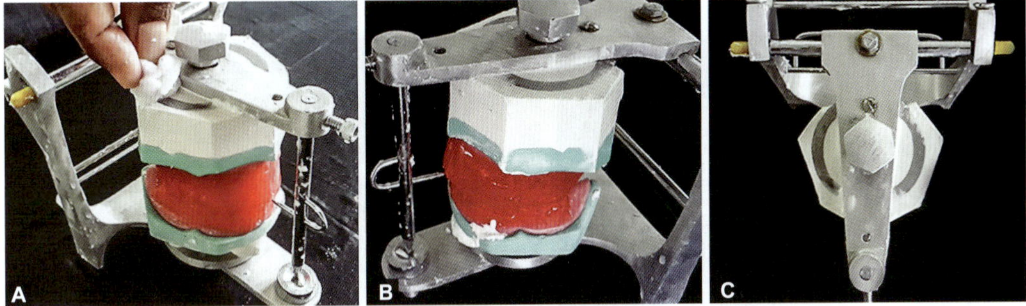

Figs. 23.11A to C: Smoothen the mounting plaster using wet cotton.

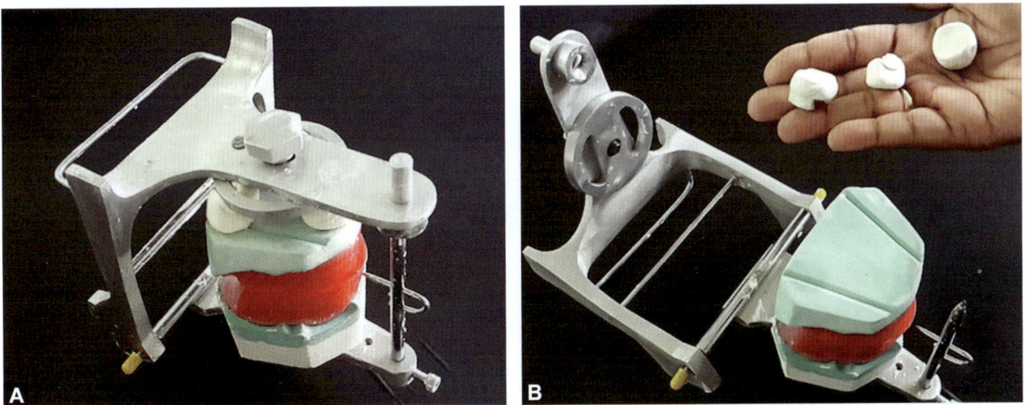

Figs. 23.12A and B: Invert the articulator for mounting mandibular cast.

Step 10

Mix plaster and pour index first and then pour remaining plaster on base. Apply some plaster on mounting ring also **(Figs. 23.14A and B)**.

Step 11

Close the lower member and follow the procedures performed during mounting of maxillary cast. Shape the mounting plaster

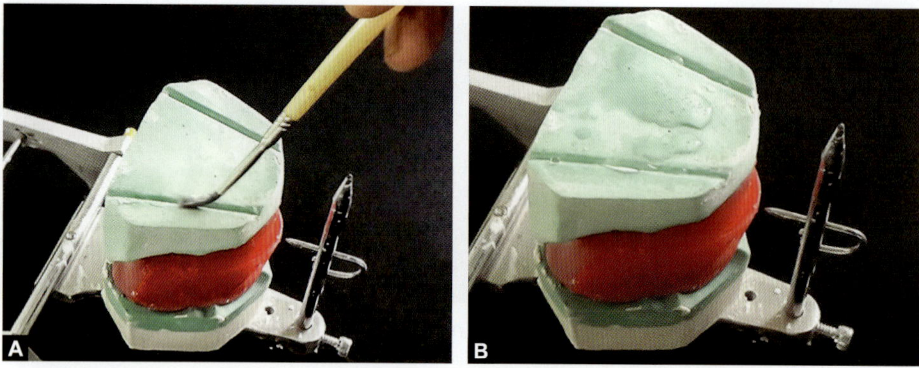
Figs. 23.13A and B: Apply petroleum jelly in index, wet the cast before placing plaster on it.

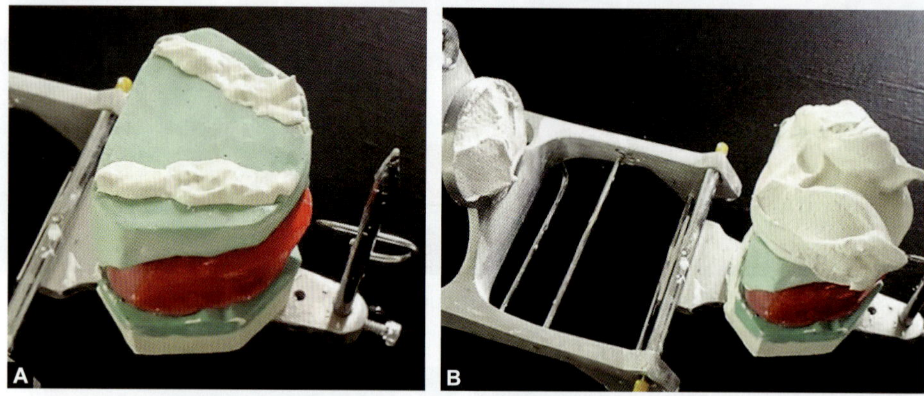
Figs. 23.14A and B: Apply mounting plaster in index and on base of the cast.

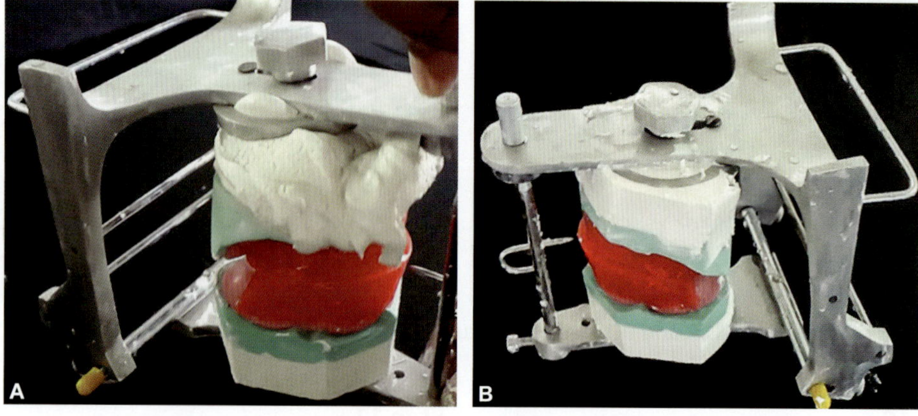
Figs. 23.15A and B: Close the lower member and shape the mounting plaster.

according to shape of cast contour (**Figs. 23.15A and B**).

Smoothen the plaster using wet cotton. Use dry cotton to clean the articulator.

Never wash articulator under tap water to clean it. This may expand mounting plaster which results in increase of vertical dimension of occlusion. If plaster expands, the vertical pin will not be in contact with anterior guide table.

Maxillary and mandibular casts mounted on mean value articulator **(Figs. 23.16A and B)**.

Extend the midline and canine lines on mounting plaster. Write name, age, sex, of the patient or roll no, and name.

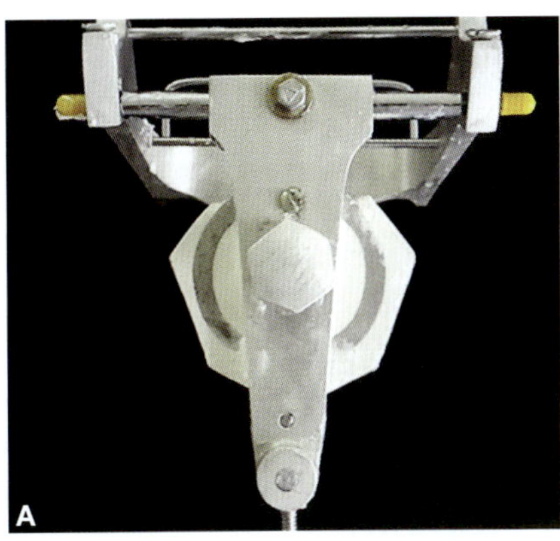

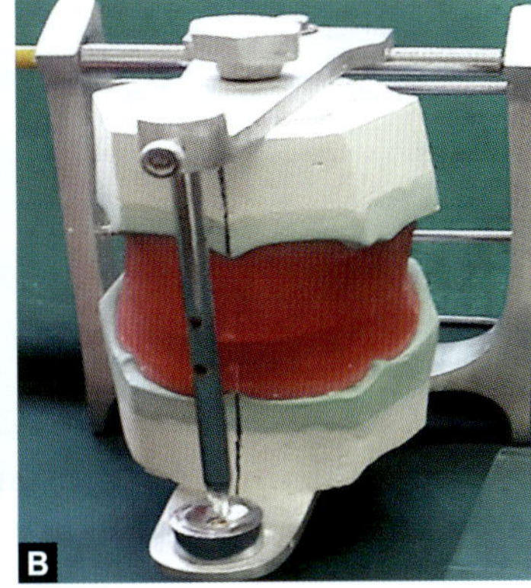

Figs. 23.16A and B: Maxillary and mandibular casts mounted on mean value articulator.

Arrangement of Artificial Teeth

Rajesh Sethuraman, Paranjay Prajapati

INTRODUCTION

Correct selection of artificial teeth and their correct arrangement is critical factor determining success and acceptance of prosthesis by patient. Varieties of artificial teeth are available in market. They are selected according to patient's need for aesthetic and other factors. This chapter describes regarding the arrangement of artificial teeth for complete denture.

SEQUENCE OF ARRANGEMENT OF TEETH

The sequence of arrangement of teeth has been shown in **Table 24.1**.

Table 24.1: Sequence of arrangement of teeth.

S. No.	*Teeth*	*Sequence*
1.	Maxillary anteriors	Right side
2.	Maxillary anteriors	Left side
3.	Mandibular anteriors	Right side
4.	Mandibular anteriors	Left side
5.	Maxillary posteriors	Right side
6.	Maxillary posteriors	Left side
7.	Mandibular posteriors	Right side
8.	Mandibular posteriors	Left side

ARMAMENTARIUM

Mean value articulator with mounted maxillary and mandibular occlusion rims on final cast **(Fig. 24.1)**.

- MacIntosh sheet
- Acrylic teeth on tooth card
- Glass plate
- Wax spatula
- Wax knife
- Lecron's carver
- Spirit lamp/burner.

Mark midline on maxillary occlusal rim with sharp instrument like carver **(Fig. 24.2)**. Extend this midline on cast and mounting plaster with pencil or marker. This will guide

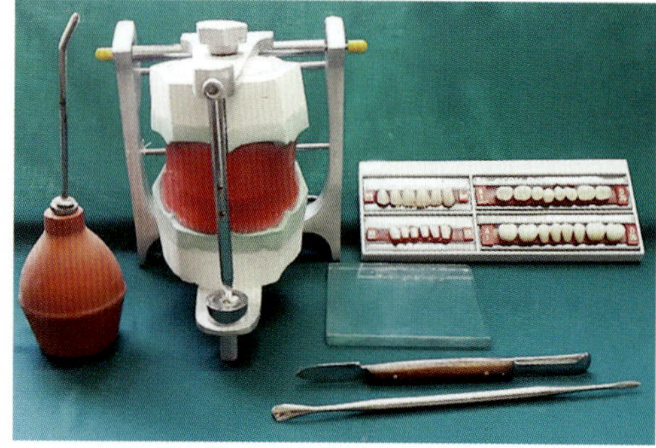

Fig. 24.1: Mounting on articulator.

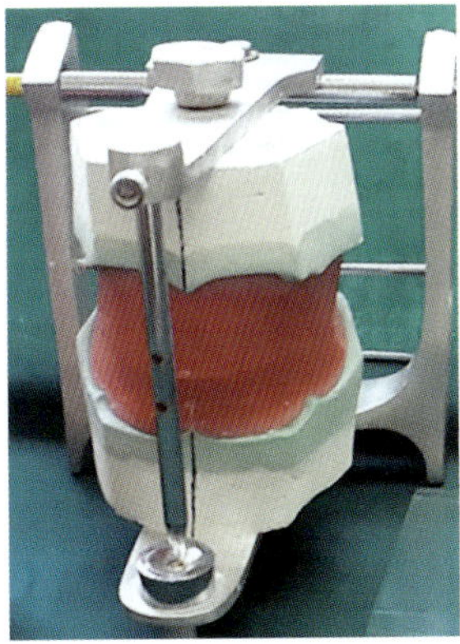

Fig. 24.2: Mark the midline on the cast using pencil or marker.

during teeth arrangement when midline on wax rim is not clear.

> While teeth arrangement, position of every tooth is finalized according to its relation with adjacent tooth, relation with glass plate (serve as occlusal plane), relation with rim contour, mesiodistal inclination, and labiolingual inclination.

ARRANGING MAXILLARY ANTERIOR TEETH

Arrangement of Maxillary Central Incisor

Step 1

Select anterior teeth according to arch shape, facial type, and other factors **(Fig. 24.3)**.

Heat wax spatula and pool wax from labial surface of maxillary occlusion rim where central incisor is to be placed **(Figs. 24.4A and B)**.

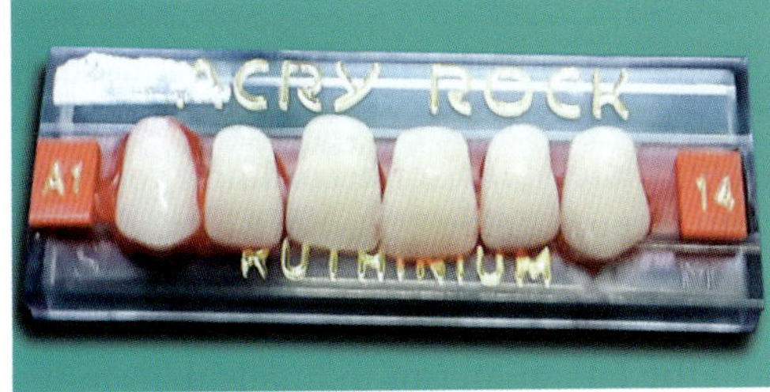

Fig. 24.3: Maxillary anterior teeth.

Step 2

Take out central incisor from tooth card **(Fig. 24.5)**. Clean carding wax from ridge lap area. Soften the wax in the area again with wax spatula. Place the central incisor in the position and set it according to the set up angulations given in **Table 24.2** and **Figures 24.6A and B**.

When viewed from front, the long axis of maxillary central incisor is positioned almost parallel to the vertical axis **(Figs. 24.7)**.

When viewed occlusally, the incisal edge of central incisor should follow the labial contour of maxillary wax rim. When viewed from side, the central incisor is sloped labially about 12–15° **(Figs. 24.8A and B)**.

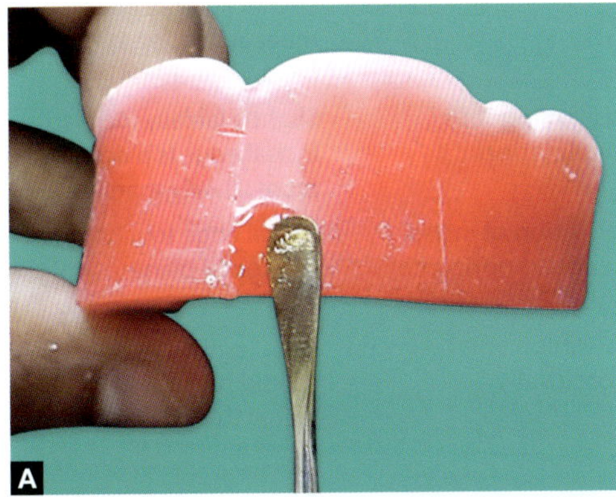

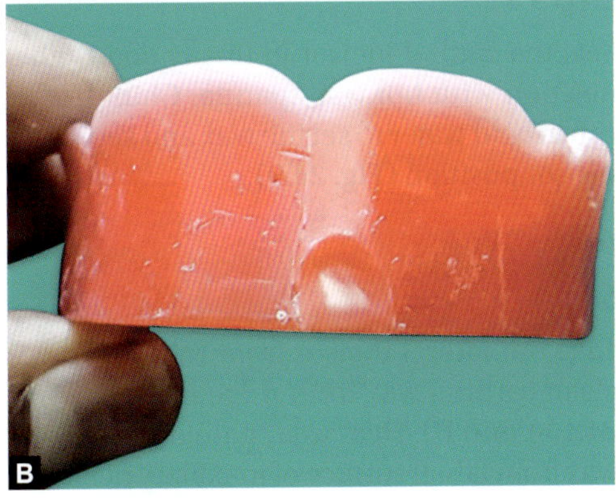

Figs. 24.4A and B: Scooping out the modeling wax in central incisor area.

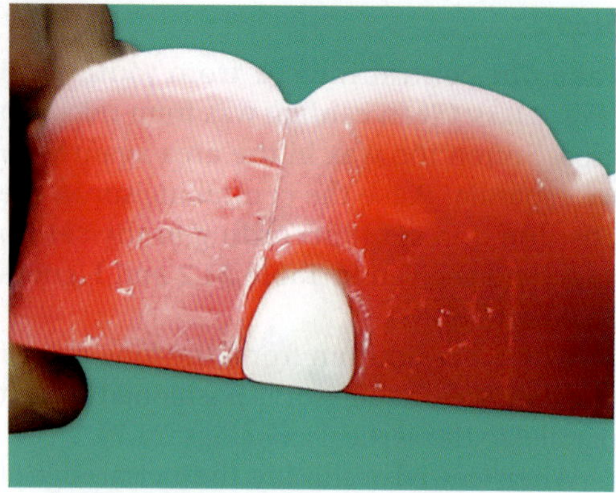

Fig. 24.5: Arranging the central incisor.

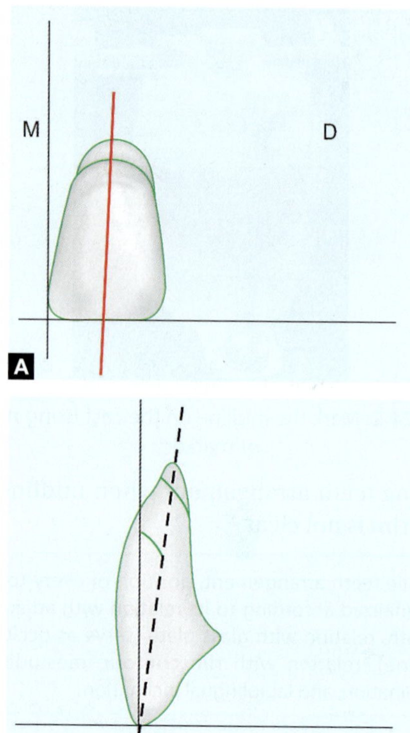

Figs. 24.6A and B: Maxillary central incisor—frontal view and side view.

Table 24.2: Maxillary central incisor arrangement guidelines.

Mesiodistal inclination	Slightly mesially inclined so that central incisors meet at midline at their incisal one-third
Labiolingual inclination	Slightly labially inclined. Incisal edge is placed more labially than neck
Relation of incisal edge to horizontal plane	Incisal edge touches the horizontal plane
Relation when viewed occlusally	Distal end of incisor should be rotated to follow the contour

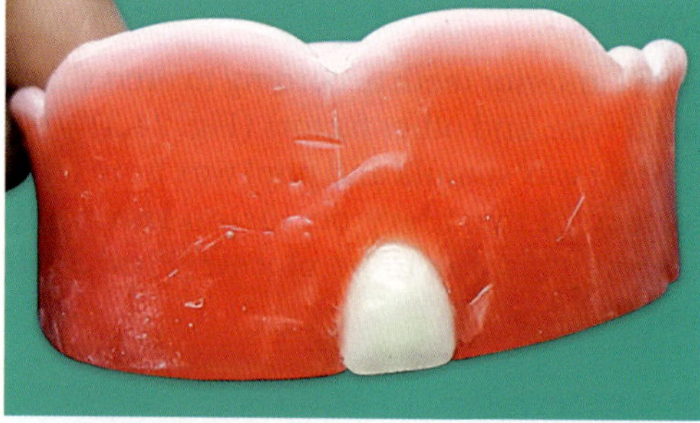

Fig. 24.7: Position of maxillary central incisor.

Step 3

Seal the central incisor in finally determined position with hot wax spatula. Chill the wax rim in cold water to set the wax and secure the incisor position **(Fig. 24.9)**.

Arrangement of Maxillary Lateral Incisor

Step 1

Take out lateral incisor from tooth card and clean carding wax from ridge lap area **(Figs. 24.10A and B)**. Heat wax spatula and remove wax from labial surface of maxillary occlusion rim in area where lateral incisor to be placed. Soften the area with hot wax spatula and arrange lateral incisor accordingly reference chart given in **Table 24.3**.

Step 2

Seal the lateral incisor in finally determined position with hot wax spatula. Put the wax rim

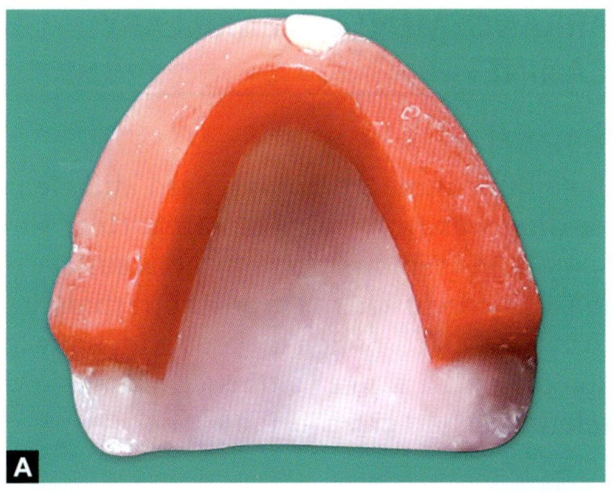

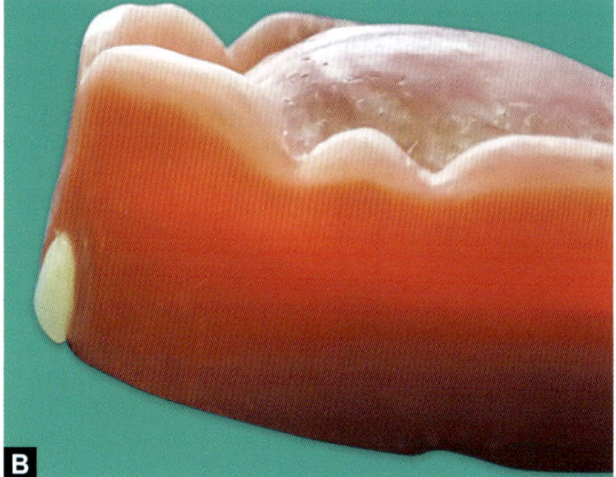

Figs. 24.8A and B: Placement of central incisor—occlusal view and side view.

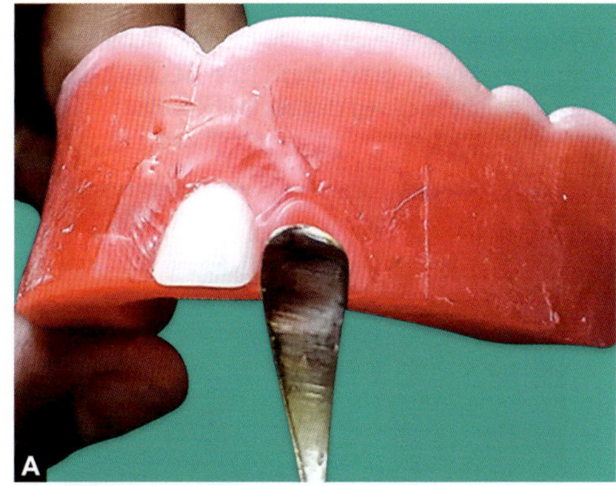

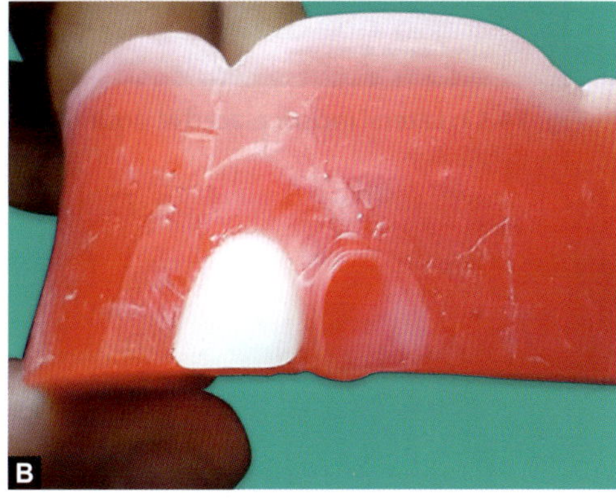

Figs. 24.10A and B: Scooping out the modeling wax in lateral incisor area.

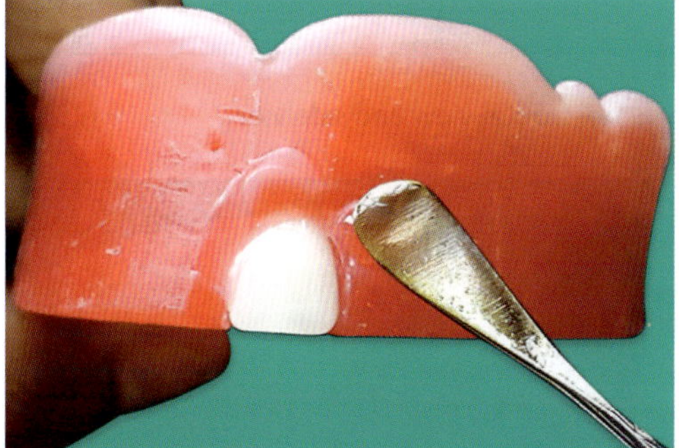

Fig. 24.9: Central incisor arranged in position.

in cold water to set the wax and tooth **(Figs. 24.11 and 24.12)**.

The incisal edge should be parallel to glass plate. Incisal edge is 1 mm above from the glass plate. The neck of the lateral incisor is inclined distally. Distal part of lateral incisor edge is rotated to follow labial contour of wax rim (**Fig. 24.13**A and B).

Table 24.3: Maxillary lateral incisor arrangement guidelines.

Mesiodistal inclination	The incisal one-third is more mesially inclined (neck distally inclined)
Labiolingual inclination	It is more mesially inclined than central incisor with neck depressed
Relation of incisal edge to horizontal plane	It is parallel to horizontal plane. Should not touch the plane. Should be 1 mm above the plane
Relation when viewed occlusally	The distal edge is more rotated to follow contour of the rim

While arranging lateral incisor focus to make incisal edge parallel to glass plate, the neck of lateral incisor will be inclined distally by default.

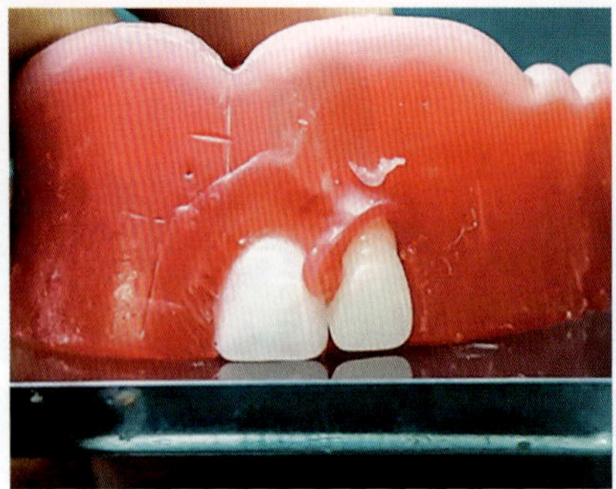

Fig. 24.11: Lateral incisor placed in position.

ARRANGEMENT OF MAXILLARY CANINE

Step 1 (Figs. 24.14 and 24.15)

Take out canine from tooth card and clean carding wax from ridge lap area. Heat wax spatula and remove wax from labial surface of maxillary occlusion rim in area corresponding to canine space. Soften the area with hot wax spatula and arrange canine accordingly the reference chart given in **Table 24.4**.

Step 2

Seal the canine in finally determined position with hot wax spatula. Put the wax rim in cold water to set the wax and tooth **(Fig. 24.16)**.

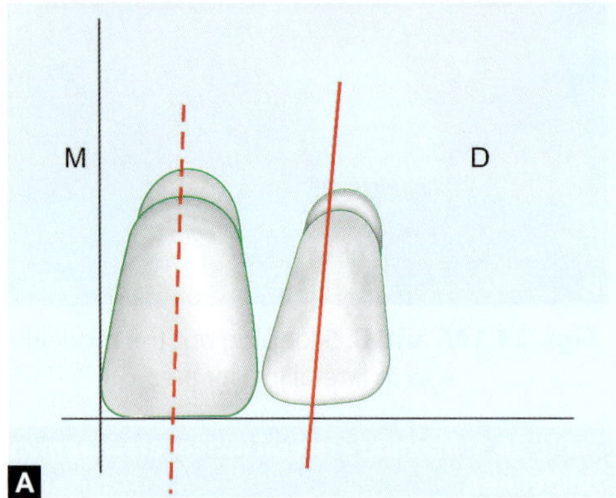

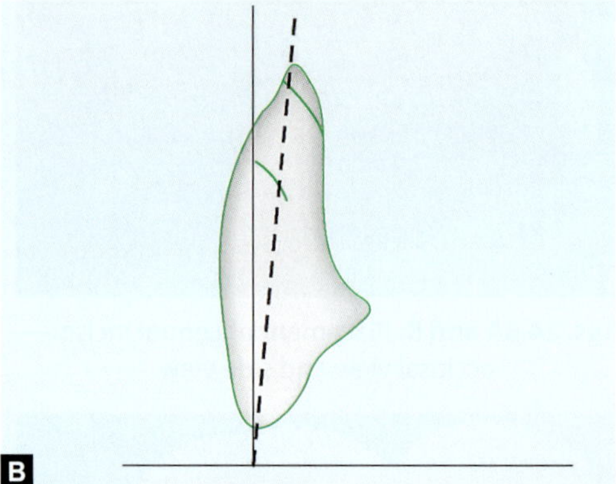

Figs. 24.12A and B: Maxillary lateral incisor—frontal view and side view.

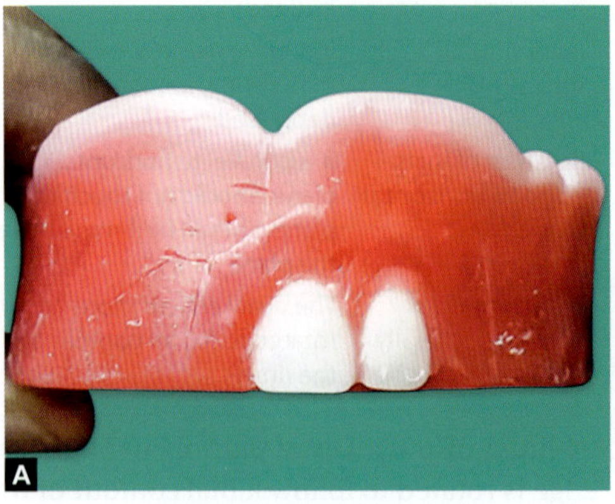

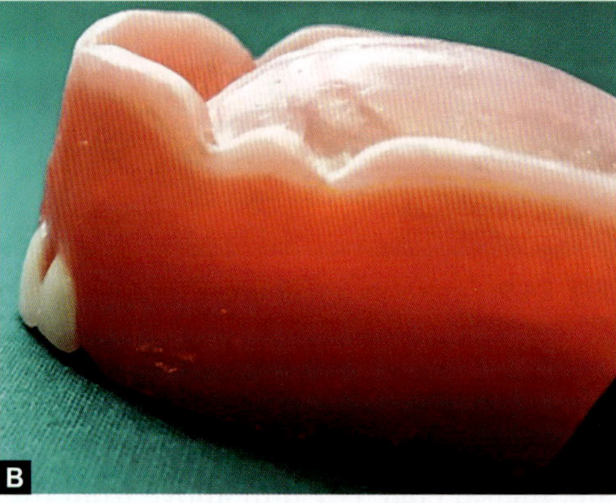

Figs. 24.13A and B: Lateral incisor in position—frontal view and side view.

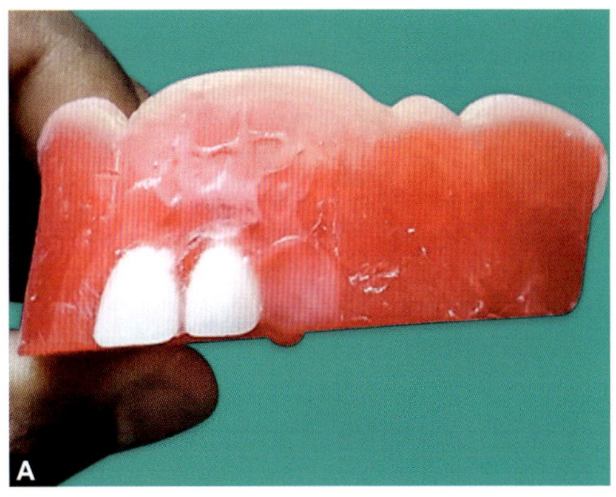
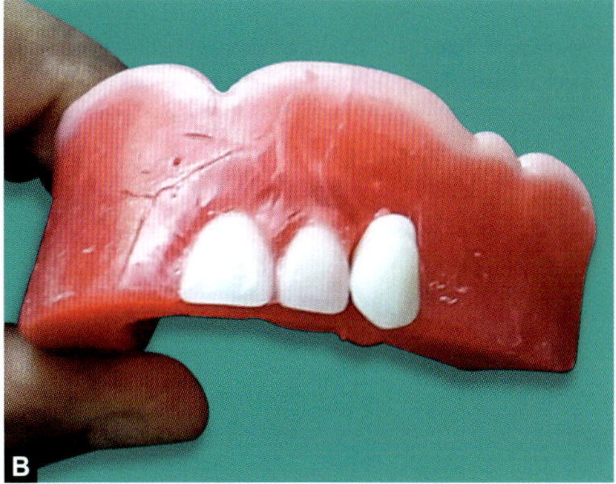

Figs. 24.14A and B: Scooping out the modeling wax in canine area and placement of canine in position.

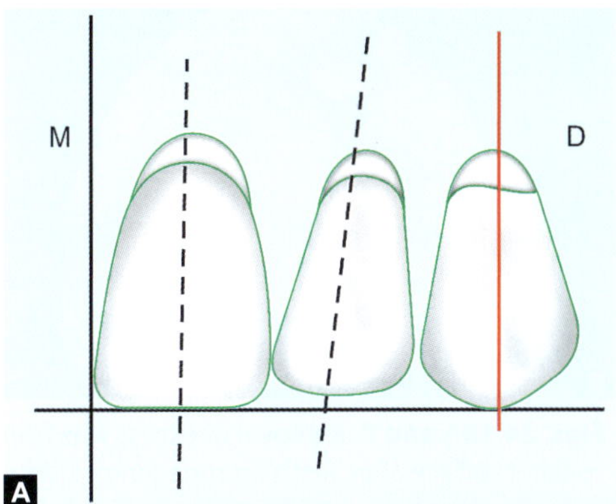

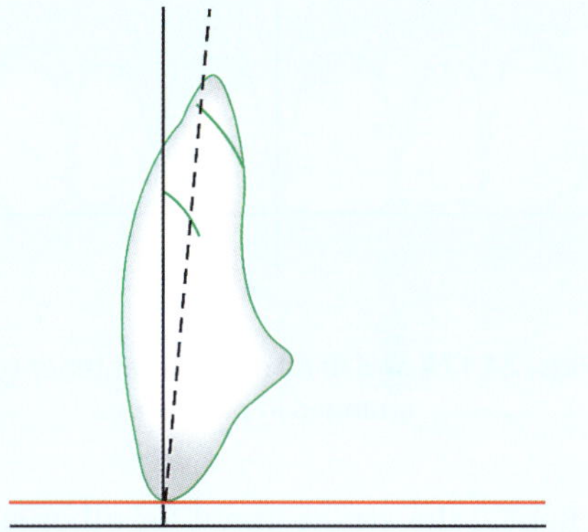

Figs. 24.15A and B: Maxillary canine—frontal view and side view.

Table 24.4: Maxillary canine arrangement guidelines.	
Mesiodistal inclination	Placed vertically with no mesial or distal inclination
Labiolingual inclination	Placed vertically upright. No specific inclination
Relation of incisal edge to horizontal plane	Tip of the canine should touch the horizontal plane
Relation when viewed occlusally	Distal half of canine is rotated to follow rim contour

When viewed from front, only mesial slope of canine is visible. The neck of canine (cervical area) is more prominent compared to centrals.

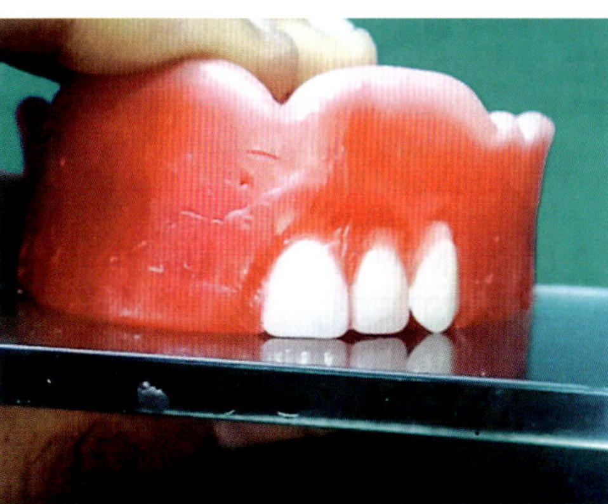

Fig. 24.16: Canine arranged in position—frontal view.

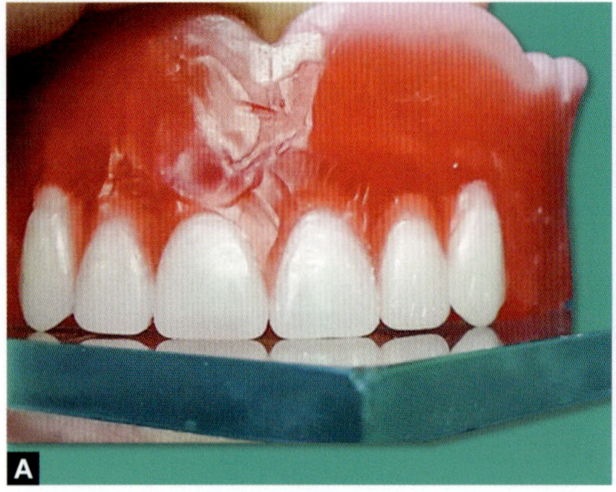
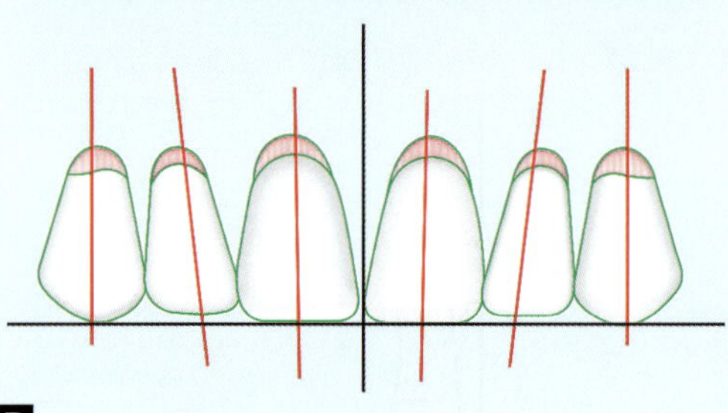

Figs. 24.17A and B: All maxillary anterior teeth arranged in position.

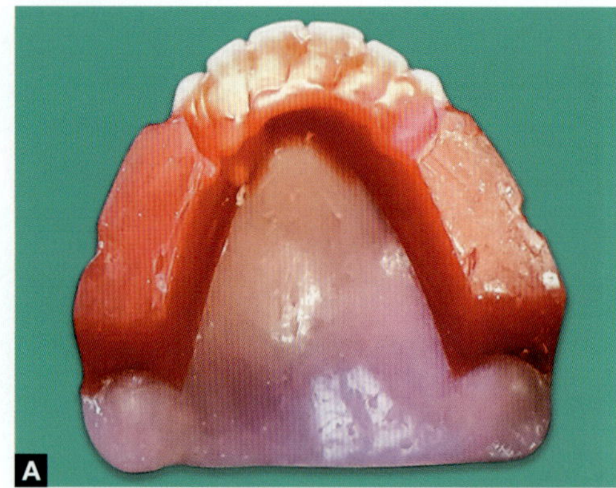
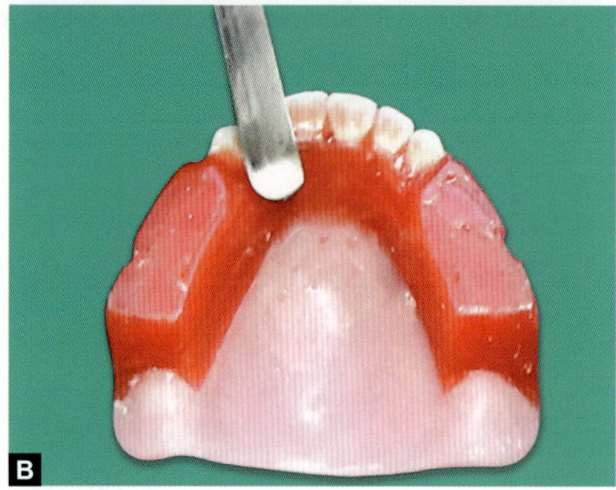

Figs. 24.18A and B: Removal of excess wax from palatal surface after teeth arranged in position.

Repeat the arrangement for other side of the arch and complete arrangement of all six maxillary anterior teeth **(Figs. 24.17A and B)**.

Remove excess wax from palatal surface. Heat the curved end of wax knife and slowly remove the wax without applying any pressure, otherwise it may change the tooth position **(Figs. 24.18A and B)**.

ARRANGEMENT OF MANDIBULAR ANTERIOR TEETH

Mandibular anterior teeth are arranged slightly lingually than maxillary anterior teeth. Vertical and horizontal overlap should be attained **(Fig. 24.19)**.

Remove the vertical pin from the articulator before arranging the mandibular anterior teeth.

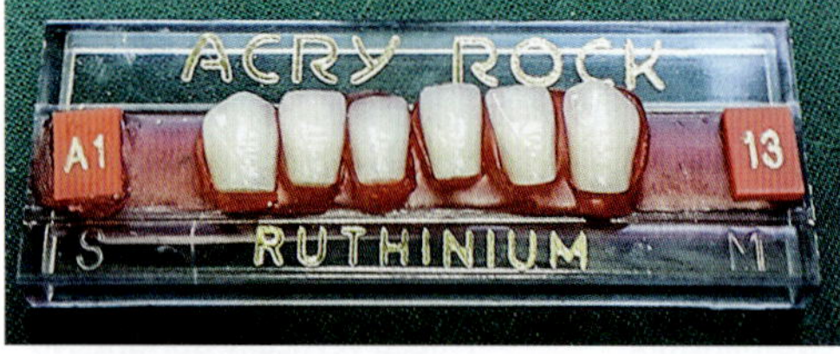

Fig. 24.19: Mandibular anterior teeth.

Arrangement of Mandibular Central Incisors

Step 1

Remove part of wax from the area and soften remaining wax. Place the central incisor so that the long axis is parallel to vertical axis when viewed from front. The mesial surface of the central incisor should coincide with the midline

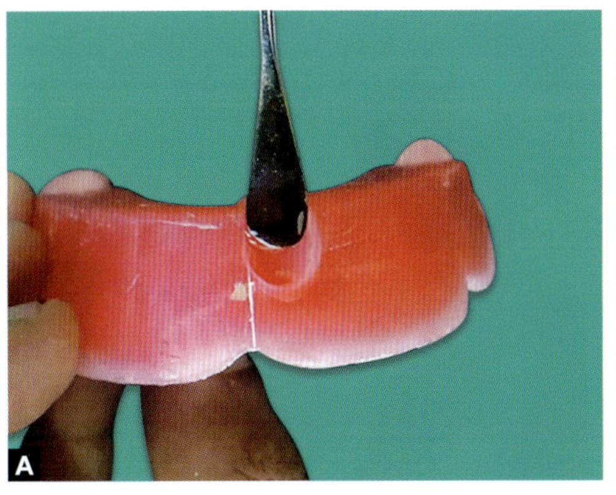

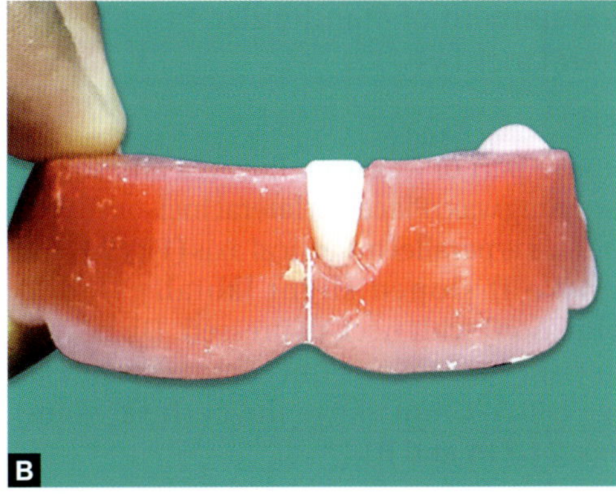

Figs. 24.20A and B: Scooping out the wax and placing mandibular central incisor.

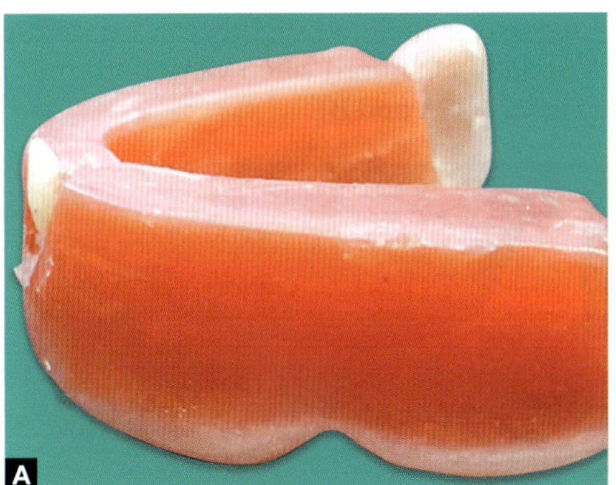

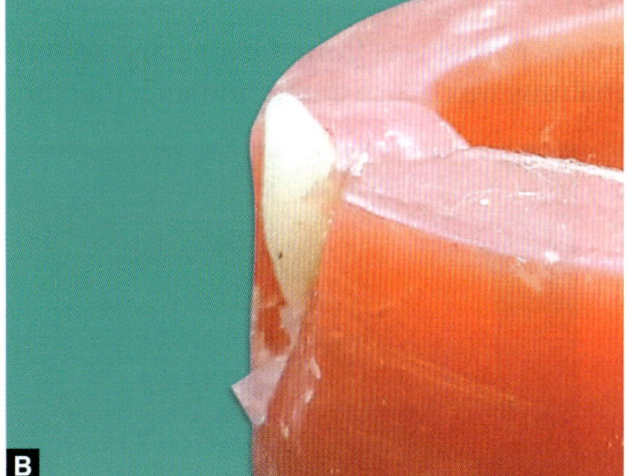

Figs. 24.21A and B: Placement of mandibular central incisor—side view.

marked on the wax occlusal rim and also with the maxillary teeth midline **(Figs. 24.20A and B)**.

Step 2

Make it sloped slightly labially (labial inclination) with neck depressed **(Figs. 24.21A and B)**.

Step 3

Place the incisal edge 0.5-1 mm above the occlusal plane **(Fig. 24.22)**.

> The incisal edges of mandibular anteriors are placed 0.5–1 mm above the occlusal plane. This is essential to create overbite.

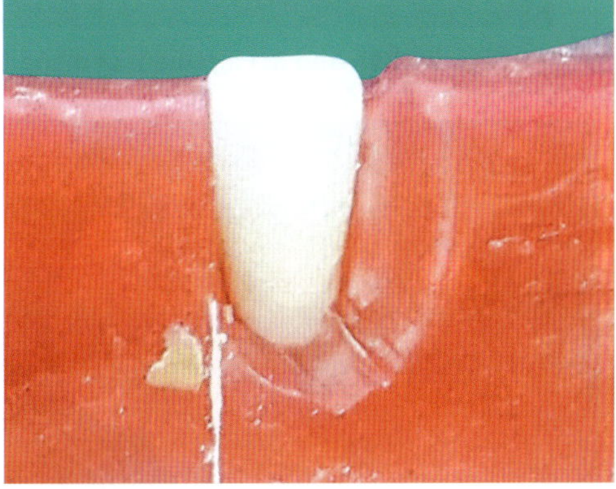

Fig. 24.22: Placement of mandibular central incisor—front view.

Arrangement of Mandibular Lateral Incisors

Step 1

Remove part of wax from the area and soften remaining wax. Place the lateral incisor so that long axis is parallel to vertical axis **(Fig. 24.23)**.

Make it sloped slight labially (labial inclination) with neck depressed. Distal end of incisor edge follows rim contour. Its incisal edge is 0.5–1 mm above the occlusal plane **(Figs. 24.24A and B)**.

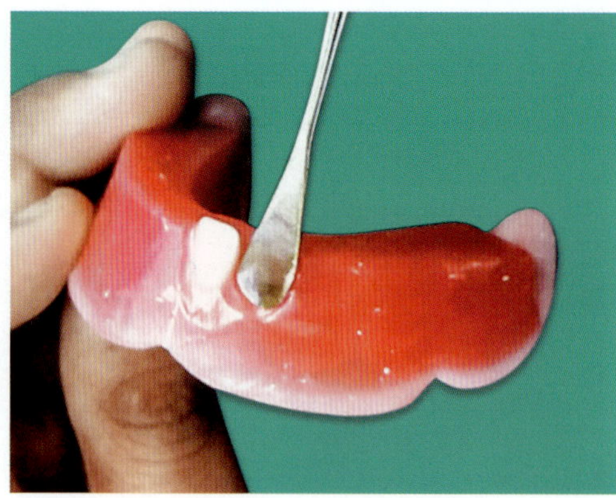

Fig. 24.23: Scoop out wax and place lateral incisor.

Arrangement of Mandibular Canine

Step 1

Remove part of wax from the area and soften remaining wax. Place the canine such that the long axis is inclined slightly toward midline (mesial inclination) when viewed from front **(Figs. 24.25A and B)**.

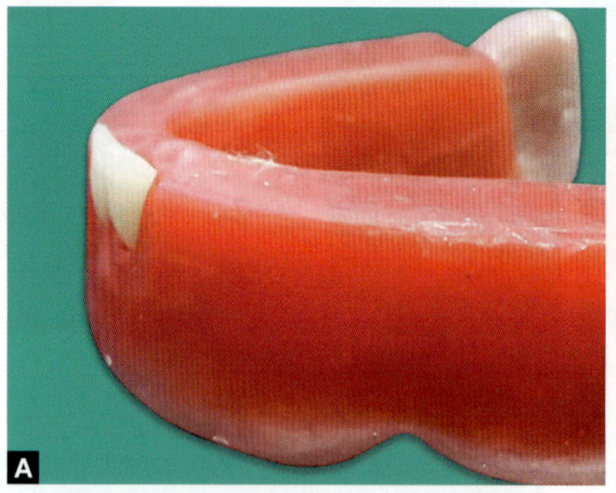

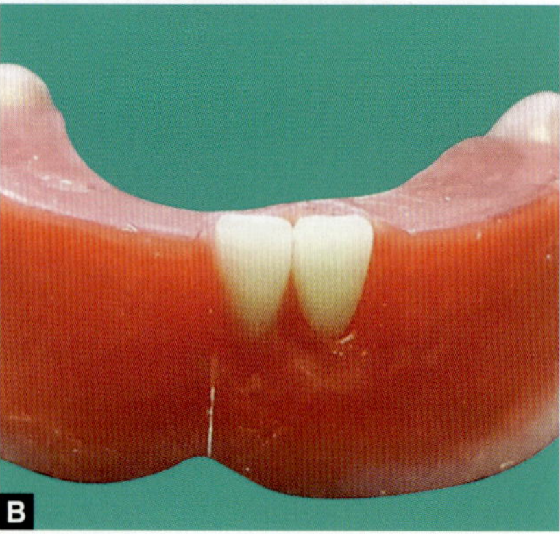

Figs. 24.24A and B: Placement of mandibular lateral incisor—side view and front view.

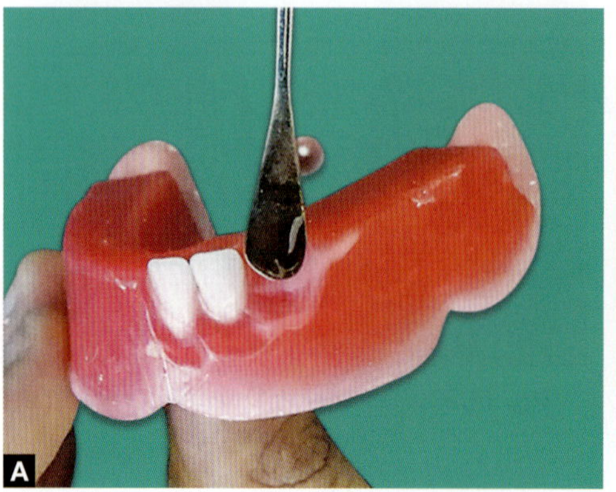

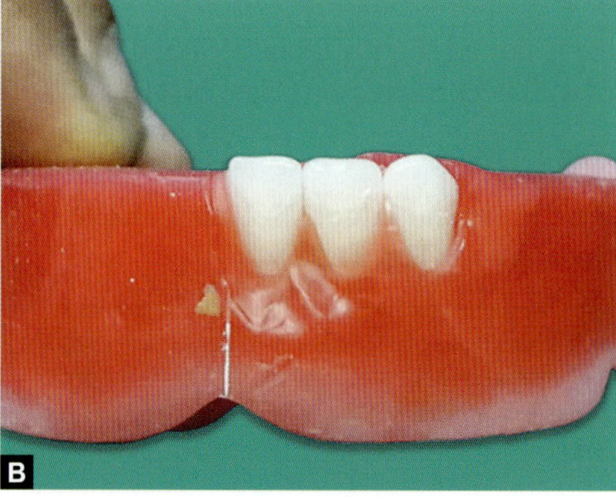

Figs. 24.25A and B: Scoop out wax and placement of canine.

Step 2

It is also slightly inclined lingually when viewed from side. Its tip is slightly more than 1 mm above the horizontal plane. It follows labial contour of the rim **(Figs. 24.26 and 24.27)**.

> Mandibular teeth when viewed occlusally should not cross land area of the cast.

Arrange all six mandibular anterior teeth accordingly. Remove wax from lingual surface of teeth **(Figs. 24.28A and B)**.

Check for overjet and overbite once the maxillary and mandibular anterior teeth are arranged.

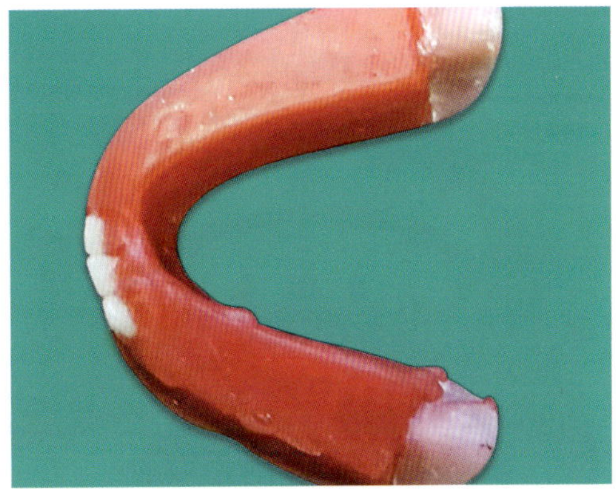

Fig. 24.26: Mandibular canine—occlusal view.

The vertical overlap between mandibular teeth and the maxillary teeth is called as over bite. It should be 0.5–1.0 mm. The horizontal overlap between the maxillary and mandibular teeth is called as overjet. It should be 1–2 mm **(Figs. 24.29A and B)**.

The overjet should be uniform from left canine to right canine **(Fig. 24.30)**.

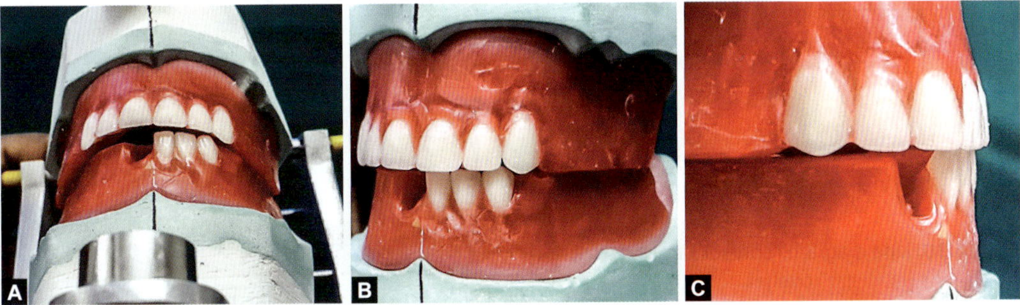

Figs. 24.27A to C: Arrangement of mandibular anterior. *Note:* Overbite, overjet and canine key of occlusion.

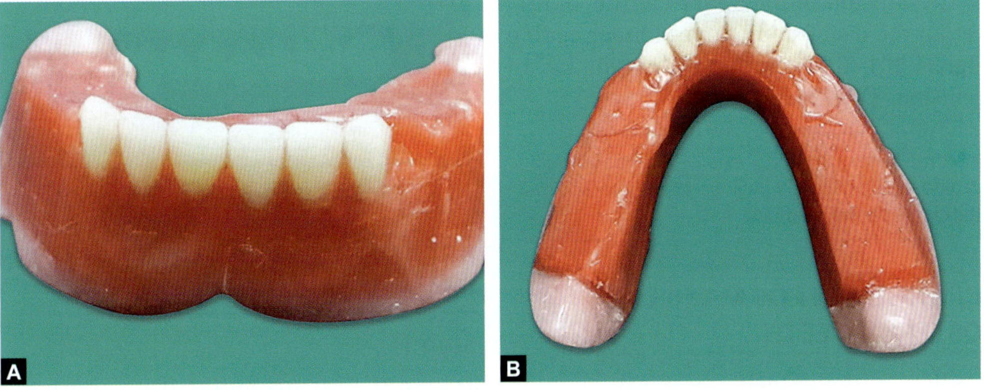

Figs. 24.28A and B: Removal of excess wax from lingual surface.

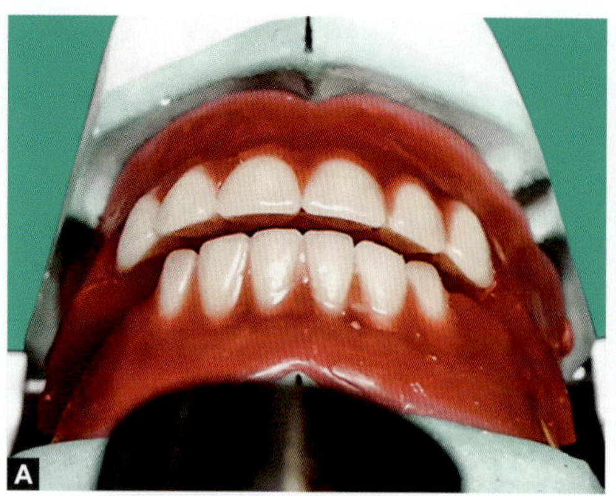

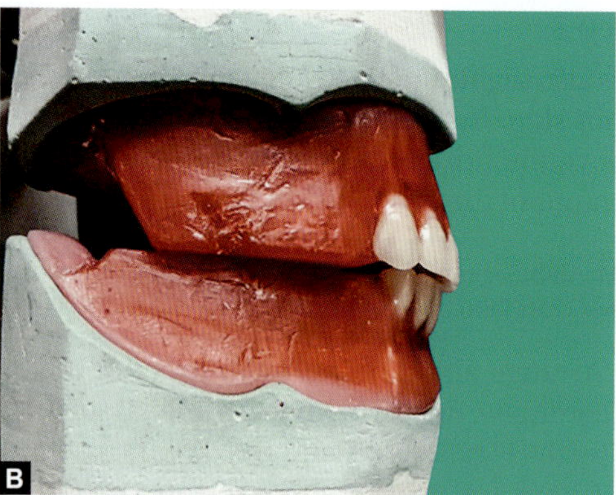

Figs. 24.29A and B: Horizontal overlap is 1–2 mm and vertical overlap is 0.5–1 mm.

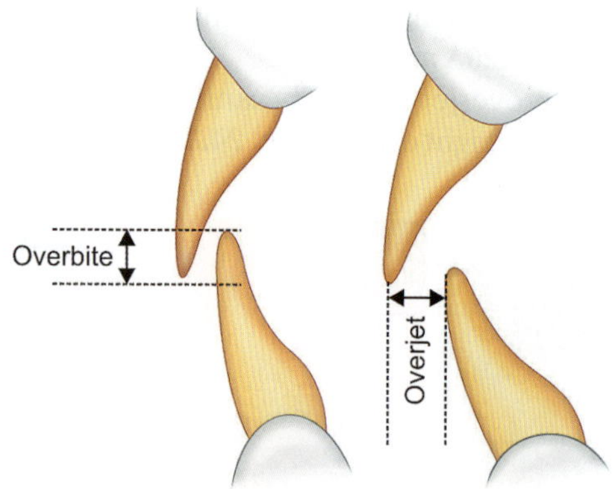

Fig. 24.30: Line diagram representing overbite and overjet.

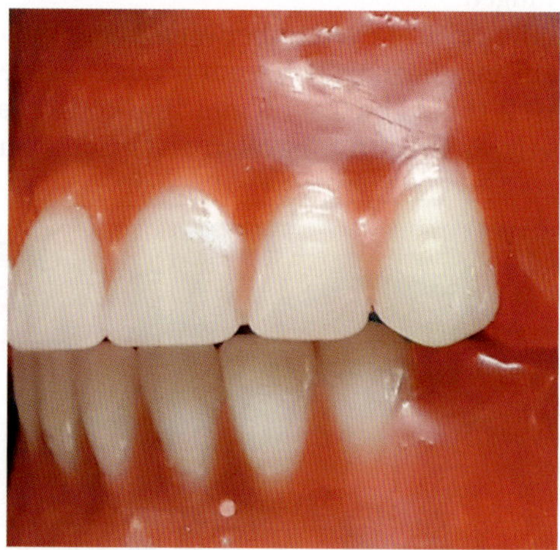

Fig. 24.31: Canine key of occlusion.

In properly arranged artificial teeth, the mesial slop of maxillary canine should overlap the distal slop of mandibular canine **(Fig. 24.30)**. This is called as "canine key of occlusion" **(Fig. 24.31)**.

> In some cases, the long axis of the mandibular canine may be slightly inclined distally to achieve the class-I canine relation.

ARRANGEMENT OF MAXILLARY POSTERIOR TEETH

Maxillary posterior teeth are shown on tooth card in **Figure 24.32**.

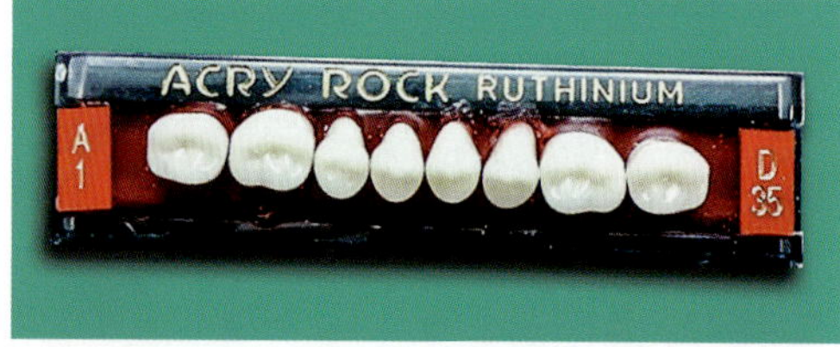

Fig. 24.32: Maxillary posterior teeth.

ARRANGEMENT OF MAXILLARY FIRST PREMOLAR

Step 1

Take out first premolar from tooth card and clean carding wax from ridge lap area

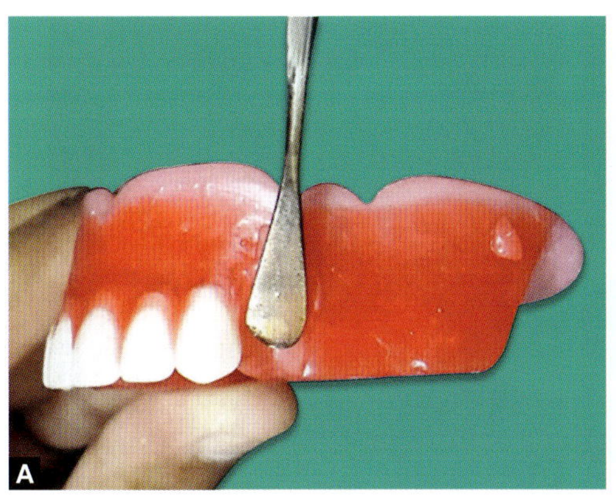

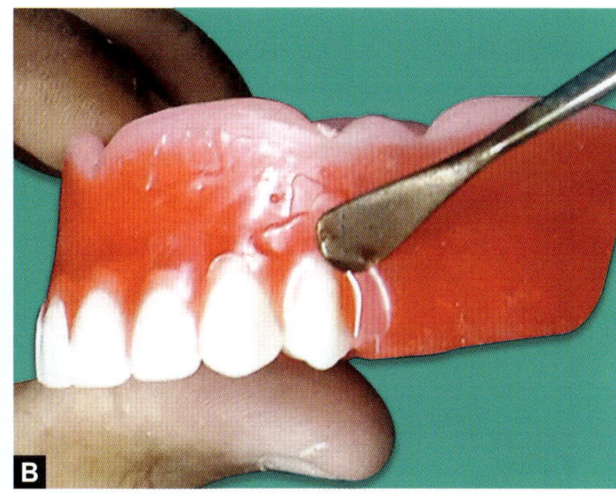

Figs. 24.33A and B: Scooping out the wax and placement of maxillary first premolar.

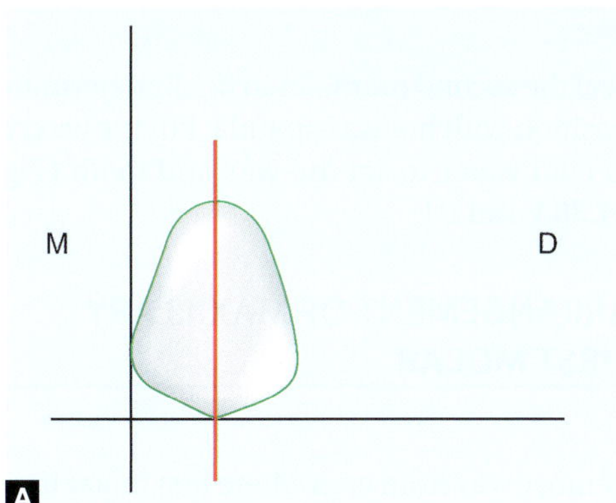

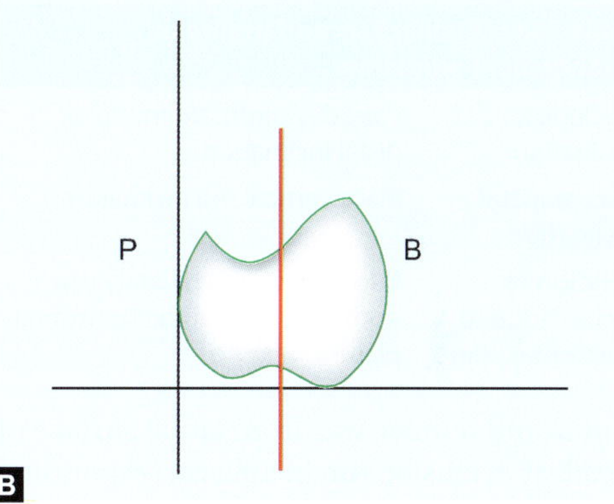

Figs. 24.34A and B: Diagrammatic representation of arrangement of maxillary first premolar.

Table 24.5: Maxillary first premolar arrangement guidelines.	
Mesiodistal inclination	Placed straight. No mesial or distal inclination
Buccopalatal inclination	Vertical. No inclination
Relation of incisal edge to horizontal plane	Buccal cusp touches the plane. The palatal cusp is 1 mm above the horizontal plane

(Figs. 24.33A and B). Heat wax spatula and remove wax from labial surface of maxillary occlusion rim in area corresponding to first premolar space. Soften the area with hot wax spatula and arrange premolar accordingly set up reference given in **Table 24.5 and Figs. 24.34A and B**.

Step 2

Seal the first premolar in finally determined position with hot wax spatula. Put the wax rim in cold water to set the wax and tooth **(Figs. 24.35A and B)**.

> When viewed occlusally, the buccal ridges of the canine and the first premolar should be flushed in one plane.

ARRANGEMENT OF MAXILLARY SECOND PREMOLAR

Step 1

Take out second premolar from tooth card and clean carding wax from ridge lap area. Heat wax

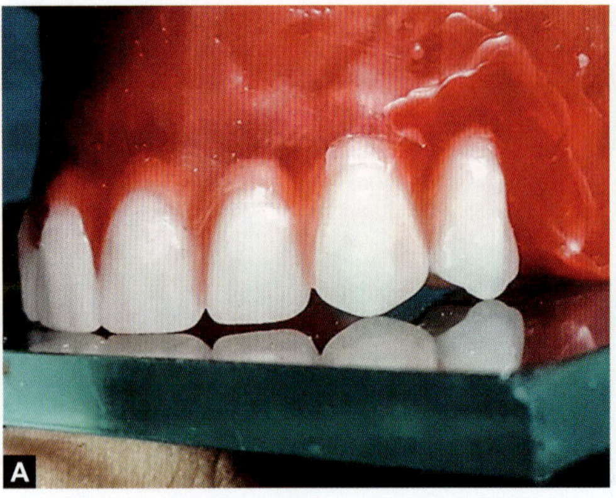
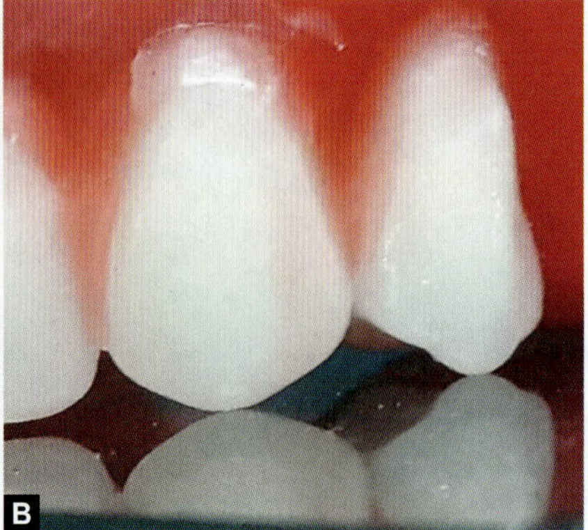

Figs. 24.35A and B: Maxillary first premolar in occlusal relation, see the palatal cusp is not in contact with glass plate.

Table 24.6: Maxillary second premolar arrangement guidelines.	
Mesiodistal inclination	Placed straight. No mesial or distal inclination
Buccopalatal inclination	Place vertical. No inclination
Relation of incisal edge to horizontal plane	Buccal cusp and palatal cusp both cusps touch the horizontal plane

spatula and remove wax from labial surface of maxillary occlusion rim in area corresponding to second premolar space. Soften the area with hot wax spatula and arrange premolar according to setup guidelines given in **Table 24.6, Figs. 24.36 and 24.37.**

Step 2

Seal the second premolar in finally determined position with hot wax spatula. Put the wax rim in cold water to set the wax and tooth **(Figs. 24.38A and B)**.

ARRANGEMENT OF MAXILLARY FIRST MOLAR

Step 1

Remove wax from area where first molar has to be arranged. Soften whole area nicely with hot wax spatula. Arrange the first molar accordingly setup guidelines given in **Table 24.7, Figs. 24.39 and 24.40.**

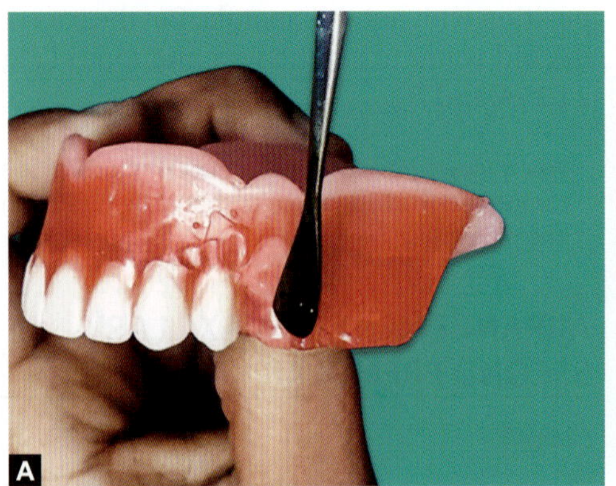
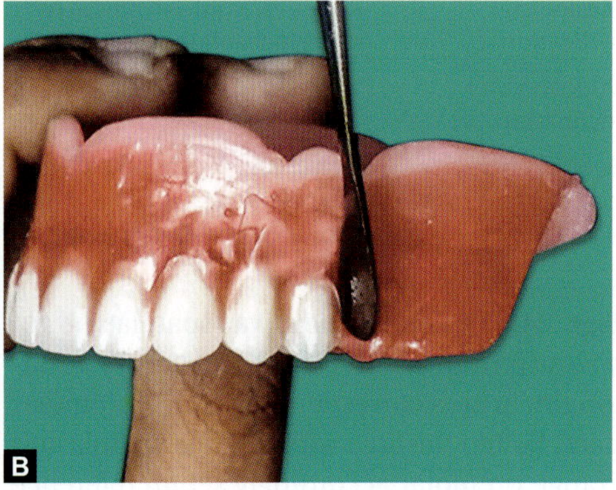

Figs. 24.36A and B: Scooping out the wax and placement of maxillary second premolar.

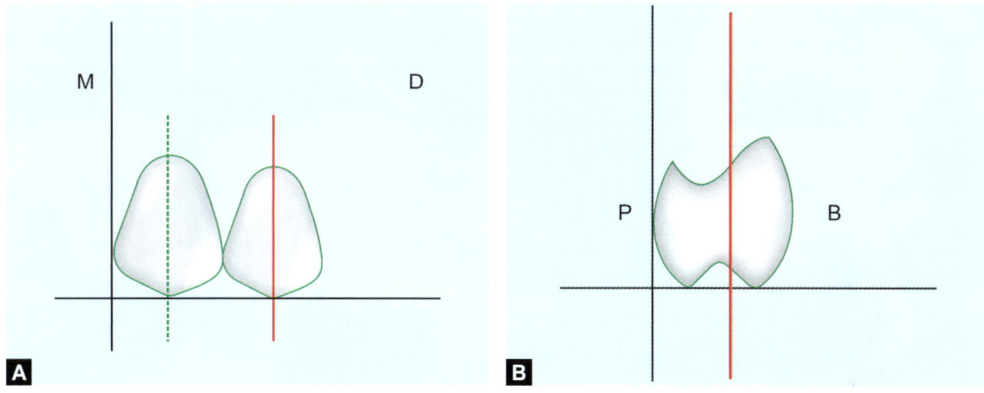

Figs. 24.37A and B: Diagrammatic representation of arrangement of maxillary second premolar.

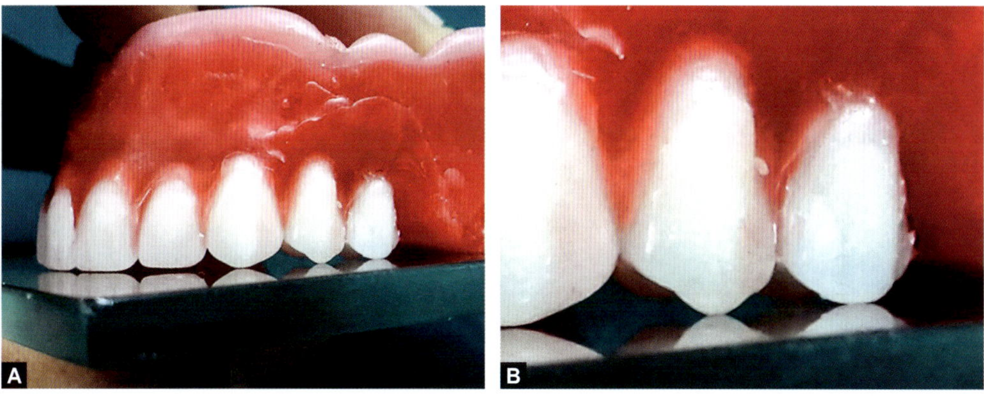

Figs. 24.38A and B: Maxillary second premolar in occlusal relation, appreciate both the palatal and buccal cusps are in contact with glass plate.

Table 24.7: Maxillary first molar arrangement guidelines.

Mesiodistal inclination	Slight distal tilt is given
Buccopalatal inclination	Slight buccal tilt is given
Relation of incisal edge to horizontal plane	❑ Only mesiopalatal cusp touches the horizontal plane ❑ Mesiobuccal cusp is 0.5 mm above the plane ❑ Distopalatal cusp and distobuccal cusps are 1 mm above the plane

Step 2

Seal the molar in finally determined position with hot wax spatula. Put the wax rim in cold water to set the wax and tooth **(Figs. 24.41A and B)**.

ARRANGEMENT OF MAXILLARY SECOND MOLAR

Step 1

Remove wax from area where second molar has to be arranged. Soften whole area nicely with hot wax spatula. Arrange the second molar accordingly given in arrangement guidelines **Table 24.8, Figs. 24.42 and 24.43.**

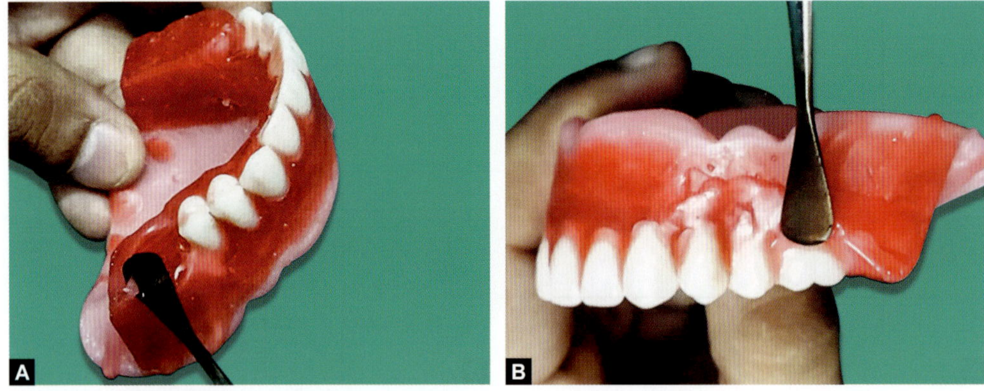

Figs. 24.39A and B: Scooping out the wax and placement of maxillary first molar.

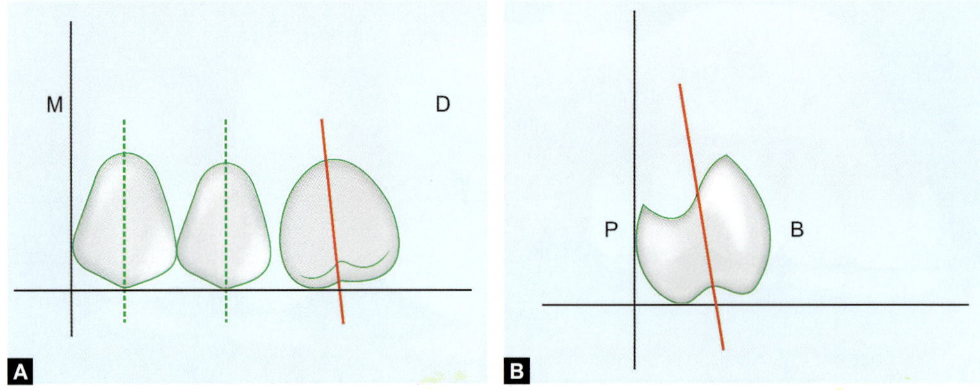

Figs. 24.40A and B: Diagrammatic representation of arrangement of maxillary first molar.

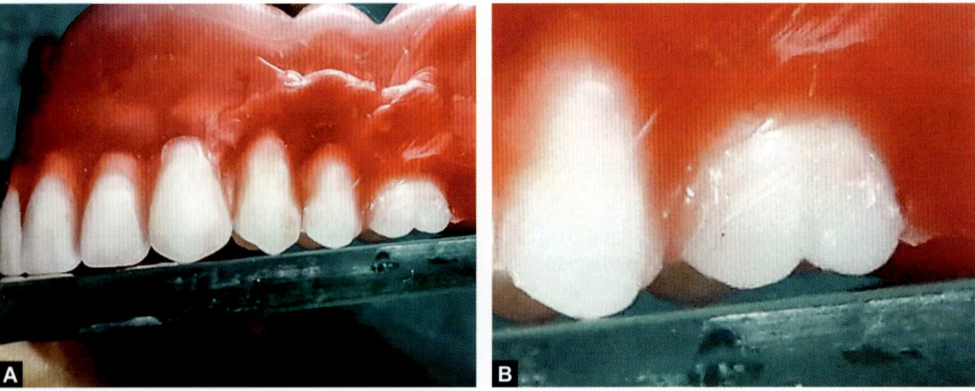

Figs. 24.41A and B: Maxillary first molar in occlusal relation, only the mesiopalatal cusp is in contact with glass plate.

Table 24.8: Maxillary second molar arrangement guidelines.

Mesiodistal inclination	Slightly more distally tilted than first molar
Buccopalatal inclination	More buccally tilted than first molar
Relation of incisal edge to horizontal plane	Arranged similar to first molar but none of the cusp touches the plane

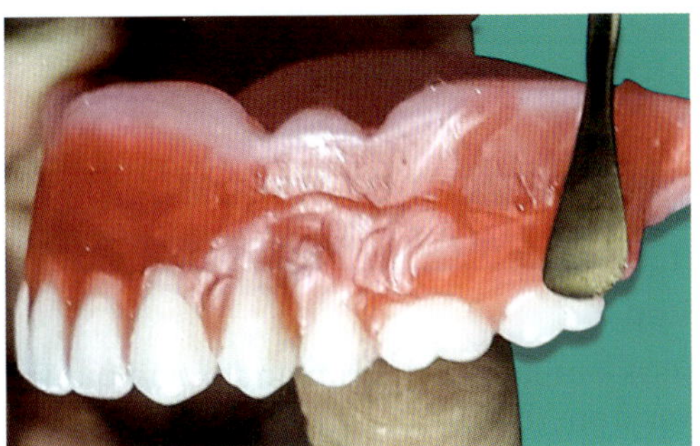

Fig. 24.42: Scooping out the wax and placement of maxillary second molar.

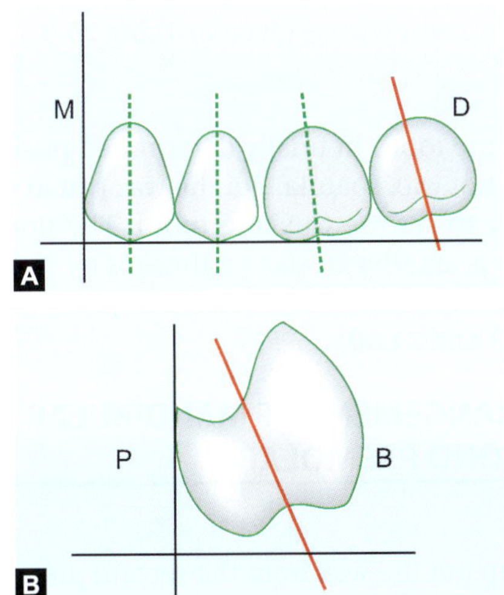

Figs. 24.43A and B: Diagrammatic representation of arrangement of maxillary second molar.

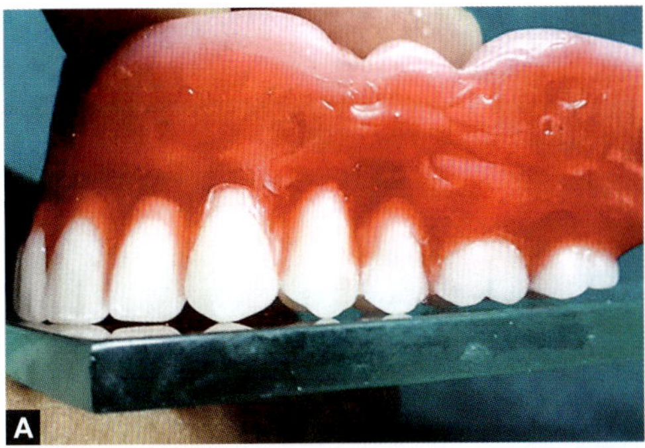

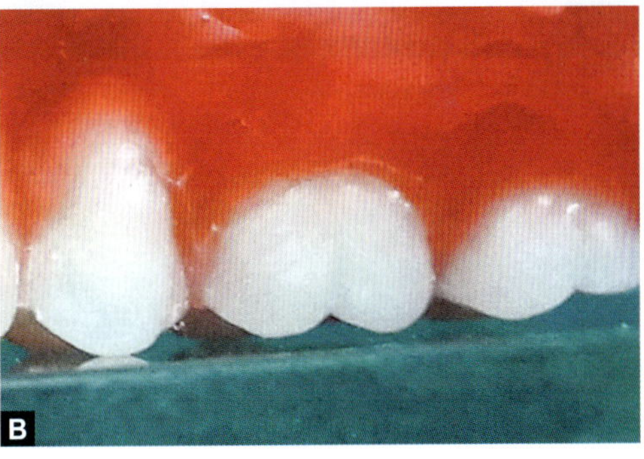

Figs. 24.44A and B: Maxillary second molar in occlusal relation, none of the cusp is in contact with glass plate.

Step 2

Seal the molar in finally determined position with hot wax spatula. Put the wax rim in cold water to set the wax and tooth **(Figs. 24.44A and B)**.

Four posterior teeth should be arranged in one line **(Figs. 24.45A and B)**.

ARRANGEMENT OF MANDIBULAR POSTERIOR TEETH

Mandibular posterior teeth should be on the crest of the ridge and in no case lingual cusp fall outside the lingual periphery. The second molar should not be higher than two-third of retromolar pad. The cusp and fossa of mandibular teeth should fit into corresponding cusps and fossa of maxillary teeth **(Figs. 24.46)**.

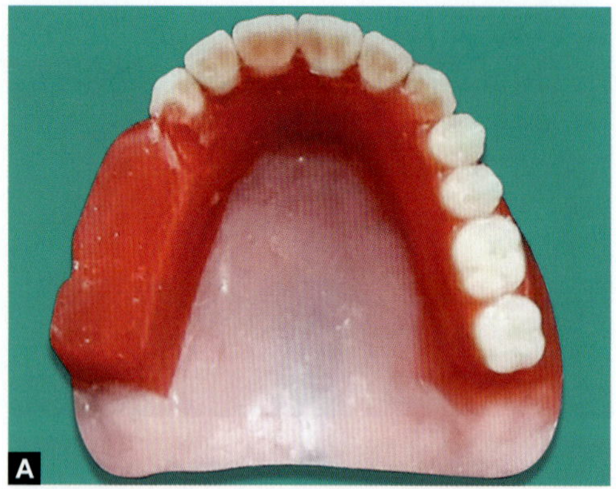

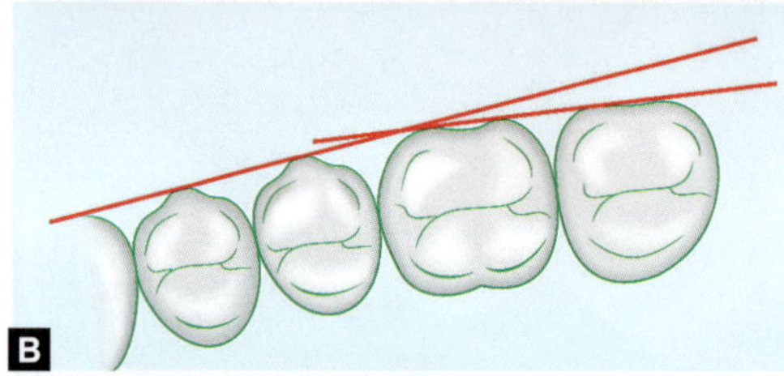

Figs. 24.45A and B: Four posterior teeth arranged in one line.

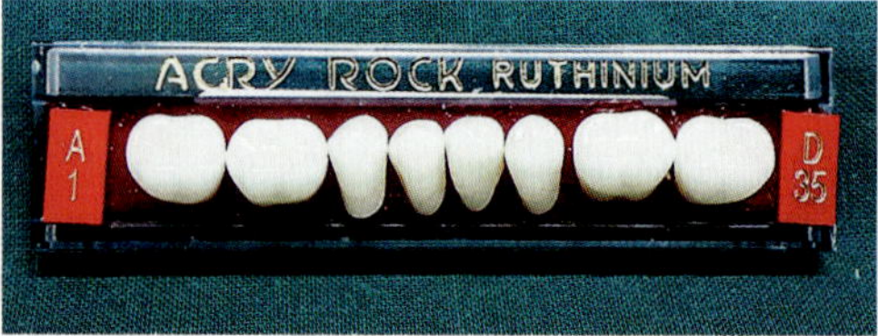

Fig. 24.46: Mandibular posterior teeth on tooth card.

Mandibular teeth should be overlapped buccally by corresponding maxillary posterior teeth. Each mandibular tooth is half a cusp mesially than opposite maxillary tooth.

Pound Triangle or Pound Lines

An imaginary line from the mesial angle of canine to the lingual border of retromolar pad **(Fig. 24.47)**.

> Lingual cusps of mandibular teeth should not be arranged beyond the pound line. Otherwise, they may restrict the tongue space.

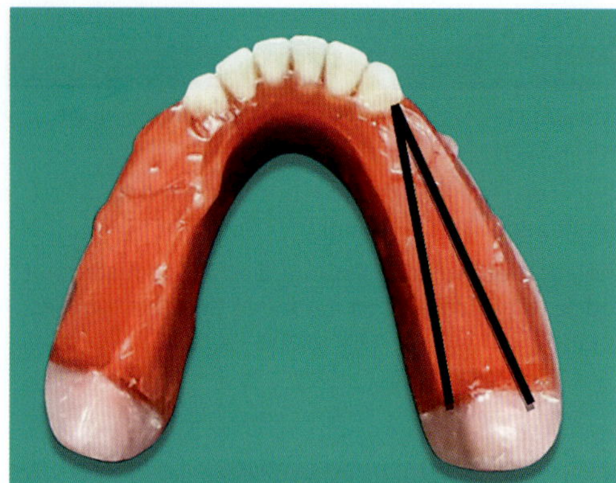

Fig. 24.47: Pound triangle or pound lines.

ARRANGEMENT OF MANDIBULAR FIRST PREMOLAR

Step 1

Mark outline on the rim and scoop out the wax from that area with hot wax spatula. The long axis of tooth is parallel to midline (placed vertically). The long axis of tooth should be inclined lingually. The buccal surface of first premolar is scarcely visible when viewed from front **(Figs. 24.48A and B)**. Arrange according to setup guidelines given in **Table 24.9**.

Step 2

Seal the tooth in finally determined position with hot wax spatula. Put the wax rim in cold water to set the wax and tooth. The lingual cusp is smaller in size so there is no lingual intercuspation when viewed lingually **(Figs. 24.49 and 24.50)**.

ARRANGEMENT OF MANDIBULAR SECOND PREMOLAR

Step 1

Scoop out the wax from the second premolar area with hot wax spatula. The long axis of tooth is parallel to midline (placed vertically). The long axis of tooth should be slightly inclined lingually **(Figs. 24.51A and B)**.

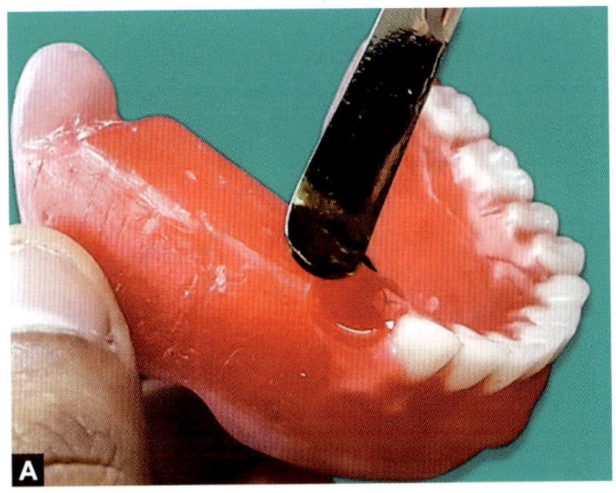

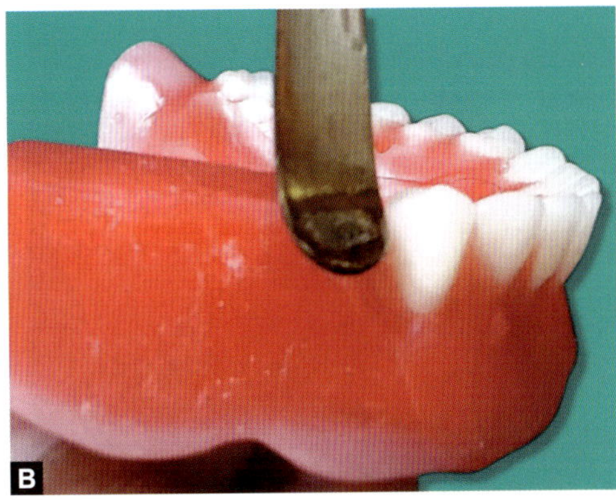

Figs. 24.48A and B: Scooping out of wax.

Table 24.9: Mandibular first premolar arrangement guidelines.

When viewed from front	Long axis parallel to vertical axis (midline)
When viewed from side	Long axis parallel to vertical axis
Relation with occlusal plane	Buccal cusp is 2 mm above the occlusal plane. The lingual cusp is below occlusal plane
Occlusal contact	Buccal cusp contacts the mesial marginal ridge of maxillary first premolar
Occlusal relation with opposite teeth	Maxillary canine and first premolar

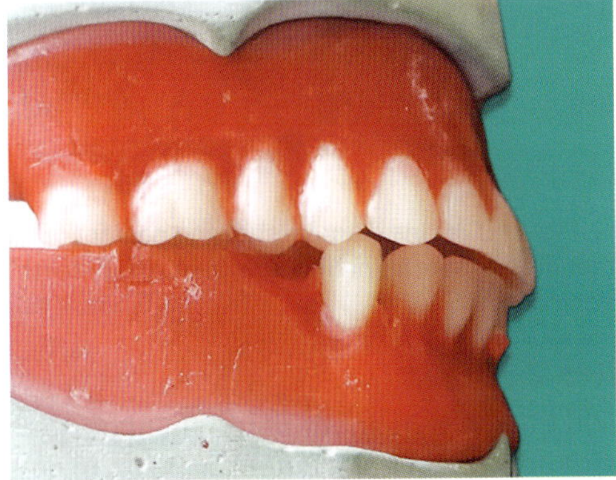

Fig. 24.49: Mandibular first premolar in occlusal with maxillary teeth.

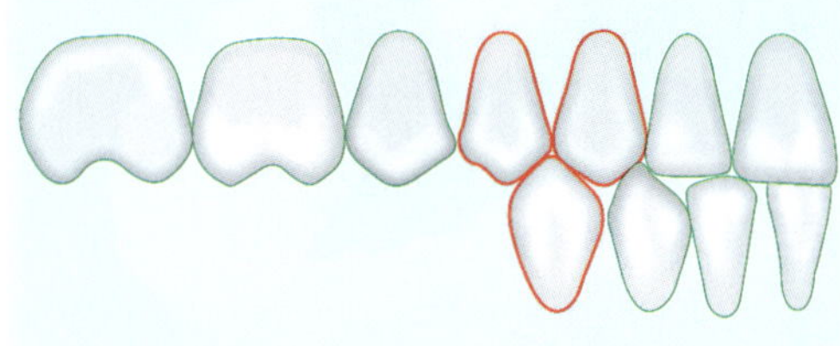

Fig. 24.50: Line diagram showing contact of mandibular first premolar with maxillary teeth.

Arrange according arrangement guidelines given in **Table 24.10**.

Step 2

Seal the tooth in finally determined position with hot wax spatula. Put the wax rim in cold water to set the wax and tooth. The mandibular second premolar is in contact with maxillary first and second premolars (**Figs. 24.52 and 24.53**).

ARRANGEMENT OF MANDIBULAR FIRST MOLAR

Step 1

Scoop out the wax from the first molar area with hot wax spatula. Place the molar such that the mesiobuccal cusp of maxillary first molar occludes with (coincide with) mesiobuccal groove of mandibular first molar. It is slightly

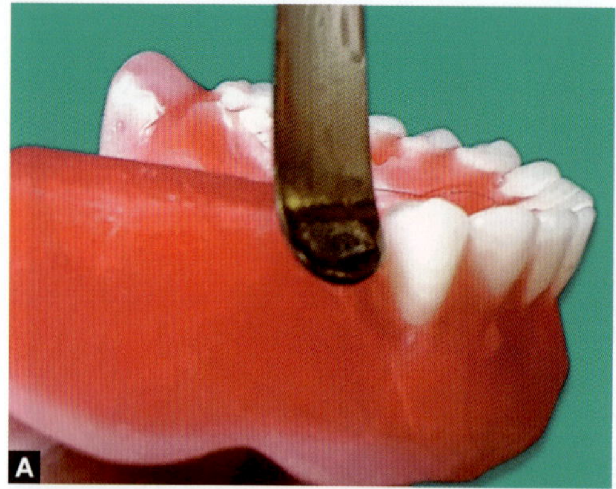

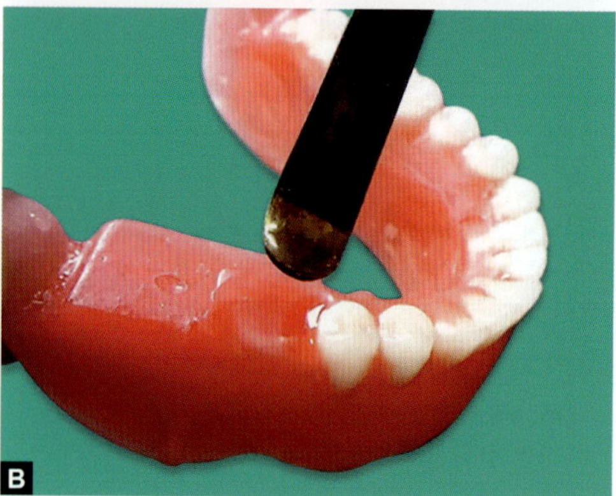

Figs. 24.51A and B: Scooping out the wax.

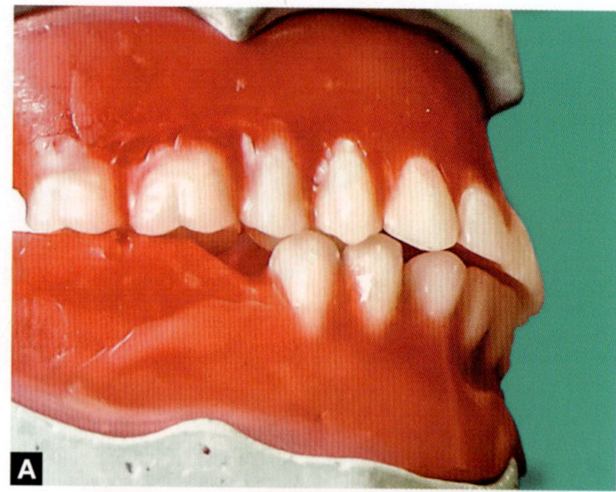

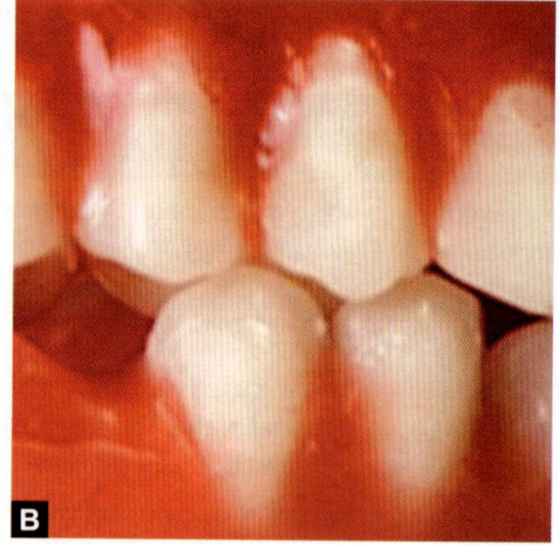

Figs. 24.52A and B: Mandibular second premolar in occlusion.

Table 24.10: Mandibular second premolar arrangement guidelines.	
When viewed from front	Long axis parallel to vertical axis (midline)
When viewed from side	Long axis parallel to vertical axis
Relation with occlusal plane	Both buccal and lingual cusps are 2 mm above the occlusal plane
Occlusal contact	Buccal cusp contacts the fossa between the two maxillary premolar
Occlusal relation with maxillary teeth	Occludes with maxillary first and second premolars

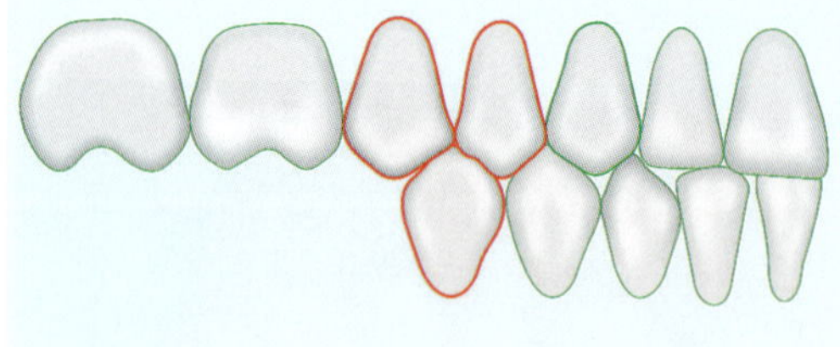

Fig. 24.53: Line diagram showing contact of mandibular second premolar with maxillary teeth.

lingually inclined (**Figs. 24.54A and B and Table 24.11**).

Step 2

Seal the tooth in finally determined position with hot wax spatula. Put the wax rim in cold water to set the wax and tooth (**Figs. 24.55 and 24.56**).

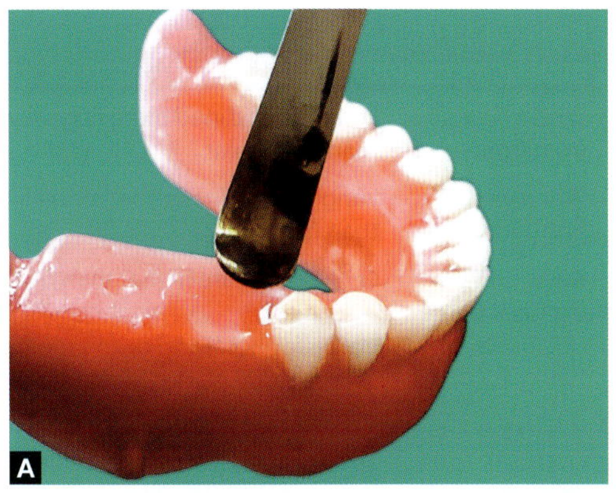

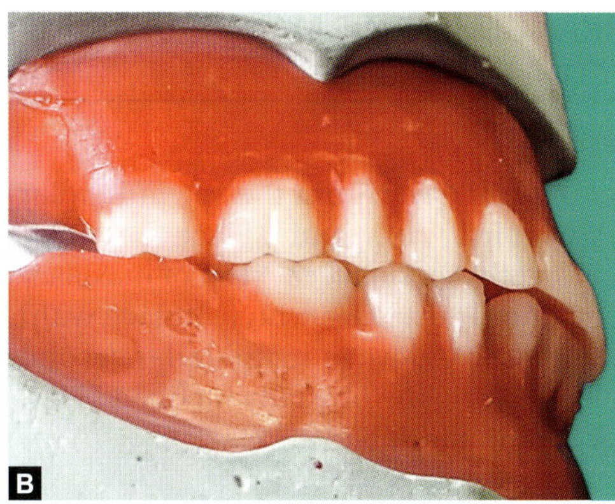

Figs. 24.54A and B: Scooping out the wax and placement of mandibular first molar.

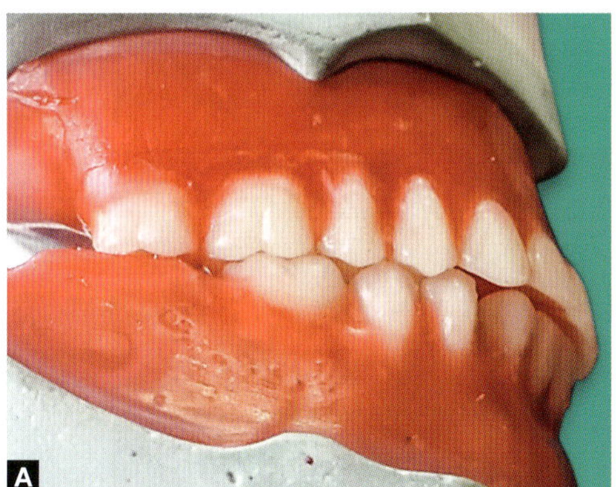

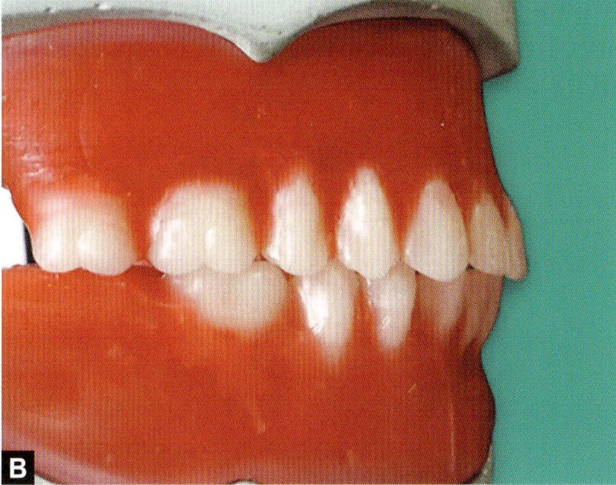

Figs. 24.55A and B: Mandibular first molar in occlusion with maxillary first molar and second premolar.

Table 24.11: Mandibular first molar arrangement guidelines.

When viewed from front	Long axis slightly inclined lingually
When viewed from side	Long axis slightly inclined mesially
Relation with occlusal plane	All cusps are higher than second premolar Distobuccal and distolingual cusps are placed higher than other cusps
Occlusal contact	The mesiobuccal cusp occludes with fossa between maxillary second premolar and first molar
Occlusal relation with maxillary teeth	With maxillary second premolar and first molar

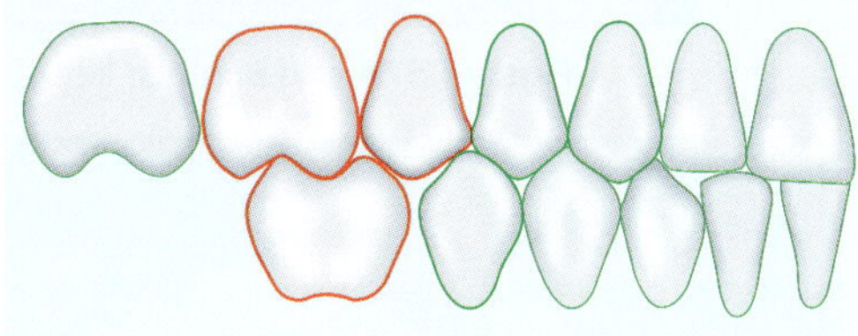

Fig. 24.56: Line diagram showing contact of mandibular first molar with maxillary teeth.

Molar key of occlusion: The mesiobuccal cusp of maxillary first molar occludes with mesiobuccal groove of mandibular first molar OR the mesiopalatal cusp of maxillary first molar occludes with central fossa of mandibular molar.

ARRANGEMENT OF MANDIBULAR SECOND MOLAR

Step 1

Scoop out the wax from the second molar area with hot wax spatula. Place the molar such that the mesiobuccal cusp of maxillary second molar occludes with (coincide with) mesiobuccal groove of mandibular second molar. It is slightly lingually inclined (**Figs. 24.57, 24.58 and Table 24.12**).

Step 2

Seal the tooth in finally determined position with hot wax spatula. Put the wax rim in cold water to set the wax and tooth (**Figs. 24.59 and 24.60**).

Table 24.12: Mandibular second molar arrangement guidelines.

When viewed from front	Long axis inclined more lingually than first molar
When viewed from side	Long axis inclined more mesially than first molar
Relation with occlusal plane	❑ All cusps are higher than first molar ❑ Distobuccal and distolingual cusps are placed higher than mesial cusps
Occlusal contact	The mesiobuccal cusp occludes between maxillary first molar and second molar
Occlusal relation with maxillary teeth	With maxillary first and second molar

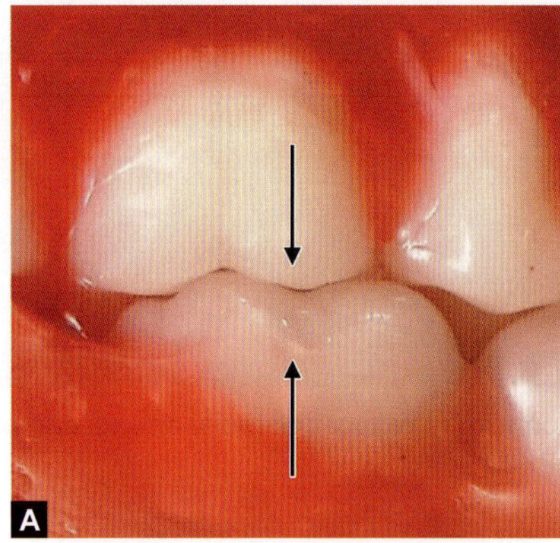

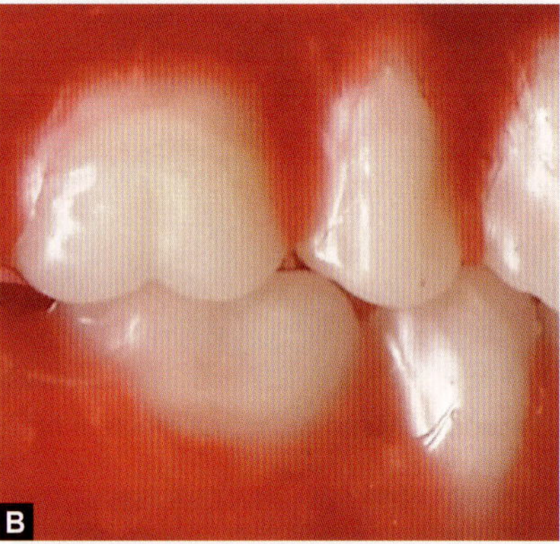

Figs. 24.57A and B: Molar key of occlusion/posterior key of occlusion.

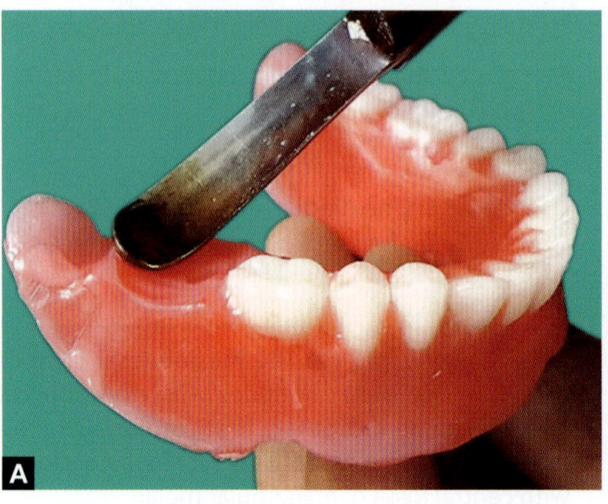

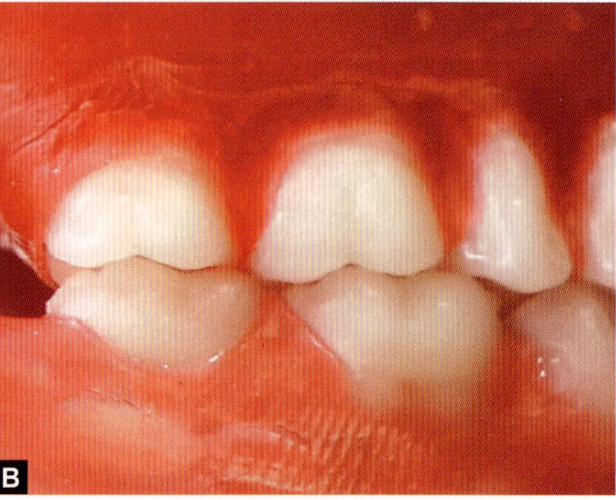

Figs. 24.58A and B: Scooping out the wax and placement of mandibular second molar.

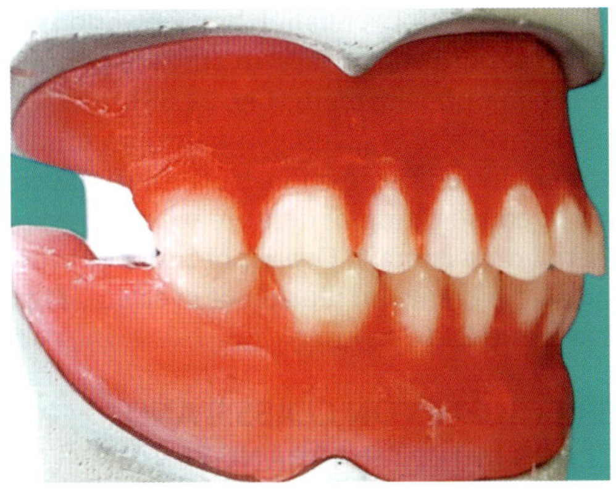

Fig. 24.59: Mandibular second molar in occlusion with maxillary first and second molar.

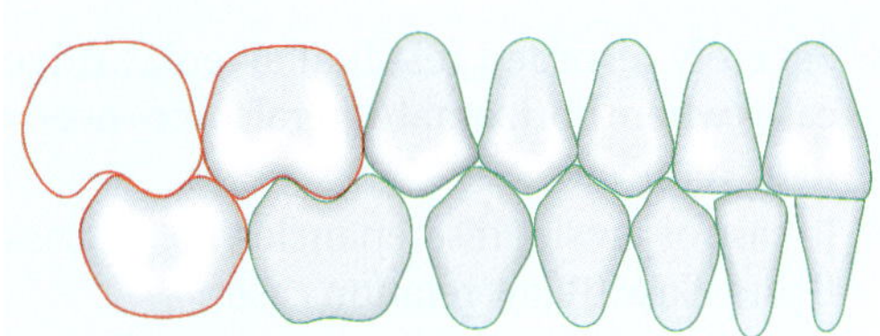

Fig. 24.60: Line diagram showing contact of mandibular first molar with maxillary teeth.

Complete arrangement of maxillary and mandibular teeth—buccal view and lingual view is shown in **Figures 24.61A and B**.

Teeth Contact

Every tooth either in maxillary arch or mandibular arch has contact with two teeth in opposite arch except mandibular central incisors and maxillary second molar. In **Figure 24.62**, teeth in red color shows one tooth contact with two opposite teeth, maxillary second molar and mandibular central incisor (green color) show contact with opposite single tooth.

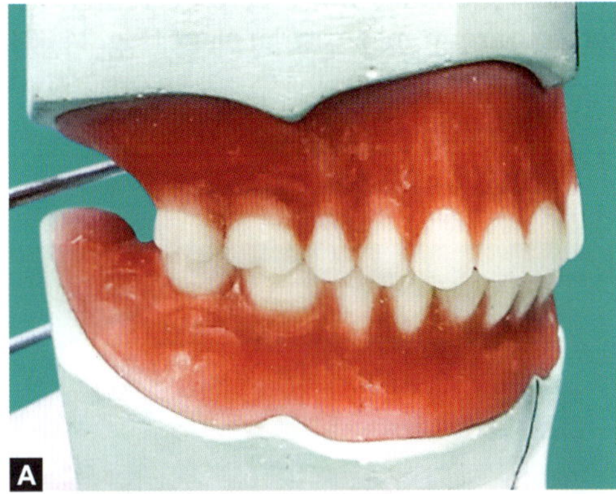

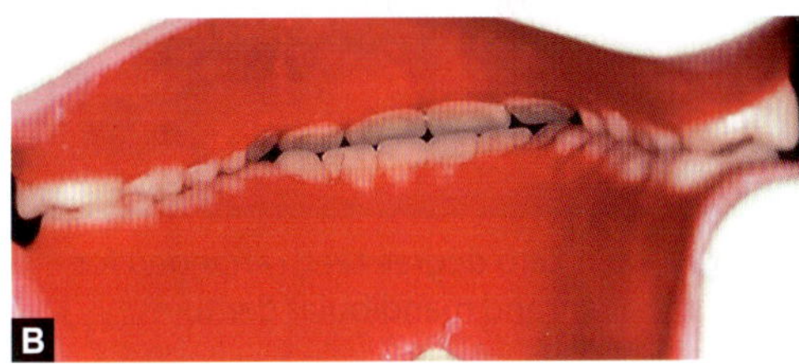

Figs. 24.61A and B: Complete arrangement of maxillary and mandibular teeth—buccal and lingual view.

TEETH ARRANGEMENT USING NONANATOMICAL (ZERO DEGREE) POSTERIOR TEETH (FIGS. 24.63 TO 24.67)

Introduction

Nonanatomical or degree teeth are arranged for some special conditions and cases where anatomical teeth are not indicated. These are cusp less teeth with flatter occlusal table which helps in reduction of lateral forces while chewing. Eliminating the lateral forces helps in improvement in denture stability.

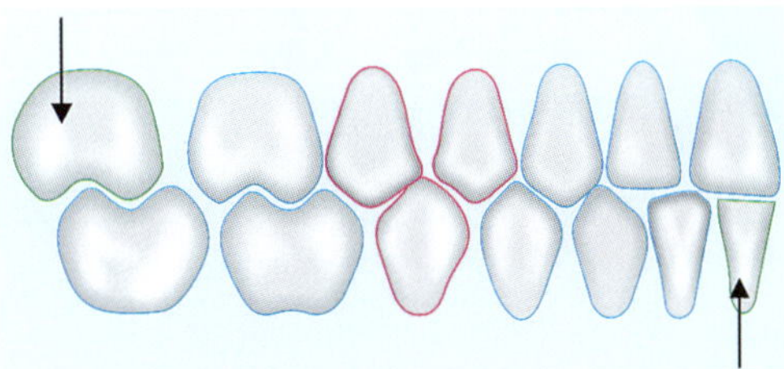

Fig. 24.62: Tooth contact with opposite teeth.

Indications

- ❖ Severely resorbed residual alveolar ridge cases where horizontal/lateral forces needs to be reduced.
- ❖ In case of jaw size discrepancies, i.e., in class II and class III jaw relation cases.
- ❖ In cases, where jaw movements are uncoordinated.

Features

Cuspless (nonanatomical/zero degree) posterior teeth are arranged on flat plane **(Fig. 24.63)**.

No compensating curves are incorporated. Teeth are arranged on a straight plane **(Fig. 24.64)**.

No cusp to fossa relation between opposite arch teeth, only surface to surface contact between opposite teeth **(Fig. 24.65)**.

No overbite is given. No anterior contact present in centric position. If overbite is given, it will cause tilting of denture when anterior teeth are in contact. Overjet of 2 mm or more is used to create an illusion of overbite **(Figs. 24.66 and 24.67)**.

BRIEF NOTES ON CLASS II AND CLASS III TEETH ARRANGEMENT

Due to discrepancy in jaw size, the arrangement of artificial teeth should be modified accordingly.

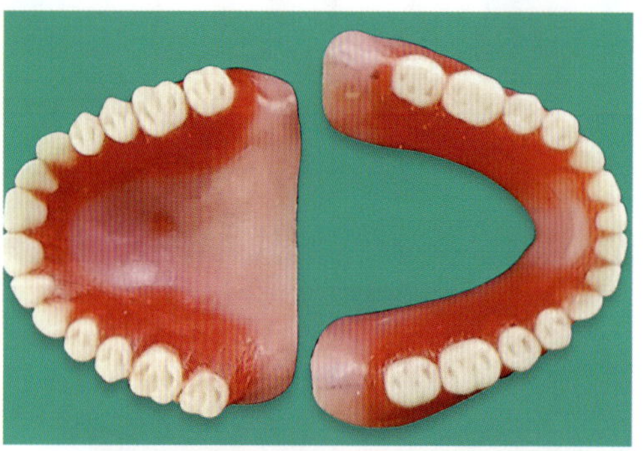

Fig. 24.63: Zero degree teeth arranged for maxillary and mandibular dentures.

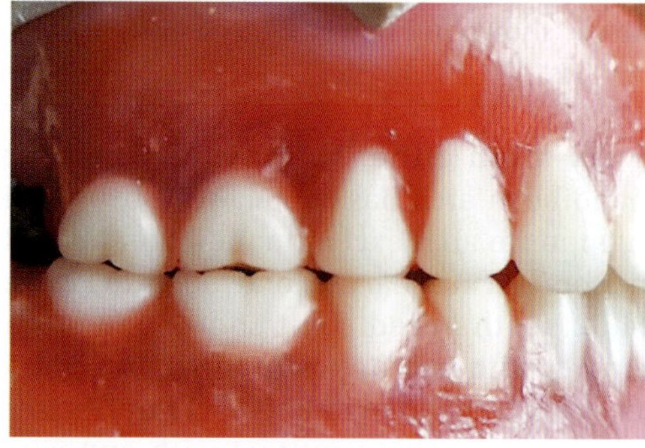

Fig. 24.65: No cusp to fossa relation between opposite teeth.

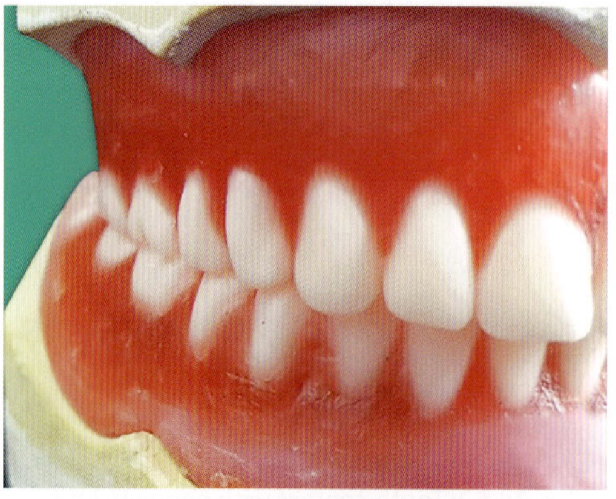

Fig. 24.64: No compensating curve given for posterior teeth arrangement.

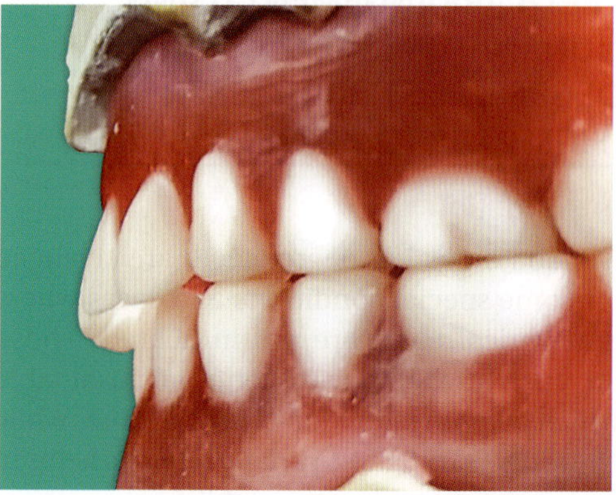

Fig. 24.66: No overbite given but overjet is given to create illusion of overbite.

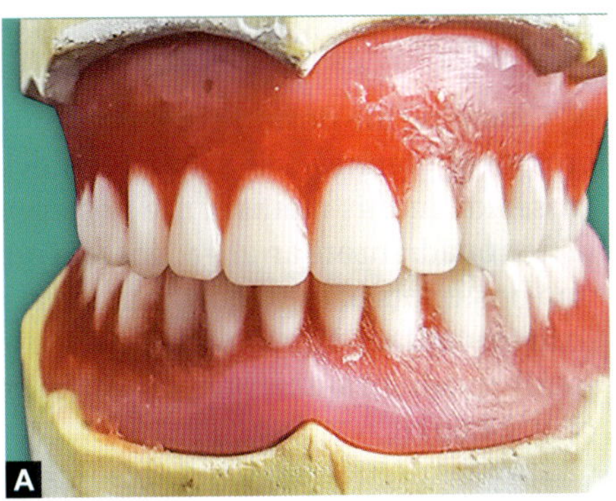

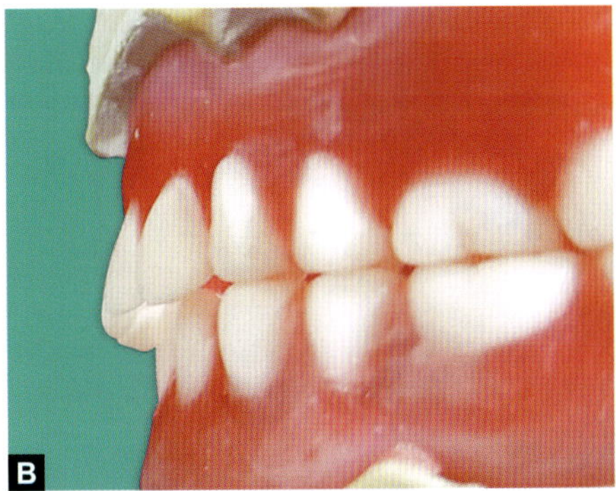

Figs. 24.67A and B: Complete arrangement of nonanatomical posterior teeth.

Class II Arrangement

In the class II relation, the mandibular ridge is smaller than maxillary ridge. The mandibular ridge is located more lingually in relation to maxillary ridge **(Fig. 24.68)**.

Teeth arrangement for class II relation has different characteristics than class I teeth arrangement as listed below:

- Horizontal overlap (overjet) increase.
- Canines are arranged more posteriorly and lingually.
- As the mandibular ridge is smaller in size, there is reduced space to arrange all the teeth. The premolars may be trimmed or one premolar bilaterally may be removed to gain space to arrange teeth on smaller size ridge.

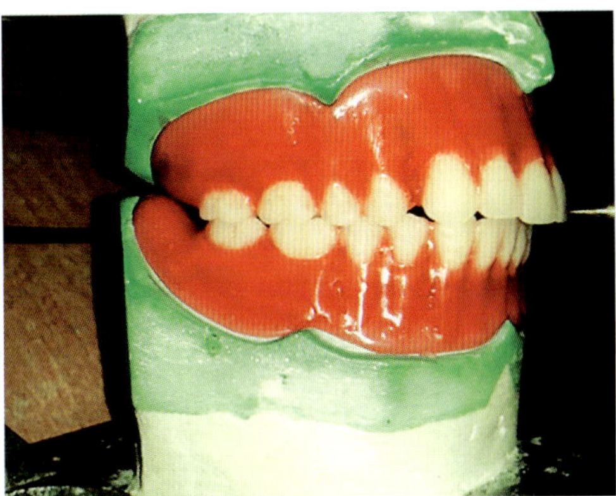

Fig. 24.68: Increased overjet in class II arrangement.

- Semianatomic or nonanatomic teeth are selected to reduce stresses on smaller and weaker ridge.
- Molars can be arranged in class II relation (the *distobuccal* cusp of the maxillary first molar occludes/falls in the *buccal groove* of the mandibular first molar) or in class I relation.
- Give space between maxillary canine and first premolar or remove one premolar from mandibular arch to overcome space discrepancy.

Class III Arrangement

In class III relationship, mandibular arch is larger than the maxillary arch. The discrepancy between ridge sizes certainly gives some problems during teeth arrangement.

The anterior teeth of opposite arch are arranged in edge-to-edge relationship. There is no overbite and overjet. The incisal edges of maxillary anterior teeth are in contact with incisal edges of mandibular anterior teeth.

Maxillary anterior teeth are arranged as far forward as required to get proper lip support.

Mandibular anterior teeth are arranged as far lingual as possible without interference to the tongue.

In class III relationship, the posterior are arranged in crossbite relationship. Crossbite relation can be achieved by horizontally

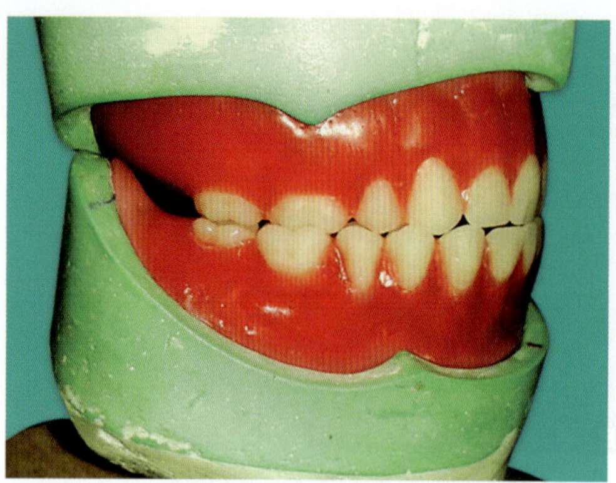

Fig. 24.69: Class III arrangement.

overlapping the buccal cusps by lower teeth.
OR

Changing the position of posterior teeth in crossover manner will help in achieving the crossbite. In this method, the posterior teeth of first quadrant are arranged in third quadrant and posteriors of third quadrant are arranged in first quadrant. Posterior teeth of second and fourth quadrant are exchanged with each other **(Fig. 24.69)**.

(*Note*: Anterior edge-to-edge relation and posterior crossbite, one premolar removed from maxillary arch.)

CHAPTER 25

Wax-up of Complete Denture

Paranjay Prajapati, YG Naveen

INTRODUCTION

Wax-up of complete denture is done to contour the polish surface of denture. Proper contouring of polished surface is important to aid in retention and stability of complete denture.

Wax up and carving contributes to esthetic by proper contouring of lost tissue, giving support to the lips and cheeks. It helps in proper phonetics. Properly made gingival embrasure helps in self-cleansing of food particles. Contouring gingival anatomy gives natural appearance to patient while talking and smiling.

ARMAMENTARIUM

- Maxillary and mandibular trial dentures
- Wax knife
- Wax spatula
- Carver
- Wax sheet
- Blow torch
- Toothbrush.

WAX-UP OF MAXILLARY COMPLETE DENTURE

Step 1

Soften the modeling wax and add it on palatal surface, buccal, and labial surface of waxed denture. Add wax to cover cervical part of labial surfaces of teeth **(Figs. 25.1A and B)**.

Step 2

Hold the roach carver at 60° angle to carve gingival margin of anterior teeth. Gingival margin is placed according to tilt of tooth as shown in **Figures 25.2A and B** to give natural contour of gingival anatomy.

Step 3

Hold the carver at approximately 45° angulation to carve the gingival margin around the posterior teeth **(Fig. 25.3)**.

Step 4

Use roach carver held at approximately 20° angle to carve the lingual surface of denture teeth. Maxillary buccal flange inclines laterally and superiorly **(Fig. 25.4)**.

Step 5

Place markings for roots on labial surface of denture as shown. Mind the tilt of cervical part (neck) of the tooth while placing the markings. The root of the tooth is in continuation with tilt of the tooth **(Fig. 25.5)**.

Step 6

Remove wax between two root markings and try to give bulge on marking areas.

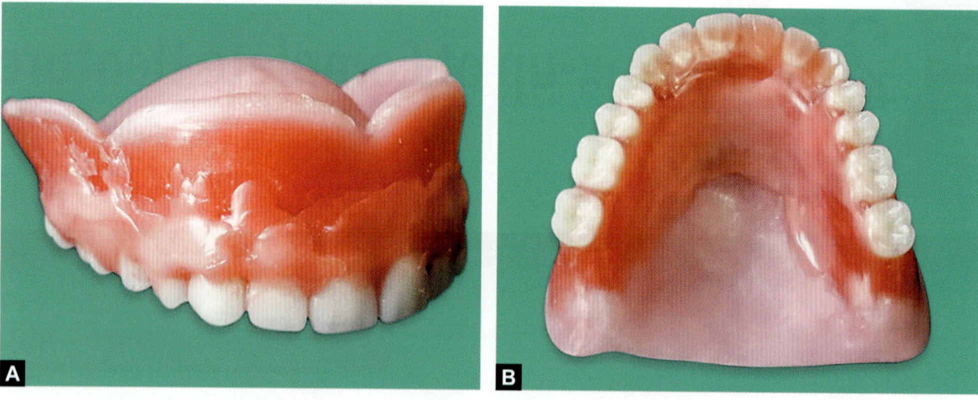

Figs. 25.1A and B: Add wax on labial, buccal, and palatal surfaces of trial denture.

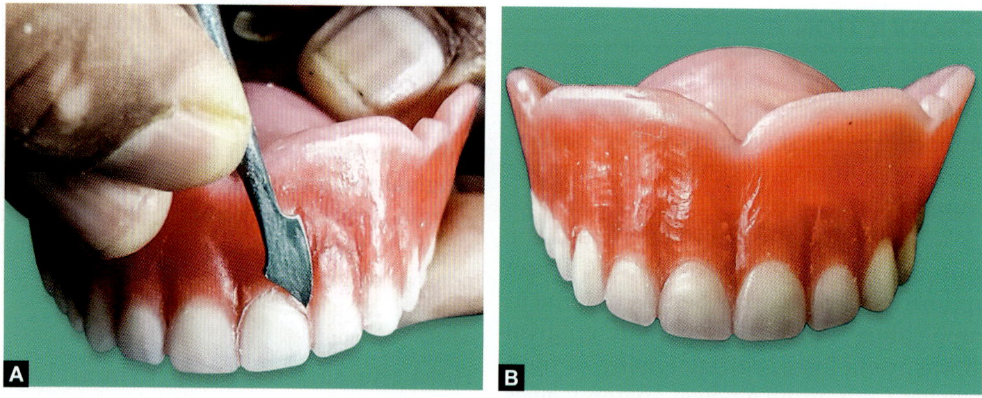

Figs. 25.2A and B: Carving the gingival margin of anterior teeth.

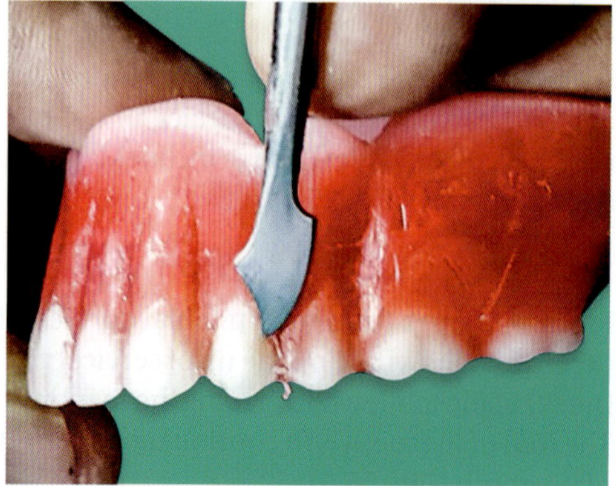

Fig. 25.3: Carving the gingival margin for posterior teeth.

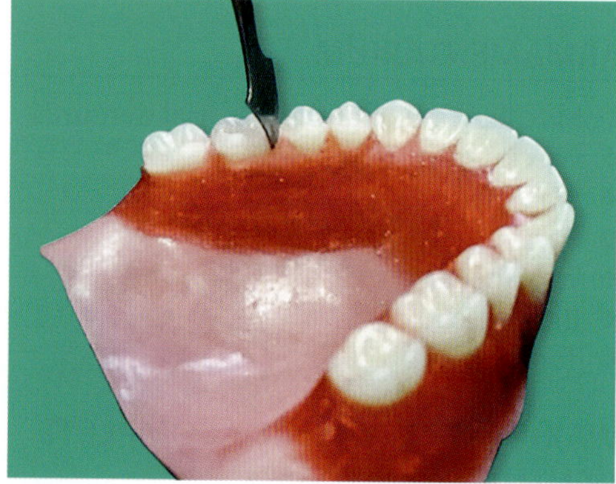

Fig. 25.4: Carving the gingival margins on palatal side.

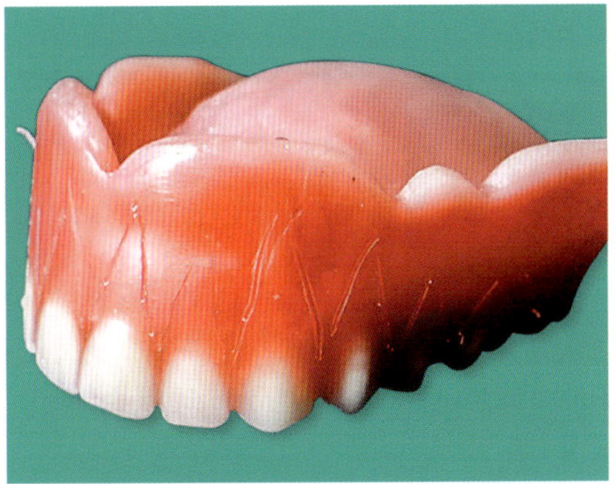

Fig. 25.5: Root markings placement.

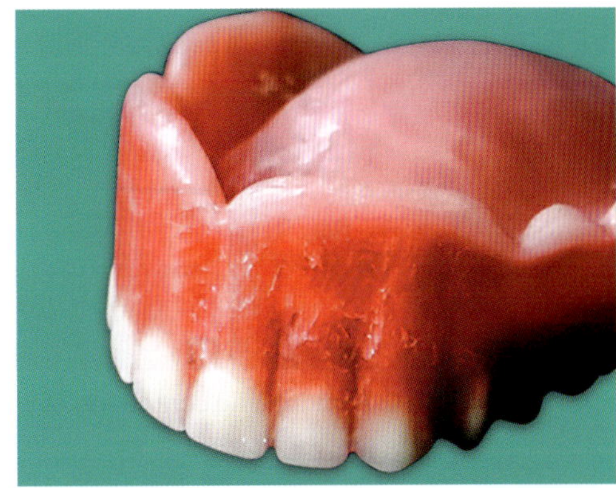

Fig. 25.7: Apical end of carving is slightly distally tilted.

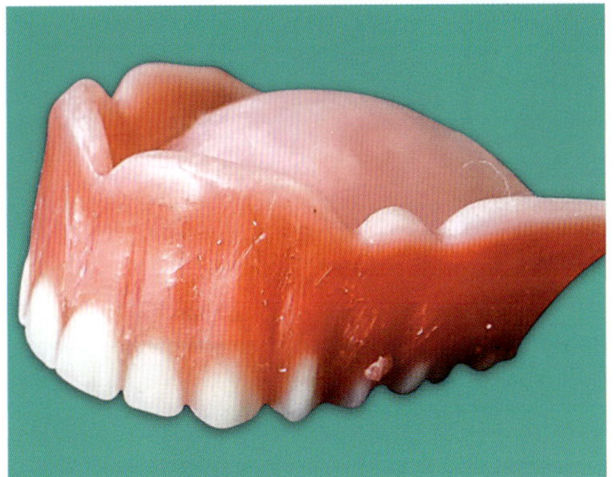

Fig. 25.6: Shaping the roots according to markings.

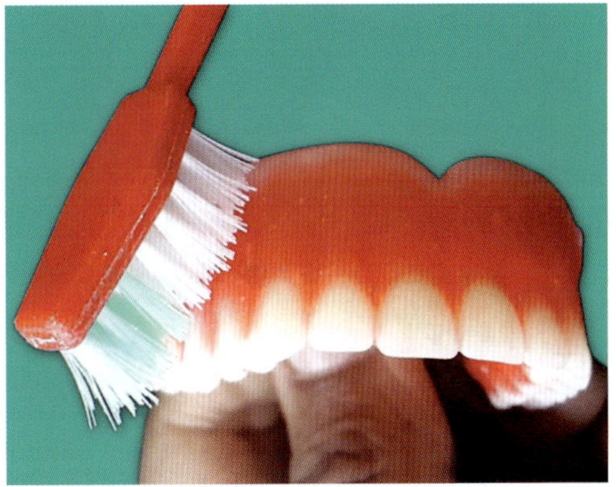

Fig. 25.8: Finishing of roots with mild pressure.

Use carver for this procedure. Roots are wider at beginning (cervical area) and become slender at apical area **(Fig. 25.6)**.

Step 7

Do not make roots till the denture borders. The root carving of central incisor is kept short of denture border. The root carving for lateral incisor is about three-fourths of the length of central incisor's root. The apical end of carving is slightly distally tilted **(Fig. 25.7)**.

Step 8

Make root carving for canine immense than that of central incisor. It is longer than central incisor. Do finishing of roots with brush by applying mild pressure **(Fig. 25.8)**.

Stippling is orange peel-like appearance of attached gingiva. In denture, stippling can be created by pressing tips of bristles of brush in wax.

Step 9

Add wax in drop shape on palatal surface between two central incisors to form the incisive papillae. Add wax in thin line along the mid palatine raphe on palatal surface and form a groove in the center and smudge it with blow torch to form midpalatine raphe **(Figs. 25.9A to C)**.

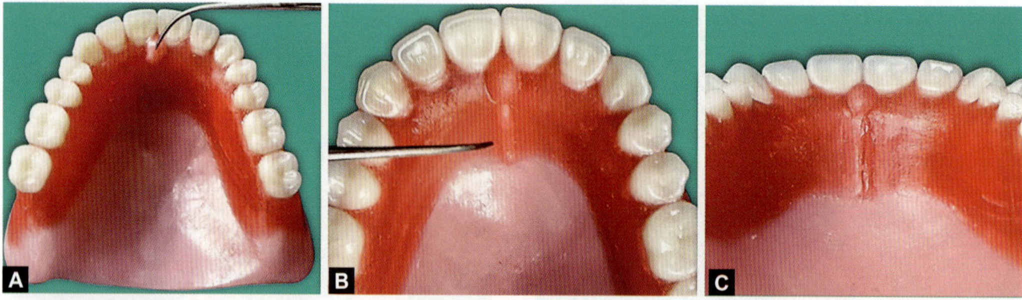

Figs. 25.9A to C: Addition and contouring of wax to make incisive papillae and midpalatine raphe.

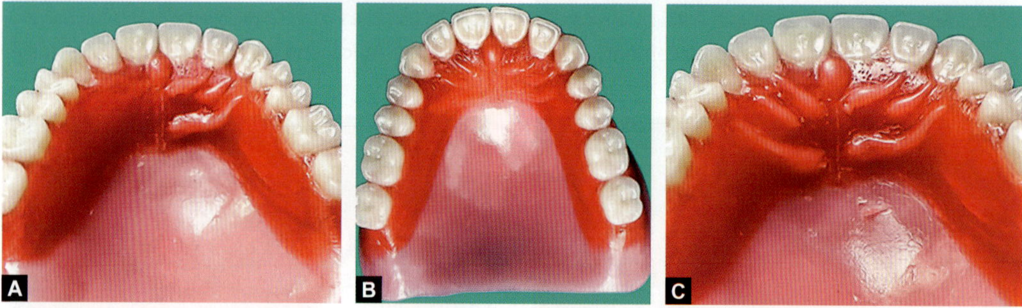

Figs. 25.10A to C: Making rugae on anterior palate.

Step 10

Form the crests and valley of rugae on both the side of midpalatine raphe in anterior palatal area. This will aid in speech **(Figs. 25.10A to C)**.

WAX-UP OF MANDIBULAR COMPLETE DENTURE

Step 1

Soften the modeling wax and add it on buccal and lingual surface of waxed denture. Add wax to cover cervical part of labial surfaces of teeth **(Fig. 25.11)**.

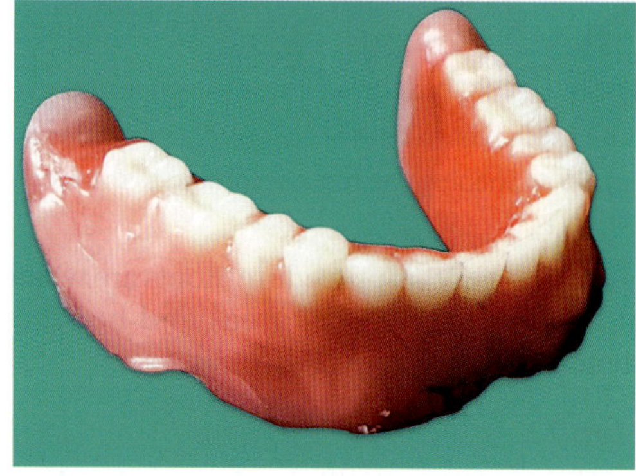

Fig. 25.11: Addition of wax on labial, buccal, and lingual surface.

Step 2

Hold the roach carver at approximately 20° to carve the gingival margin. Shape the interdental papillae and gingival bulge similar to maxillary denture **(Figs. 25.12A to C)**.

Step 3

Place markings for roots on labial surface of denture as shown. The mandibular teeth roots markings are placed vertically **(Fig. 25.13)**.

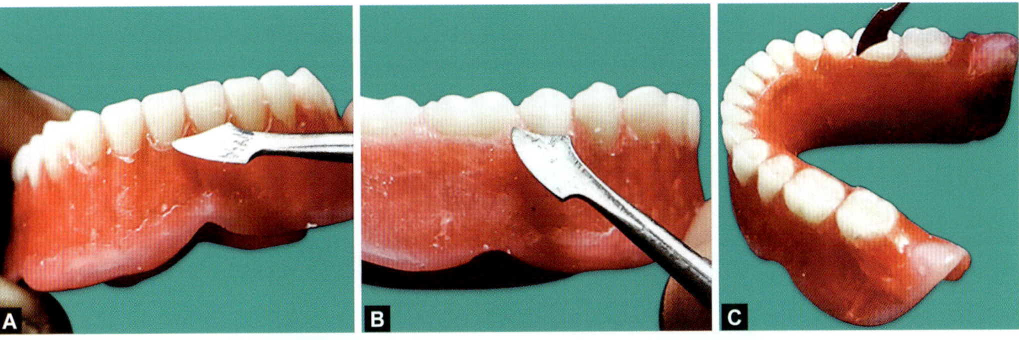

Figs. 25.12A to C: Carving the gingival margins for anterior teeth.

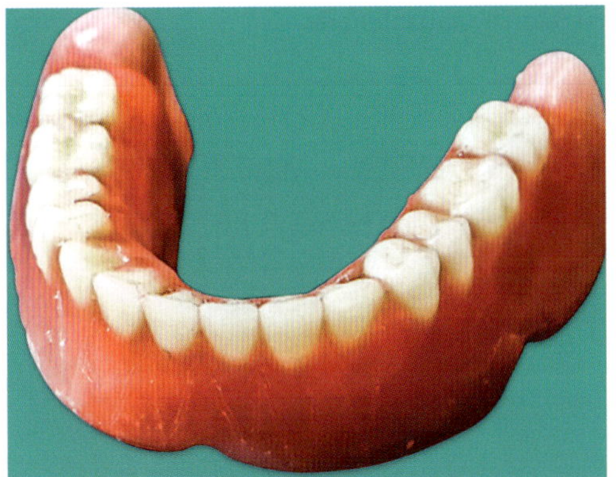

Fig. 25.13: Marking the roots on mandibular trial denture.

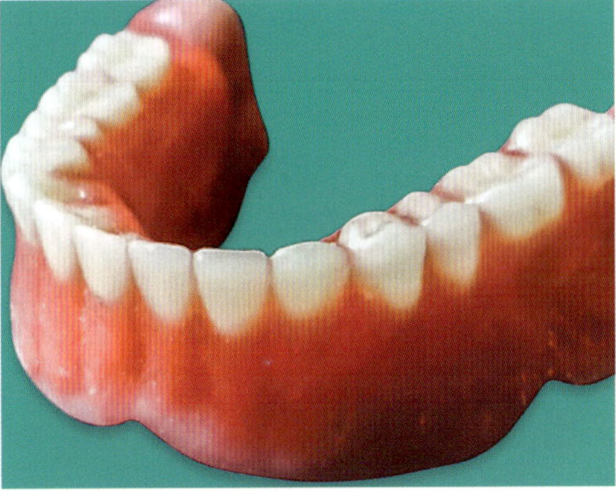

Fig. 25.14: Shaping the roots on trial denture.

Step 4

Remove wax between two root markings and try to give bulge on marking areas. Use carver for this procedure. Roots are wider at beginning (cervical area) and become slender at apical area **(Fig. 25.14)**.

Step 5

Wax the distolingual area of the lingual flange to blend it with retromylohyoid area. Shape the lingual flange as inclined plane to accommodate tongue **(Fig. 25.15)**.

Step 6

Make shallow depression in molar area of mandibular denture. Mandibular buccal flange should incline laterally and inferiorly. Lingual flange should incline medially and inferiorly **(Fig. 25.16)**.

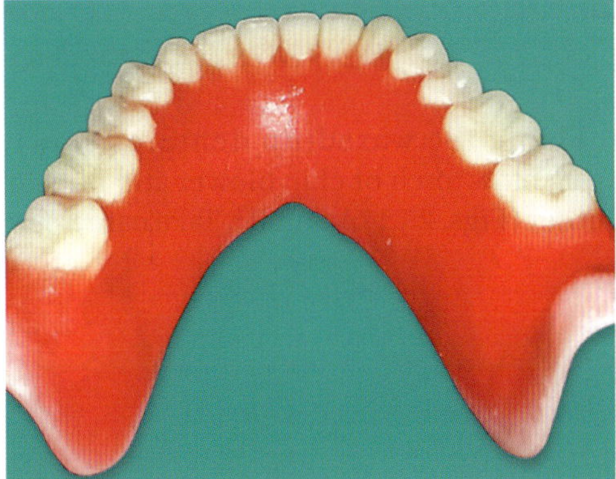

Fig. 25.15: Distobuccal area of lingual flange merged with retromylohyoid area.

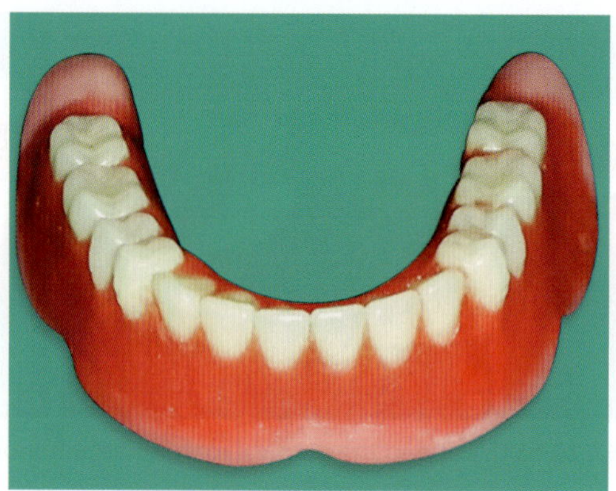

Fig. 25.16: Buccal flange inclines laterally and inferiorly.

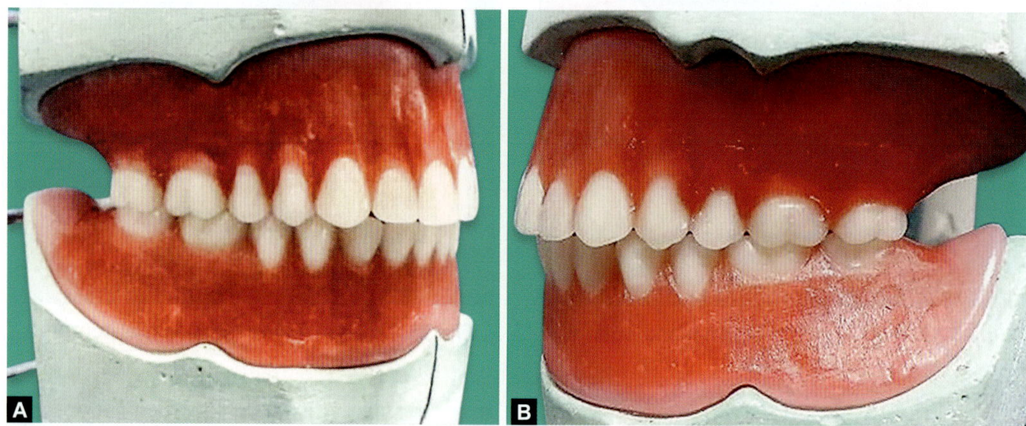

Figs. 25.17A and B: Waxed-up maxillary and mandibular dentures.

Flame the waxed-up dentures slowly using blow torch or chip blower and Bunsen burner **(Figs. 25.17A and B)**. Take care not to overheat and melt the wax. Use toothbrush lightly to give stipple appearance of attached gingival.

Processing of Waxed-up Denture

Paranjay Prajapati, Sneha Kulkarni

INTRODUCTION

The complete denture processing includes flasking procedure, dewaxing (wax elimination) procedures, and curing procedures.

FLASKING PROCEDURE

Step 1 (Fig. 26.1)

Seal the maxillary and mandibular waxed up denture on respective casts. Take care not to disturb the root morphology carved on denture and avoid overfill till the land area. After sealing, close the articulator and re-evaluate the occlusion.

Step 2 (Figs. 26.2 and 26.3)

Safely demount the casts along with sealed try-in denture from mounting plaster of articulator. The indexing should not be fractured while demounting the casts.

Step 3 (Figs. 26.4A and B)

Select the flask that is accurately fitting with its parts without rocking and gap in between parts. Put the cast with sealed try-in denture in the flask and make sure that teeth on trial denture are not projecting out of flask height. There should be equal clearance between cast and wall of the flask.

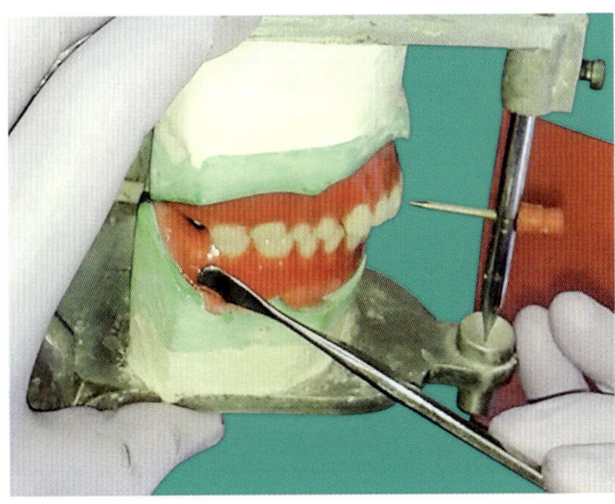

Fig. 26.1: Sealing of waxed-up dentures with casts.

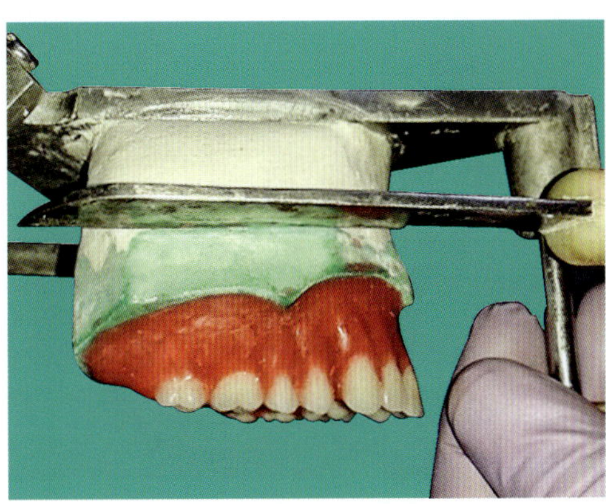

Fig. 26.2: Demounting the cast.

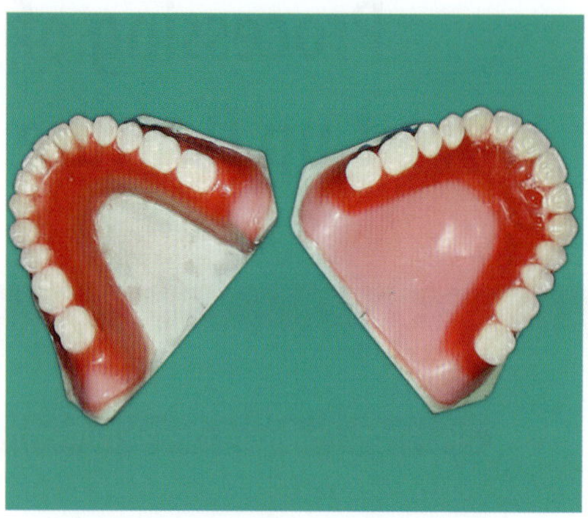

Fig. 26.3: Sealed maxillary and mandibular trial denture on casts.

Step 4 (Fig. 26.5)

Put the casts in slurry water for 5–10 minutes. The casts will take up slurry water hence it will not absorb water from investing plaster. This is required for good union between cast and investing plaster.

If cast absorbs water from investing plaster, it results in weak bonding between them. Mix dental plaster according to recommended water-powder ratio. Manipulate it to make smooth and creamy mixture.

Step 5 (Fig. 26.6)

Pour the smooth, creamy mixture into the base of the flask till two-third of its height.

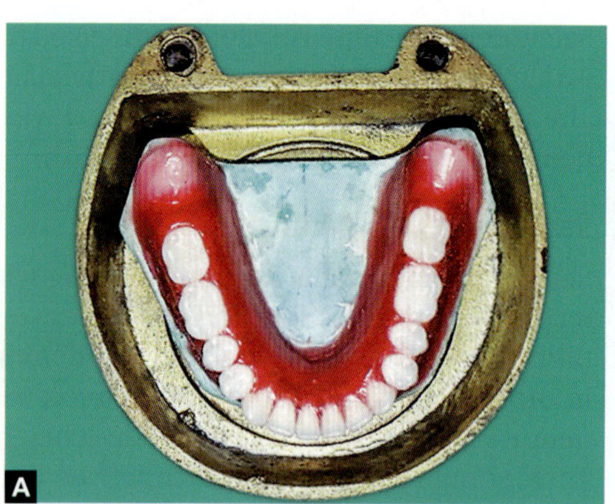

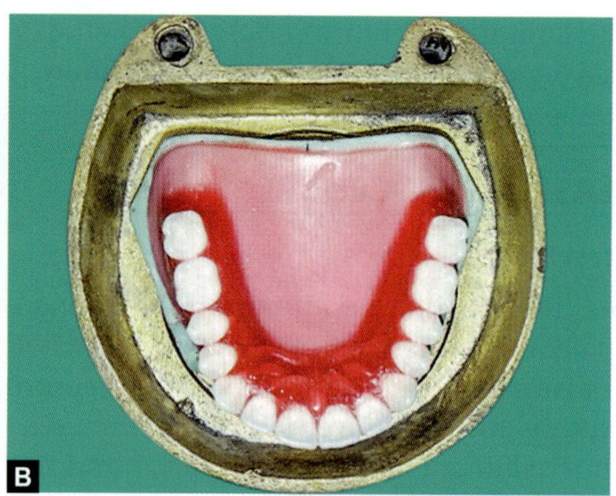

Figs. 26.4A and B: Checking clearance of casts in denture flask.

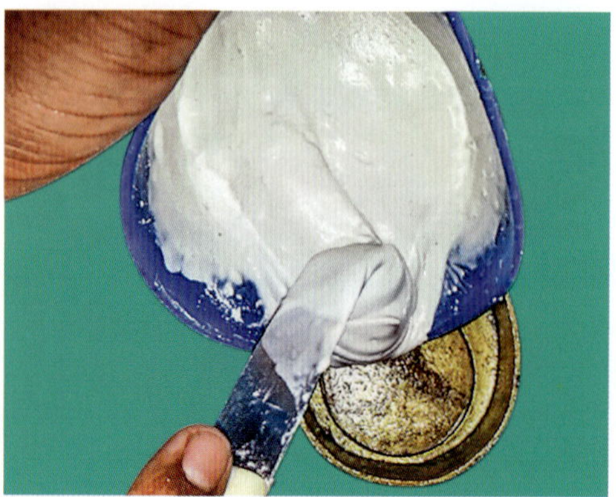

Fig. 26.5: Pouring dental plaster in base of the flask.

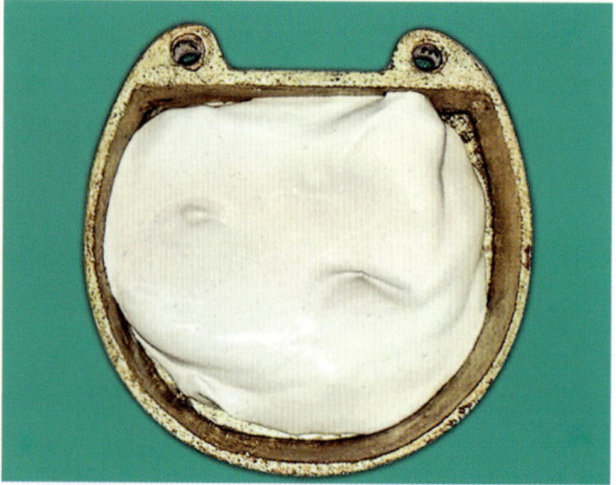

Fig. 26.6: Pour flask till two-third of its height.

Pouring the investing plaster into base of the flask is called as first pour.

Step 6 (Figs. 26.7A and B)

Remove the cast from slurry water and place it in the center of the flask over the investing plaster in such a way that occlusal plane is parallel to base of the flask.

Step 7 (Figs. 26.8 and 26.9)

Smooth the investing plaster around the cast with spatula. Add or remove the plaster as needed. The investing plaster should merge with land area of the cast. There should be inclined surface of investing plaster, starting from land area of the cast to the rim of the flask. Make sure that there is no undercuts in

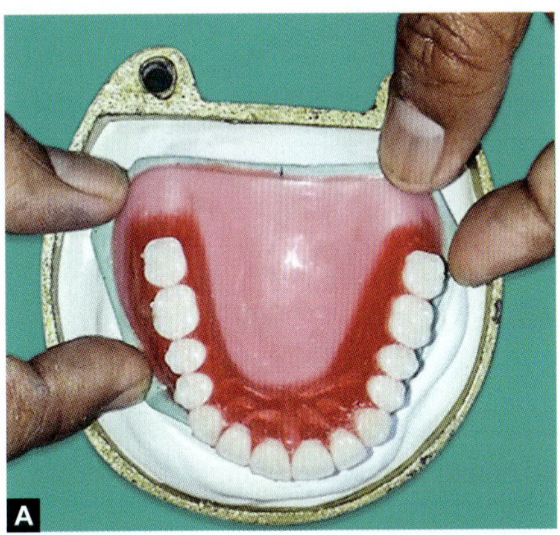

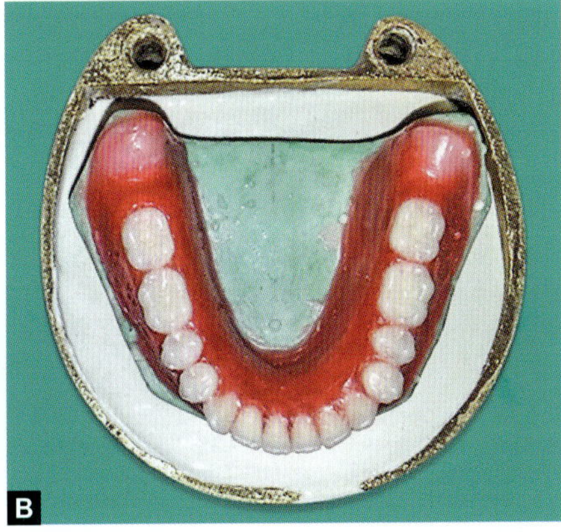

Figs. 26.7A and B: Placement of casts in center of the first pour.

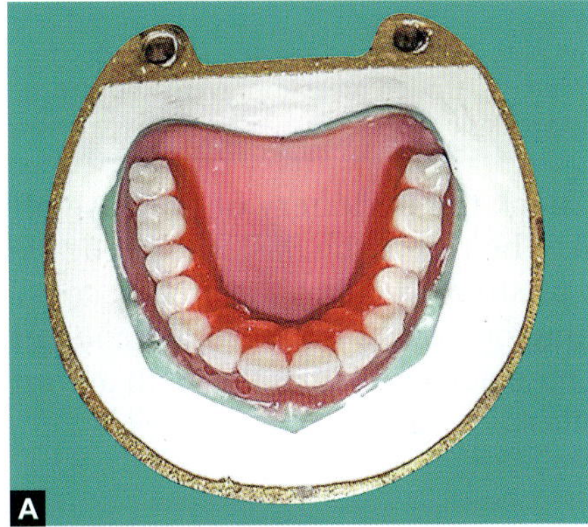

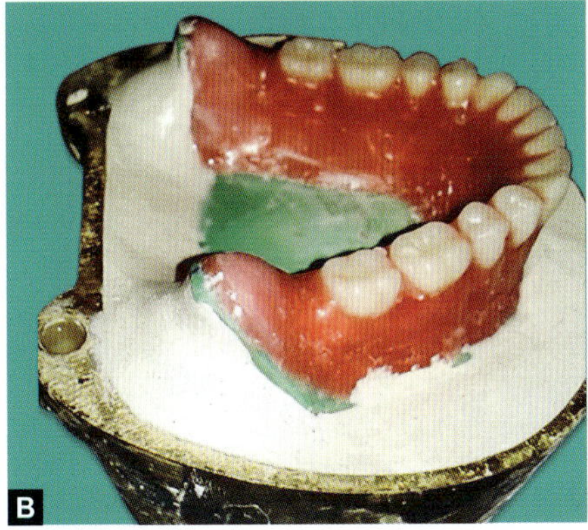

Figs. 26.8A and B: Smooth the investing plaster around the cast with spatula.

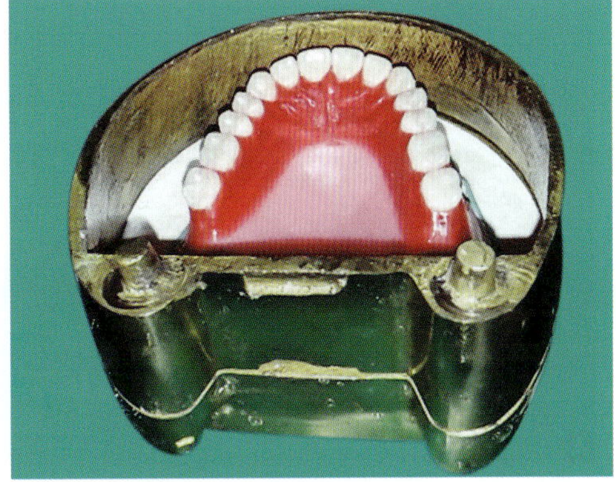

Fig. 26.9: Place the counter and check that the teeth are within height of the flask.

this slope. The heal area of mandibular cast should form a slop at 45° to the rim of the flask. Smooth the investing plaster with wet cotton.

> This part of investing plaster should be free of undercuts. Undercuts will prevent separation of parts of flask.

Check the periphery of the base of the flask. The rim of the flask should be clean. Any plaster on this area will prevent complete seating of parts of flask. Put the counter on the base and check that the teeth are within the flask.

Step 8 (Figs. 26.10A and B)

Apply cold mould seal (separating medium) on first pour. Take care not to apply separating medium on denture base and artificial teeth. Some separating medium may stains acrylic teeth.

Step 9 (Figs. 26.11A and B)

Assemble counter part of flask on base part. Make sure both parts are seating perfectly without any gap in between. Manipulate dental stone according to recommended water powder ratio till it become smooth and creamy mixture.

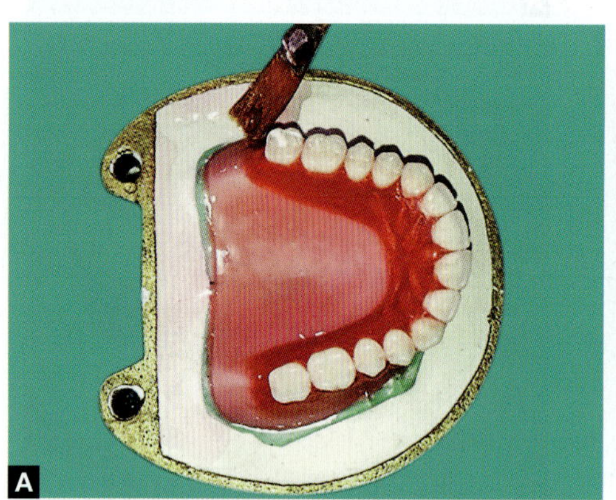
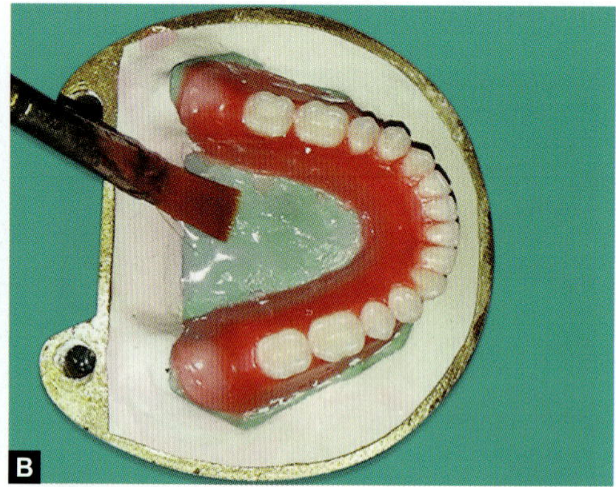

Figs. 26.10A and B: Application of cold mould seal on first pour.

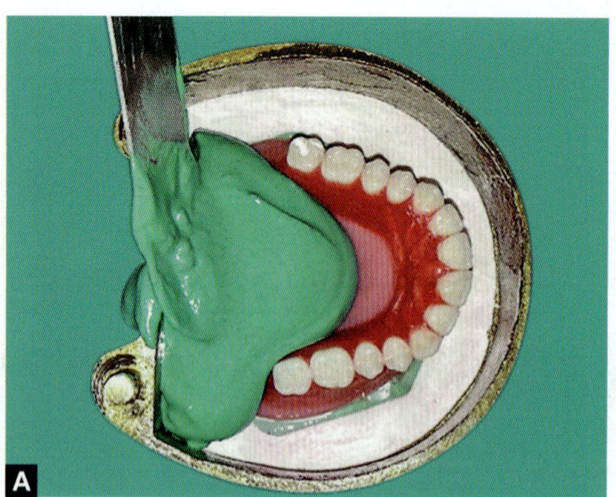
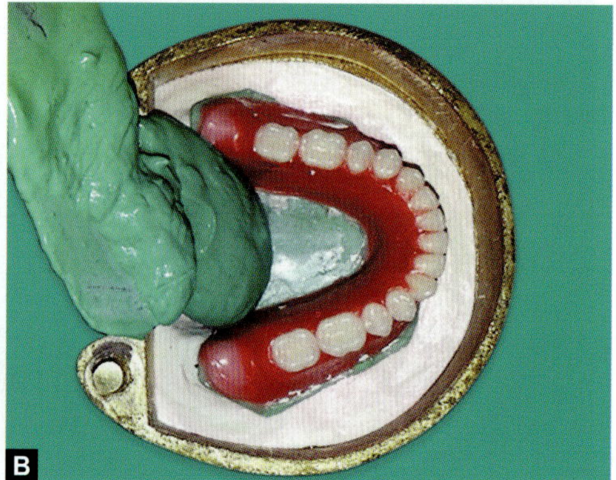

Figs. 26.11A and B: Pouring dental plaster as second pour.

Pour it into flask from one side till it cover all area and reach to other side. Vibrate flask and make sure that dental stone flows and fills all areas without air incorporation.

Step 10 (Figs. 26.12A and B)

Fill the dental stone till incisal and occlusal surfaces. Clean incisal and occlusal surfaces with finger/cotton to expose them.

> This part of flask pouring is called as second pour.

Step 11 (Figs. 26.13A and B)

Manipulate dental plaster according to recommended water-powder ratio till it becomes smooth and creamy mixture. Pour it on exposed incisal and occlusal surface to fill the top surface of flask.

> This part of pouring is called as third pour. Three pour techniques enable easy removal of denture after curing.

Step 12 (Figs. 26.14A and B)

Make sure that, the rim of the flask is clean of any material. Put the lid on the counter of the flask and press it nicely. The excess material will come out from vent holes provided on the lid. Clean any excess material flown out from the flask.

> In two pour technique, the second and third pour is replaced by single pour.

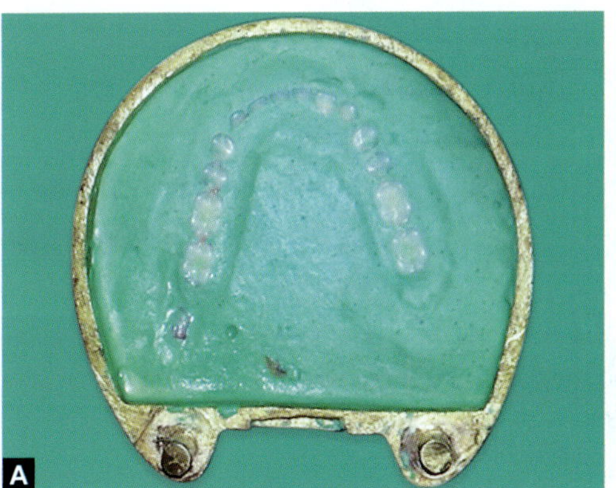

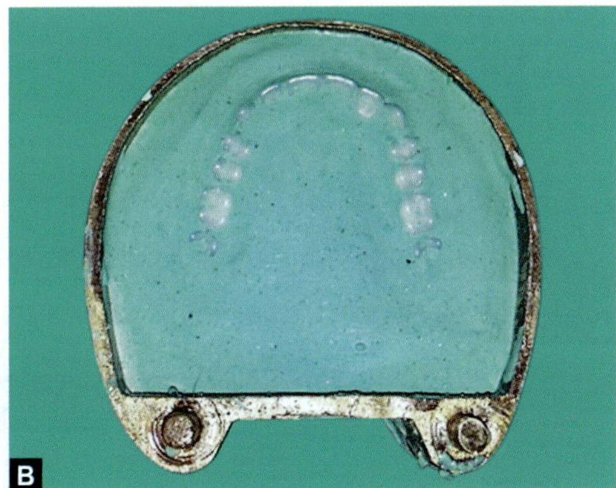

Figs. 26.12A and B: Exposure of incisal and occlusal surfaces.

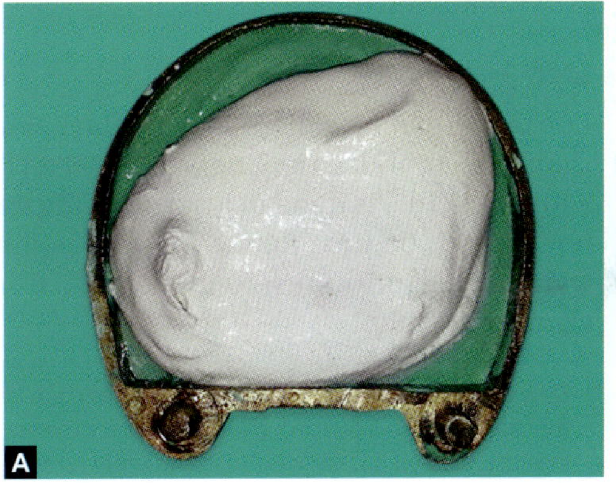

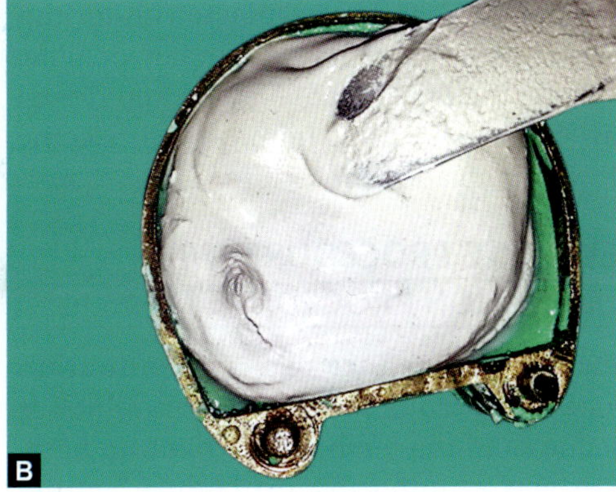

Figs. 26.13A and B: Pouring dental plaster as third pour.

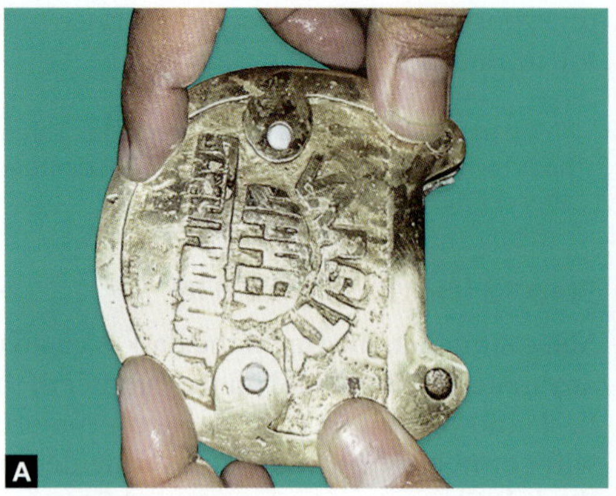
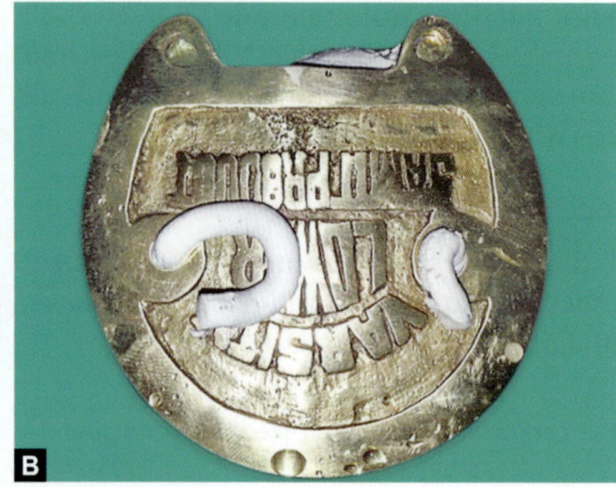

Figs. 26.14A and B: Placement of lid on the flask.

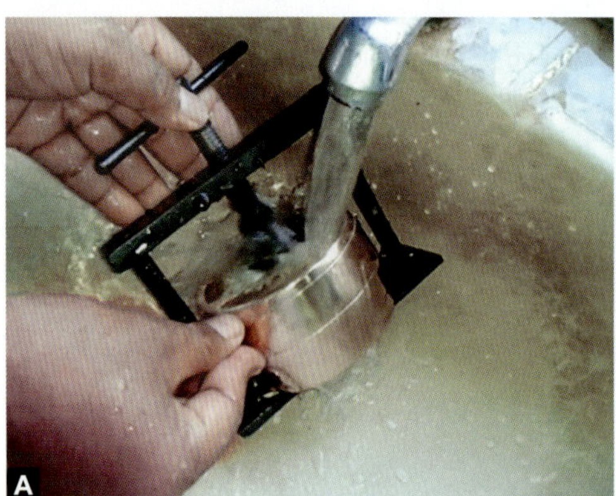
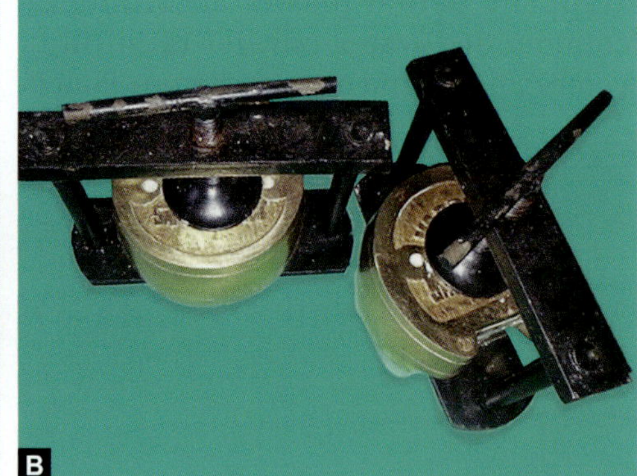

Figs. 26.15A and B: Cleaning the flasks under tap water.

Step 13 (Figs. 26.15A and B)

Put flask into clamp assembly and tighten it properly. Wash excess plaster under tap water. Flasking procedure is completed. Allow investing materials (dental stone and dental plaster) to set for 20–30 minutes before going for wax elimination procedure.

DEWAXING PROCEDURE (WAX ELIMINATION PROCEDURE)

Dewaxing procedure or wax elimination procedure is done to remove wax, which is used to hold the teeth on the denture base. After wax elimination procedure, empty space (mould) is created in which acrylic resin is filled (wax is replaced by acrylic resin). Complete elimination of wax is required to avoid contamination of acrylic.

Step 1

Loosen the clamp slightly. Put flask with clamp assembly into boiling water (100°C) for 5 minutes. This is done to just soften the wax not to melt the wax. Remove it from boiling water after 5 minutes. Remove flask from clamp assembly.

> Dewaxing for longer time will lead to dispersion of the wax into the investing plaster. Once it disperse into the plaster, it is difficult to completely remove the wax.

Step 2 (Figs. 26.16A and B)

Place plaster knife on joint between base part and counter part of the flask. Hit slowly on plaster knife with rubber hammer to open flask.

> Be careful while opening the flask. Molten wax may burn skin. Safety precautions should be practiced during this exercise. Use eyewear, heavy duty gloves to protect yourself from boiling water and steam.

Step 3 (Figs. 26.17A and B)

Carefully remove temporary record base.

Wash out molten wax with hot water mixed with soap water. Continue to pour hot water till elimination of all traces of wax. Finally wash it with clean hot water **(Figs. 26.18 and 26.19)**.

> Soap water will react with gypsum and form a membrane impermeable to wax. This prevents wax from dispersion in investing dental plaster.

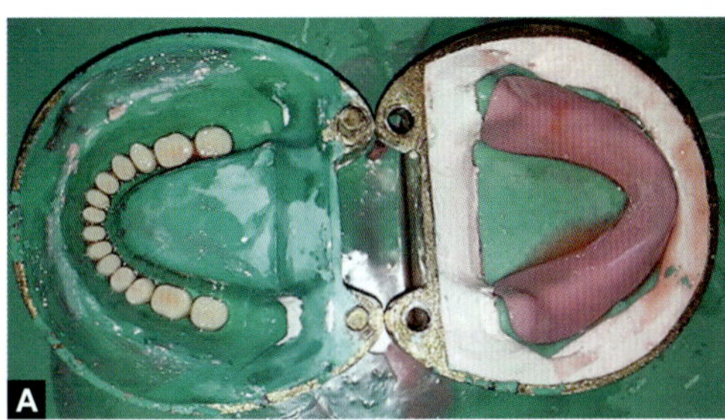

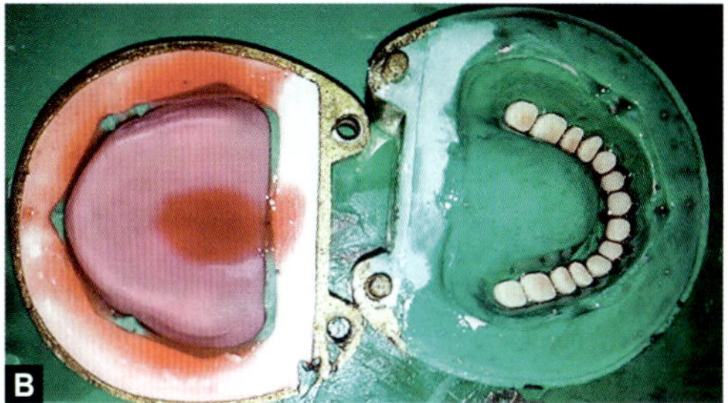

Figs. 26.16A and B: Opening of flasks after dewaxing procedure.

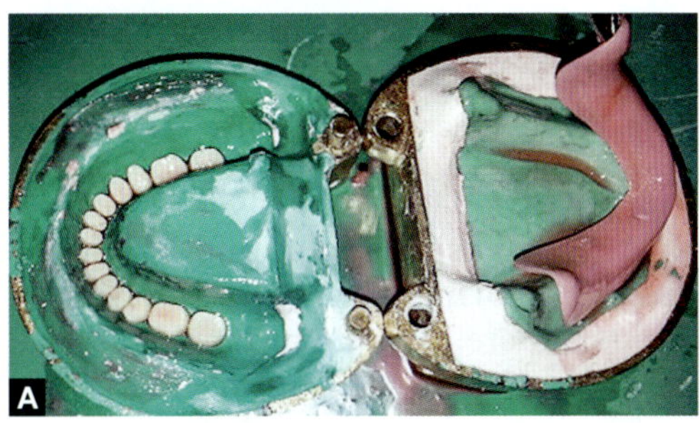

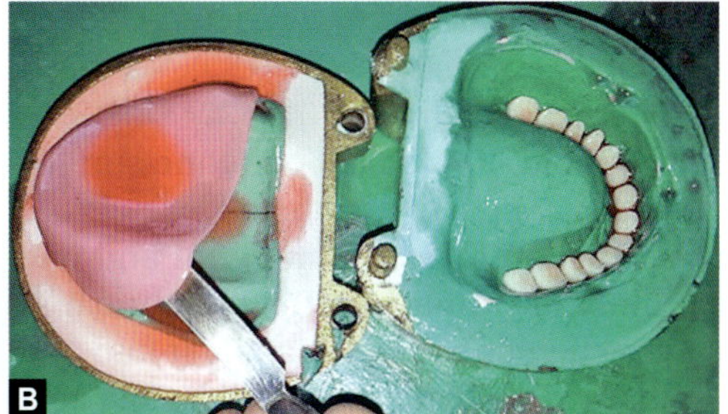

Figs. 26.17A and B: Removal of temporary record base.

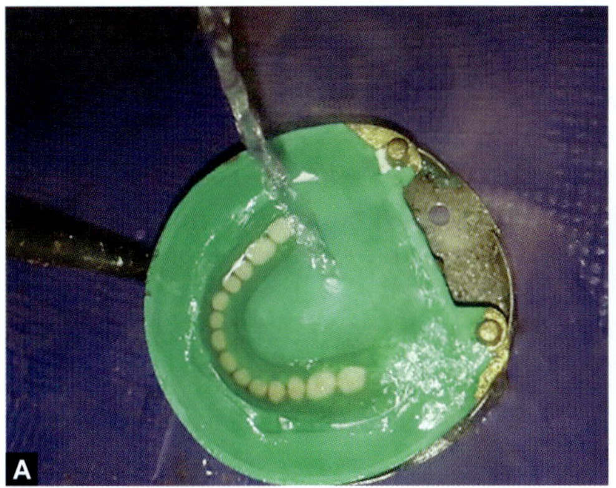

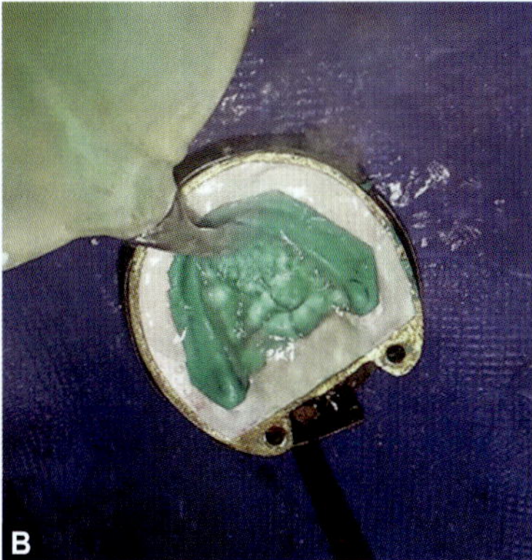

Figs. 26.18A and B: Wax elimination with hot water.

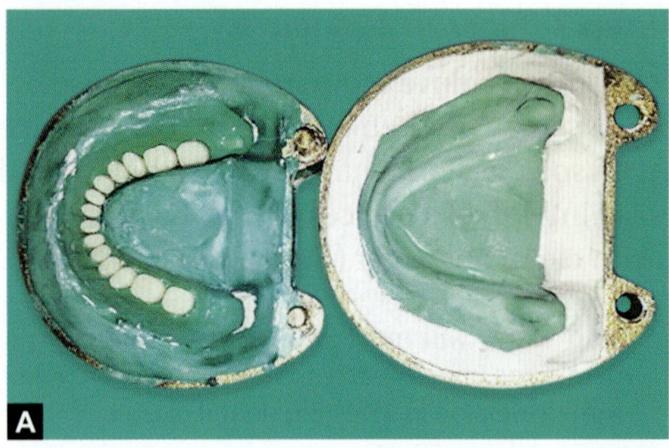
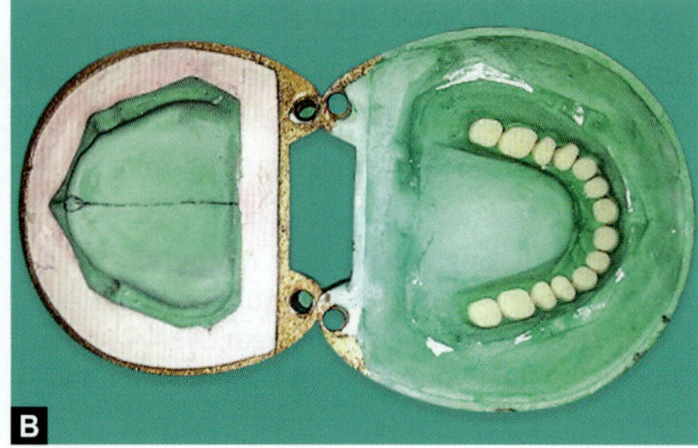

Figs. 26.19A and B: Complete removal of wax.

PACKING THE ACRYLIC RESIN IN THE MOULD

Armamentarium (Fig. 26.20)

- Heat cure acrylic resin (polymer and monomer)
- Cold mould seal
- Painting brush
- Wax knife
- Dappen dish/dish
- Cellophane sheets
- Porcelain jar with lid.

Apply cold mould seal on stone surface in the flask. Apply two to three coats of cold mould seal on investing material and one coat on casts. Apply it with clean brush in one direction only. Do not apply it into and fro motion. Do not apply it on ridge lap area of teeth. Allow the flask to cool down to room temperature before packing procedure **(Figs. 26.21A to D)**.

> Apply one coat of cold mould seal immediately after dewaxing procedure when the flask and investment plaster is still warm. Apply second coat immediately before packing the acrylic resin.

> Apply cold mould seal in one direction only. If applied into and fro motion, it removes formed thin layer of calcium alginate which is separating layer.

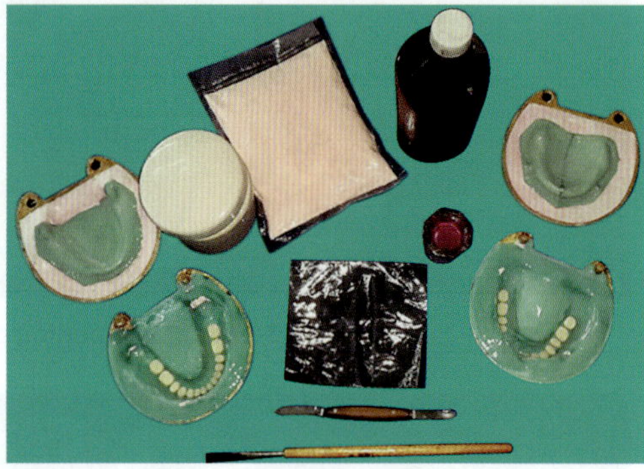

Fig. 26.20: Armamentarium of the acrylic resin in the mould.

Acrylic resin is supplied as polymer (powder) and monomer (liquid). Polymer and monomer are mixed in recommended ratio, i.e. 3:1 by volume or 2:1 by weight.

There are five physical stages of resin manipulation like wet sand stage, stringy stage, dough-like stage, and stiff or plastic stage. The ideal stage to pack resin into mould is dough stage.

Wet Sand Stage (Fig. 26.22)

In the first stage of resin manipulation, the material is grainy in consistency.

Stringy Stage (Fig. 26.23)

This is the second stage of resin manipulation. In this stage, material is sticky in consistency.

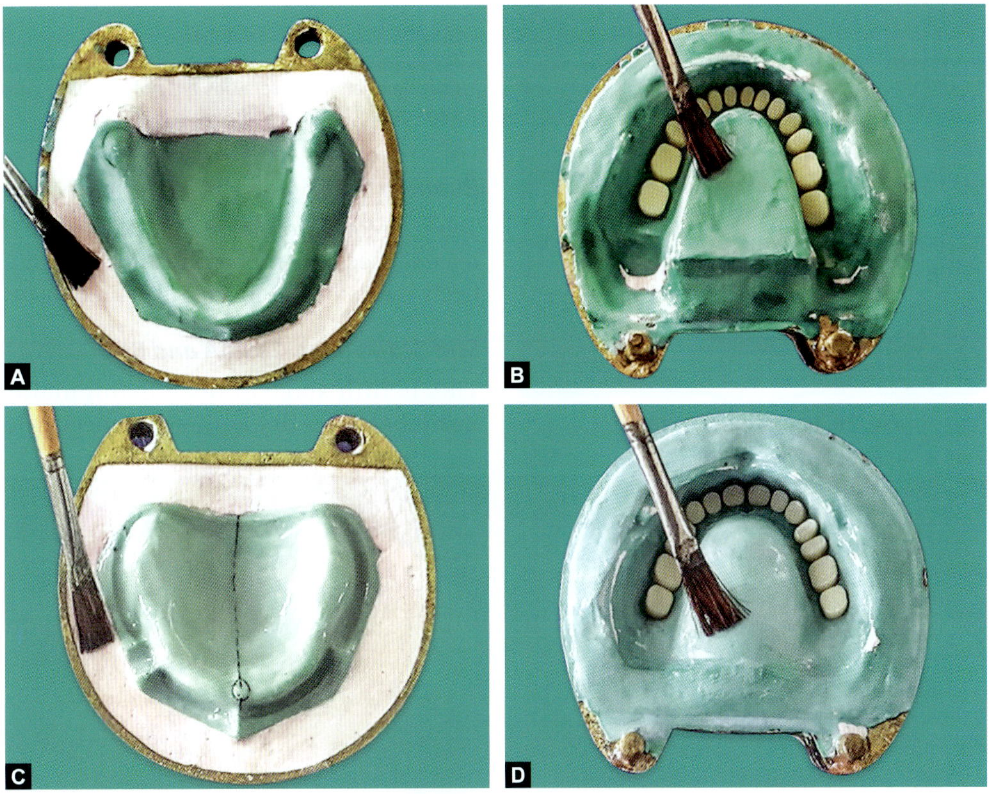

Figs. 26.21A to D: Application of cold mould seal before packing the acrylic resin.

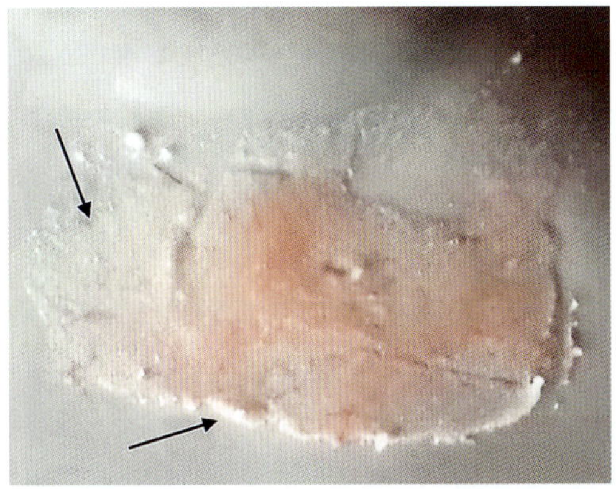

Fig. 26.22: Wet sand stage (Arrows).

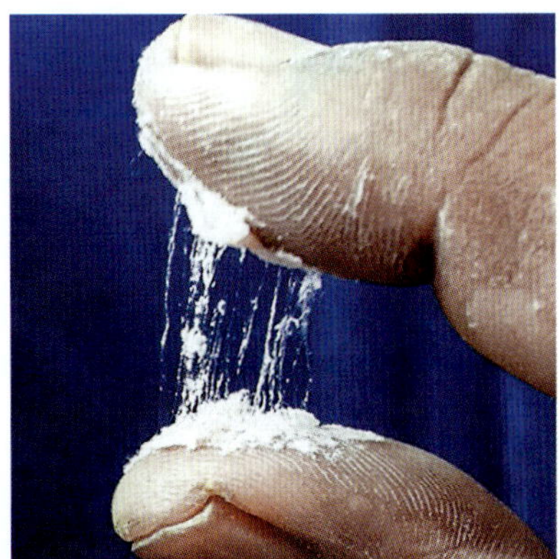

Fig. 26.23: Stringy stage.

Dough-like Stage (Fig. 26.24)

It is the third stage of resin manipulation. Material in this stage has no stickiness. It becomes pliable and can be easily separated from the porcelain jar. Manipulation is easy in this stage. Material in this stage can flow easily and can be molded according to desired shape.

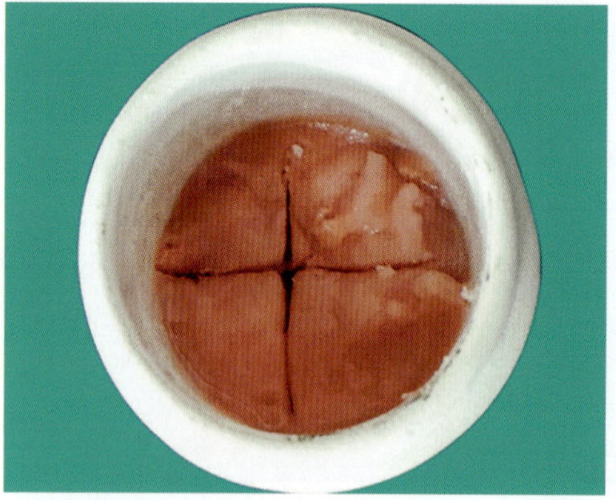

Fig. 26.24: Dough-like stage.

How to check dough-like stage?
Try to separate material in two or more sections in porcelain jar. If the sections are not merging with each other than it is in dough-like stage.

Rubbery Stage (Figs. 26.25A and B)

This is the fourth stage of resin manipulation. The material becomes rubbery and no longer flows freely and cannot be molded in desired shape.

Stiff Stage (Figs. 26.26A and B)

This is fifth stage of resin manipulation. Resin becomes dry and resists mechanical

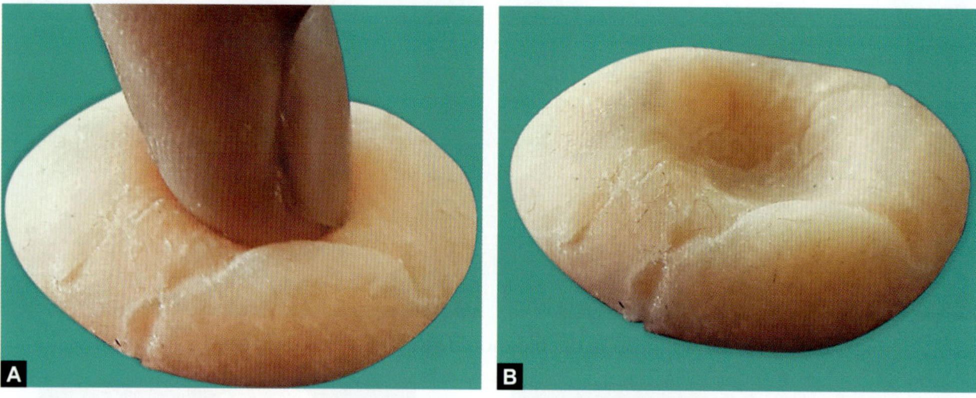

Figs. 26.25A and B: Rubbery stage—excess pressure needed to manipulate rubber consistency.

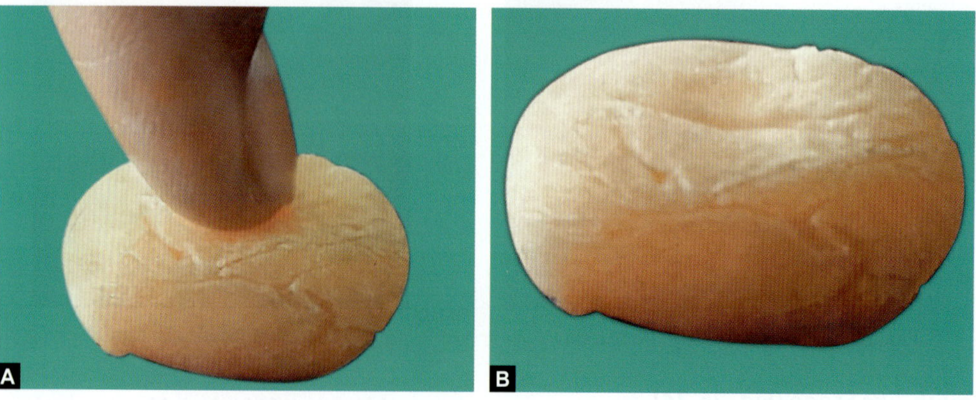

Figs. 26.26A and B: Stiff stage becomes dry that cannot be molded.

deformation. It cannot be molded in desired shape.

Measuring the Polymer and Monomer by Volume (Figs. 26.27 and 26.28)

Take a dappen dish to measure quantity of polymer and monomer by volume. Take one dappen dish full of monomer and shift it into the porcelain jar. Take polymer full of dappen dish three times and shift it in porcelain jar to mix with monomer. Close the porcelain jar with lid.

This will prevent evaporation of monomer and so prevent any change in polymer monomer ratio.

> Take correct volume of polymer and monomer. Excess monomer increases the polymerization shrinkage and less monomer results in porosity.

Step 1 (Figs. 26.29 and 26.30)

Remove the acrylic resin from the jar when it reaches the stringy stage or early dough stage. Kneading is done to improve handling characteristics. Packing is done when it is in dough-like stage. Wear gloves to avoid contamination of resin. Adapt the resin in the mould of the flask. Place the wet cellophane sheet over the acrylic resin.

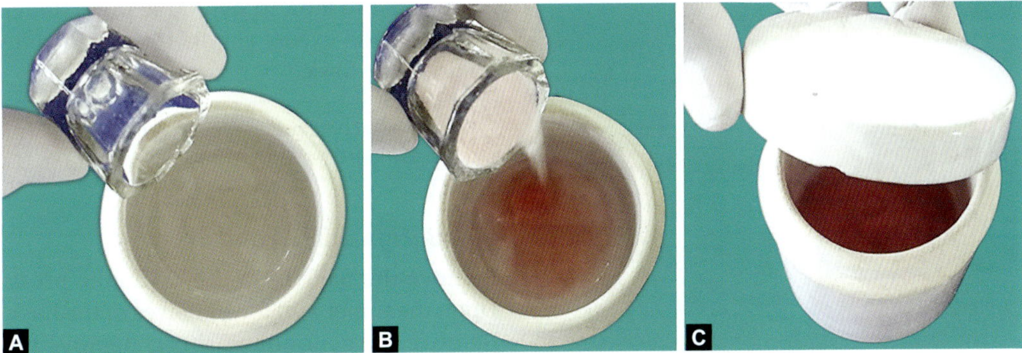

Figs. 26.27A to C: Take monomer and polymer in porcelain jar.

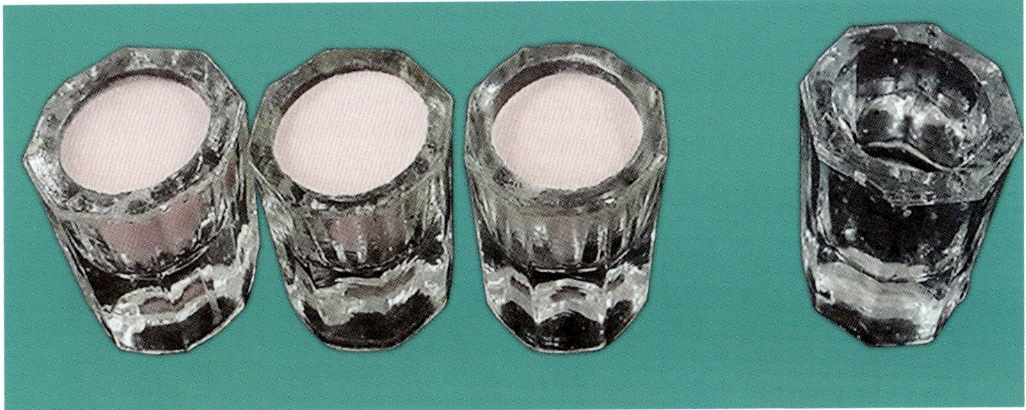

Fig. 26.28: Measuring correct polymer to monomer ratio (3:1) by volume.

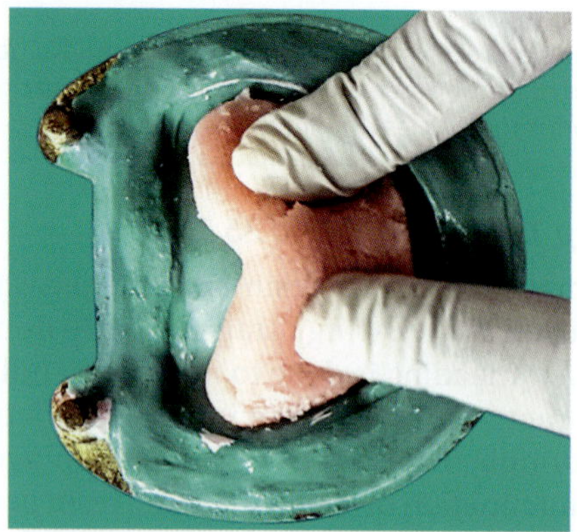

Fig. 26.29: Packing acrylic in the mould.

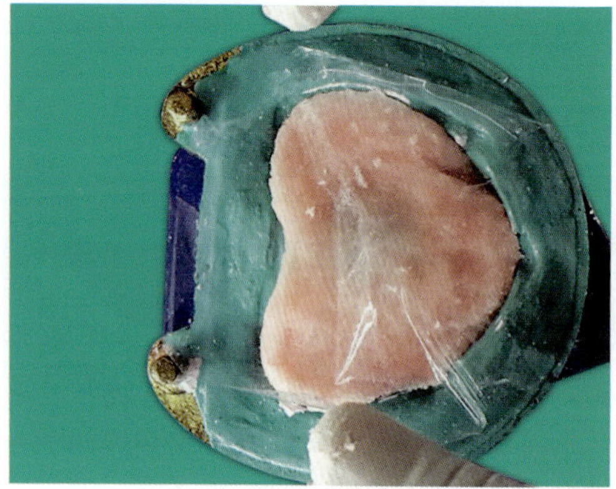

Fig. 26.30: Cover the acrylic with cellophane sheet.

Step 2 (Fig. 26.31)

Place the second half of the flask over the wet cellophane sheet and close it. Make sure that two halves of flasks are in correct contact.

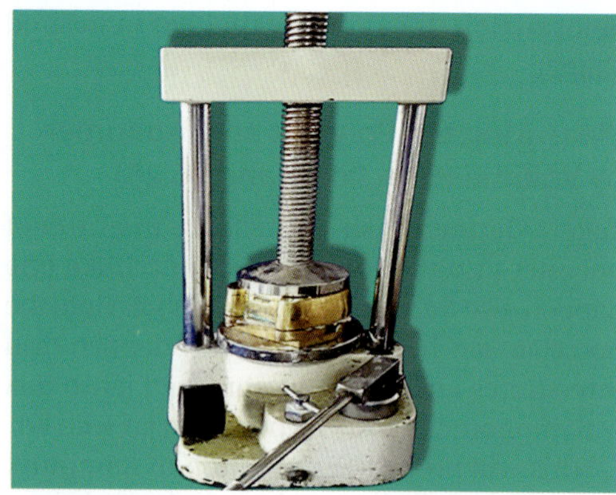

Fig. 26.31: Compress the flask under hydraulic press.

Compress the flask in hydraulic press under 1,500 psi. The excess acrylic resin will come out from the flask.

> The excess acrylic resin coming out from flask is called as "flash".

Step 3 (Figs. 26.32A and B)

Remove the flask from the hydraulic press. Open the upper and lower halves of the flask. Remove the cellophane sheet. Remove the excess material with a blunt knife without making scratch on the plaster surface. Repeat the procedure till all excess material is removed.

> This procedure of removing excess material is known as "trial closure".

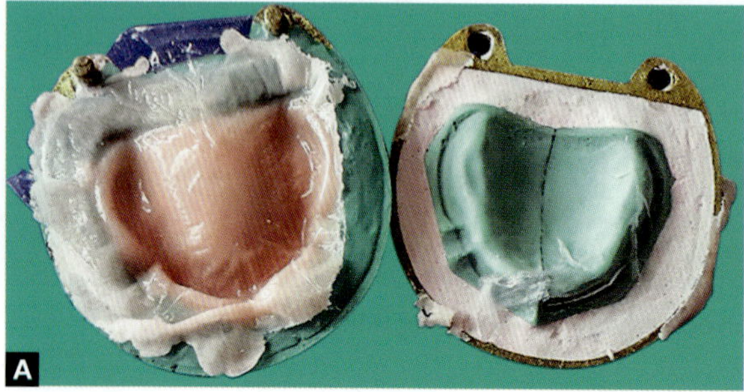

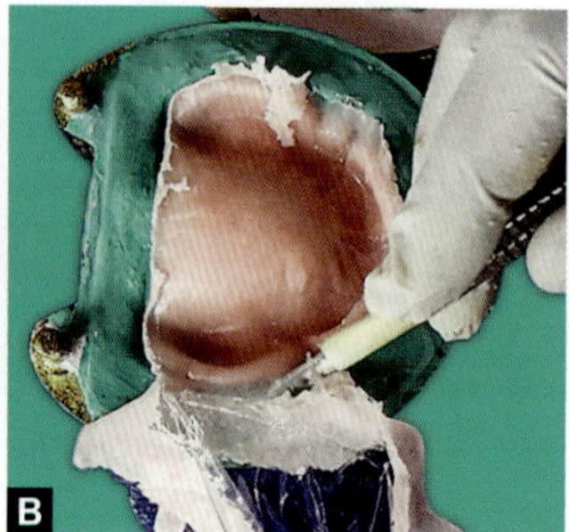

Figs. 26.32A and B: Removal of flash with blunt knife.

Step 4 (Figs. 26.33A and B)

Apply another coat of separating medium on the stone surface before final closure of flask. Do not place cellophane sheet during final closure.

Step 5 (Fig. 26.34)

Tighten the flask in hydraulic press under 3,500 psi. Then transfer flask in manual bench press. The flask is kept in bench press for 30 minutes before heat processing under water bath. This is called as "bench curing". Remove flask from manual press and place in clamps.

> *Bench curing:* A stage of resin processing that allows a chemical reaction to occur under the conditions present in the ambient environment.

HEAT PROCESSING/CURING/ POLYMERIZATION

Heat processing of acrylic resin is done in water bath. The laboratory equipment used for acrylization procedure is called as "acrylizer unit" **(Fig. 26.35)**. This unit has temperature and time controlling system.

The curing cycle/polymerization cycle is technical term for the heating process used to polymerize the resin. It controls the temperature for definite time for polymerization. There are two types of curing cycles depending upon the duration and temperature. They are short curing cycle and long curing cycle.

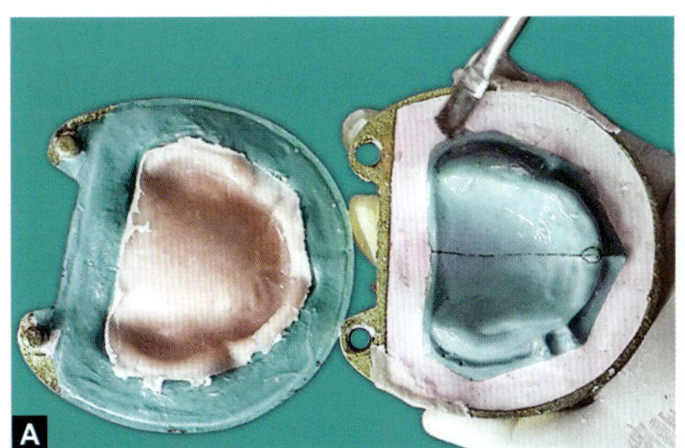

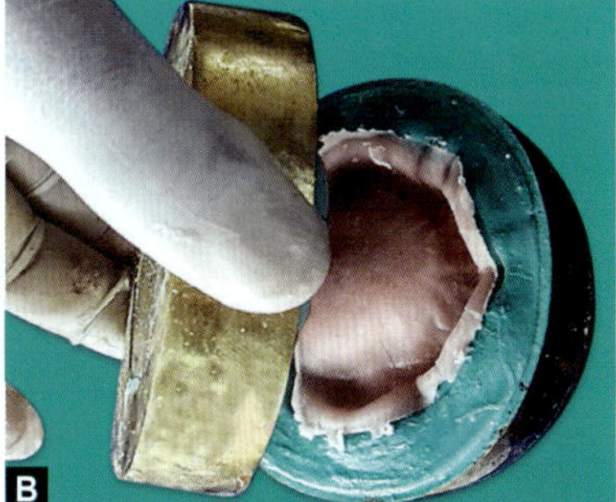

Figs. 26.33A and B: Apply one coat of cold mould seal on the cast and proceed for final closure.

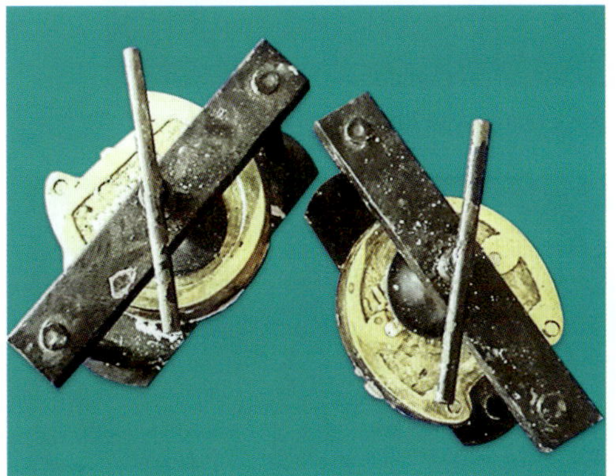

Fig. 26.34: Flasks placed in clamps.

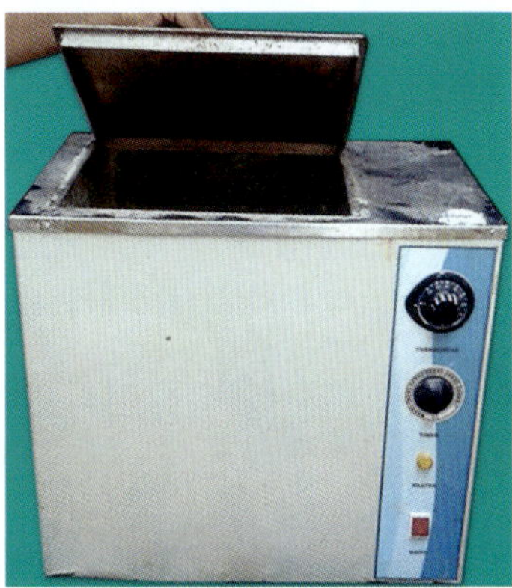

Fig. 26.35: Acrylizer unit for polymerization of heat cure acrylic resin.

Short Curing Cycle

In this curing cycle, flask are kept in water bath at 74°C for 1.5 hours and then temperature is raised till 100°C and maintained for 1 hour.

Long Curing Cycle

In this cycle, the temperature is kept at 74°C for 8–9 hours.

> The boiling point of monomer is 100.8°C. Temperature rise beyond this will lead to boiling of monomer resulting in denture porosity.

The flask after heat processing should be left in the water bath for slow cooling till the room temperature. Sudden cooling of flask can result in warpage of denture due to differential thermal contraction of resin and investing gypsum products. Ideally it should be cooled for overnight.

DEFLASKING PROCEDURE

Deflasking is separation of flask in two parts after curing procedure.

Step 1

Remove the flask from the clamps. Try to open the flask (base and counterparts of the flask) by engaging the curved end of wax knife or use plaster knife as shown in **Figures 26.36A and B**.

Step 2 (Figs. 26.37A and B)

The counterpart of the flask is open from both the side. Slowly tap the outer surface of the counter to loosen and break the investment plaster.

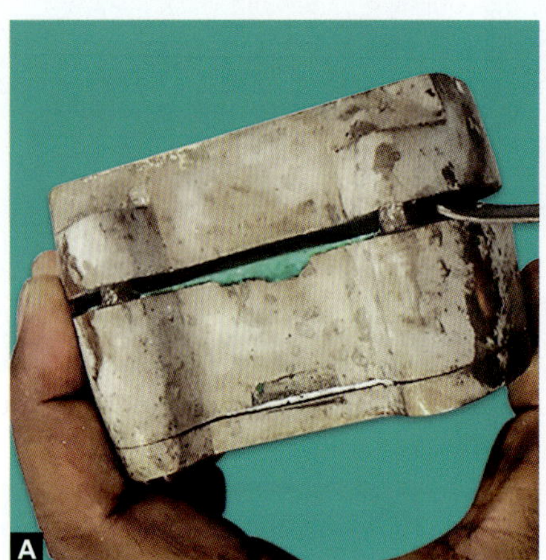

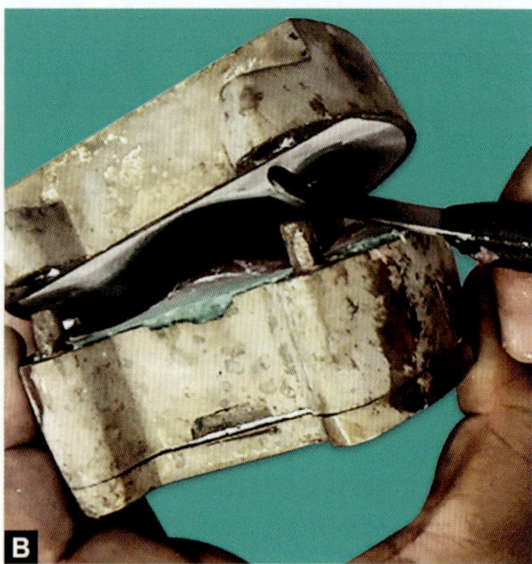

Figs. 26.36A and B: Opening of denture flask using wax knife or plaster knife.

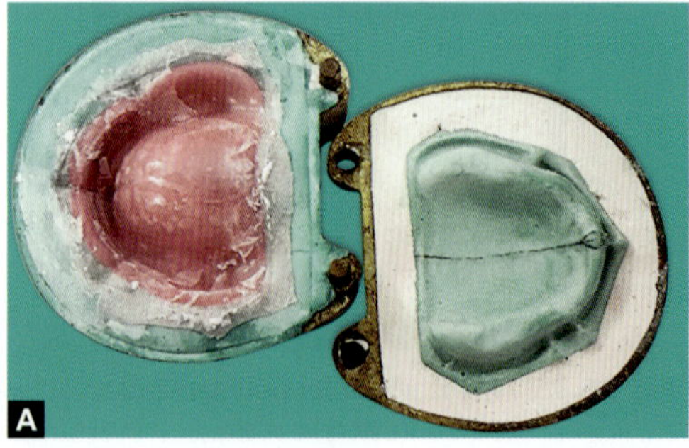

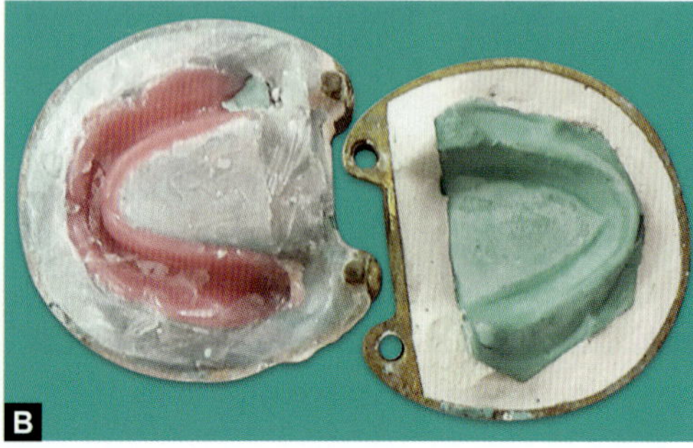

Figs. 26.37A and B: Opening of flasks.

Step 3 (Fig. 26.38)

Retrieve the denture carefully from the investment plaster.

REMOUNT PROCEDURE AND SELECTIVE GRINDING

Objective

There are chances of alteration in teeth position during waxing, packing, and processing procedures. These alterations in teeth position may lead to occlusal discrepancy and premature contacts.

To correct these altered position of teeth and to obtain a smooth even contact of the teeth in centric and eccentric positions, remounting and selective grinding procedure is done.

Processing Errors

During flasking and processing changes in the occlusion may occur due to several possible causes called processing errors.

Processing errors are due to following reasons:

- Dimensional changes in the wax after setting up of the teeth can cause teeth movement.
- During the curing process of heat cure acrylic resin, acrylic resin expands and contracts.

  It expands as the polymerizing temperature is reached then starts to contract (polymerization shrinkage).

  Then as it cools to room temperature it contracts again.

  The total effect of this dimensional change is a slight shrinkage which may change the position of the teeth.
- The expansion of the investing material during the processing may change teeth position.
- The pressure of the flask press during packing affects teeth position.

In order to correct these errors, the dentures are returned to the articulator after deflasking.

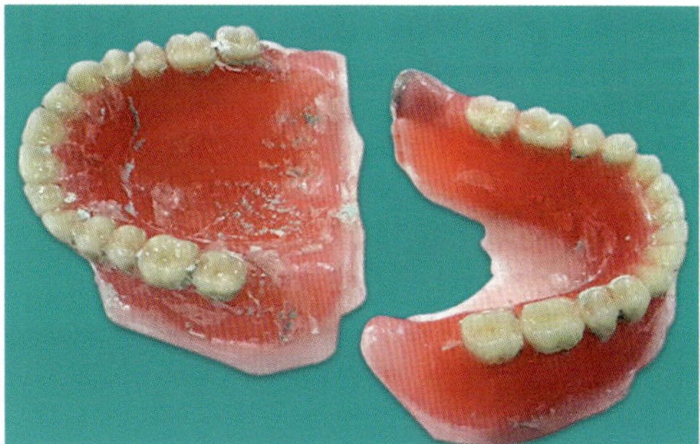

Fig. 26.38: Maxillary and mandibular dentures retrieved from investment.

The casts are repositioned on the original plaster mountings using the indexing (notch indexing or groove indexing) in the base of the cast.

If the incisal pin does not touch the incisal guide table after remounting it means that the occlusal vertical dimension has been changed and must be re-established. Selective grinding is exercised to re-establish vertical dimension of occlusion.

Selective Grinding

Selective grinding is carried out using articulating paper to mark the area of premature contacts.

Red articulating paper is used to mark centric occlusion contacts and blue articulating paper for the eccentric occlusion contacts. Grinding of premature contacts is done with small green or diamond stones.

As a rule in selective grinding the centric holding cusps or functional cusps are not altered. In maxillary arch palatal cusps are functional cusps and in mandibular arch buccal cusps are functional cusps.

These cusps are essential to maintain the recorded vertical dimension. So, if interference exists, reduce either upper buccal cusps or lower lingual cusps to establish the correct vertical dimension of occlusion. This is called BULL rule.

BULL rule: **B**uccal **U**pper and **L**ower **L**ingual (cusps to be reduced during selective grinding procedure)

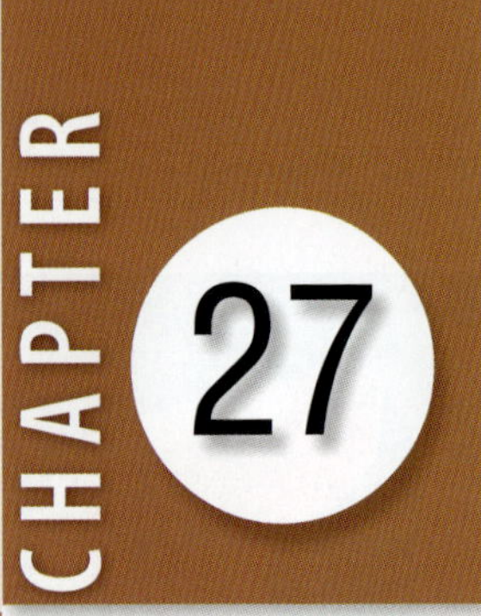

Finishing and Polishing of Complete Denture

Paranjay Prajapati, Jignesh Chaudhari

INTRODUCTION

Finishing is removal of gross surface roughness. It is usually done with laboratory bur, aluminum oxide acrylic trimmer, and sand paper. Polishing is done to smoothen the surface and to give luster or polish to the surface.

FINISHING THE DENTURE

Step 1 (Figs. 27.1A and B)

Remove the mounting plaster from denture surface. Take care while removing plaster from the impression surface. Sharp BP blade can be used to remove investing plaster/stone from interdental areas.

Step 2

Use tungsten carbide laboratory bur mounted on micromotor straight handpiece to trim excess material from borders of dentures **(Fig. 27.2)**.

Use fine tungsten carbide laboratory bur to finish the flanges. Do not apply excess pressure while finishing, it may cause indentation on surface of denture flanges **(Figs. 27.3A and B)**.

Step 3 (Fig. 27.4)

Use straight fissure bur or small round bur to remove investing plaster from interdental areas. Make appropriate notches in frenum areas to relieve frenum. The notch for labial frenum is long and narrow and notches for

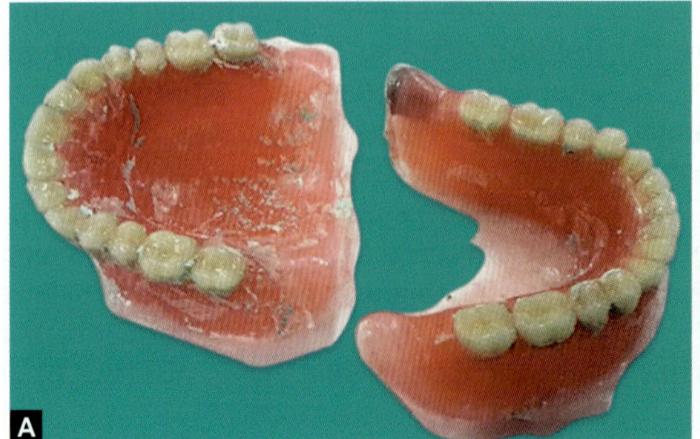

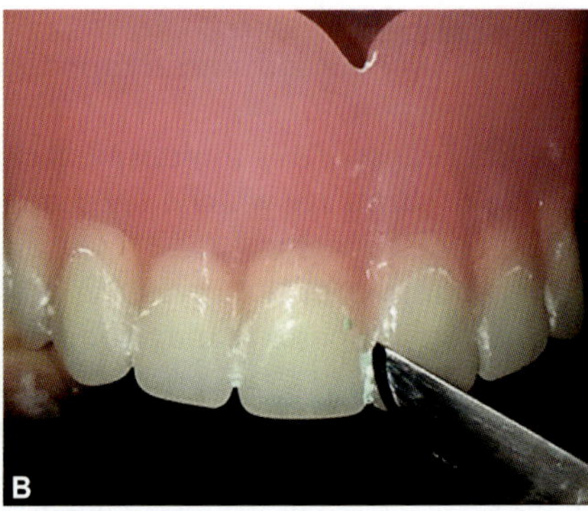

Figs. 27.1A and B: Remove mounting plaster from denture surface.

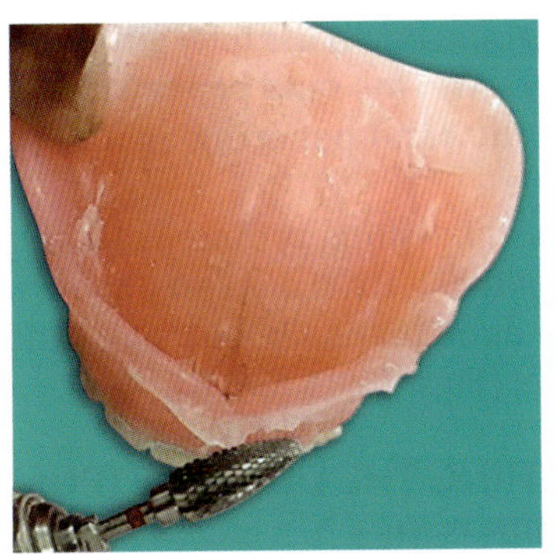

Fig. 27.2: Trimming excess material from denture borders.

lingual and buccal frenum are wider and shallow.

Step 4 (Fig. 27.5)

Smoothen the flanges and borders using aluminum oxide mounted acrylic trimmer. Take care of root morphology while trimming. Follow the contour of root bulges.

Step 5 (Fig. 27.6)

Use rubber point mounted on straight hand-piece to remove scratches from the denture surface.

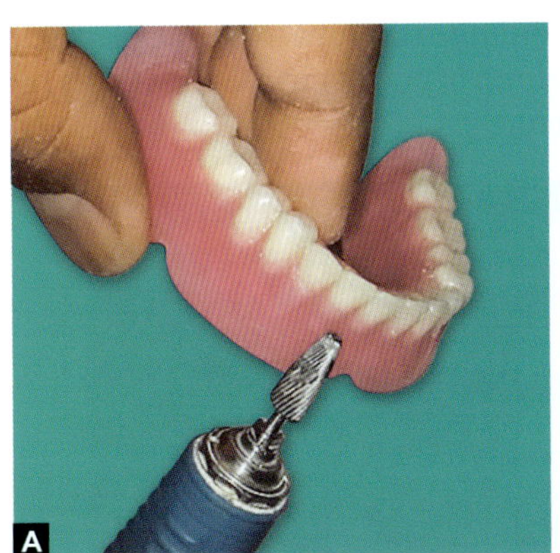

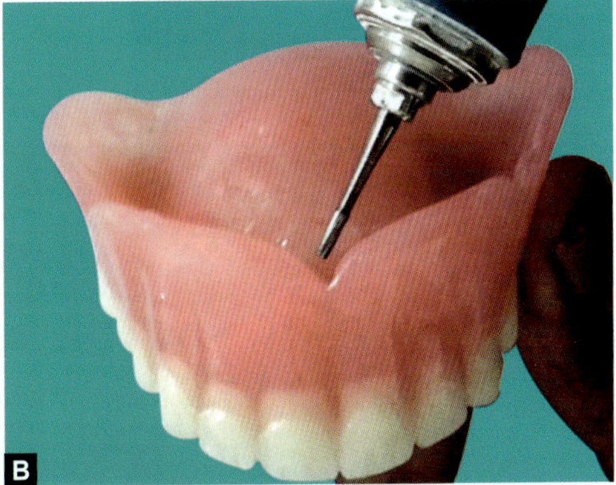

Figs. 27.3A and B: Finishing of denture using fine tungsten carbide laboratory bur.

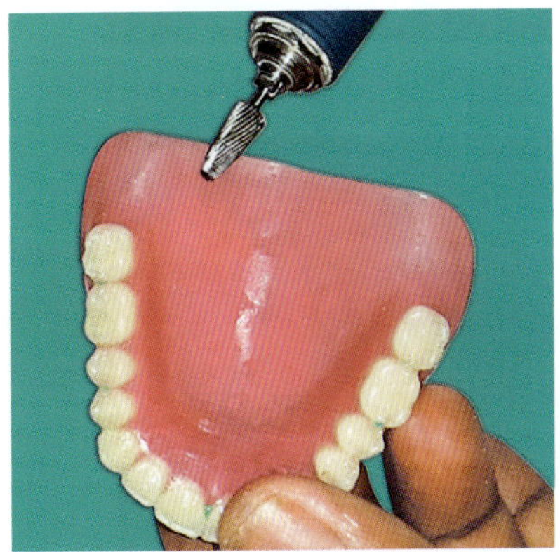

Fig. 27.4: Use straight fissure bur to create notch for frenum.

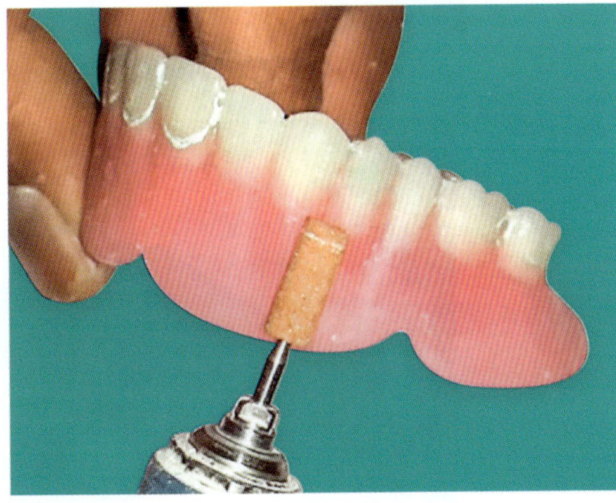

Fig. 27.5: Use of aluminum oxide acrylic trimmer for finishing.

Step 6 (Figs. 27.7A and B)

Use sand papers of various grit sizes to smoothen the polish surface of denture. Start sand papering with coarse sand paper (80–100 number) and finally use finer grit size (250–300 number). Wet the sand paper with water and repeat the sand papering again (wet sand papering).

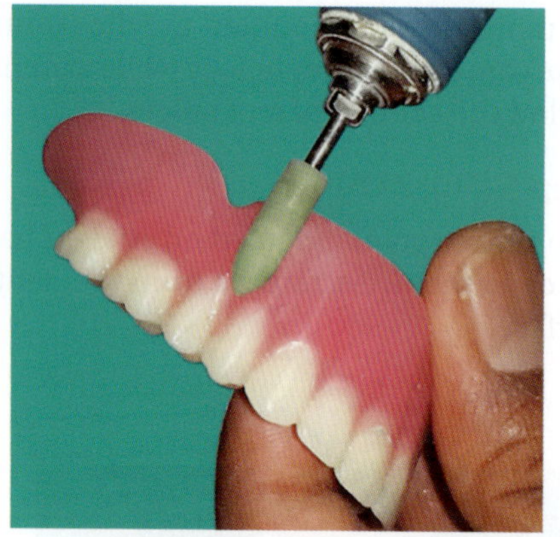

Fig. 27.6: Use rubber point to remove scratches.

At last, finishing is done with fine emery paper of 1,000–1,200 numbers. Sand papering can be done manually or using sand paper mandrel **(Figs. 27.8A and B)**.

POLISHING THE DENTURE (PUMICING THE DENTURE)

Polishing of denture is done on flanges, borders, and on palate. Do not finish or polish tissue surface of denture. For polishing of denture, polishing buff and rag wheel are used according to the area to be polished. Pumice in the form of powder or cake is used as polishing agent.

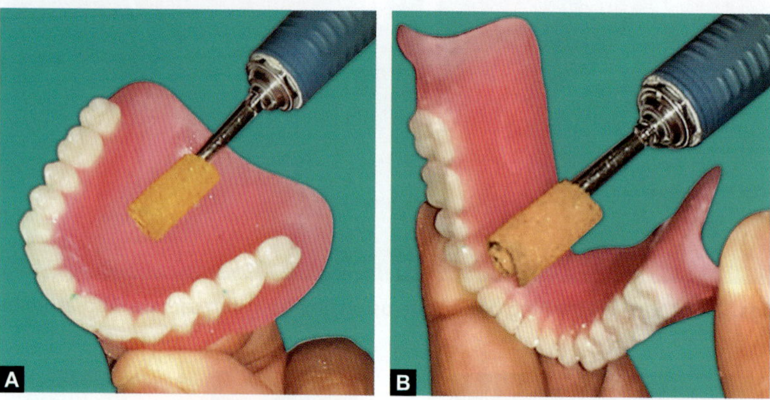

Figs. 27.7A and B: Use of sand paper for finishing of dentures.

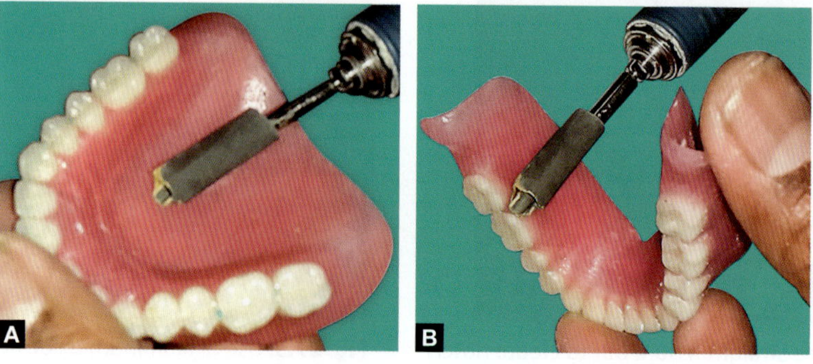

Figs. 27.8A and B: Use of emery paper for final finishing.

Step 1 (Figs. 27.9A and B)

Add pumice powder in water to make slurry. Use copious amount of pumice slurry with polishing buff to polish the denture. Polish the surface in various directions to give shine. Use appropriate pressure while polishing.

Step 2 (Figs. 27.10A and B)

Use laboratory motor driven rag wheel to polish areas where polishing is not possible with polishing buff. Use rag wheel to polish lingual flange of mandibular denture and palatal surface of maxillary denture.

Wash the denture with clean water and dry it. Examine for scratches on the surface. If scratches are found, repeat the polishing with slurry. Use pumice cake with polishing buff and rag wheel to give high polish to the denture. Examine for scratches if any.

Step 3

Lightly use clean cotton buff without pumice to give high luster to denture. This will also remove pumice from denture surface **(Figs. 27.11A to C)**.

Step 4

Use soap water and soft bristle toothbrush to clean any residue of polishing agent from denture surface.

Wash the denture with water. Polishing of denture is completed. Store the denture in water **(Figs. 27.12 to 27.14)**.

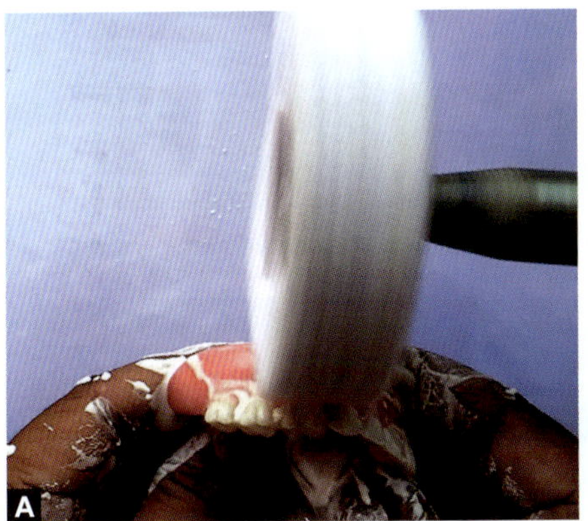

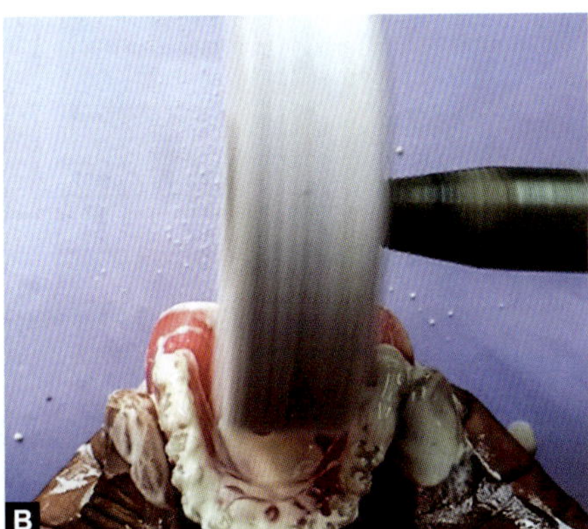

Figs. 27.9A and B: Use copious pumice slurry to polish the denture.

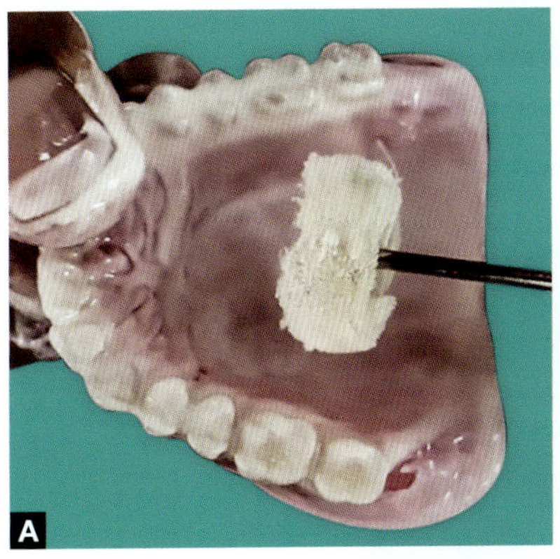

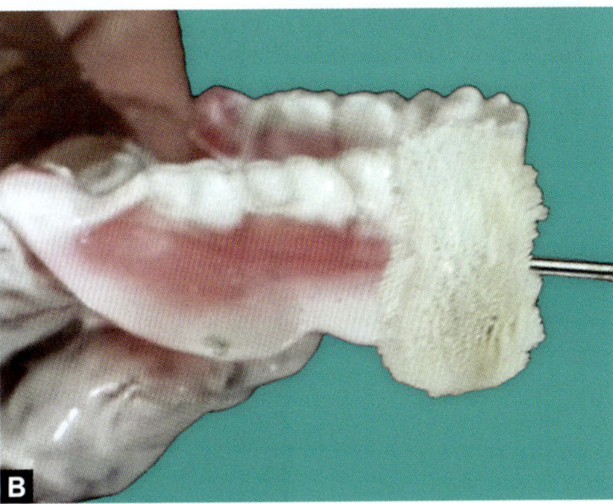

Figs. 27.10A and B: Polishing with laboratory motor driven rag wheel.

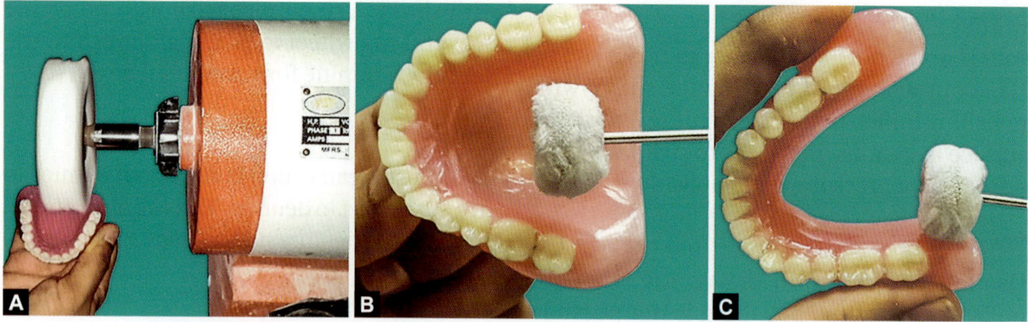

Figs. 27.11A to C: Use clean cotton buff without pumice to give high polish.

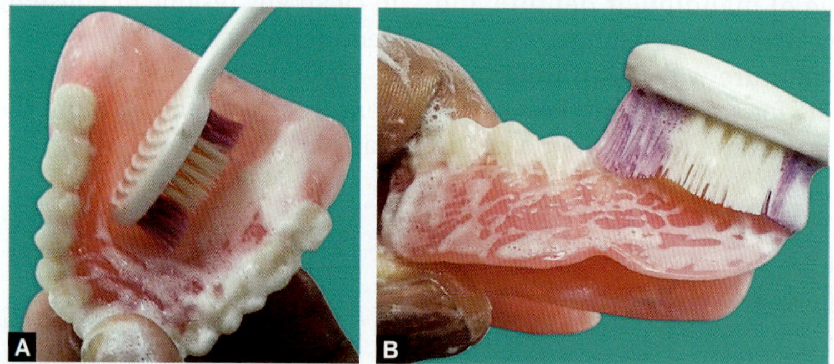

Figs. 27.12A and B: Removal of any residue of polishing agent using soap water.

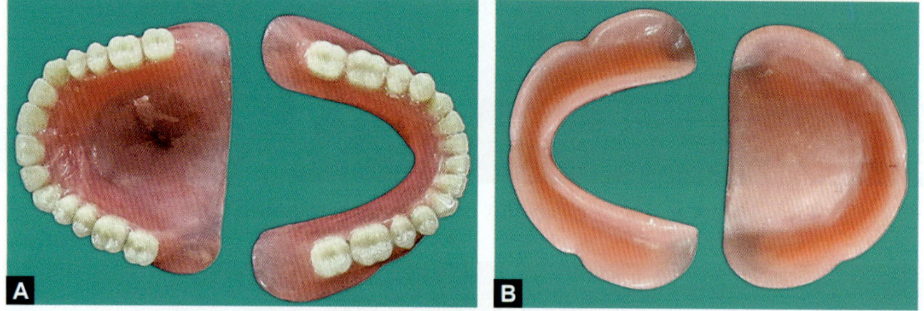

Figs. 27.13A and B: Finished and polished dentures—polished surface and tissue surface.

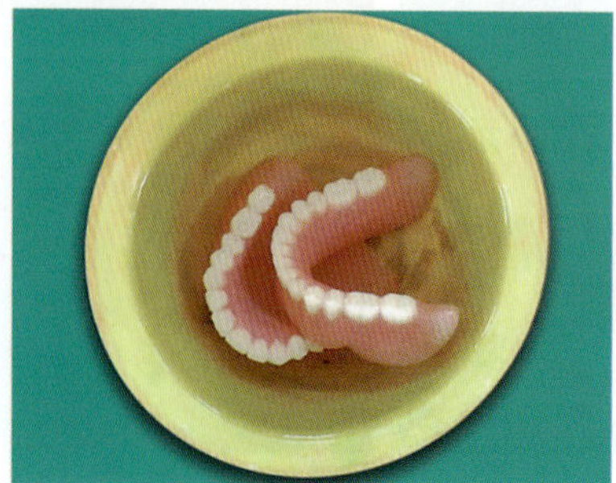

Fig. 27.14: Store dentures in water.

CHAPTER 28

Repair of Fractured Denture

JR Patel, Jignesh Chaudhari

INTRODUCTION

Complete denture fracture is frequently encountered problem. The fracture results due to sudden drop of denture by patient during removal or washing. Fractured denture is repaired using autopolymerizing acrylic resin.

Repair of fracture denture involves mainly two steps:

1. Preparation of working cast.
2. Repair of fracture denture.

PREPARATION OF WORKING CAST

Fracture maxillary and mandibular dentures at midline are shown in **Figures 28.1A and B**.

Step 1 (Fig. 28.2)

Assemble the fracture segments of denture at fracture line and add drop of cyanoacrylate to temporarily hold them together.

Step 2 (Figs. 28.3A and B)

Use wooden toothpicks or matchsticks to stabilize fragments of fracture denture **(Figs. 28.3A and B)**. Place toothpicks on occlusal surface and seal them with sticky wax.

Step 3

If any undercut is present block it with modeling wax and apply petroleum jelly all over the tissue surface **(Fig. 28.4)**.

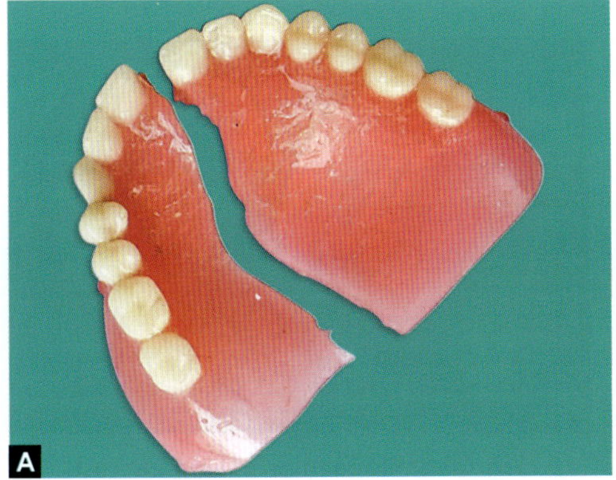

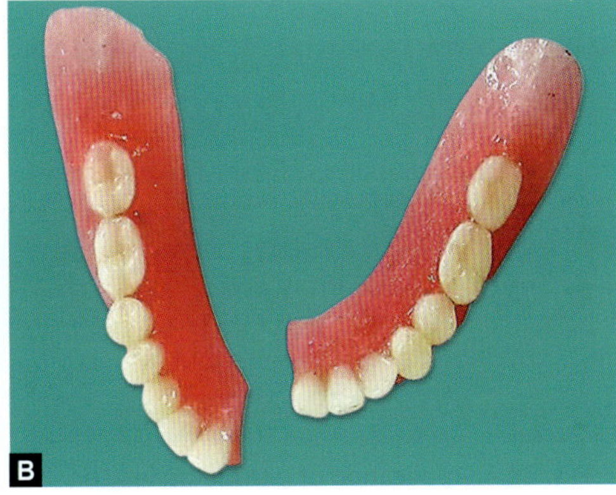

Figs. 28.1A and B: Fractured maxillary and mandibular dentures.

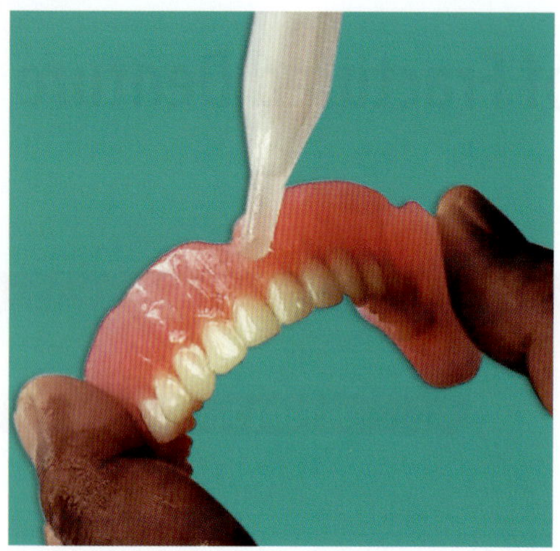

Fig. 28.2: Add drop of cyanoacrylate to temporarily join the fragments.

Step 4 (Fig. 28.5)

Mix dental plaster in creamy consistency and pour it on tissue surface till the height of borders. Pour remaining plaster on tile and invert the denture on it to form the working cast. Do not cover borders on polished surface. Make adequate thickness of base of the working cast. Allow plaster to set completely. Once it is set, remove the denture from the cast for repair.

REPAIR OF FRACTURE DENTURE

Step 1

Remove toothpicks or matchsticks. Separate the fracture components. Trim the fracture edges by 2 mm and form the bevel for proper adaptation of acrylic resin. This is done to

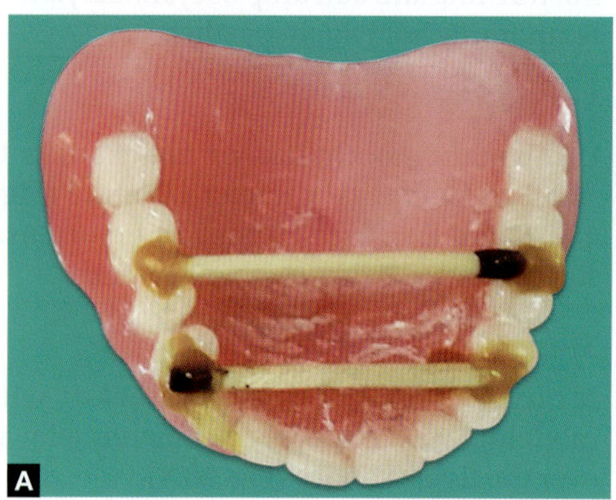

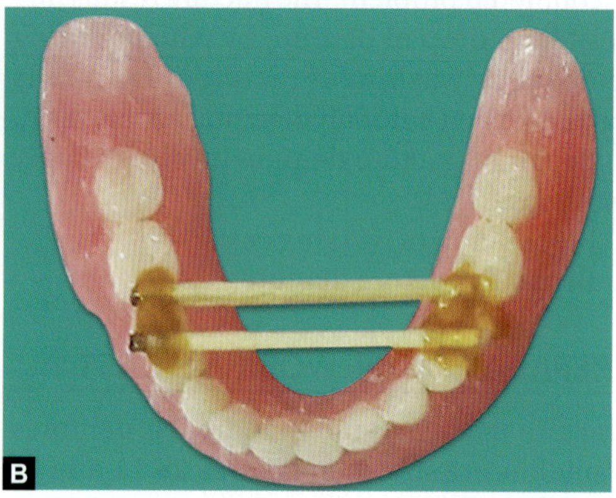

Figs. 28.3A and B: Stabilization of fragments using matchsticks and sticky wax.

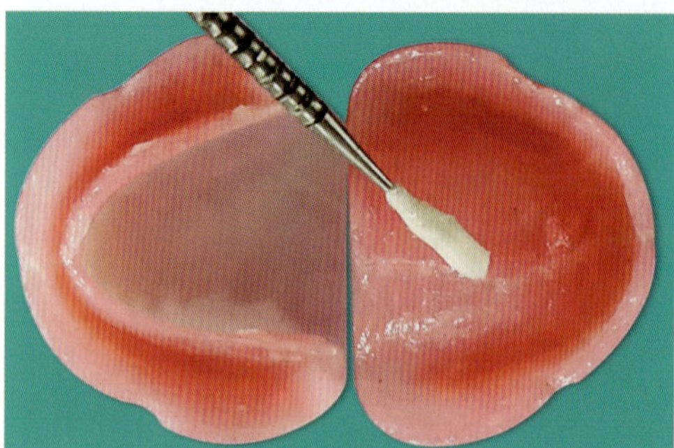

Fig. 28.4: Application of petroleum jelly on impression surface.

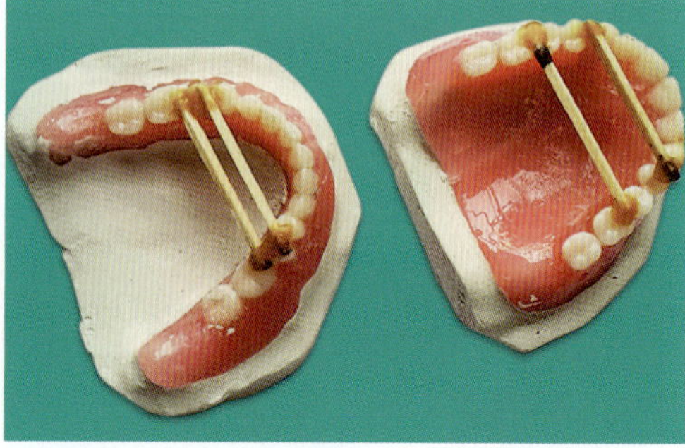

Fig. 28.5: Preparation of working casts.

create space to fill repair resin and join the fracture components.

Make grooves on lingual surface of mandibular denture. The grooves should cross the fracture line. Place wrought wire in the grooves. The wire is used to reinforce the broken denture (**Figs. 28.6A and B**).

For maxillary denture, make dumbbell-shaped grooves along the fracture line (**Figs. 28.7A to C**).

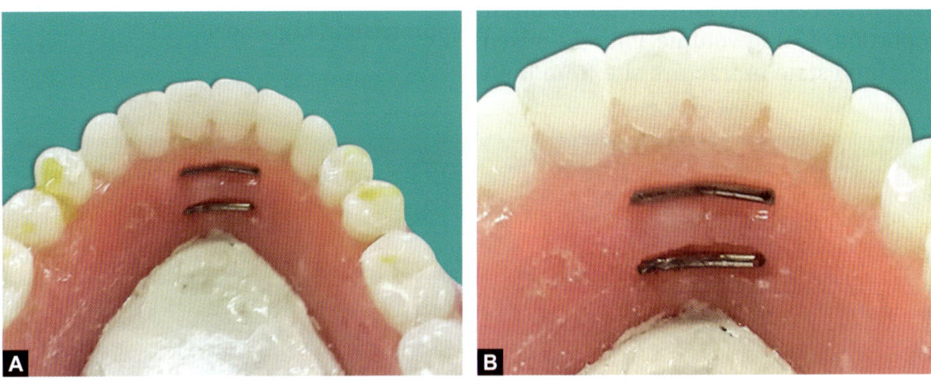

Figs. 28.6A and B: Reinforcing mandibular denture with wrought wire.

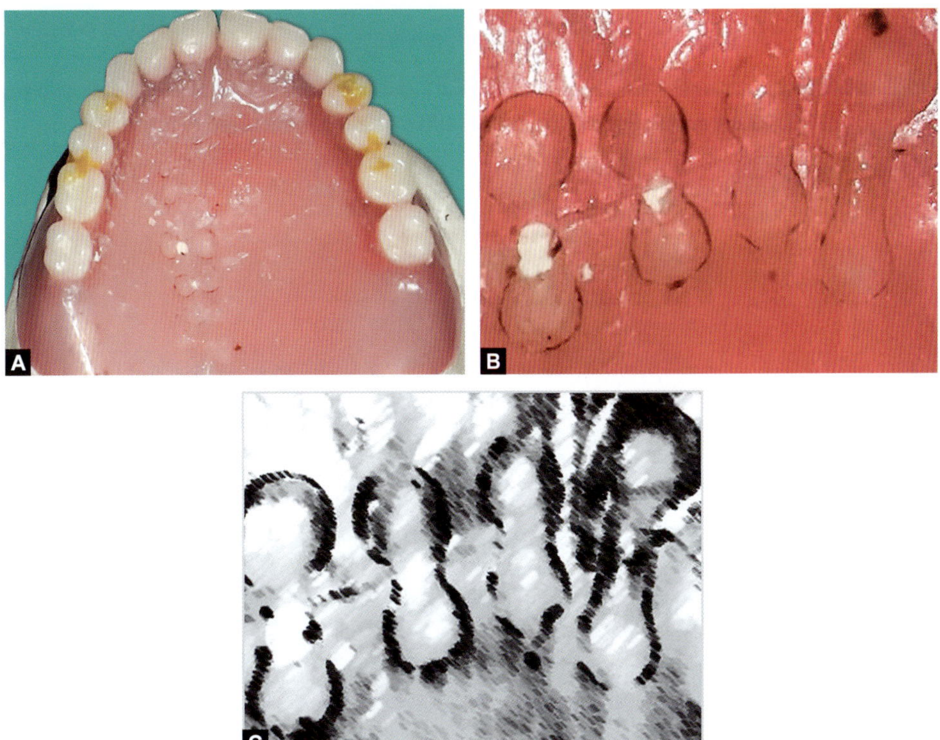

Figs. 28.7A to C: (A) Dumbbell-shaped grooves along the fracture line; (B) Dumbbell-shaped grooves; (C) Reformed picture to visualize the grooves.

Step 2 (Figs. 28.8A and B)

Apply cold mould seal on working cast in the region of fracture. Use unidirectional strokes. Allow it to dry completely. Place the components of denture on the working cast.

Mix polymer and monomer in porcelain jar in proportion of 3:1 by volume. Pour the mixed resin in fluid state in fracture site from both labial and lingual side. Allow it to polymerize completely.

Remove the denture from the working cast. Trim the excess resin from labial and lingual side using acrylic trimmer and do finishing with sand paper or emery paper. Polish it using pumice and rag wheel.

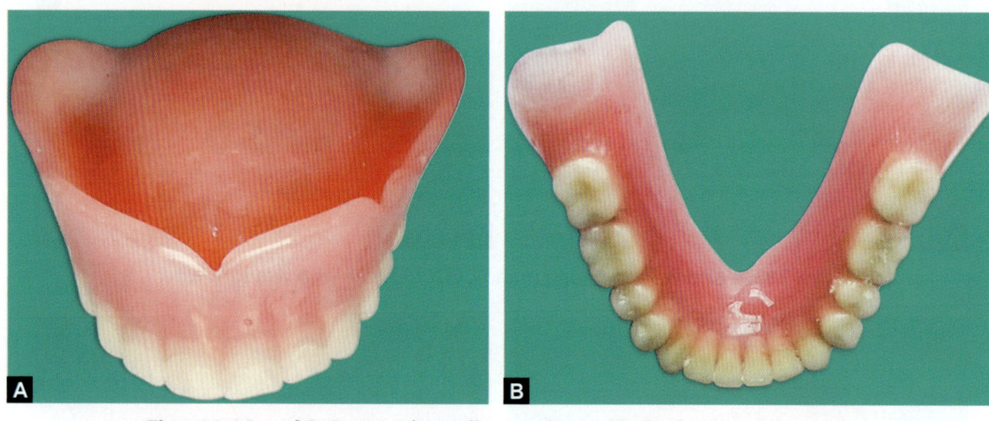

Figs. 28.8A and B: Repaired maxillary and mandibular fractured dentures.

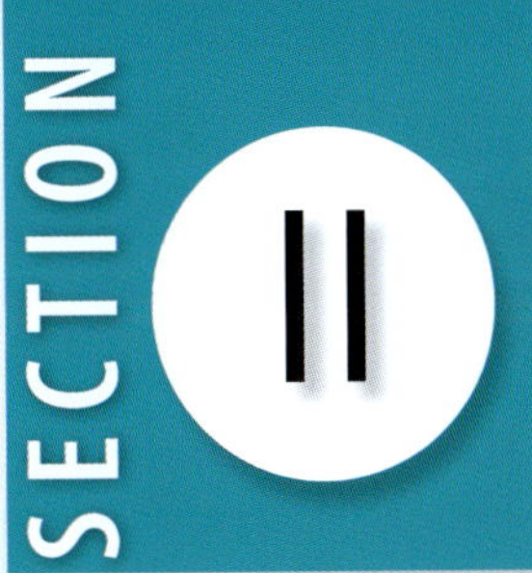

Removable Partial Denture

Section Outline

CHAPTER 29

Removable Partial Denture

Paranjay Prajapati, Jignesh Chaudhari

INTRODUCTION

Loss of tooth/teeth is serious event in terms of compromise in esthetic, phonetics, and masticatory efficiency. If some teeth are missing, they can be replaced with partial denture. The partial dentures can be of two types, i.e., one which can be removable and the other one is fixed. Present chapter is about removable partial denture. Fixed partial denture will be discussed in Chapter 39.

DEFINITIONS

- **Partial denture:** Prosthesis that replaces one or more, but not all of the missing natural teeth and supporting structures. It is supported by the teeth and/or the mucosa or implants. It may be removable or fixed.
- **Removable partial denture:** A partial denture that can be removed and replaced in the mouth by the patient.
- **Retention:** Resistance to removal from the tissues or teeth.
- **Abutment:** A tooth that supports a partial denture.
- **Retainer:** A component of a partial denture that provides retention to the partial denture.

TREATMENT OBJECTIVES OF REMOVABLE PARTIAL DENTURE

- Improve mastication.
- Restore esthetics and phonetics.
- Preserve remaining teeth and supporting structures.
- Restore health, comfort, and quality of life.

Indications for Removable Partial Denture

- Long edentulous span, when fixed partial denture is contraindication.
- No posterior abutment available for a fixed prosthesis.
- Esthetic problem due to excessive alveolar bone loss.

Classification of Partially Edentulous Arch

Paranjay Prajapati, Jignesh Chaudhari

INTRODUCTION

Partially edentulous arch can be classified by various classifications. Any partially edentulous condition can be classified by several classifications. The present chapter deals with commonly used classification. A brief discussion is presented about the rules which are applied to classify the particular partially edentulous condition.

IDEAL REQUIREMENTS OF CLASSIFICATION

- It should be universally acceptable.
- It should differentiate between types of support available, i.e., tooth supported or tissue supported partial denture.
- The classification should help the operator/technician to design the partial denture.
- It should permit easy visualization of partially edentulous arch.

Various classifications are proposed to classify partially edentulous arch. The most accepted classification is one proposed by Edward Kennedy in 1925. This is the most popular classification.

This classification is based on common occurrence of particular condition, i.e., loss of posterior teeth is more common, so condition where posterior teeth are missing is classified as class I.

KENNEDY'S CLASSIFICATION

- **Class I:** Bilateral edentulous area located posterior to the remaining natural teeth **(Fig. 30.1)**.
- **Class II:** Unilateral edentulous area located posterior to the remaining natural teeth **(Fig. 30.2)**.
- **Class III:** Unilateral edentulous area bounded anteriorly and posteriorly by the natural teeth **(Fig. 30.3)**.

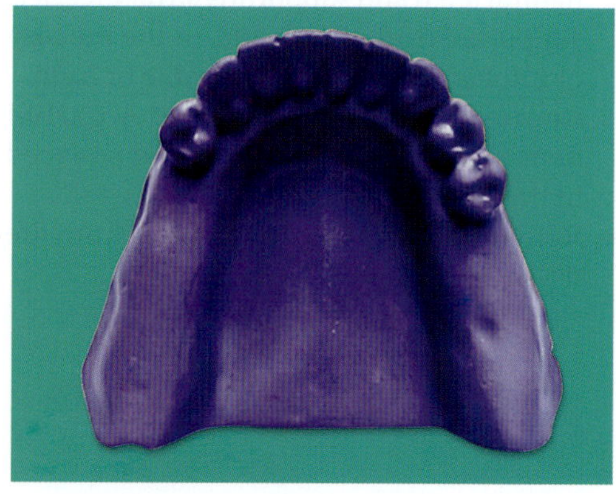

Fig. 30.1: Kennedy's classification—Class I.

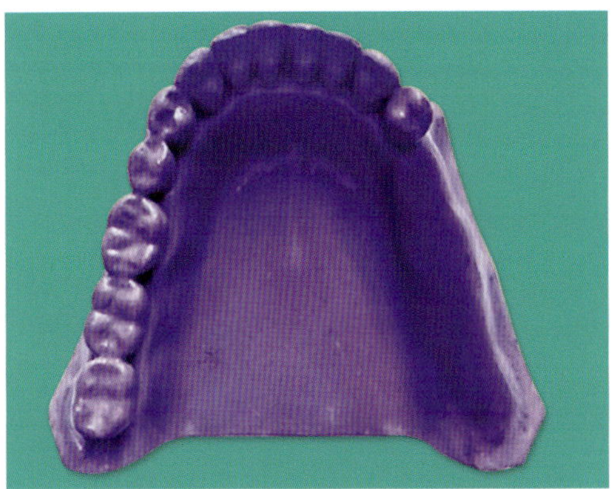

Fig. 30.2: Kennedy's classification—Class II.

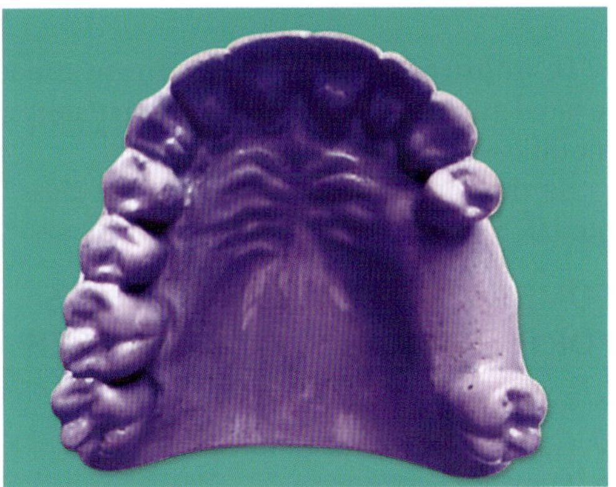

Fig. 30.3: Kennedy's classification—Class III.

- **Class IV:** Single edentulous area located anterior to the remaining natural teeth and crossing the midline **(Fig. 30.4)**.

  Applegate expanded the classification of Kennedy by adding two more class to the classification as under.

1. **Class V:** An edentulous area bounded anteriorly and posteriorly by natural teeth but in which the anterior abutment (if lateral incisor is the anterior abutment) is not suitable for support.
2. **Class VI:** In edentulous area, in which the teeth adjacent to the space are capable of total support of the required prosthesis. This does not require any tissue support.

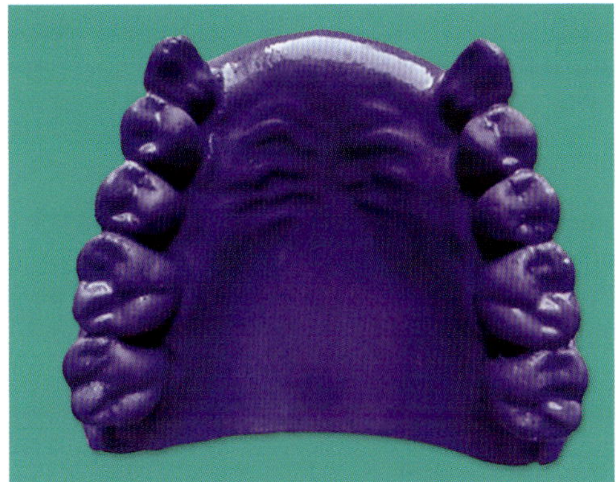

Fig. 30.4: Kennedy's classification—Class IV.

It would occur in young adult for whom a fixed partial denture is recommended.

APPLEGATE'S RULES FOR APPLYING THE KENNEDY CLASSIFICATION

- **Rule 1:** Classification should follow rather than precede mouth preparations or extraction.
- **Rule 2:** If the third molar is missing and not to be replaced, it is not considered in the classification.
- **Rule 3:** If the third molar is present and to be used as an abutment, it is considered in the classification.
- **Rule 4:** If the second molar is missing and not to be replaced, it is not considered in the classification.
- **Rule 5:** The most posterior edentulous area determines the classification.
- **Rule 6:** Edentulous areas other than those determining classification are called modification spaces.
- **Rule 7:** The extent of the modification is not considered, only the number (modification gives idea about additional edentulous spaces other than one which determines the classification. It does not give idea about number of missing teeth).
- **Rule 8:** There is no modification space in Class IV.

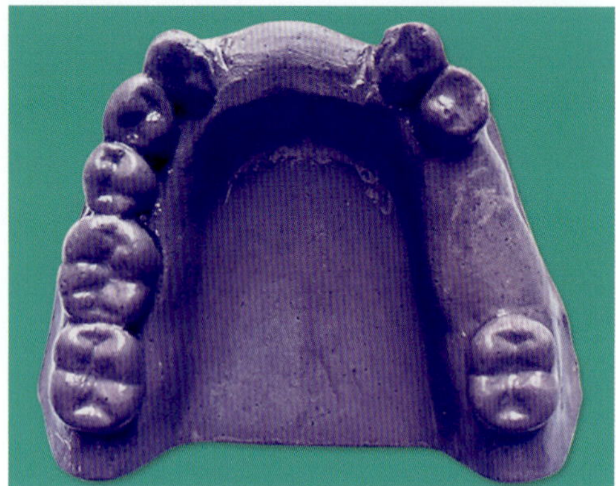

Fig. 30.5: Class III mod I partial edentulous condition.

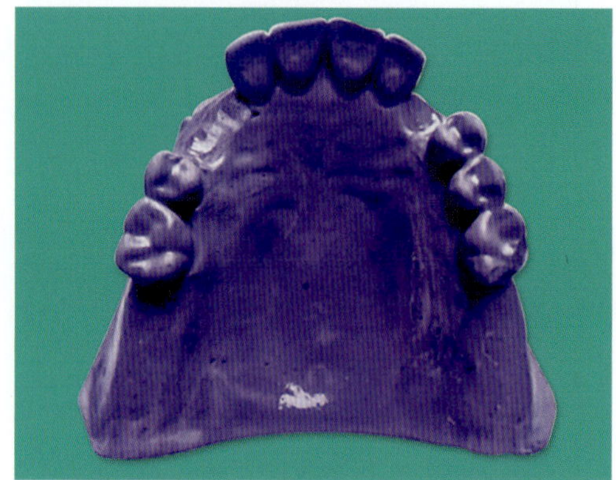

Fig. 30.6: Class II mod II partial edentulous condition.

How to Classify the Condition?

- **Class III, mod I:** First of all, calculate the number of partially edentulous areas. There are two partial edentulous areas present in the cast. The most posterior partial edentulous area is bounded anteriorly and posteriorly by remaining natural teeth so classified as class III and there is one additional partially edentulous area located in anterior section. That will be considered as modification **(Fig. 30.5)**. So, the condition is classified as class III, mod I.
- **Class I, mod II:** Four partially edentulous areas are present on the cast. The most posterior area is located bilaterally giving the classification as class I.

In addition, there are two more areas located anteriorly which will be designated as modifications **(Fig. 30.6)**.

So, the condition can be classified as class I, mod II.

SOME COMMON CLASSIFICATIONS FOR PARTIALLY EDENTULOUS ARCH

- Cummer's classification
- Godfrey's classification
- Mauk's classification
- Bailyn's classification
- Neurohr's classification
- Beckett's classification
- Friedman's classification
- Skinner's classification
- Swenson's classification
- ACP classification.

Components of Acrylic Partial and Cast Partial Denture

Paranjay Prajapati, Jignesh Chaudhari

INTRODUCTION

Partially edentulous arches can be restored with removable partial dentures. Acrylic partial denture used as temporary or interim prosthesis. Cast partial denture is definitive removable partial denture.

COMPONENTS OF ACRYLIC PARTIAL DENTURE

Acrylic partial denture has following components **(Fig. 31.1)**.

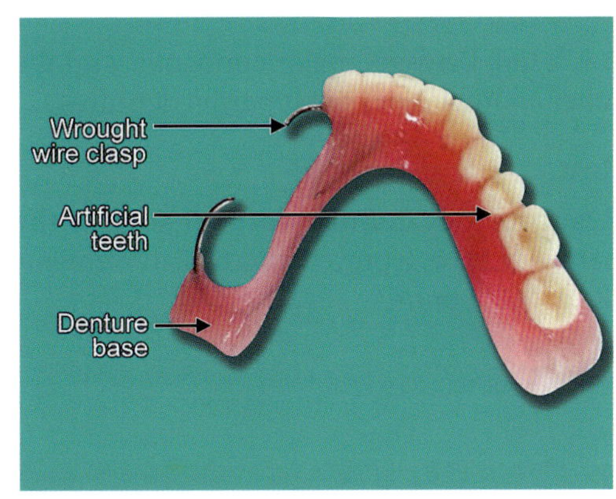

Fig. 31.1: Acrylic partial denture.

Denture Base

It supports the other components of partial denture. It helps in achieving support from denture foundation. It is made up of heat cure acrylic resin. It is 2–3 mm in thickness. Its extension in interdental areas helps in retention of partial denture.

Artificial Teeth

They are attached with denture base. They replace missing natural teeth.

Wrought Wire Clasp

It is attached with denture base. It is usually "C" clasp made up of 19 gauge wrought wire. It provides retention to acrylic partial denture.

COMPONENTS OF CAST PARTIAL DENTURE

Cast partial denture has following components **(Fig. 31.2)**.

Major Connector

The unit of a cast partial denture that connects the various parts of the denture. Its main functions are to provide unification and rigidity to the denture. It helps in equal distribution of occlusal load along the prosthesis and foundation. All components are attached directly or indirectly to major connector.

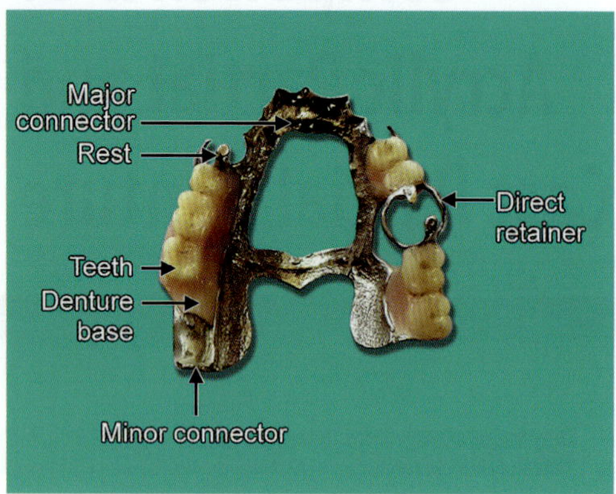

Fig. 31.2: Cast partial denture.

Minor Connector

It is a link between major connector and the other components of cast partial dentures.

Rest

Rest provides definite vertical stop to the partial denture. It prevents vertical movements of partial denture.

Direct Retainer

It provides retention to partial denture.

Indirect Retainer

Mainly indicated in distal extension cases. It provides additional retention and prevents movement of partial denture around fulcrum lines.

Denture Base

It helps in achieving support from foundation area. Made up of processed acrylic resin.

Artificial Teeth

Replaces missing teeth and restores their function in terms of esthetic, phonetics, and mastication.

CHAPTER 32

Maxillary Major Connectors

Paranjay Prajapati, Jignesh Chaudhari

INTRODUCTION

Major connector unites all other components with it and gives unified unit which act as single unit as a removable partial denture. Selection of major connector varies according to missing teeth and their location. This chapter focuses on brief review on maxillary major connectors and their indication.

MAJOR CONNECTOR

The component of a removable partial denture that connects the parts (of RPD) located on one side of the dental arch to those on the other side.

Its main functions are to provide unification and rigidity to the denture.

Selection of major connector for particular edentulous maxillary arch:

- If remaining natural teeth are periodontally weak the required support should be taken from palate. For this, full palatal major connector should be used.
- If remaining natural teeth are periodontally sound and little support is required then palatal strap or double palatal bar can be used.
- If torus present and inoperable then use horseshoe, closed horseshoe major connector.
- Avoid use of palatal bar because of its greater bulk and interference with tongue, speech.
- For anterior teeth replacement, horseshoe or closed horseshoe can be used.
- Major connectors in the maxillary arch should terminate 4.0 mm or more from the free gingival margin.

MAXILLARY MAJOR CONNECTORS

Palatal Bar (Single Posterior Palatal Bar) Major Connector (Fig. 32.1)

Indications

- Used when one or two teeth to be replaced.
- Used with class III edentulous condition.

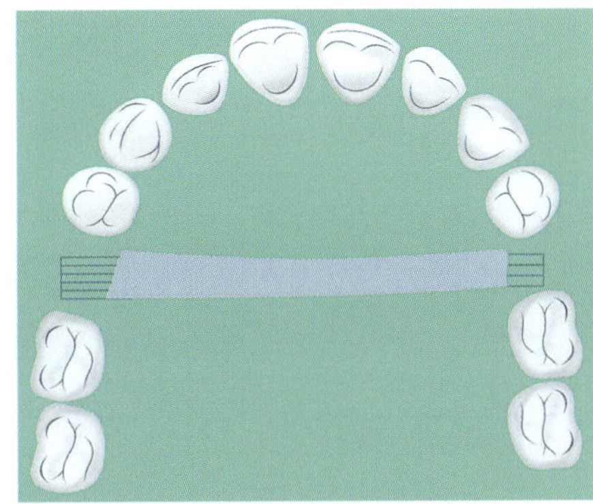

Fig. 32.1: Palatal bar (single posterior palatal bar) major connector.

- Requires strong abutment.
- When present tori are noninterfering.

Advantages

- It was widely used earlier.
- Simple design configuration.

Disadvantages

- It is very bulky.
- Interfere with tongue movement.
- Interfere with speech.
- Cannot be used for replacement of multiple teeth.

Palatal Strap Major Connector (Fig. 32.2)

Indications

- For short edentulous span.
- Bilateral edentulous space.
- Tooth supported partial denture.

Advantages

- Less interference with tongue movements.
- More degree of resistance.
- Even distribution of load.

Disadvantages

- More palatal coverage than palatal bar.
- More tissue reaction.

Anteroposterior (Double Palatal) Bar Major Connector

Indications

- Used with periodontally strong abutments.
- Used with U-shape palate.
- Class-I partially edentulous condition.

Advantages

- It offers excellent rigidity
- Offers less palatal coverage
- It can be used when multiple missing teeth to be replaced

Disadvantages

- Not for high vault palate.
- Offers little support.
- Bulk of metal interferes with tongue.
- Speech may get altered temporarily.

U-shaped Palatal Major Connector (Horseshoe-shaped Major Connector) (Fig. 32.3)

Indications

- Indicated for class I and class IV conditions.
- When tori is present and inoperable.
- If tori extends till posterior part of hard palate.

Advantages

- Derives support and indirect retention from palatal tissue.

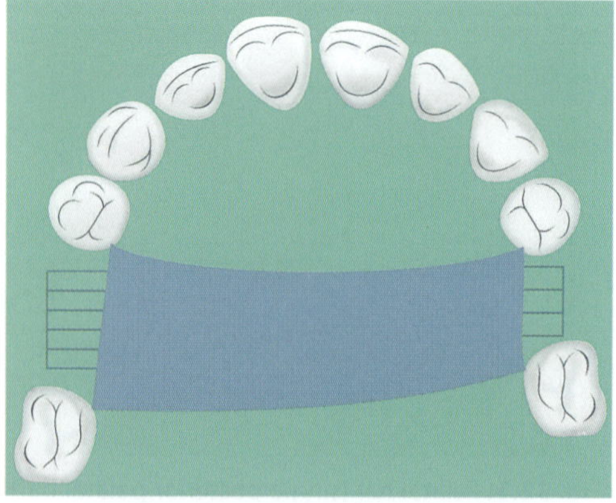

Fig. 32.2: Palatal strap major connector.

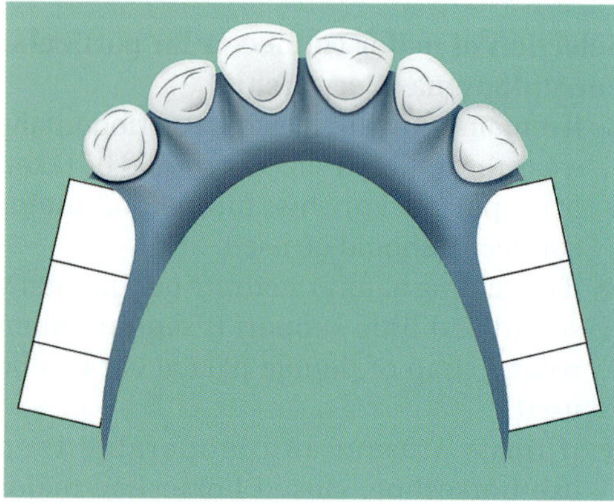

Fig. 32.3: U-shaped palatal major connector.

- When several anterior teeth are being replaced.

Disadvantages

- When used in distal extension cases, it may flex during mastication due to posterior open ends.
- Need excess bulk in rugae.
- May interfere with speech.

Anteroposterior Strap Major Connector (Fig. 32.4)

Indications

- Indicated for class I and class II conditions with sound abutments.
- Long edentulous span in class I with modification.
- Class-IV condition when anterior teeth to be replaced with removable partial denture.
- Inoperable tori but not extending till posterior part of palate.

Advantages

- Can be used for most of the partially edentulous conditions.
- Anterior and posterior straps closed by longitudinal metal extensions give circular configuration which gives rigidity to major connector.

Disadvantages

- Not indicated when abutment teeth have reduced periodontal support.
- Interfere with speech.
- Not indicated with high arch palate.

Full Palatal Plate (Complete Palate Coverage) Major Connector (Fig. 32.5)

Full palatal plate major connector is of three types:

1. Full metal palate.
2. Full acrylic palatal connector.
3. Metal acrylic combination.

Indications

- When many teeth are missing.
- Long class I edentulous condition with modification.
- When need to take support from palate.
- In cleft palate cases.
- When remaining teeth are not sound periodontally to provide support.

Advantages

- Advantages of metallic denture base.
- Good support and rigidity.

Disadvantages

- Adverse tissue reaction.
- Problem in speech.

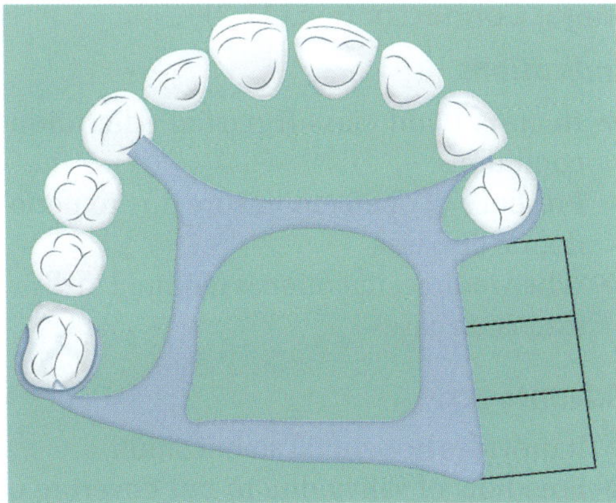

Fig. 32.4: Anteroposterior strap major connector.

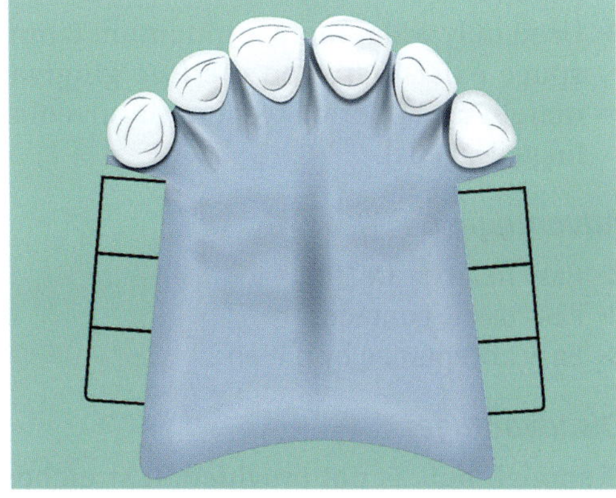

Fig. 32.5: Full palatal plate (complete palate coverage) major connector.

CHAPTER 33

Mandibular Major Connectors

Paranjay Prajapati, Rajesh Sethuraman

INTRODUCTION

Compared to maxillary arch mandibular arch has lesser surface area. The designs of mandibular major connectors are different than maxillary one. This chapter describes in brief about types of mandibular major connectors their indications, advantages, and disadvantages.

MANDIBULAR MAJOR CONNECTORS

Mandibular Lingual Bar Major Connector (Fig. 33.1)

Indications

- Indicated for Kennedy's class I and class II conditions.
- Used only when there is minimum 8 mm space exists between the free gingival margin and floor of the mouth (alveolar lingual sulcus).

Advantages

- Easy to fabricate.
- Less tissue contact.
- Easy acceptance by patient.

Disadvantages

If enough bulk is not provided, it stretches during use (will not be rigid).

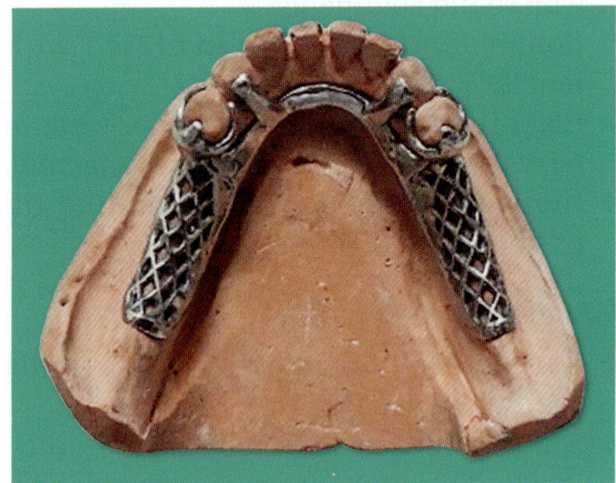

Fig. 33.1: Mandibular lingual bar major connector.

Double Lingual Bar (Kennedy Bar) Major Connector (Fig. 33.2)

Indications

- In class I and class II partial edentulous conditions.
- Presence of open embrasure due to periodontal diseases.
- When indirect retention is required in distal extension cases.

Advantages

- It provides horizontal stabilization.
- Free flow of saliva due to not covering of gingival margins and interproximal areas.

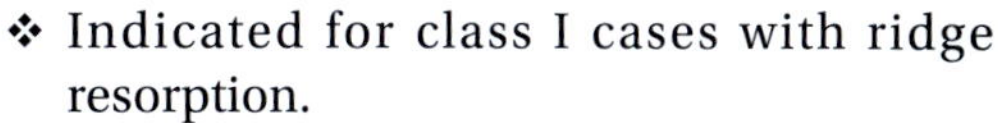

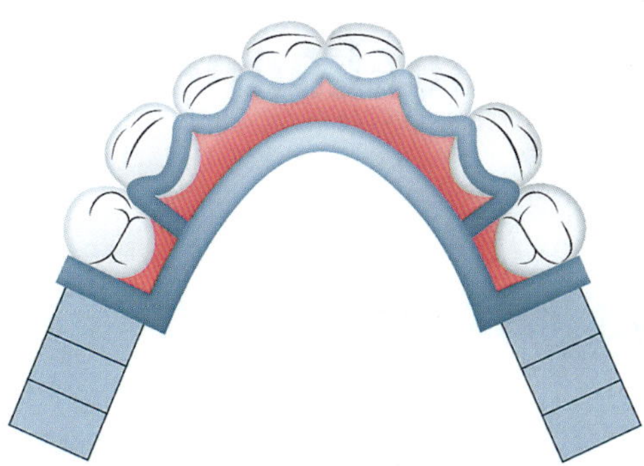

Fig. 33.2: Double lingual bar (Kennedy bar) major connector.

- Gingival margin receives natural stimulation.

Disadvantages

- Greater bulk
- More tongue interference
- Food entrapment.

Mandibular Lingual Plate Major Connector (Fig. 33.3)

Indications

- When space between free gingival margin and floor of the mouth is less than 8 mm.
- When remaining teeth are periodontally compromised.
- Indicated for class I cases with ridge resorption.

Advantages

- Provides greater support and stabilization.
- Provides indirect retention.
- Patient is more comfortable with this major connector than bar type.
- Ease in phonetics.

Disadvantages

- Irritation to soft tissue.
- Decalcification of enamel.

Mandibular Labial Bar (Fig. 33.4)

Indications

- When remaining anterior teeth are lingually inclined.
- When mandibular tori present and designing a lingual major connector is not possible.
- In severe lingual undercut condition.
- Sometime for replacement of anterior teeth.

Advantages

Only available simple design to be used when anterior teeth are tilted lingually.

Disadvantages

Bulk of labial bar may distort the lower lip.

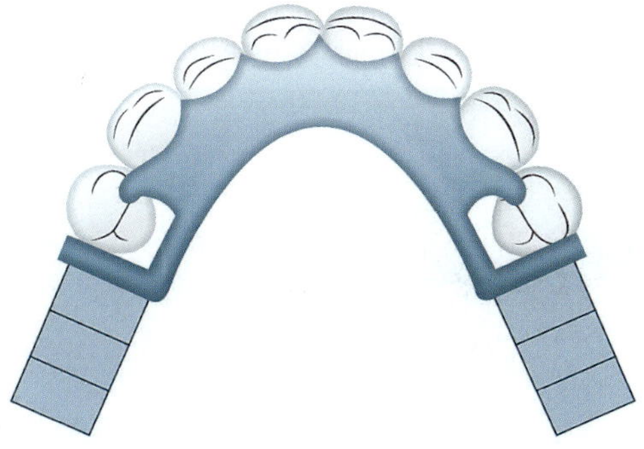

Fig. 33.3: Mandibular lingual plate major connector.

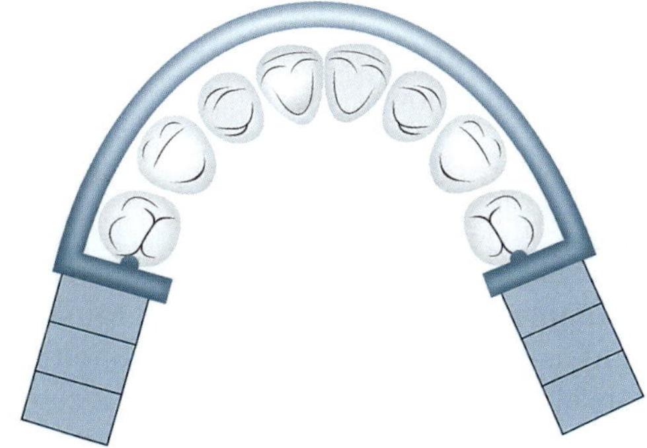

Fig. 33.4: Mandibular labial bar.

CHAPTER 34

Minor Connectors

JR Patel, YG Naveen

INTRODUCTION

Minor connector is a connecting link between major connector and other components. It connects various components with major connector and also helps the major connector in distributing stress. Different types of minor connectors are discussed in this chapter.

FUNCTIONS

- The primary function is to provide link between the components (of removable partial denture) and major connector.
- It helps in distribution of masticatory load and stress (in association with major connector).

TYPES

There are four types of minor connectors. These are as follows:

Minor Connector Joining Clasp Assembly to the Major Connector (Fig. 34.1)

This type of minor connector joins the clasp assembly to the major connector. Must be rigid as they support active component of partial dentures (retentive clasp). Located on proximal surfaces of teeth adjacent to edentulous areas.

Minor Connector Joining Indirect Retainer to Major Connector (Fig. 34.2)

Minor connector that joins indirect retainer or auxiliary rests to major connectors generally arises from the major connector. They should form a right angle with major connector but the junction should have gentle curve.

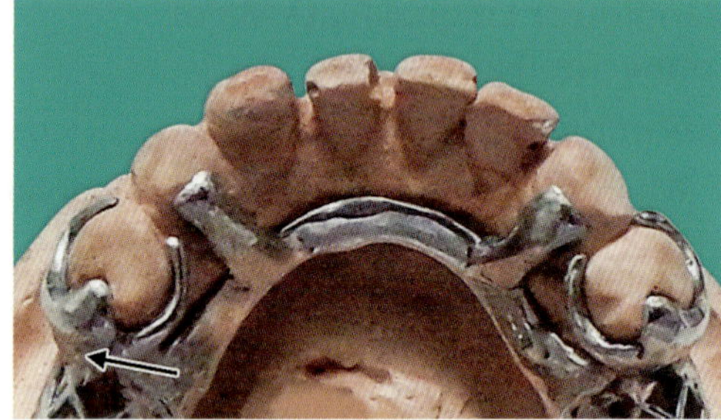

Fig. 34.1: Minor connector joining clasp assembly to the major connector.

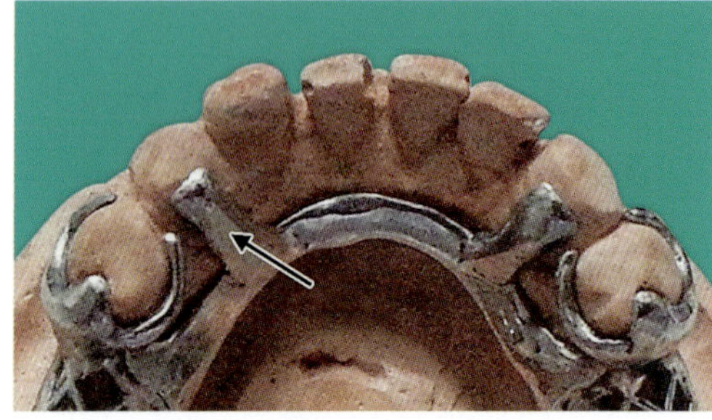

Fig. 34.2: Minor connector joining indirect retainer to major connector.

Minor Connector Joining Denture Base to Major Connector

Lattice Work Construction (Figs. 34.3A and B)

It consists of two longitudinal struts of metal. Struts positioned buccally and lingually to residual ridge. The length of lattice work extends two-thirds of total edentulous span. The horizontal strut placed in between longitudinal struts to join them. This is commonly used with class I and class II partially edentulous condition.

Advantages:

- Used to replace multiple teeth.
- Provide strongest attachment between denture base and major connector.
- Reline of denture is easy.
- More space available for placement of teeth.

Mesh Construction (Figs. 34.4A and B)

It is a metal sheet with small holes. Used when multiple teeth to be replaced. Commonly used in Kennedy's class I and class II partial edentulous conditions. It requires more pressure to pack acrylic resin. It does not provide strong attachment between mesh and acrylic as holes are smaller. It requires good interarch space.

Nail-head, Wire, or Bead Connector (Fig. 34.5)

It is metallic plate which rest directly on edentulous ridge. Acrylic is attached with beads, wires present on superior surface of this type of connector. This is used to replace one or two teeth. Used in class III condition. Better soft tissue response. Weakest attachment between acrylic and metal. Difficult to reline it.

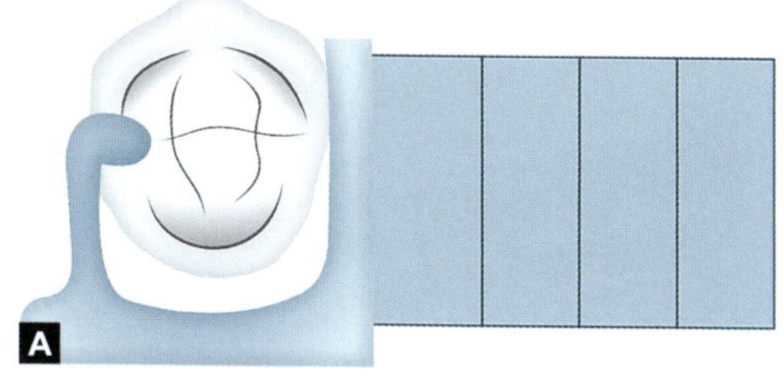

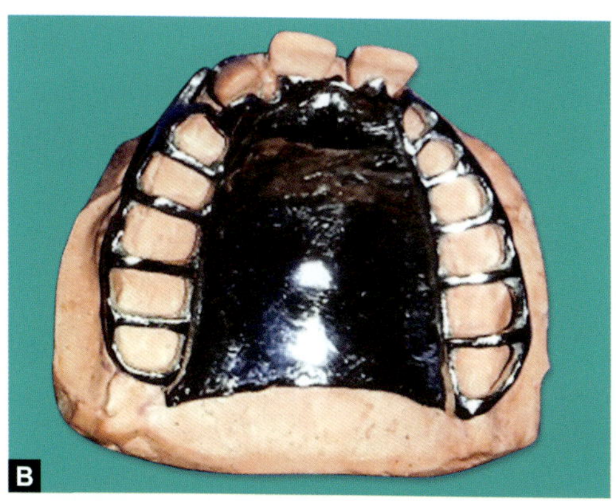

Figs. 34.3A and B: Minor connector joining denture base to major connector (lattice type minor connector).

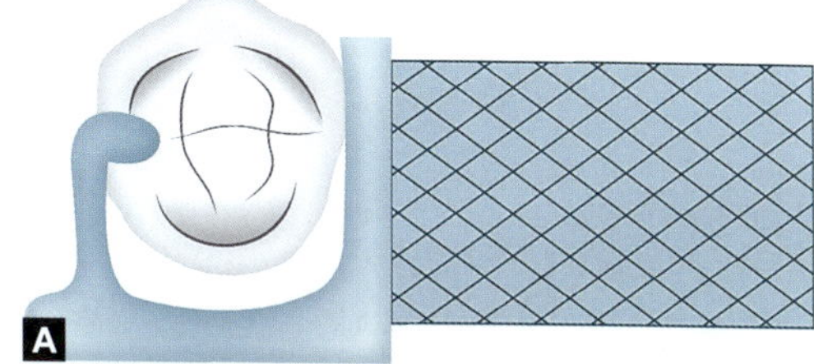

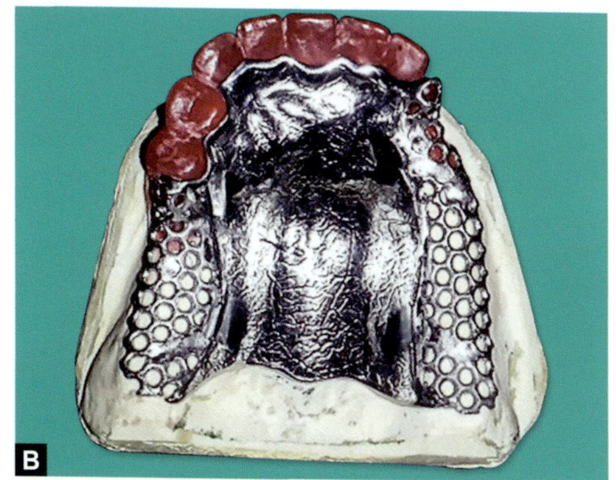

Figs. 34.4A and B: Minor connector joining denture base to major connector (mesh type minor connector).

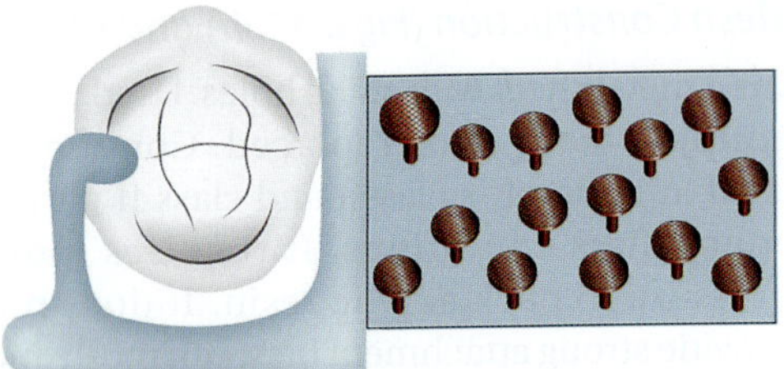

Fig. 34.5: Minor connector joining denture base to major connector (nail head type minor connector).

An Approach Arm of Bar Type Clasp (Fig. 34.6)

This is the only flexible minor connector. This connects terminal of bar clasp with major connector.

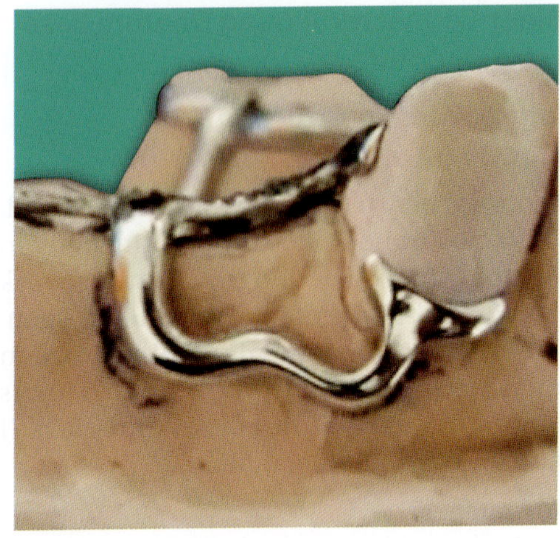

Fig. 34.6: Approach arm of bar type clasp.

CHAPTER 35

Direct and Indirect Retainers

Rajesh Sethuraman, Paranjay Prajapati

RETAINERS

Retainer provides retention to removable partial denture. There are various types of retainer designs; operator selects one according to the requirement of partially edentulous condition. Retainer is also known as clasp assembly. Retention of removable partial denture can also be achieved by precision attachments. This chapter presents brief review about various clasp assembly design and their indications.

DIRECT RETAINER

Definition

Direct retainer is component of removable partial denture, which provides retention to prosthesis and prevents its displacement against path of insertion.

Types

There are two types of retainer based on their design and mechanism of achieving retention (**Flowchart 35.1**).

Flowchart 35.1: Types of retainer.

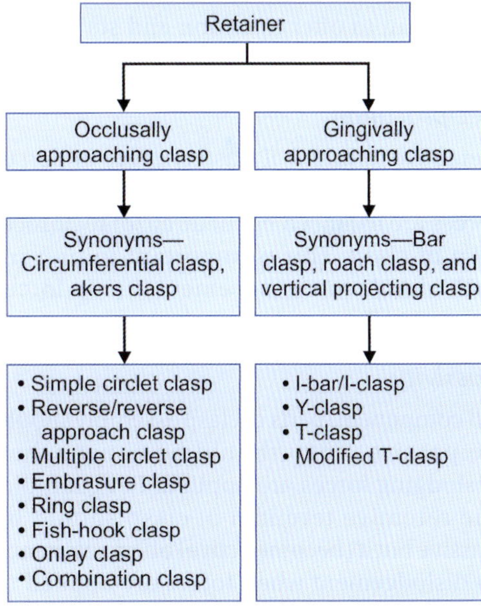

Requirements/Objectives of Clasp Design

Retention

It is resistance offered by prosthesis to dislodgement forces acting against its path of insertion. It is inherent property of retainer. It prevents dislodgement of prosthesis. It holds prosthesis to the foundation area. Retention is provided by retentive terminal of clasp by engaging the undercut present on tooth. Retention decreases as the flexibility of clasp increases.

Support

Support is provided by rest of clasp assembly. It is the characteristic of prosthesis to resist movement of prosthesis toward foundation.

Stability

This is the quality of prosthesis to resist its movements against lateral or horizontal forces applied to it. Rigid components of clasp assembly provide stability. Rest and minor connector also contribute to stability.

Encirclement

Each clasp assembly or retainer should be designed in such a way that it encircles abutment tooth more than 180°. This is important to offer retention and stability by retainer.

Reciprocation

Retentive terminal of clasp engages undercut and it apply forces when get activated. These forces are balanced by (neutralize) reciprocal arm of clasp. This is important to prevent orthodontic tooth movement due to forces generated by retentive terminal.

Passivity

All component/parts of clasp assembly should be passive. They should be active when dislodging forces are applied. For example, the retentive terminal of clasp should be passive but it (become active) offers resistance to dislodgement when forces are applied to dislodge the prosthesis.

Parts of Direct Retainer (Clasp Assembly)

Parts of Circumferential Clasp

The six parts of circumferential clasp are as follows **(Fig. 35.1)**:

1. Rest
2. Body
3. Shoulder
4. Reciprocal arm

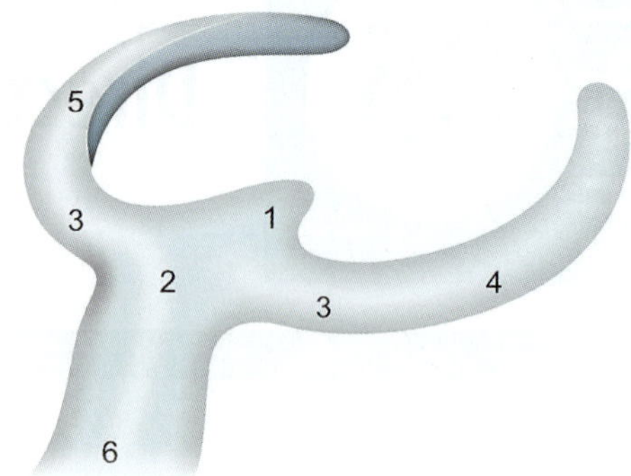

Fig. 35.1: Parts of circumferential clasp.

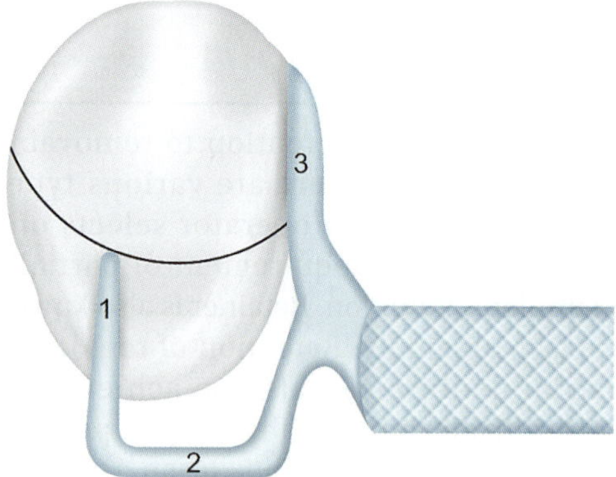

Fig. 35.2: Parts of bar clasp.

5. Retentive arm
6. Minor connector.

Parts of Bar Clasp

The three parts of bar clasp are as follows **(Fig. 35.2)**:

1. Retentive terminal (clasp terminal).
2. Approach arm (minor connector).
3. Proximal plate.

Factors Affecting Flexibility of Clasp

- **Length of the clasp:**
  - Increase in length.
  - Increases in flexibility.
- **Diameter of clasp arm:**
  - Increase in diameter.
  - Decrease in flexibility.

- **Crosssection form of clasp arm:**
    - *Round cross-section*: More flexibility (wrought wire).
    - *Half round section*: Less flexibility (cast clasp/circumferential).
- **Materials used:**
    - Cast gold alloys are more flexible than Cr-Co alloys.
    - Wrought alloys are more flexible than cast alloys.

Circumferential Clasp

Simple Circlet Clasp (Fig. 35.3)

Indication: Indicated for tooth supported removable partial denture.

Advantages:
- Easy to construct/fabricate.
- Most versatile clasp design.
- Easy to repair.

Disadvantages:
- Covering more amount of tooth surface.
- Changes the tooth morphology due to more coverage.
- Not esthetically accepted on anterior teeth.
- Adjustment in occlusogingival direction is not possible.

Ring Clasp (Fig. 35.4)

Indication: Tilted or tipped molars.

Advantages:
- Good coverage of tooth surface.
- Occlusal rest prevents tooth movements.

Disadvantages:
- Large amount of tooth surface covered by metal.
- Unesthetic.

Embrasure Clasp (Fig. 35.5)

Indications:
- For class II and class III conditions.
- Given on arch side opposite to edentulous space.

Advantages:
- Better retention.
- Use single embrasure for two clasps.

Disadvantage: More susceptible to fracture.

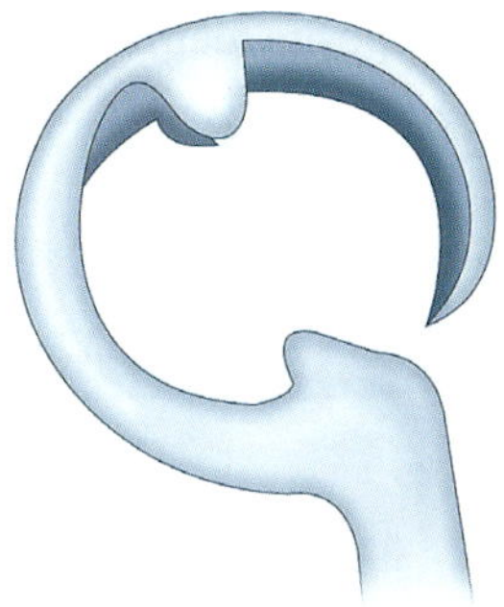

Fig. 35.4: Ring clasp.

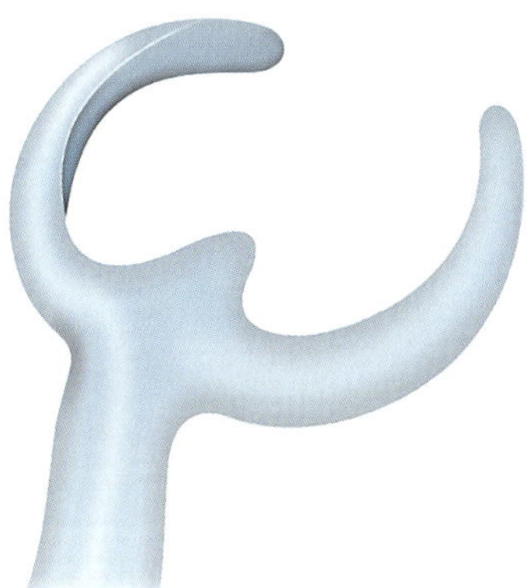

Fig. 35.3: Simple circlet clasp.

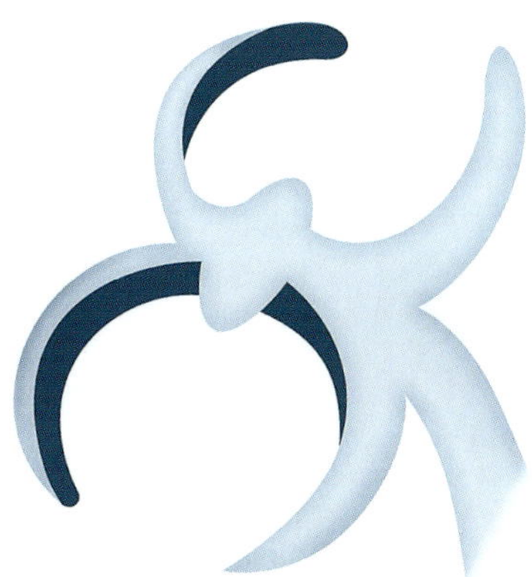

Fig. 35.5: Embrasure clasp.

Fish-hook or Hairpin Clasp (Fig. 35.6)

Indication: Used when retentive undercut is on lingual side.

Advantage: Good option to use in lingual undercut.

Disadvantages:
- ❖ Need more amount of tooth structure.
- ❖ Cannot be used on smaller crowns.
- ❖ Esthetically not acceptable.

Onlay Clasp (Fig. 35.7)

Indication: When occlusal surface of abutment teeth is below occlusal plane.

Advantage: Used to increase occlusal height of abutment tooth.

Disadvantages:
- ❖ Tooth should be caries resistance.
- ❖ Can abrade opposite teeth.

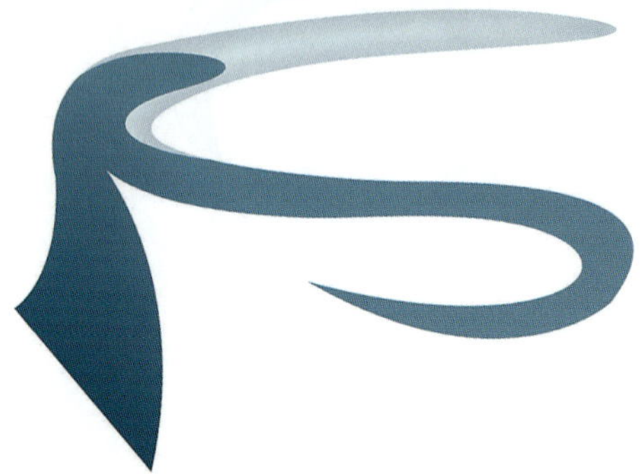

Fig. 35.6: Fish-hook or hairpin clasp.

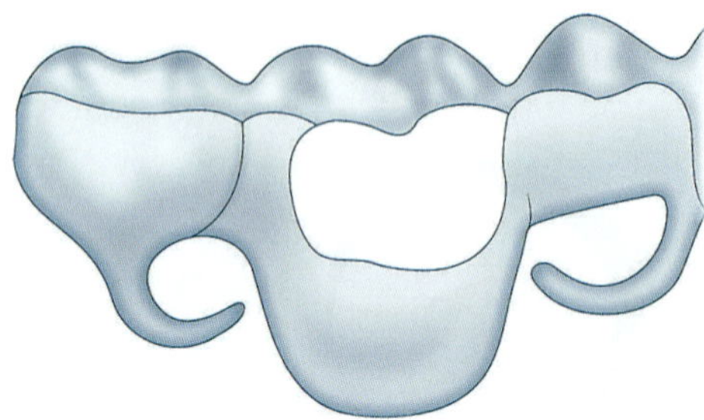

Fig. 35.7: Onlay clasp.

Combination Clasp (Fig. 35.8)

Retentive arm is made up of wrought wire and reciprocal arm is made up of cast metal.

Indications:
- ❖ Distal extension cases (mainly long span class I cases).
- ❖ On abutment near to edentulous space.

Advantages:
- ❖ Minimum surface contact.
- ❖ Wrought wire combines with cast reciprocating arm, act as stress equalizer.
- ❖ Helps to dissipate torquing forces.

Disadvantages:
- ❖ Difficult fabrication.
- ❖ Easy to fracture.
- ❖ Easy distortion.

Bar Clasp

I-bar (Fig. 35.9)

Indications:
- ❖ In esthetic region (on anterior teeth).
- ❖ Distal extension cases.

Advantages:
- ❖ Covers minimum tooth surface.
- ❖ Less visibility of metal part.
- ❖ Esthetic.

Disadvantage: Encirclement is compromised.

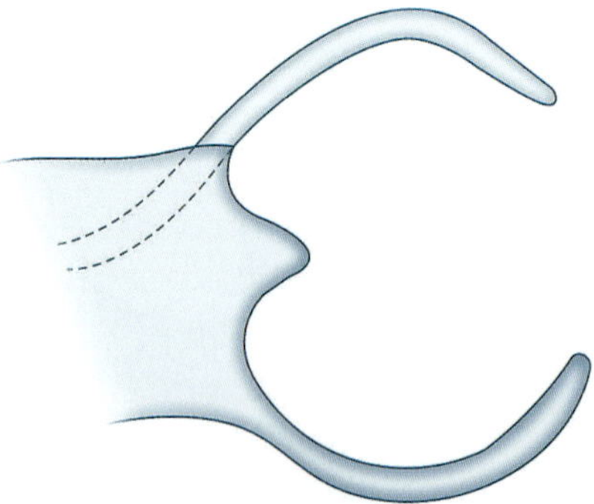

Fig. 35.8: Combination clasp.

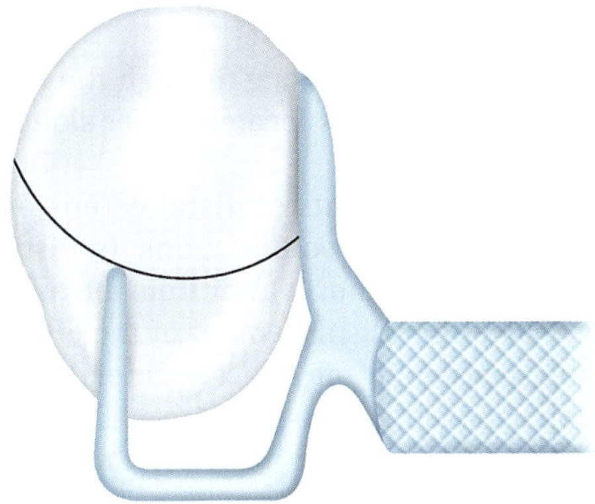

Fig. 35.9: I-bar.

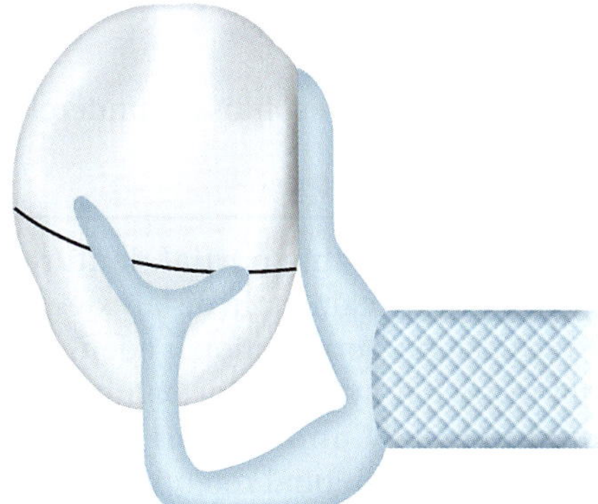

Fig. 35.10: Y-bar.

Y-bar (Fig. 35.10)

Indication: When height of contour on facial side is higher on mesial than distal side.

Advantage: Minimum tooth coverage.

Disadvantages:
- Esthetically superior to Aker clasp.
- Reduces torquing forces.

T-bar (Fig. 35.11)

Indications:
- Used in tooth supported denture where undercut is located adjacent to edentulous space.
- Undercut on the distobuccal surface of abutment.

Advantages:
- Minimum tooth coverage.
- Esthetically superior.

Disadvantages:
- Cannot be used over soft tissue undercut.
- Not used on terminal abutment.

Modified T-bar (Fig. 35.12)

Indication: In esthetic zone.

Advantage: Least tooth coverage.

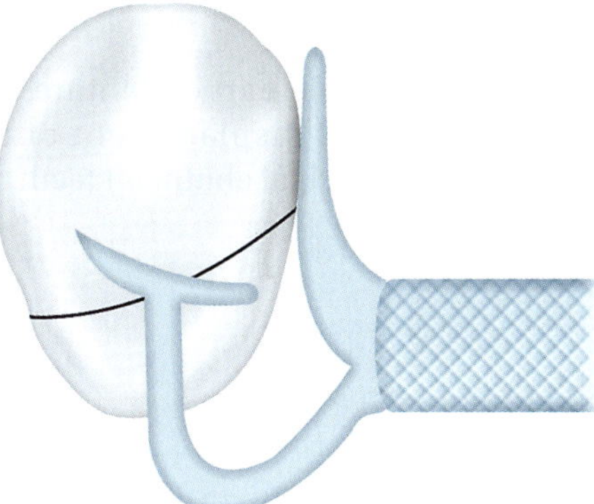

Fig. 35.11: T-bar.

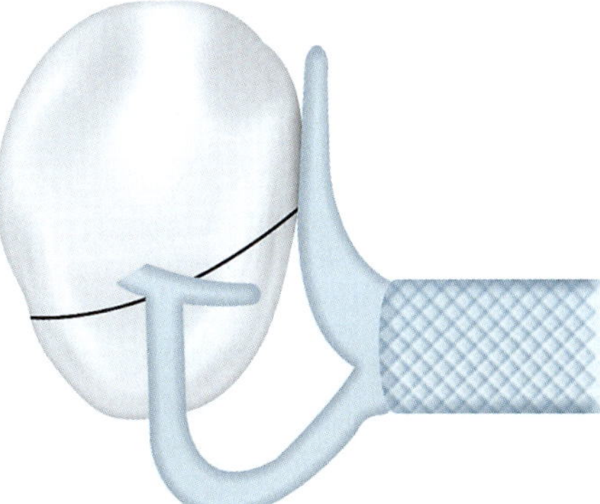

Fig. 35.12: Modified T-bar.

Disadvantages:

- Lesser encirclement.
- Cannot be used over soft tissue undercut.

INDIRECT RETAINERS

Retention in removable partial denture is provided by direct retainers. In distal extension cases, the posterior termination is edentulous and not restricted by posterior natural teeth (Kennedy's class I and class II). In such situation, some additional retentive features required to prevent movement of partial denture. These additional components are indirect retainer.

Definition

A part of a removable partial denture that prevents rotational displacement of the denture around principal abutment teeth.

Fulcrum Line

It is imaginary line passing through the two most distal abutments located either side of the arch.

Vertical movements of distal extension bases can occur in two directions. In distal extension, denture moves away from the ridge tissues via either displacement of the entire denture (resisted by the direct retainers), or a rotational movement around an axis. This axis passes through the most posterior abutment teeth and is called the fulcrum line.

Forms of Indirect Retainers

- Auxiliary occlusal rest
- Canine rest
- Canine extension from occlusal rest
- Cingulum bars
- Linguoplate major connector Rugae area.

Rest and Rest Seat

JR Patel, YG Naveen

INTRODUCTION

Rest is part of partial denture framework and rest seat is prepared on tooth surface to accommodate rest. If abutment tooth is restored then the rest seat can be prepared on restoration. This chapter briefly describes the rest and rest seat.

DEFINITION

Rest

Part of removable partial denture which transfer forces along the long axis of abutment teeth.

Rest Seat

The prepared recess in a tooth or restoration created to receive the occlusal, incisal, cingulum, or lingual rest.

FUNCTIONS OF REST

- It transfers the masticatory load to the abutment teeth.
- It provides definite vertical stop to the partial denture.
- It prevents impingement on soft tissue.
- Maintain the clasp in proper position.
- To prevent extrusion of abutment teeth.
- To provide positive reference seats in rebasing and/or impression procedures.

TYPES OF REST

Primary Rest

It is part of direct retainer assembly. It provides definite vertical stop to the prosthesis and prevent its displacement toward the tissue. It also transfers lateral and horizontal forces applied on partial denture to the abutment tooth. This load can be absorbed by the fibers of the periodontal ligaments without damaging the ligaments or bone.

Auxiliary Rest

It is used for indirect retention in distal extension cases (class I and class II). It is also called secondary rest. It prevents movement of partial denture around the fulcrum.

REST AND REST SEAT FORM

Occlusal Rest (Fig. 36.1)

- The outline of an occlusal rest seat is a rounded triangular shape.
- Apex of rest is located toward the center of the tooth.
- The base of the triangular shape is at the marginal ridge.

- Rest should be approximately one-third the buccolingual width of the tooth.
- The marginal ridge must be lowered and rounded to permit a sufficient bulk of metal to prevent fracture of the rest from the minor connector (1–1.5 mm).
- Occlusal rest seat should be shallow and saucer-shaped. The floor of the rest seat should be inclined toward the center of the tooth, should be less than 90°. This helps to direct the occlusal forces along the long axis of the tooth **(Fig. 36.2)**.

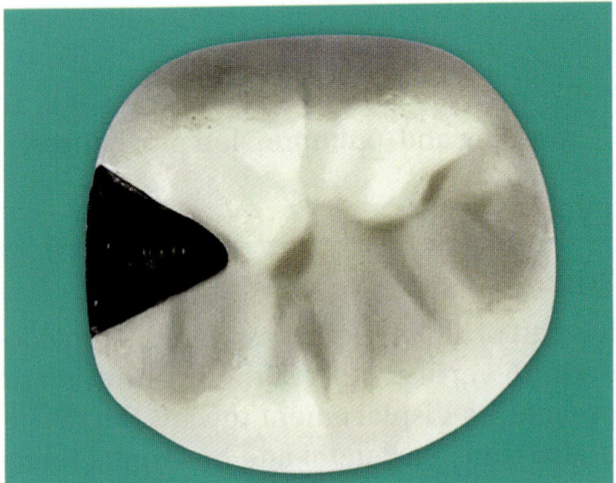

Fig. 36.1: Occlusal rest.

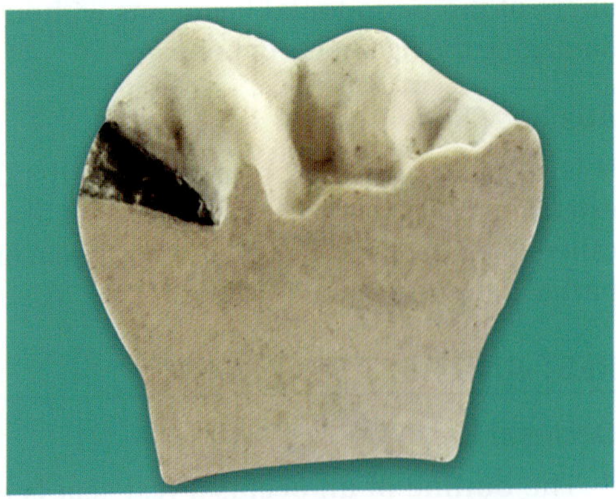

Fig. 36.2: Floor of rest seat inclined toward center and should be less than 90°.

Cingulum or Lingual Rest (Figs. 36.3A and B)

- Used primarily on maxillary canines.
- If in case canine is missing then multiple incisors are used to receive cingulum rest.
- It is more esthetical than incisal rest.
- Less chances of breakage and distortion.

Incisal Rest

- Commonly used on mandibular canine.
- Positioned near incisal edge of abutment tooth.
- For esthetic reason, it is placed on distoincisal surface of tooth.

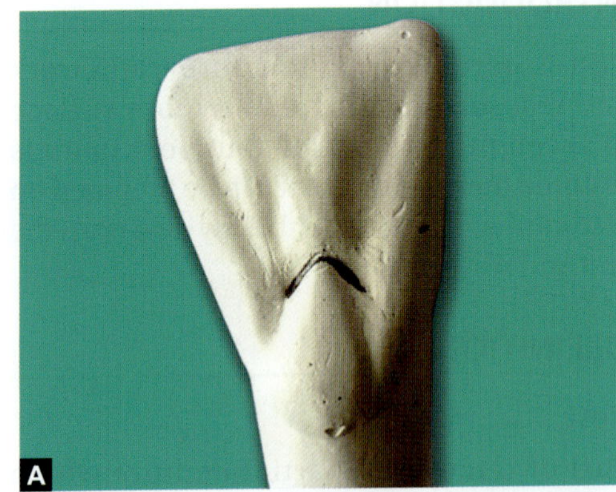

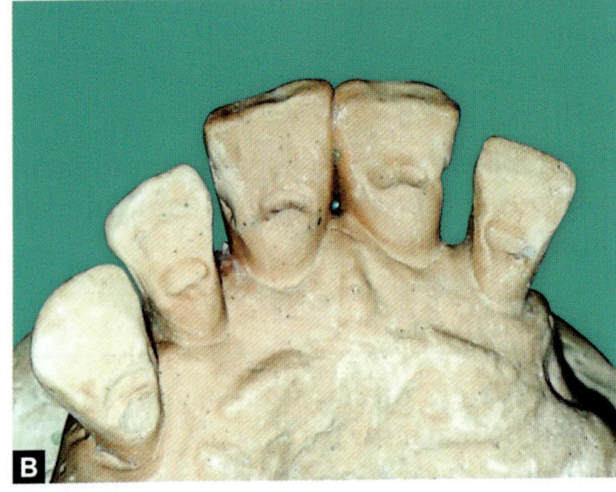

Figs. 36.3A and B: Cingulum or lingual rest.

CHAPTER 37

Survey Lines and Surveyor

Paranjay Prajapati, Rajesh Sethuraman

SURVEY LINES

The line produced on a cast by a surveyor marking the greatest prominence of contour. It marks the highest point on tooth contour. It is marked with carbon marker attached with surveyor. It has various configurations and can be changed by changing the tilt of a cast.

CLASSIFICATION OF SURVEY LINES

Any abutment tooth near to partial edentulous space can be divided in two parts. Blatterfein divided the abutment tooth into two halves by a vertical line passing through center of tooth. The part of tooth near to edentulous space was termed as *near zone* and area away from edentulous space was termed as *far zone* **(Fig. 37.1)**.

Based on their relation with far and near zone, survey lines are classified as:

- ❖ High survey line
- ❖ Low survey line
- ❖ Medium survey line
- ❖ Diagonal survey line.

High Survey Line (Fig. 37.2)

It is located in occlusal third in both near and far zones. It is seen on inclined teeth. It can be changed by tilting the cast. Wrought wire clasp or ring clasp is advocated.

Low Survey Line (Fig. 37.3)

This type of survey line is located in gingival third in both far zone as well as in near zone. It is seen on opposite side to tilted tooth. Better to change contour by tilting the cast.

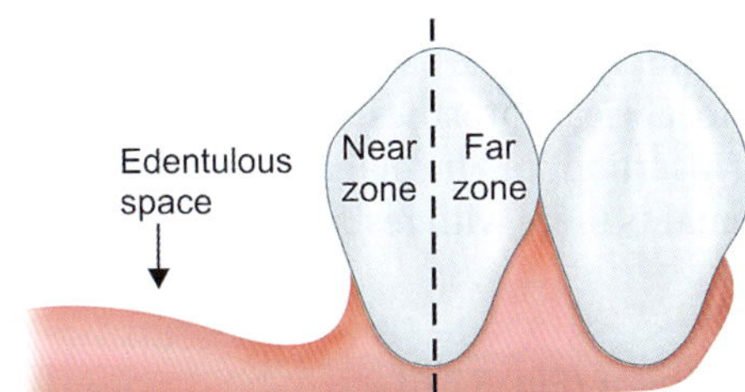

Fig. 37.1: Near zone and far zone of abutment tooth.

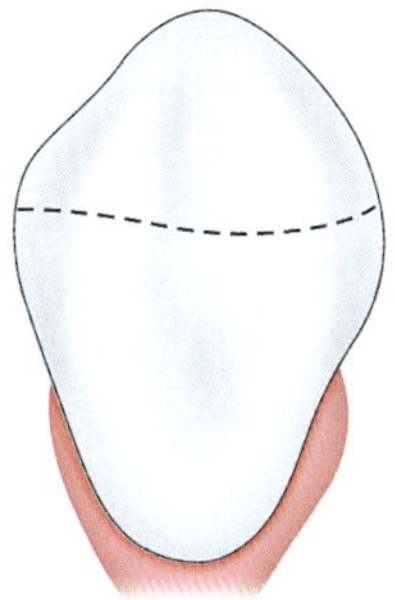

Fig. 37.2: High survey line.

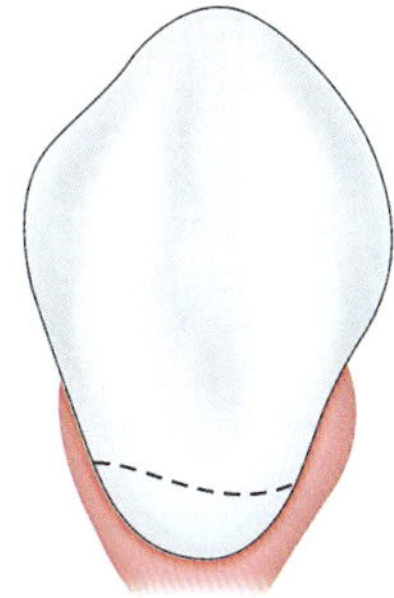

Fig. 37.3: Low survey line.

Medium Survey Line (Fig. 37.4)

It starts or travels from middle third of the tooth in the near zone to gingival third of the tooth in far zone. It is ideal survey line, used with circumferential clasp and bar clasp.

Diagonal Survey Line (Fig. 37.5)

It runs from occlusal third in near zone to the gingival third in far zone. It is commonly seen on buccal surface of canine and premolars. Circumferential, hairpin, modified T-bar, and "T"-bar clasp can be used.

SURVEYOR

Any partial edentulous arch is blend of remaining natural teeth and partial edentulous spaces. This is unique about partially edentulous arch as it has both dentulous and edentulous characteristics. The all remaining natural teeth may not have similar angulation so it is difficult to fabricate prosthesis. The problem with partially edentulous condition is to fabricate prosthesis which has single path of insertion, can be placed easily on arch, and remains there with resistance to removal.

Definition

Surveyor (Fig. 37.6)

A paralleling instrument used in construction of a dental prosthesis to locate and delineate the contours and relative positions of abutment teeth and associated structure.

Types

Most commonly used surveyors are:
- Ney surveyor (horizontal arm is fixed).
- Williams surveyor (horizontal arm is split and connected).
- Jelenko surveyor (horizontal arm can swivel).

Parts of Surveyor (Fig. 37.7)

Surveying Platform

It is metal platform or base parallel to floor on which cast holder and vertical arm are attached. It is the base of surveyor on which other parts of surveyor are fixed.

Surveying Table

It consists of cast holder and base. The base is attached on platform and on it the cast holder is fixed. Cast is placed on cast holder for surveying. The holder is attached to platform with ball and socket mechanism which allow tilting of the cast.

Vertical Arm

It is attached to the platform and supports the horizontal arm.

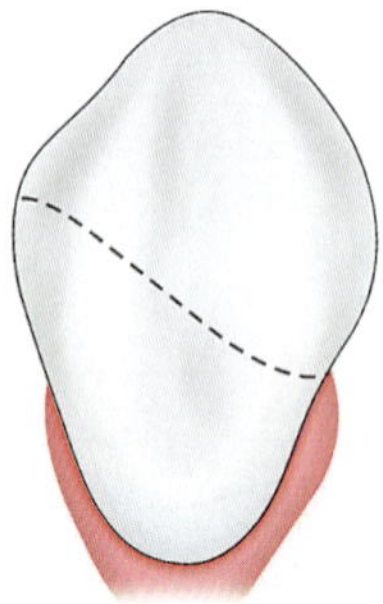

Fig. 37.4: Medium survey line.

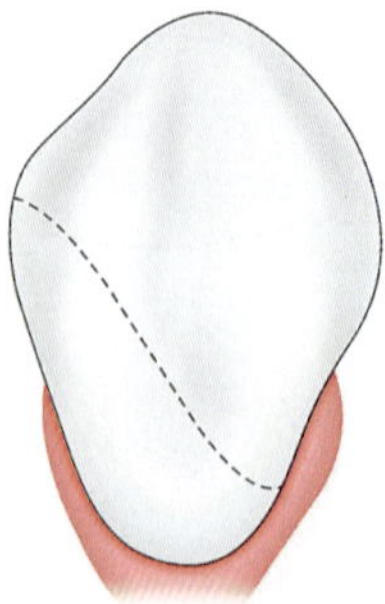

Fig. 37.5: Diagonal survey line.

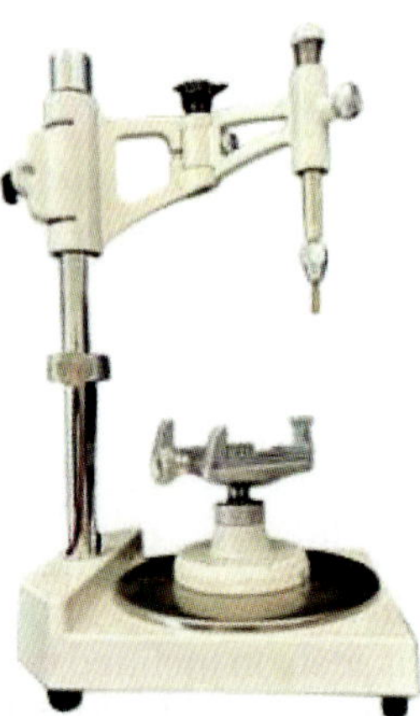

Fig. 37.6: Surveyor.

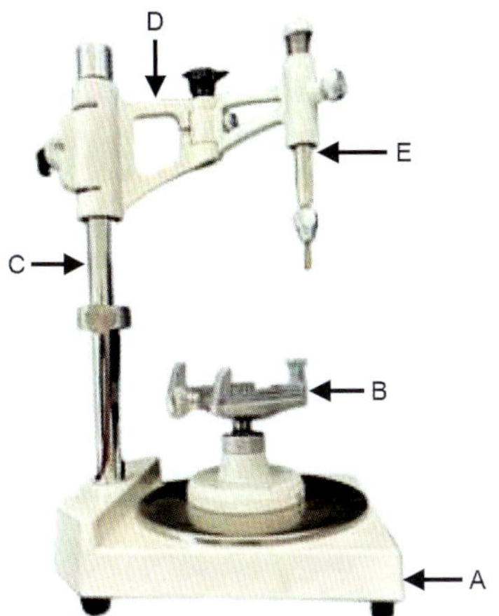

Fig. 37.7: Parts of surveyor; A. surveying platform, B. surveying table, C. vertical arm, D. horizontal arm, E. surveying arm.

Horizontal Arm

It is attached with vertical arm at right angle and surveying arm is attached with it.

Surveying Arm

It drops vertically from the free end of horizontal arm. It can be moved up and down vertically. On free end (lower end), the mandrel is attached which holds surveying tools and carbon marker.

Surveying Tools

Analyzing Rod (Fig. 37.8)

It is a metal rod to be used for surveying. It helps in determining relative parallelism between abutments. It helps in determining the height of contour.

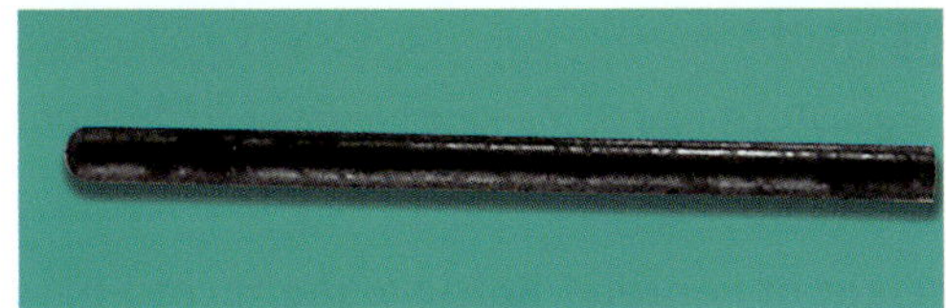

Fig. 37.8: Analyzing rod.

Carbon Marker (Fig. 37.9)

It is a carbon lead of around 2 mm diameter similar to pencil lead. It is used to mark survey lines on teeth. The free end of carbon marker is circular in Ney surveyor and triangular in Jelenko surveyor.

Undercut Gauge (Fig. 37.10)

Used to determine size and location of undercuts. Usually it comes as 0.001, 0.002, and 0.003 inch sizes.

Wax Trimmer (Fig. 37.11)

Used for trimming out the excess wax from block out area to make them parallel to the path of insertion.

Purposes/Uses of Surveyor

- Surveying the diagnostic cast
- Surveying the master cast
- Tripoding
- Contouring the wax pattern
- Contouring the crowns
- Placing internal attachments and rests.

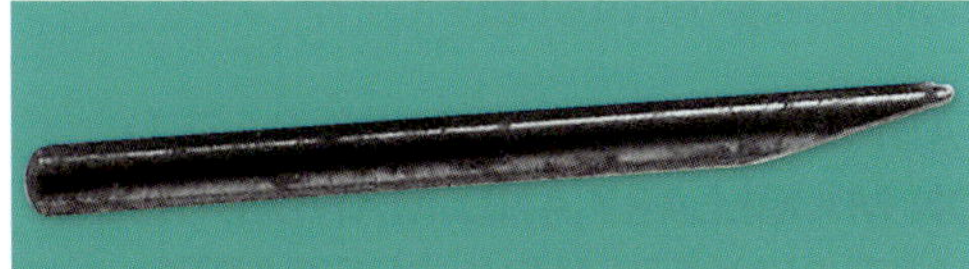

Fig. 37.9: Carbon marker.

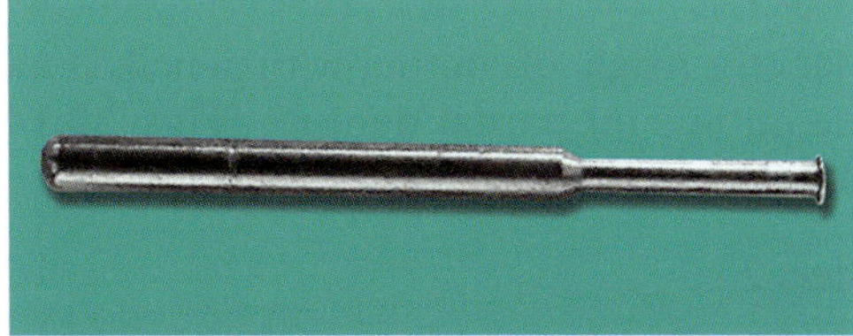

Fig. 37.10: Undercut gauge.

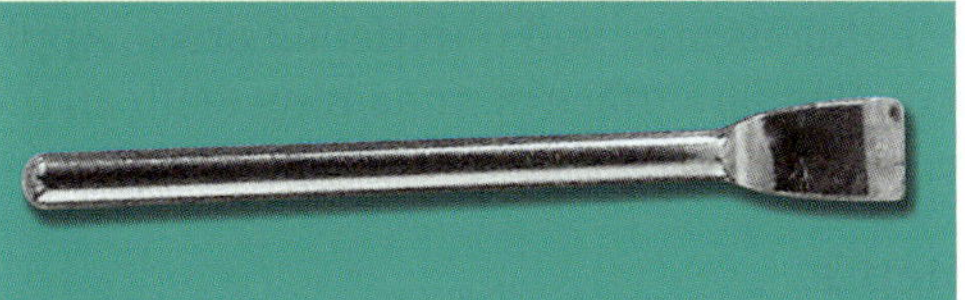

Fig. 37.11: Wax trimmer.

CHAPTER 38 Fabrication of Removable Partial Denture

Paranjay Prajapati, YG Naveen

INTRODUCTION

Complete denture is fabricated to replace all missing teeth and associated structures. Removable partial denture is fabricated to restore partially edentulous arches.

The basic procedures and principles for fabrication of removable partial denture are similar to that of complete denture. In this chapter, the fabrication of removable partial denture is given in brief.

FABRICATION OF RECORD BASED ON MAXILLARY AND MANDIBULAR PARTIALLY EDENTULOUS CASTS

Step 1

Mark the height of contour with pencil. Draw the outline for partial denture **(Figs. 38.1A and B)**.

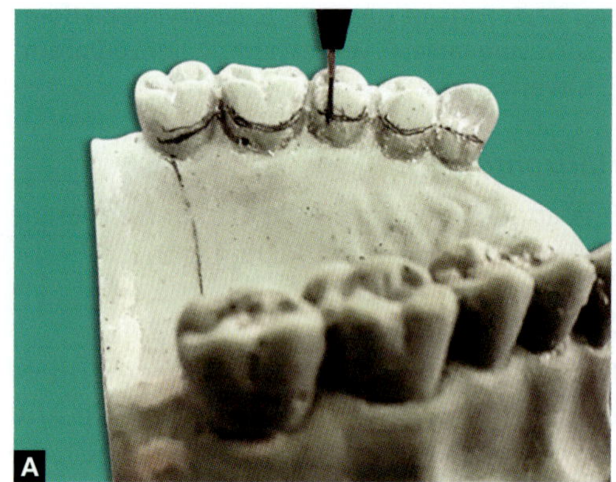

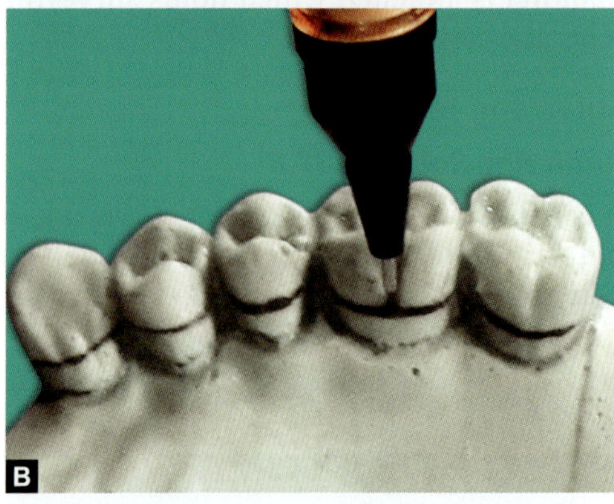

Figs. 38.1A and B: Marking height of contour on remaining teeth.

Step 2

Mark outline for making record base **(Figs. 38.2A and B)**. Apply cold mould seal on the edentulous area and interdental areas. Apply it on lingual surface of remaining teeth on the cast. Allow it to dry.

Step 3

Make record base with self-cure acrylic resin. Cover the remaining teeth on cast till the height of contour. Retrieve the record base slowly from the cast. Trim the excess acrylic resin from borders and smoothen the borders.

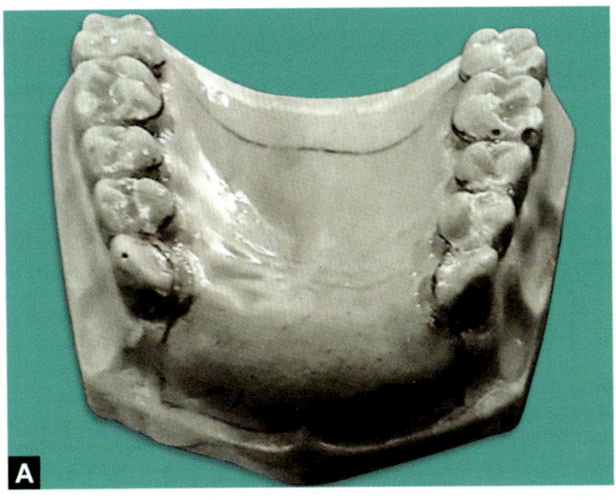

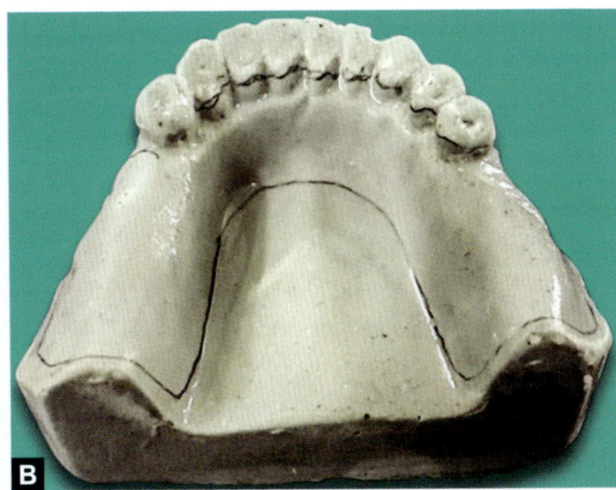

Figs. 38.2A and B: Marking outline and application of cold mould seal.

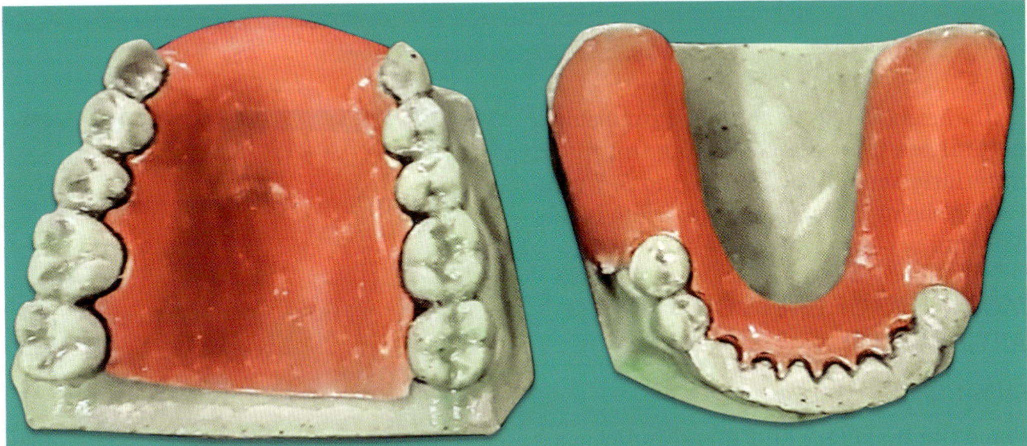

Fig. 38.3: Fabrication of record base for removable partial denture.

Extend the mandibular record base till the retromolar pads bilaterally **(Fig. 38.3)**.

FABRICATION OF OCCLUSION RIMS

Step 1 (Fig. 38.4)

Soften the wax sheet on Bunsen burner and fold it to make a roll of it. Take care not to entrap the air while making the wax roll.

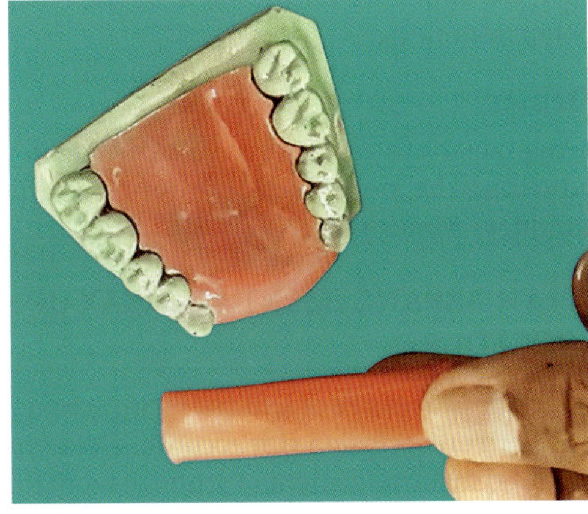

Fig. 38.4: Make wax roll of modeling wax.

Step 2 (Fig. 38.5)

Cut the wax roll according to the length of the edentulous span. Adapt the wax roll on denture base in edentulous area. Heat the wax knife and seal the wax on the record base.

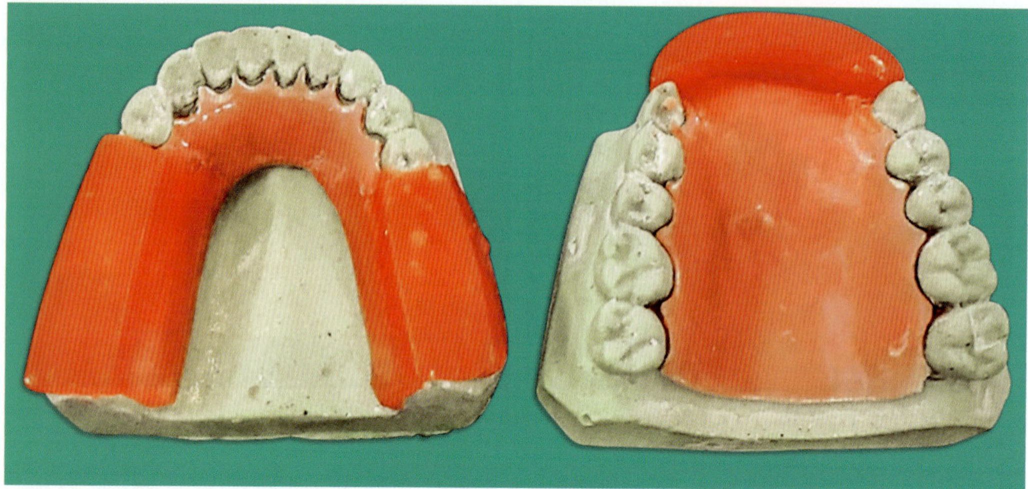

Fig. 38.5: Fabrication of occlusal rims.

The height is adjusted according to remaining natural teeth on the cast using hot plate. Anteriorly keep the width around 5–7 mm. Place it slightly labially. Posterior width is kept 8–10 mm.

MOUNTING OF CASTS ON ARTICULATOR

Step 1 (Fig. 38.6)

Place the maxillary and mandibular casts together. The remaining teeth on each cast should be in occlusion with teeth on opposite cast. Do indexing on the base of the casts before mounting.

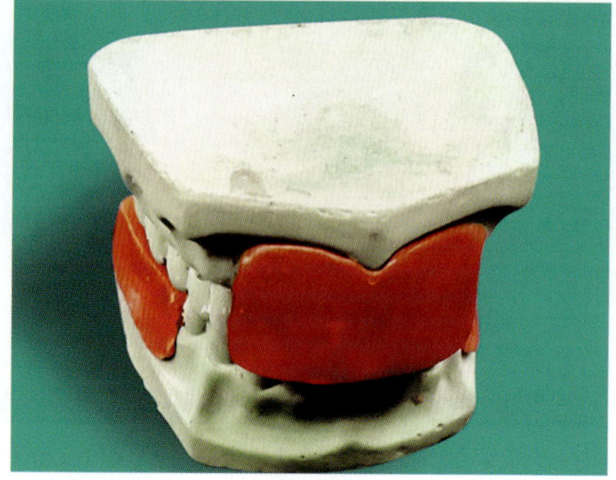

Fig. 38.6: Placing casts in occlusion.

Step 2

Articulate the casts on mean value articulator following the steps used for mounting the complete denture casts **(Figs. 38.7A to C)**.

TEETH ARRANGEMENT AND WAX UP PROCEDURE

Select the proper size of artificial teeth. Arrange the teeth on occlusion rim according to steps followed for arrangement of artificial teeth for complete denture. Make sure that artificial teeth are arranged with proper overjet and overbite along with proper occlusal contacts **(Figs. 38.8A to C)**.

Do the wax up according to the steps followed for complete denture wax up procedure.

PROCESSING OF REMOVABLE PARTIAL DENTURE

The flasking is done according to the standard procedure used for complete denture **(Fig. 38.9)**.

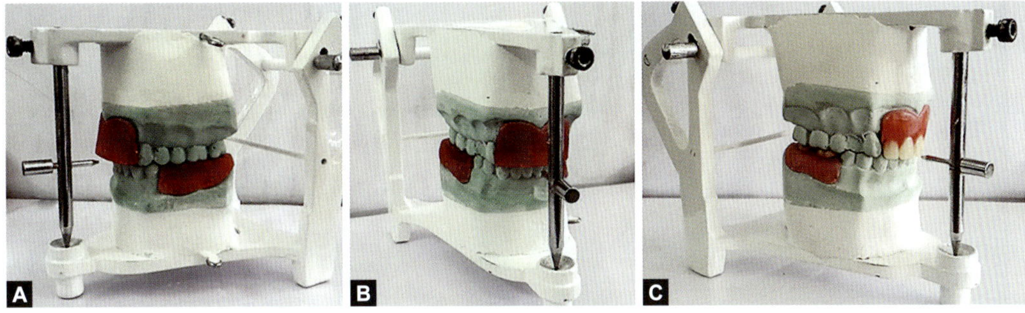

Figs. 38.7A to C: Mounting casts on mean value articulator.

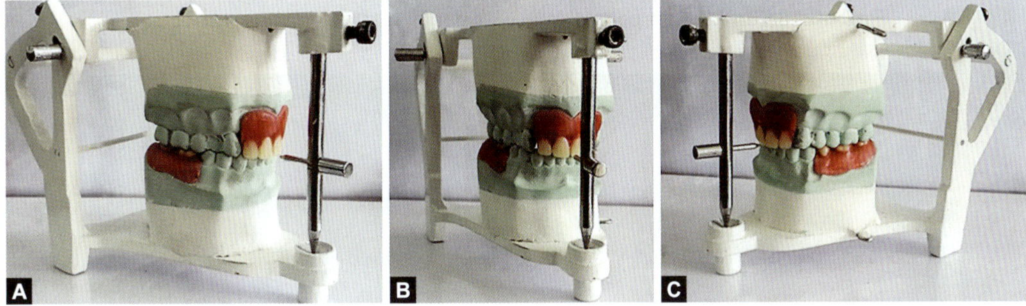

Figs. 38.8A to C: Teeth arrangement.

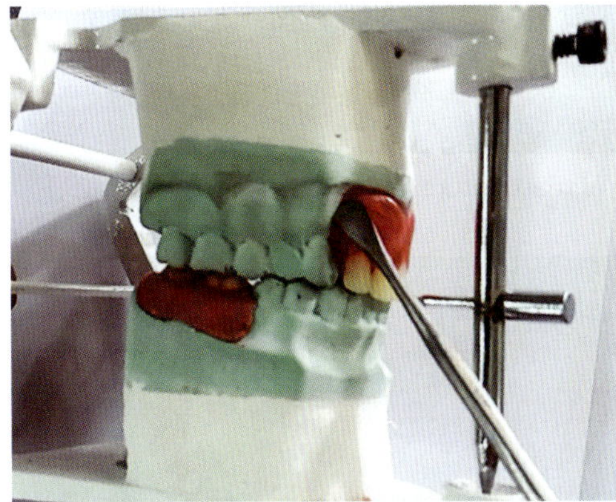

Fig. 38.9: Sealing of trial denture on the cast.

Select appropriate flasks. Pour creamy mixture of investing plaster on base of the flask and place cast in the center. Keep occlusal plane parallel to the base of the flask.

Make sure that there is no undercut in first pour. Make it sloping toward the rim of the flask. Heal of the mandibular cast should be at 45° **(Figs. 38.10A and B)**.

> Cover the remaining natural teeth on cast with plaster of first pour. This is done to eliminate undercuts created due to inclination of teeth.

Apply separating medium in unidirectional manner. Pour the second pour till the incisal edges and occlusal surfaces. Mix dental plaster and pour the third pour. Place the flasks on clamps and tighten them completely. Wax elimination is done by following the steps for complete denture wax elimination procedure **(Fig. 38.11)**.

Pack acrylic resin in dough stage and proceed for acrylization procedure. Remove flask after acrylization and open them to retrieve cured partial denture **(Fig. 38.12)**.

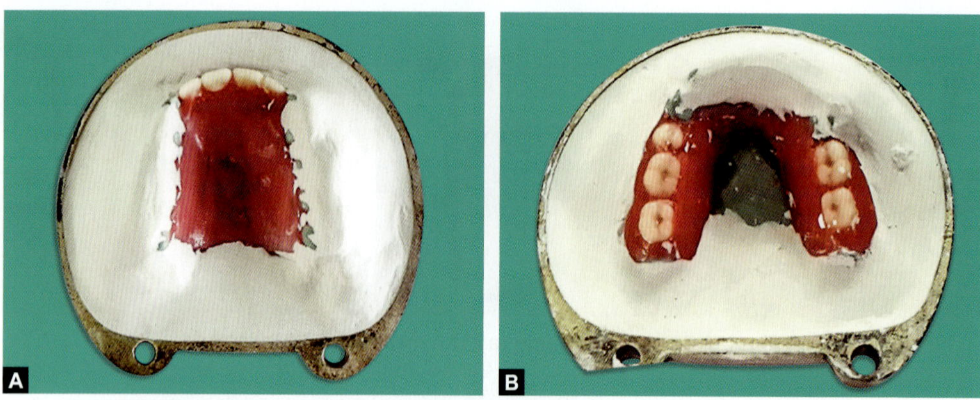

Figs. 38.10A and B: First pour is done with dental plaster with no undercuts.

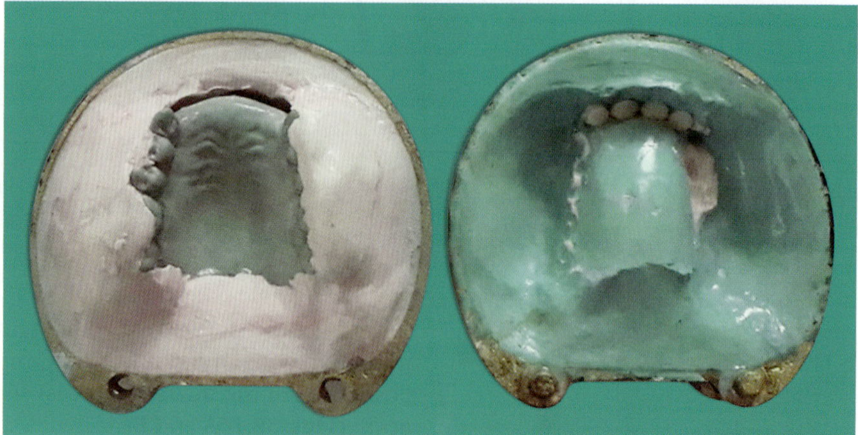

Fig. 38.11: Dewaxing of trial denture.

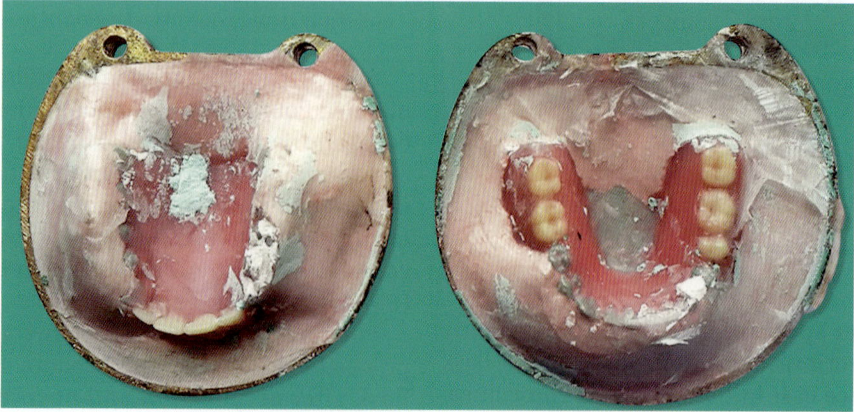

Fig. 38.12: Acrylization of removable partial dentures.

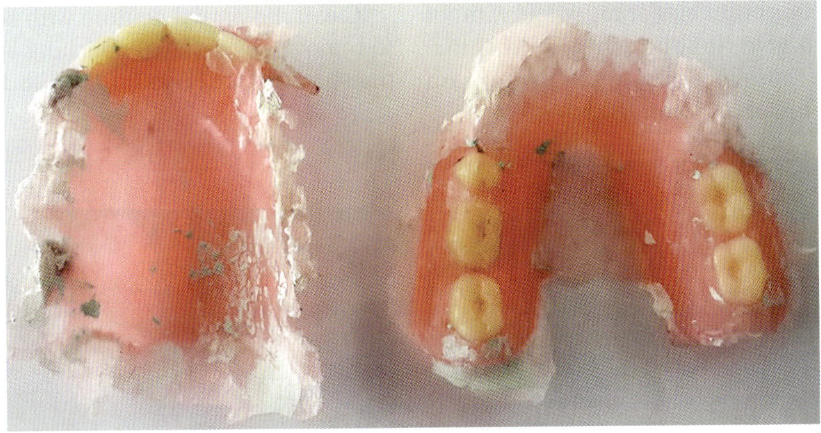

Fig. 38.13: Removable partial dentures retrieved from flasks.

Carefully retrieve the removable partial dentures from flasks. Trim excess material from borders and peripheries **(Fig. 38.13)**.

Finishing of removable partial denture is done using sand paper and emery paper **(Fig. 38.14)**.

Polishing (pumicing) is done using pumice powder or pumice cake. Use rag wheel to polish palatal surface of maxillary partial and lingual surface of mandibular partial denture **(Figs. 38.15A and B)**.

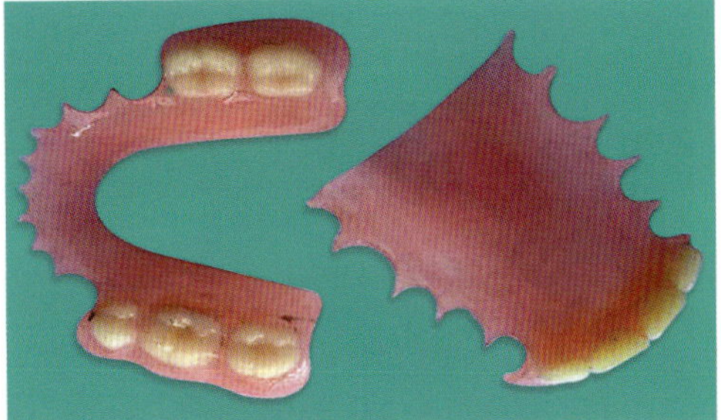

Fig. 38.14: Finished maxillary and mandibular partial dentures.

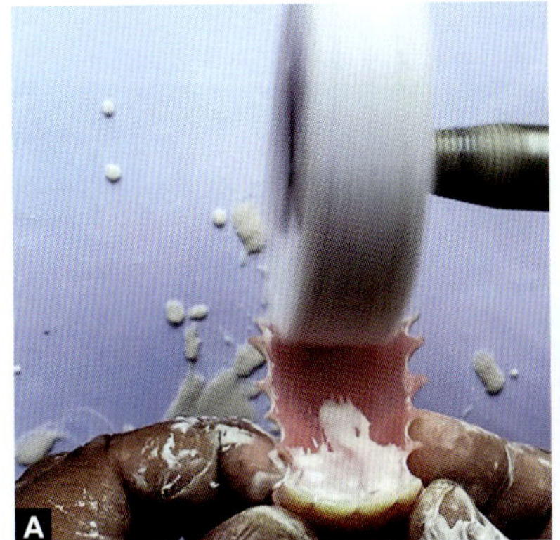

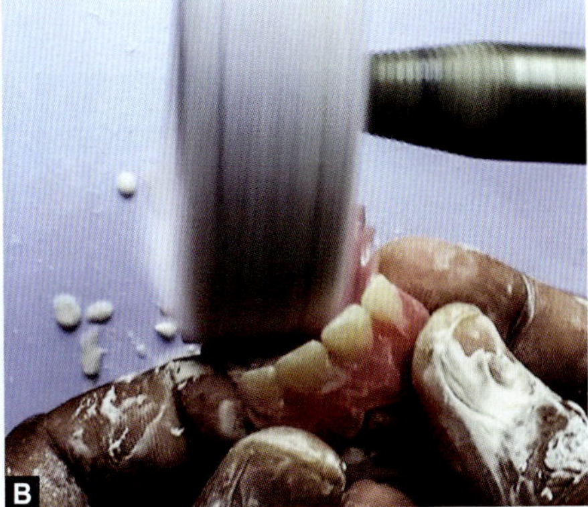

Figs. 38.15A and B: Polishing of maxillary and mandibular partial denture.

Use clean cotton buff or rag wheel without pumice to give final polishing and shine. This will remove any pumice present on surface **(Figs. 38.16A and B)**.

Clean the partial denture with soap water to remove any residual polishing agent from polished surface **(Figs. 38.17 to 38.19)**.

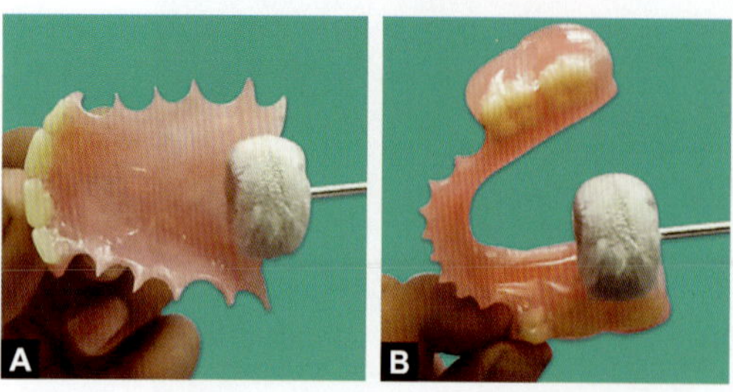

Figs. 38.16A and B: Use clean cotton buff or rag wheel to clean pumice from surface and give final luster.

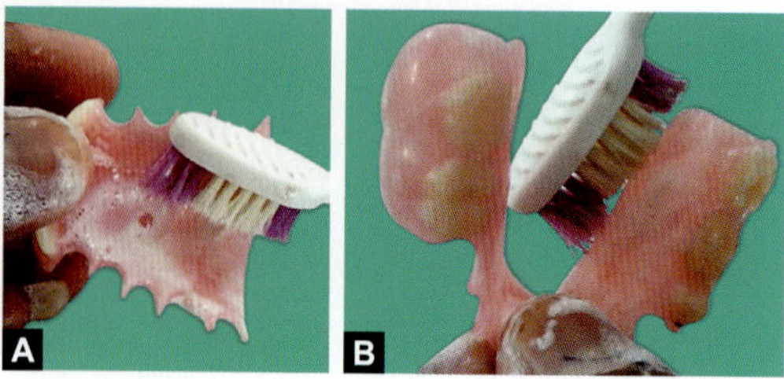

Figs. 38.17A and B: Cleaning with soap water.

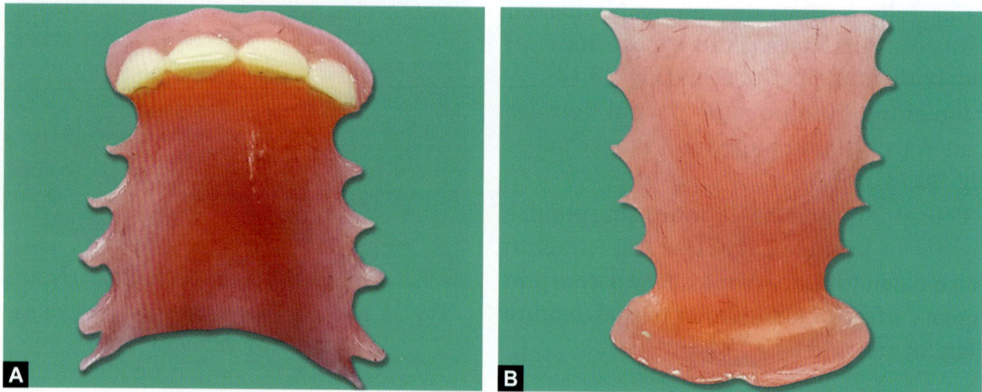

Figs. 38.18A and B: Polished surface and tissue surface of maxillary partial denture.

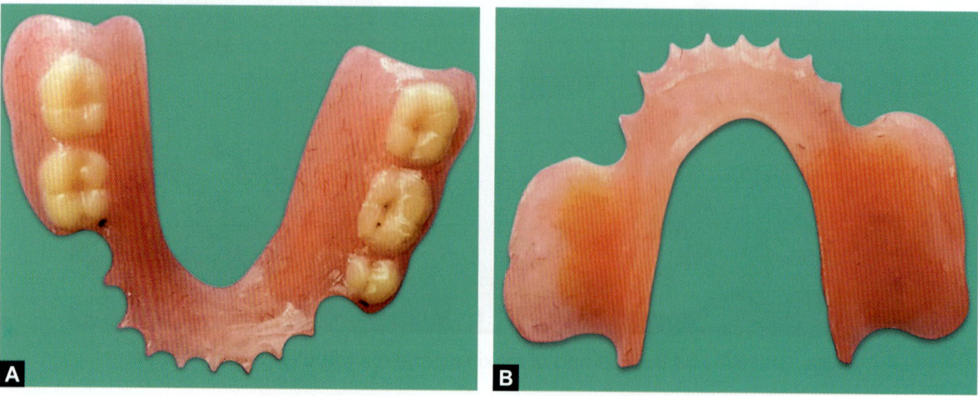

Figs. 38.19A and B: Polished surface and tissue surface of mandibular partial denture.

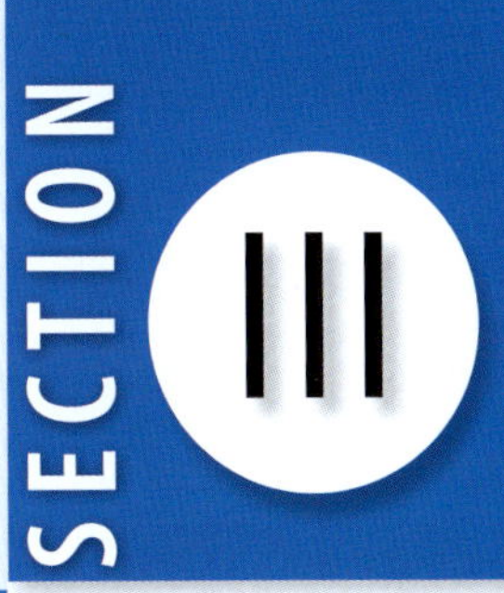

Fixed Partial Denture

Section Outline

CHAPTER 39

Fixed Partial Denture

Paranjay Prajapati, Rajesh Sethuraman

INTRODUCTION

Fixed partial denture or fixed dental prosthesis is a type of prosthesis which is fixed on prepared tooth surface. The abutments on which fixed partial denture is fixed are prepared by removing some of the tooth surface to achieve parallelism between abutments. This chapter introduces the fixed partial denture and its indications and contraindications.

DEFINITION

Fixed Prosthodontics

The branch of prosthodontics concerned with the replacement and/or restoration of teeth by artificial substitutes that are not readily removed from the mouth.

Fixed prosthodontics involves crown and fixed partial denture.

Crown

Replacement of missing tooth structure by surrounding all surfaces of tooth.

Fixed Partial Denture (Bridge Prosthesis)

A partial denture that is cemented or otherwise securely retained to natural teeth, tooth roots, or dental implant abutments that provide primary support for the prosthesis.

PARTS OF FIXED PARTIAL DENTURE (FIG. 39.1)

There are three parts of fixed partial denture **(Fig. 39.1)**:

1. Retainer
2. Pontic
3. Connector.

TYPES OF CROWN

Complete/Full Crown or Full Veneer Crown

It is a type of restoration which covers all surfaces of the tooth (occlusal, mesial, distal, buccal, and lingual).

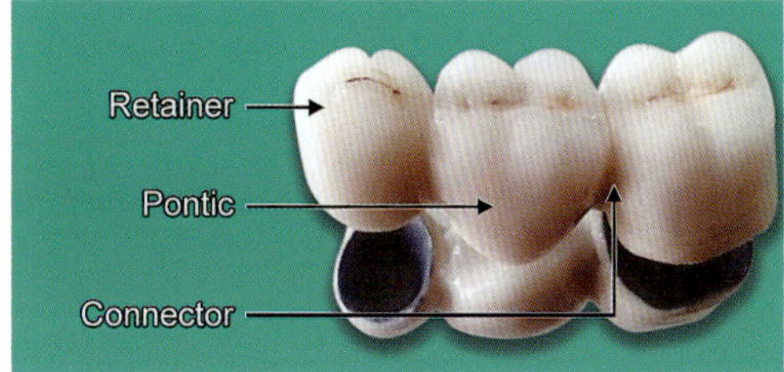

Fig. 39.1: Parts of fixed partial denture.

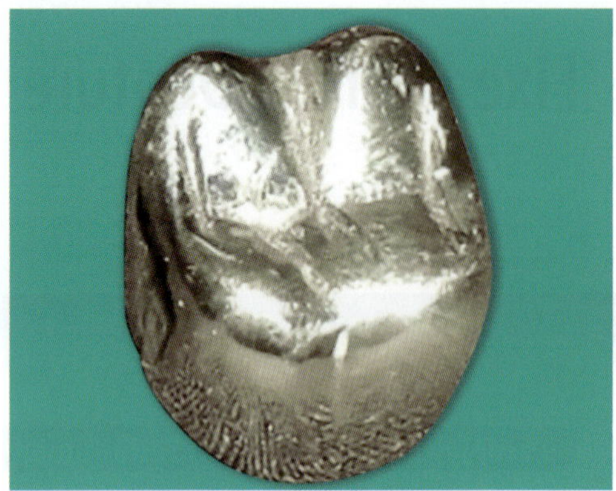

Fig. 39.2: All metal crown.

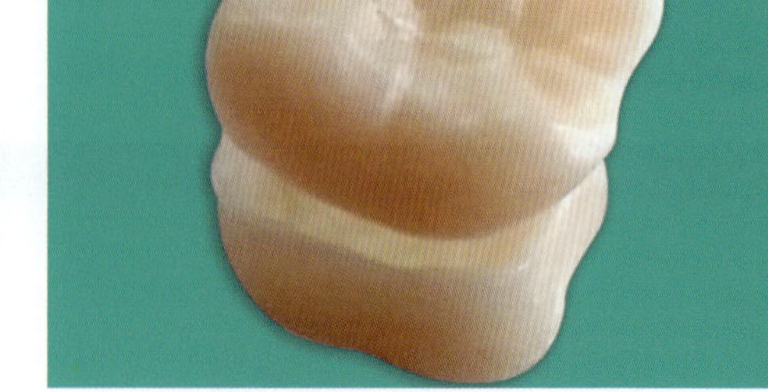

Fig. 39.3: All ceramic crown.

All Metal Crown (Fig. 39.2)

Made up of precious or nonprecious metal.

All Ceramic Crown (Fig. 39.3)

- Entirely fabricated of ceramic material.
- Used for esthetic replacement.

Metal with Ceramic (Porcelain Fused to Metal) (Fig. 39.4)

It is a combination of metal and porcelain materials. Metal substructure on which ceramic material is layered.

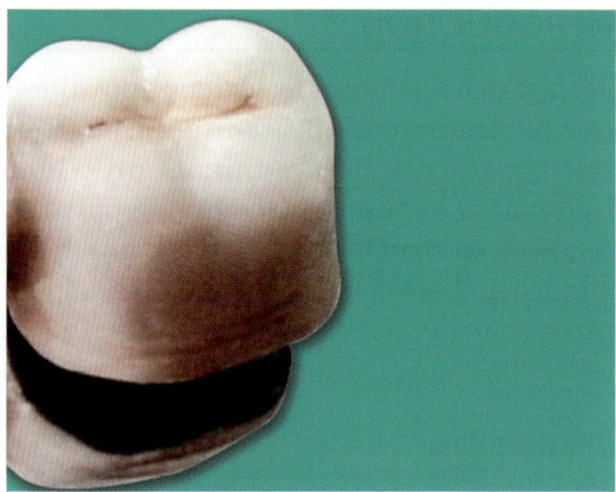

Fig. 39.4: Metal with ceramic (porcelain fused to metal).

Partial Veneer Crown

An extracoronal restoration that covers only part of the clinical crown is considered to be a partial veneer crown.

- Anterior third-fourths crown
- Posterior seven-eighths crown
- Posterior mesial half crown.

CHAPTER 40

Principles of Tooth Preparation: A Brief Overview

Paranjay Prajapati, Rajesh Sethuraman

INTRODUCTION

The success of fixed prosthodontics depends on the design of tooth preparation. Tooth preparation to receive cast restoration is based on principles of tooth preparation.

RATIONALE OF TOOTH PREPARATION

- Tooth preparation is done to receive the prosthesis.
- It is done to make the walls parallel or tapered and to device the path of insertion for prosthesis.
- Tooth preparation is done to achieve adequate retention and resistance form.
- To establish an adequate finish line as endpoint of restoration.

PRINCIPLES OF TOOTH PREPARATION

The principles governing the tooth preparation to receive fixed restorations are discussed as under.

Preservation of Tooth Structure

- The fixed prosthesis, must replace the lost tooth structure, but at the same time, it should not excessively reduce the remaining tooth structure.
- Making depth orientation grooves, before actual reduction prevents excessive tooth preparation.
- Prefer partial veneer crowns to save tooth structure wherever possible.
- Tooth preparation should be done under adequate coolant.
- Supragingival finish lines required less tooth preparation compared to subgingivally finish lines.

Retention and Resistance

Retention

It is the ability of the preparation to prevent the removal of restoration along its path of insertion (vertical forces).

Resistance

It is the ability of the preparation to prevent dislodgement of the restoration by forces directed in an apical/oblique/horizontal direction and to prevent any movement of the restoration under occlusive forces.

Factors Affecting Retention

Degree of taper: The prepared opposite walls should have tapered configuration. The preparation of opposite walls has a taper of

6° (3° on either side). To achieve desired amount of tapered on the wall, diamond point of known taper is used.

If the given taper is more, there will be reduction in the retention.

Total surface area of the cement film: Retention is directly proportional to available cementing area. If more tooth surface is available, the retention achieved will be more compared to lesser tooth surface. Molar will have greater retention than anteriors and premolars due to more surface area available for cementation on molars.

Roughness of the surface: Rough surface gives more retention compared to smooth surface. This is due to increase in surface area and micromechanical retention as a result of surface roughness. The prepared tooth cannot be made rough, so tissue surface of crown or prosthesis is made rough to get advantages of increased retention.

Factors Affecting Resistance

Length of the preparation: During tooth preparation minimum height of tooth should be maintained. Minimum length of abutment tooth should be 3–3.5 mm for adequate resistance and retention. If less crown height is available, than operator should place the finish line subgingivally to attain more length of prepared tooth.

Prevention of rotation around vertical axis: Resistance to rotation around vertical axis is core feature to achieve resistance. To prevent rotation of the crown around the vertical axis grooves, retentive boxes and retentive pins can be incorporated in tooth preparation.

Structural Durability

The preparation should be so designed that the restoration will have adequate bulk of metal or porcelain to withstand occlusal forces. The contours should be such that they prevent periodontal and occlusal problems. The functional cusp (palatal cusp in maxillary arch and buccal cusp in mandibular arch) should be reduced more compared to nonfunctional cusp to provide more bulk of material. Functional cusp bevel is indicated for this purpose. If functional cusp bevel is not given, then the resultant casting or restoration will be weaker.

If reduction is inadequate, it results in weak restoration, occlusal discrepancy, and easy perforation of restoration. The occlusal surface preparation should follow the tooth anatomy. The inclined planes of cusp should be maintained. Cusp tips should be rounded after preparation.

Marginal Integrity

The success of a restoration depends upon the adaptation of the margins to the finish line. For the success of restoration, the margins should extend up to the tooth line of preparation. It should closely adapt to the cavosurface of finish line. It should maintain a continuous contact with the finish line. An acute angle should be given at the margin for better adaptation. The finish line should follow the contour of gingival margin.

Preservation of Periodontium

During tooth preparation there should be no trauma to periodontal tissue. Preserve gingival integrity during tooth preparation. If finish line is to be placed subgingivally, it should not encroach upon gingival tissue.

Finish Lines

Finish line is termination of prepared tooth on which the restoration seats. Finish lines can be classified according to their shape and according to their location of placement.

Finish Lines According to Location

The finish lines according to location are given in **Table 40.1**.

Finish Lines According to Shape

The finish lines according to shape are described in **Table 40.2**.

Table 40.1: Finish lines according to location.

Supragingival finish line	Placed 0.5–1.0 mm above the gingival margin
Equigingival finish line	Placed at the level of gingival margin
Subgingival finish line	Placed below gingival margin. Placed in gingival sulcus. Indicated for esthetic zone

Table 40.2: Finish lines according to shape.

Finish line	*Configuration*	*Indications/advantages*
Chamfer	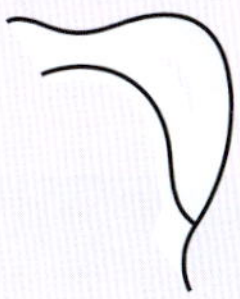	❑ Allows a slip joint and provides adequate bulk ❑ Tooth reduction needed is not much ❑ Especially used for gold restorations or metal restorations ❑ Easy to establish ❑ Can be easily burnished
Shoulder	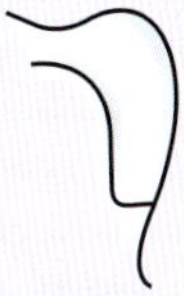	❑ For all porcelain jacket crown ❑ For porcelain fused to metal restoration especially on labial surface ❑ The wide ledge provides resistance to occlusal forces and minimizes stresses that may fracture porcelain
Beveled shoulder	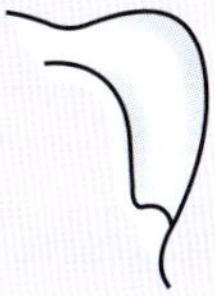	❑ It is a modified type of shoulder finish line ❑ The angle of the bevel improves marginal adaptation ❑ It forms an obtuse angle with the axial wall ❑ Especially indicated on labial finish line of porcelain fused to metal restorations
Heavy chamfer	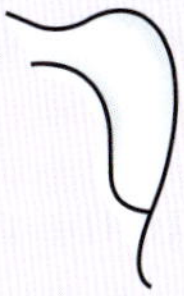	❑ Angle with a large-radius rounded internal angle ❑ The heavy chamfer provides better support for a ceramic crown than does a conventional chamfer, but it is not as good as a shoulder
Knife edge	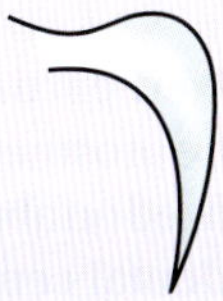	❑ Minimum tooth preparation ❑ For metal restoration ❑ Not widely used ❑ Indicated for tilted tooth ❑ In case of gingival recession

Pontic, Retainers, and Connectors

Paranjay Prajapati, Rajesh Sethuraman

INTRODUCTION

Fixed partial denture has three parts namely: (1) pontic, (2) retainer, and (3) connector **(Fig. 41.1)**. This chapter deals with types and characteristics of each components of fixed partial denture.

PONTIC

Definition

An artificial tooth on a fixed dental prosthesis that replaces a missing natural tooth restores its function and usually fills the space previously occupied by the clinical crown.

This replaces the missing natural tooth crown and its functions. It may be made up of acrylic, metal, ceramic and combination of metal, and ceramic and metal with acrylic.

Classification

Pontics are classified on the basis of material of fabrication and method of fabrication and based on contact with mucosa **(Flowchart 41.1)**.

RETAINER

Definition

Fixed dental prosthesis retainer: The part of a fixed dental prosthesis that unites the abutment(s) to the remainder of the restoration.

Or

A component of fixed partial denture which support and fixes the prosthesis on abutments.

Retainer will be fixed on abutment (prepared tooth/teeth) with dental cement or any other mechanism. This helps the prosthesis to be fix in its position. Retainer can be of various types as given in classification.

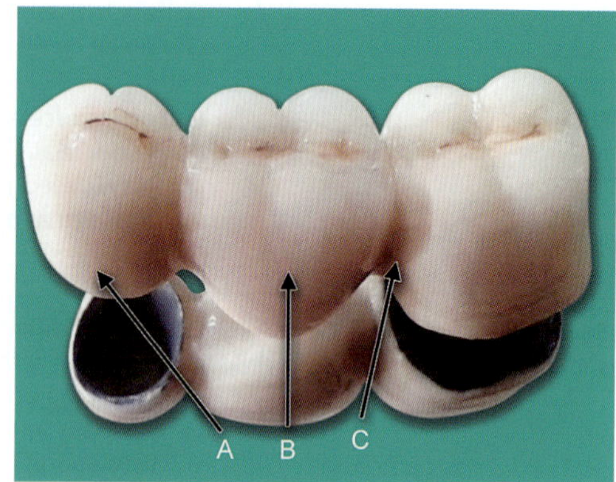

Fig. 41.1: Parts of fixed partial denture: A, retainer; B, pontic; C, connector.

Classification

The classification of retainers is given in **Flowchart 41.2**.

Flowchart 41.1: Classification of pontic.

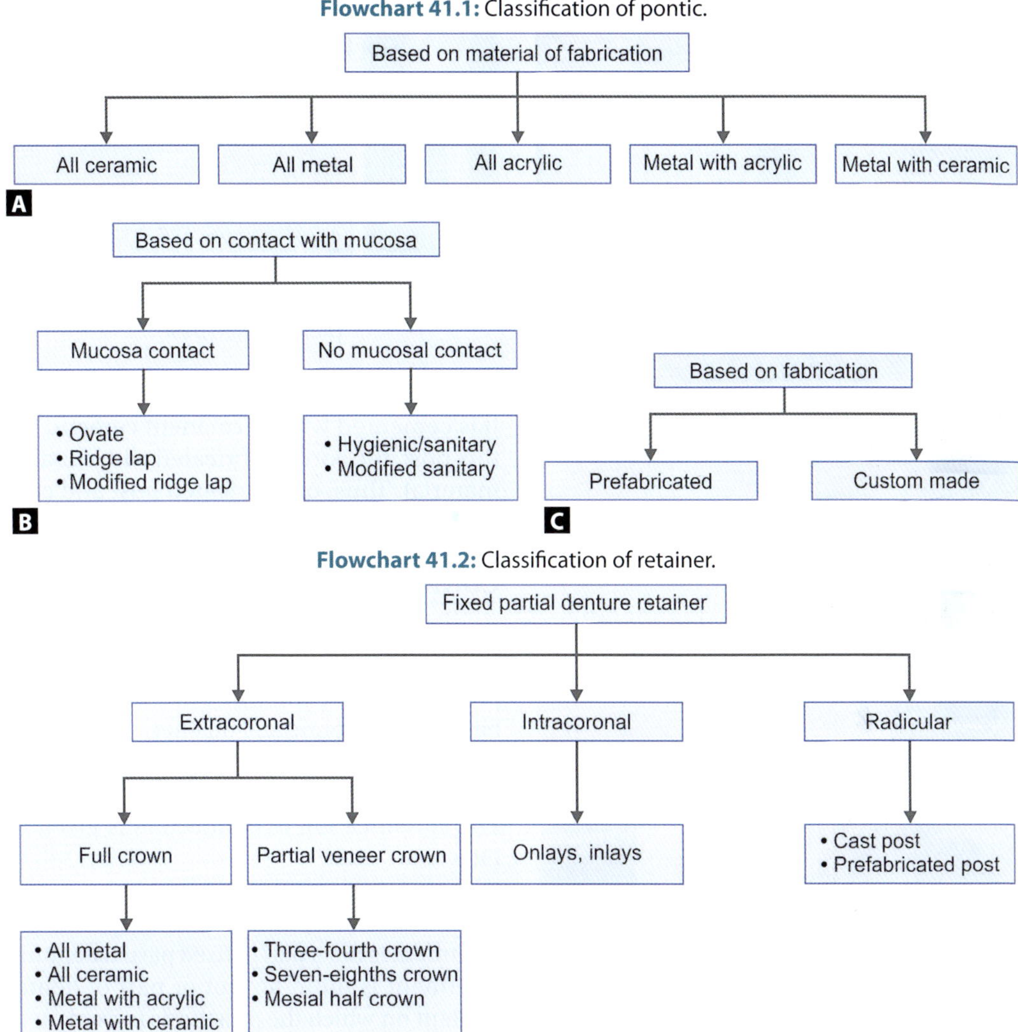

Flowchart 41.2: Classification of retainer.

Intracoronal Retainers

Inlays: This is a type of dental restoration which is made outside the oral cavity and does not cover the full occlusal surface. This type of restoration confines to the prepared cavity particularly made for it.

Onlays: This kind of restoration may cover one or more cusps with adjoining occlusal surface. It may cover the entire occlusal surface but other surfaces are not covered by it (in full crown all the surfaces of tooth are covered).

Radicular Retainers

When the amount of remaining coronal tooth structure is not sufficient to provide adequate support for prosthesis, radicular retainers are used. They are used with endodontically treated tooth. It is also known as post and core (**Figs. 41.2 and 41.3**).

Cast post: It is custom cast post, which has core part attached with post. Post and core are made up of same material (one piece).

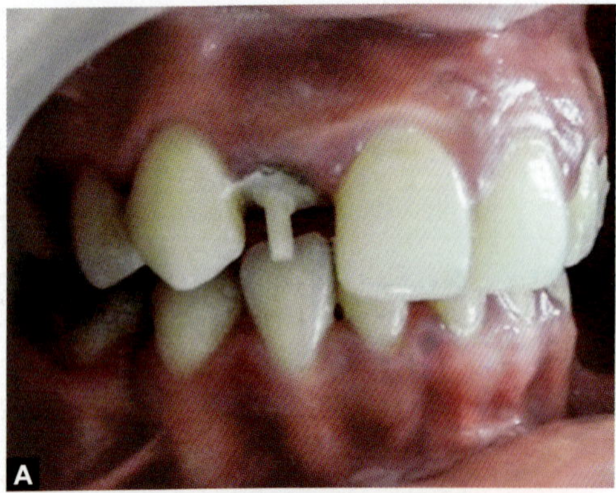

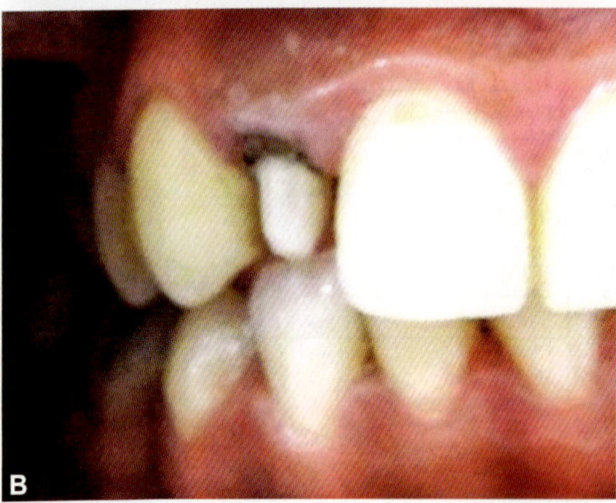

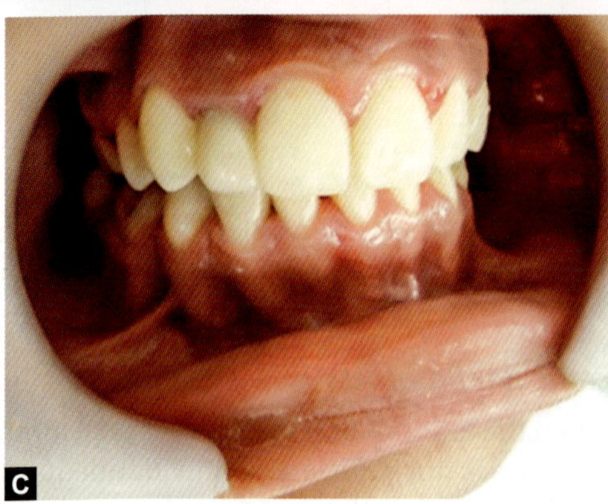

Figs. 41.2A to C: Use of prefabricated post.

Prefabricated post: They are available in various designs and materials. The post is inserted in root canal (after preparing post space) according to the diameter of canal. It is placed as apical as possible in root canal

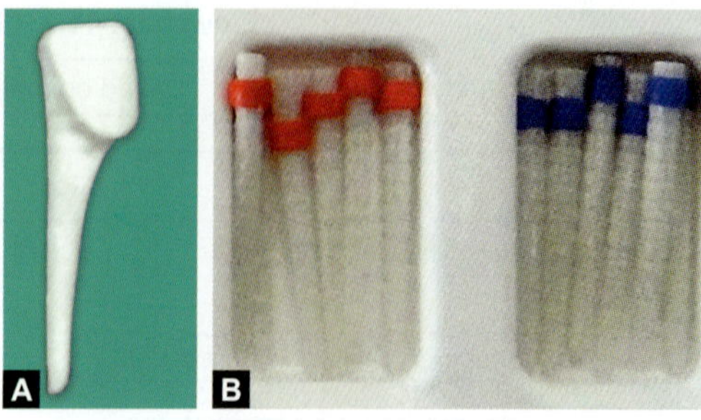

Figs. 41.3A and B: Cast post and core, and prefabricated post.

to attain maximum retention and support. It is cemented with permanent cement. On this post, the core is fabricated with suitable material. Thus, prefabricated post and core are two separate units but joined together.

CONNECTORS

Connector is a part of fixed partial denture. It connects the pontic with the retainer. It provides connection or link or continuity between the pontic and retainer.

Classification

The classification of connectors is given in **Flowchart 41.3**.

Abutment

Abutment is not a part of fixed partial denture. Abutment is tooth or root or part of dental implant on which the prosthesis is fixed.

Flowchart 41.3: Classification of connectors.

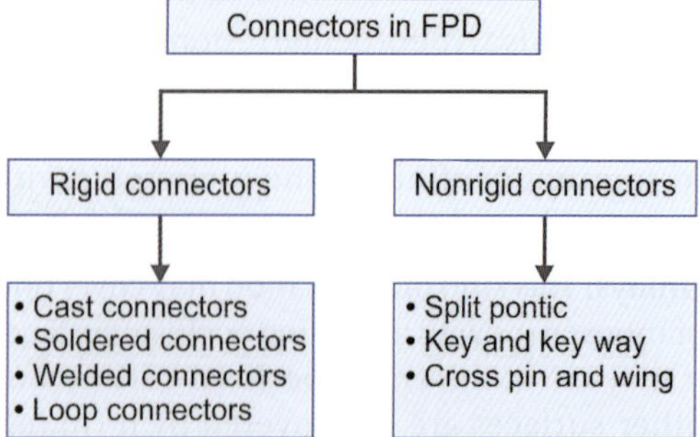

CHAPTER 42

Tooth Preparation to Receive all Ceramic Crown

Paranjay Prajapati, Rajesh Sethuraman

INTRODUCTION

All ceramic crowns are considered as esthetic option for anterior restoration. The preparation to receive all ceramic crowns needs more amount of tooth reduction compared to other available options. This chapter describes stepwise tooth preparation to receive all ceramic crown restoration.

TOOTH PREPARATION

The stepwise preparation of maxillary central incisor to receive all ceramic crowns is given here.

Incisal Reduction

Depth of preparation (amount of tooth preparation): 2 mm.

Instrument: Flat-end tapering diamond.

Place depths orienting grooves or depth cuts on the incisal edge. Place three cuts on incisal edge, one on mid-incisal region and one each at the junction of each proximal surface **(Figs. 42.1A and B)**.

Remove remaining tooth structure from incisal edge using small wheel diamond or flat-end tapering diamond **(Figs. 42.2A and B)**.

Labial Reduction

Depth of preparation (amount of tooth preparation): 1.5 mm.

Instrument: Flat-end tapering diamond.

The labial surface of incisor can be divided in two planes. These are located at different angulation thus labial surface is prepared in two planes **(Figs. 42.3A to C)**.

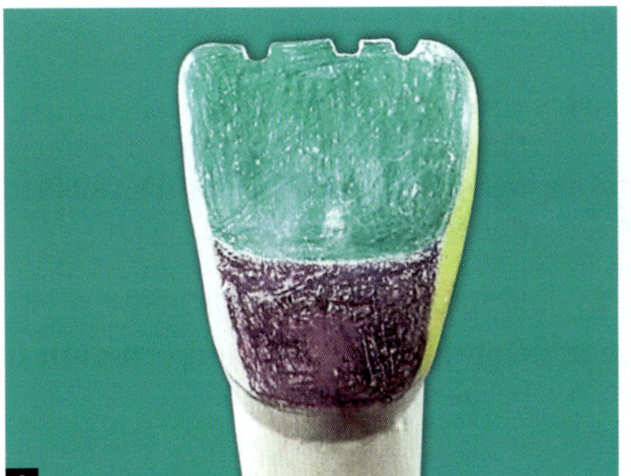

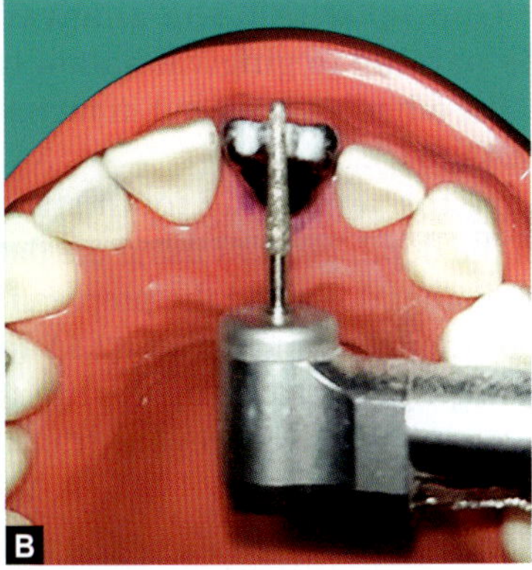

Figs. 42.1A and B: Place depth orientation grooves on incisal edge.

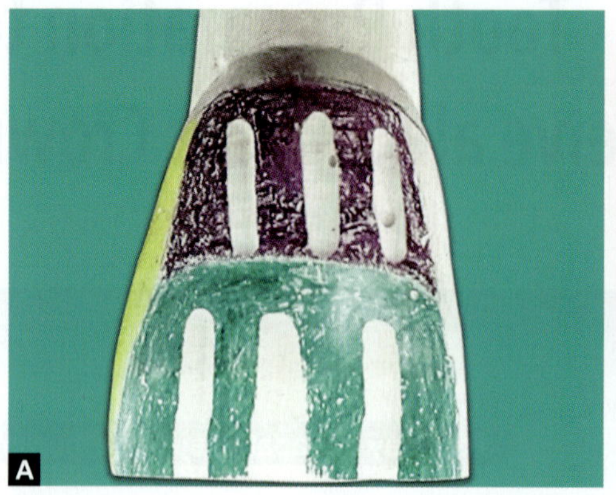

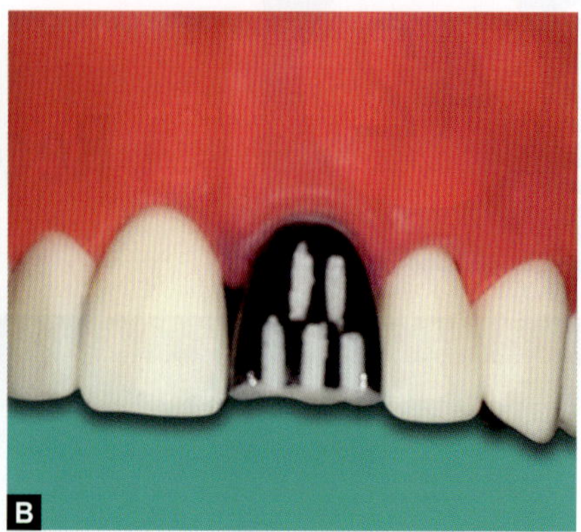

Figs. 42.2A and B: Reduction of incisal edge.

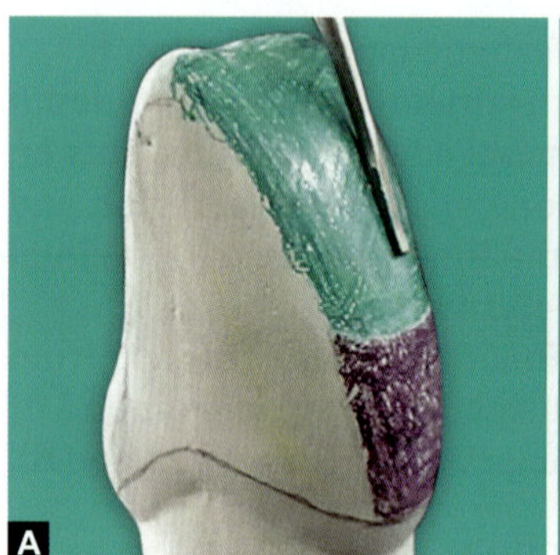

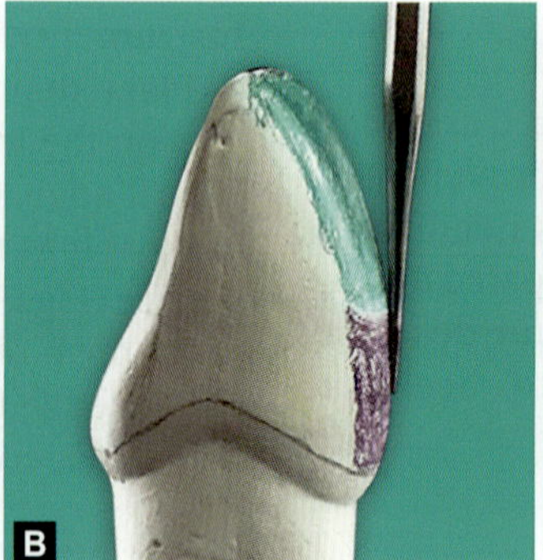

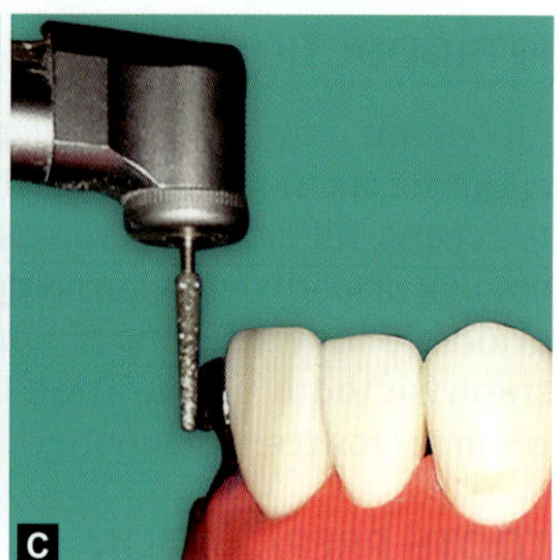

Figs. 42.3A to C: Two planes of labial surface of central incisors.

Prepare the labial surface of maxillary incisor in two planes. Place the depth orientation grooves by sinking flat-end tapering diamond up to 1.2 mm which after finishing will produce a depth of 1.5 mm.

Place the depth orienting grooves in two planes. One set within the gingival half and it is parallel to gingival half of labial surface. The other set is placed in incisal half **(Figs. 42.4A to C)**.

Remove the remaining tooth structure between the depth grooves using the flat-end tapering diamond. Extend the preparation to the facioproximal line angle **(Figs. 42.5A and B)**.

Follow gingival contour during tooth preparation. This will prevent trauma to interdental papillae and limit the preparation in gingival sulcus.

A shoulder finish line is produced by flat-end tapered diamond. Shoulder finish line can be placed subgingival (recommended for anterior teeth) or equigingival **(Figs. 42.6A and B)**.

Lingual Reduction

Lingual reduction is done in two parts. Axial reduction is done first and then tooth reduction done from lingual fossa.

Lingual Axial Reduction

Depth of preparation (amount of tooth preparation): 1.5 mm.

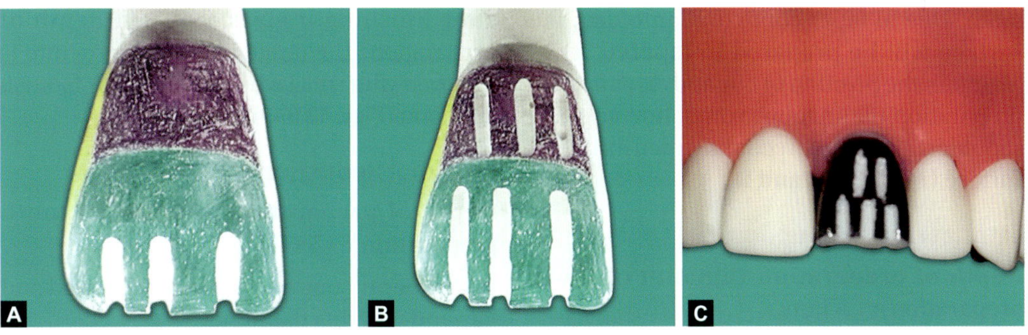

Figs. 42.4A to C: Placement of depth orienting grooves in two planes.

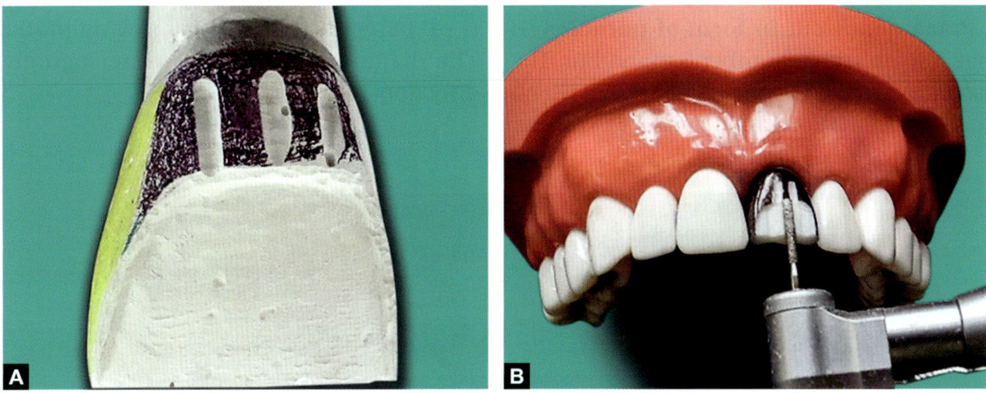

Figs. 42.5A and B: Removal of tooth structure between the grooves.

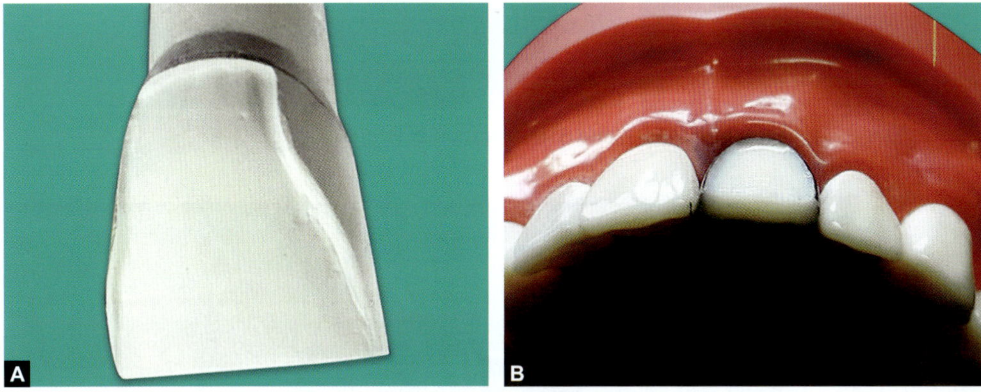

Figs. 42.6A and B: Shoulder finish line on labial surface.

Instrument: Flat-end tapering diamond.

Lingual axial reduction will prepare cervical portion of lingual surface of tooth. This surface should be given taper of 3–5° with cervical part of labial surface. Place flat-end taper diamond straight against this surface and prepare the tooth. Due to taper configuration of bur, the surface will be prepared in tapered style. Maintain the position of bur and extend tooth preparation till linguoproximal line angle. A shoulder finish line is recommended in lingual surface (**Figs. 42.7A and B**).

Lingual Fossa Reduction

Depth of preparation (amount of tooth preparation): 1.5 mm.

Instrument: Number 6 round bur and wheel diamond or football diamond.

Place depth cut in form of potholes in lingual fossa with a number 6 round bur. The diameter of round bur should be 1.8 mm which produces depth cuts of approximately 1–1.2 mm after finishing it gives required depth of preparation. The remaining tooth structure is removed with small wheel diamond or football diamond (**Figs. 42.8A to C**).

Proximal Reduction

Depth of preparation (amount of tooth preparation): 1.5 mm.

Instrument: Long thin tapering diamond and flat-end tapering diamond.

Long thin tapering diamond is used to prepare proximal tooth surface. The access is prepared using a vertical sawing motion. The diamond should follow incisogingival direction.

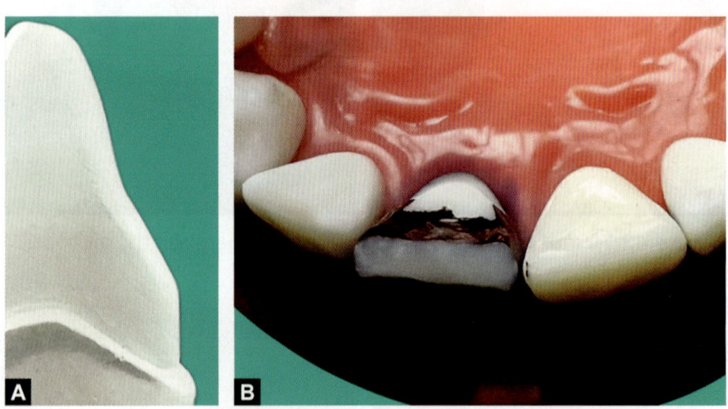

Figs. 42.7A and B: Preparation of lingual surface.

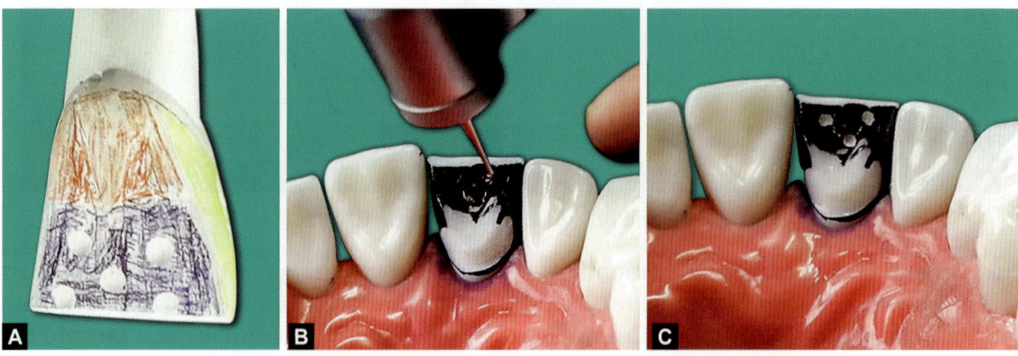

Figs. 42.8A to C: Depth orientation using number 6 round bur.

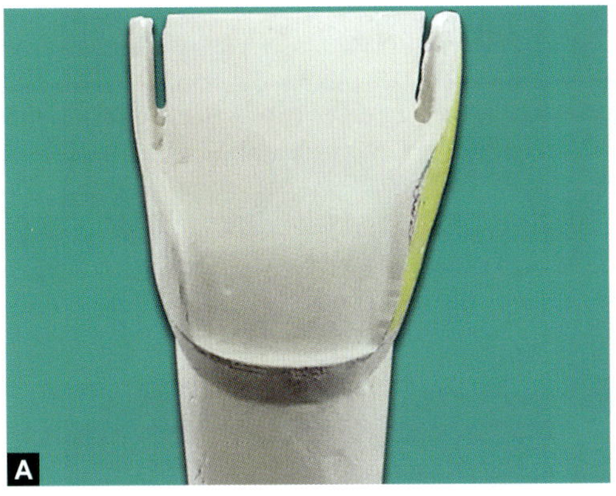

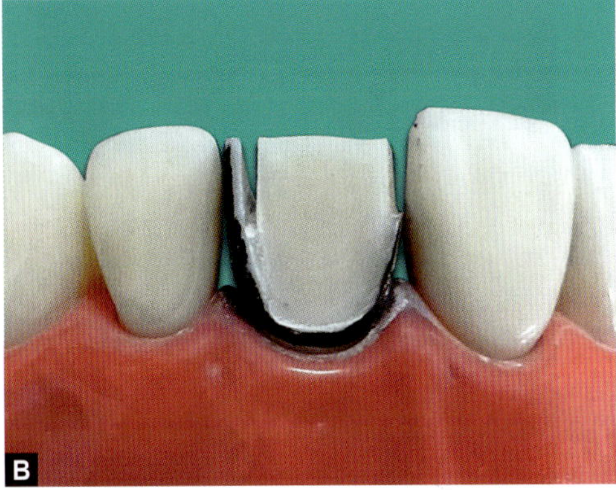

Figs. 42.9A and B: Formation of enamel lip.

This motion will cut the tooth surface proximally. The cut is through proximal enamel and produce the enamel lip **(Figs. 42.9A and B)**.

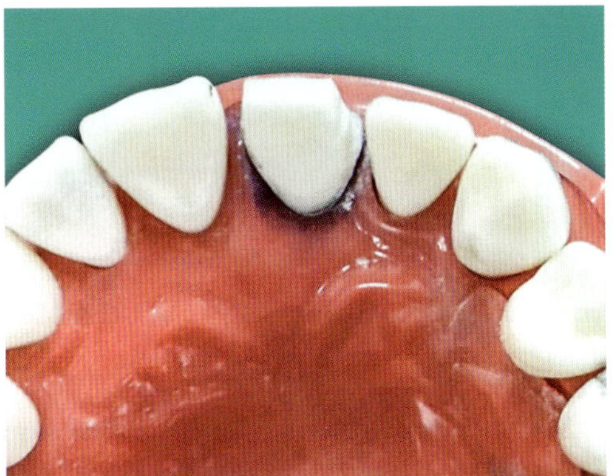

Fig. 42.10: Join labial and lingual preparation in proximal area.

Remove enamel lip by any hand instrument or by diamond point. Use flat-end tapering diamond to join facial and lingual preparation through proximal area. This produces proximal surface with taper of 3–5°. Produce smooth shoulder in proximal area following the gingival contour **(Fig. 42.10)**.

Prepared tooth to receive all ceramic crown **(Figs. 42.11A to C)**.

FINISHING OF PREPARATION

Make all the point and line angles rounded to prevent stress concentration and fracture.

Axial surface can be finished with yellow collar fine grit diamond. The shoulder can be

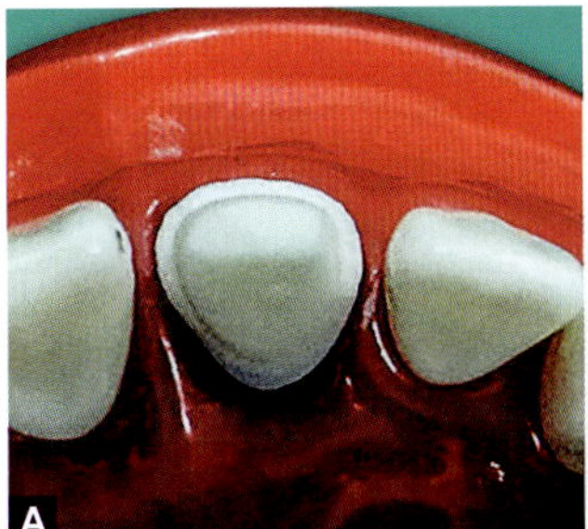

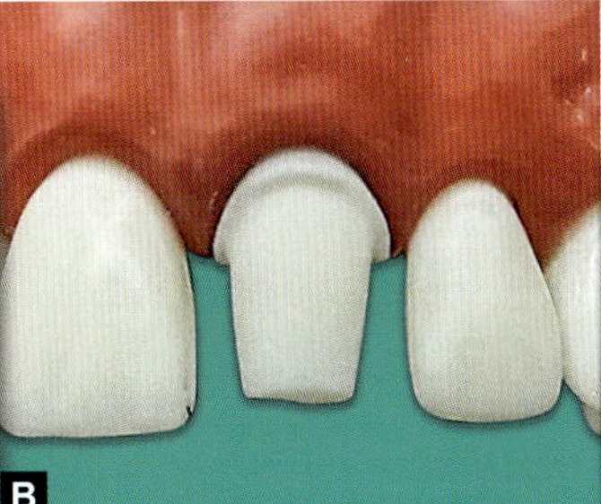

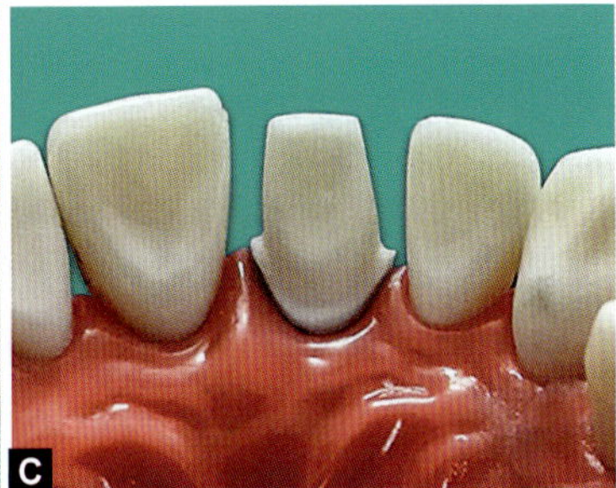

Figs. 42.11A to C: Prepared maxillary central incisor—occlusal view, labial view, and lingual view.

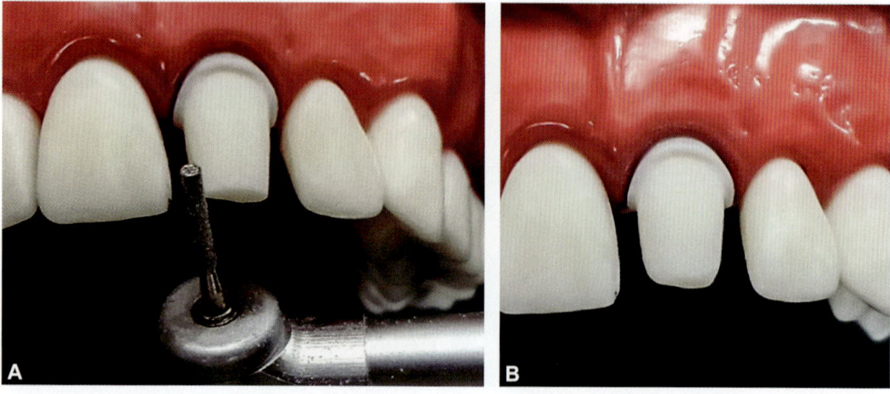

Figs. 42.12A and B: Make all the point and line angles rounded.

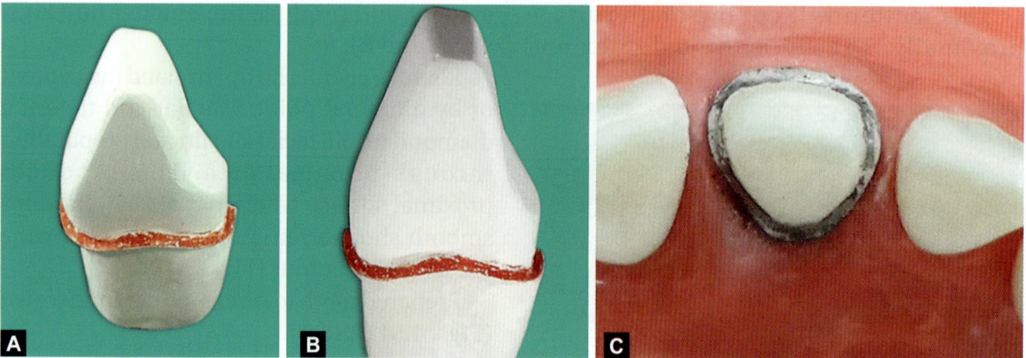

Figs. 42.13A to C: Tooth preparation and shoulder finish line—side view and top view.

finished with end cutting diamond where only tip has fine diamonds and sides are noncutting **(Figs. 42.12A and B)**.

See the shoulder finish line on labial side, proximal side, and lingual side **(Figs. 42.13A to C)**.

CHAPTER 43

Tooth Preparation to Receive all Metal Crown

Paranjay Prajapati, Rajesh Sethuraman

INTRODUCTION

The preparation to receive all metal crown needs less amount of tooth reduction. This chapter describes stepwise tooth preparation to receive all metal crown restoration on mandibular molar.

TOOTH PREPARATION

The stepwise preparation of maxillary central incisor to receive porcelain fused metal (PFM) crown is given here.

Occlusal Reduction

Depth of preparation (amount of tooth preparation): 1 mm on nonfunctional cusp and 1.5 mm on functional cusp.

Instrument: Round-end tapering diamond.

Depth orienting grooves or depth cuts of 1 mm are placed on the occlusal grooves. Round diamond or bur of 2 mm diameter can also be used for placing depth cuts on occlusal surface **(Figs. 43.1 and 43.2)**.

Place depth cuts on triangular ridges from cusp tip to base **(Fig. 43.3)**.

Remove tooth structure between the depth cuts. Follow the contour and anatomy during tooth preparation **(Fig. 43.4)**.

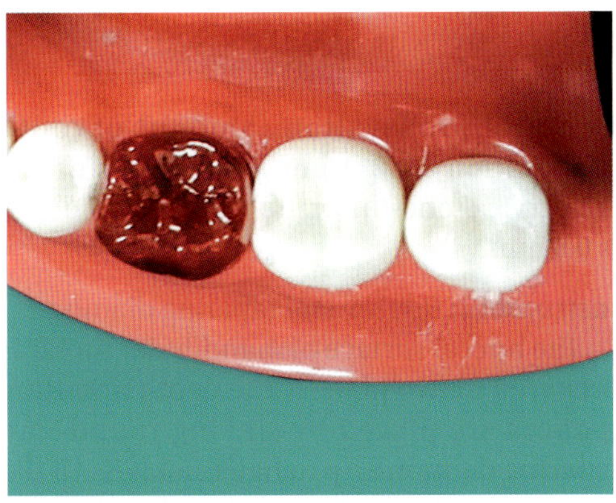

Fig. 43.1: Depth orienting grooves.

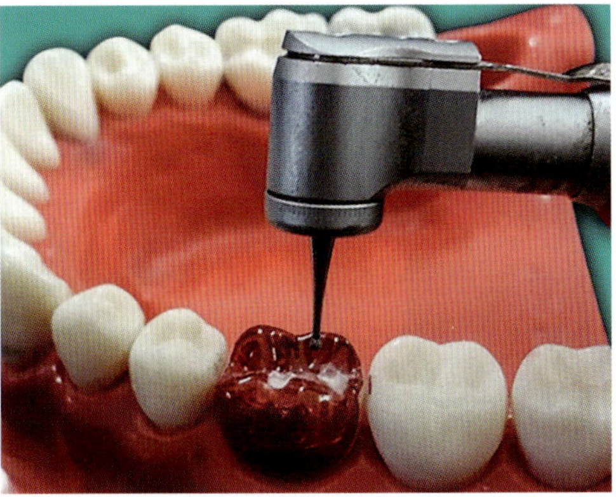

Fig. 43.2: Placing depth cuts.

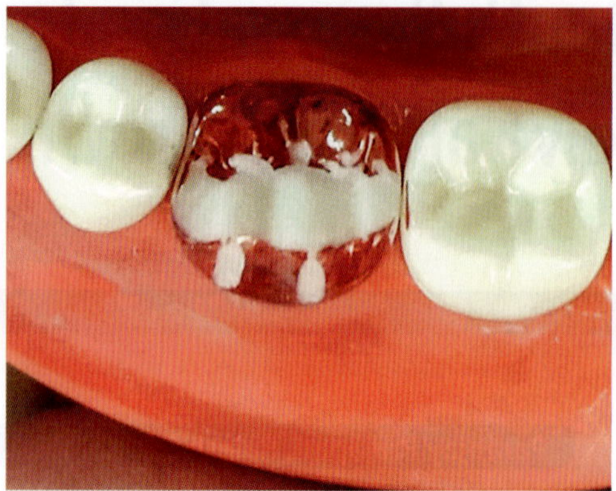

Fig. 43.3: Depth cuts on triangular ridges.

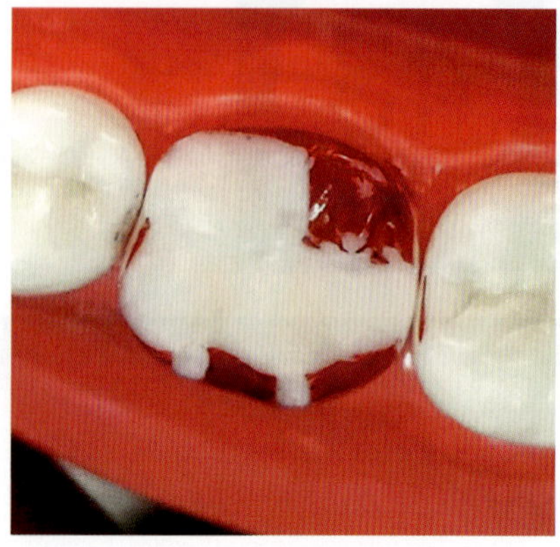

Fig. 43.4: Remove tooth between the grooves.

Axial Reduction: Buccal and Lingual Preparation

Depth of preparation (amount of tooth preparation): 0.8–1 mm on buccal surface. On cervical one-third, the preparation depth is 0.5 mm.

Instrument: Round-end tapering diamond.

The buccal surface of mandibular molar is prepared in two planes. The depth orienting grooves are placed by sinking round-end tapering diamond up to half thickness (if the diameter of bur is 2 mm, then it will place depth-orientation grooves of 1 mm by sinking the bur by half thickness) **(Figs. 43.5A and B)**.

The depth orienting grooves are placed in two planes. One within the gingival half and it is parallel to gingival half of axial surface. The other is placed in occlusal half.

The remaining tooth structure between the depth grooves is then removed using the round-end tapering diamond. Extend the preparation proximally 1 mm beyond the contact point **(Fig. 43.6)**.

Follow gingival contour during tooth preparation. This will prevent trauma to interdental papillae.

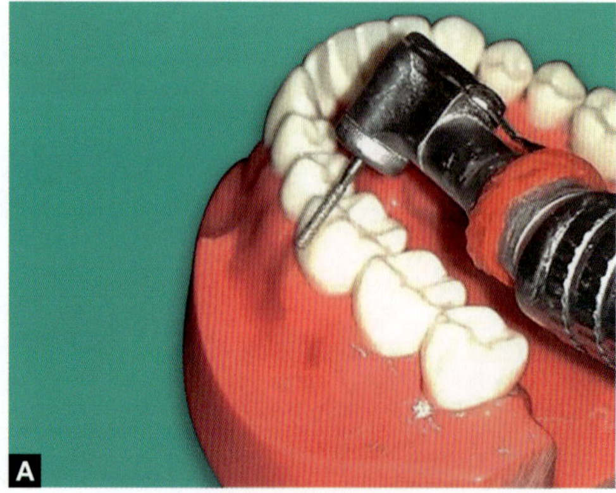

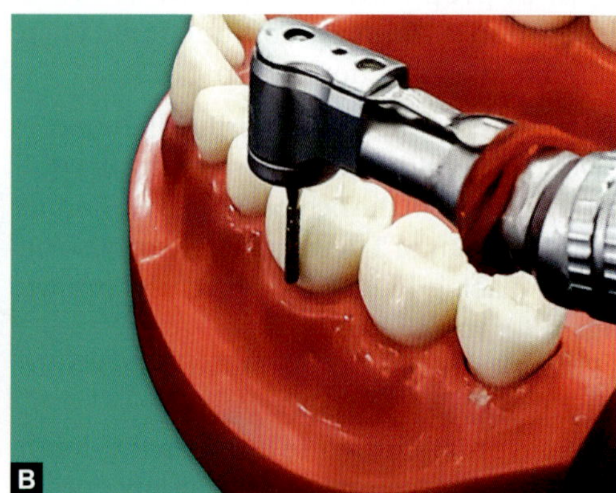

Figs. 43.5A and B: Two planes on buccal surface of mandibular molar.

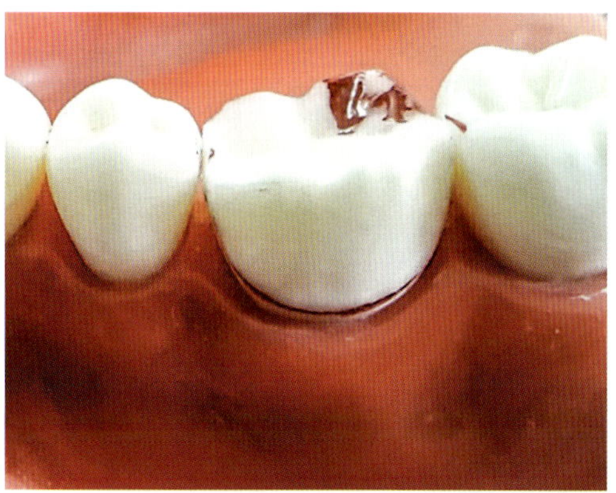

Fig. 43.6: Remove tooth structure between grooves on buccal surface.

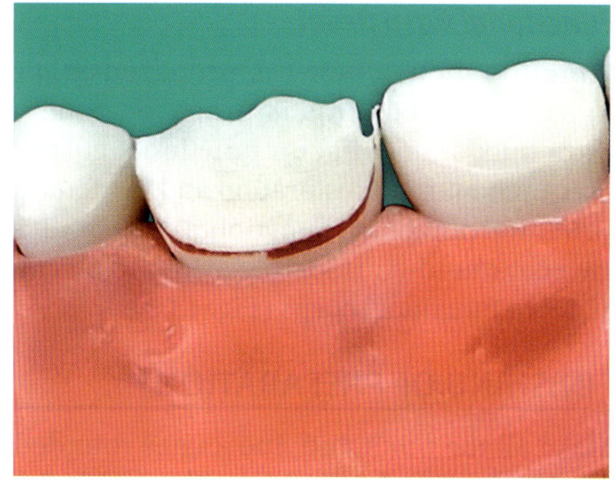

Fig. 43.7: Enamel lip preparation.

Preparing the buccal surface with round-end tapering diamond produces necessary taper of 3–5°.

Proximal Reduction

Depth of preparation (amount of tooth preparation): 0.8–1 mm.

Instrument: Long thin tapering diamond and round-end tapering diamond.

Long thin tapering diamond is used to prepare proximal tooth surface. The access is prepared using a vertical sawing motion. The diamond should follow incisogingival direction. This motion will cut the tooth surface proximally. The cut is through proximal enamel and produce the enamel lip **(Fig. 43.7)**.

Remove enamel lip by any hand instrument or by diamond point. Use round-end tapering diamond to join facial and lingual preparation through proximal area. This produces proximal surface with taper of 3–5°. Produce smooth chamfer in proximal area following the gingival contour **(Figs. 43.8A and B)**.

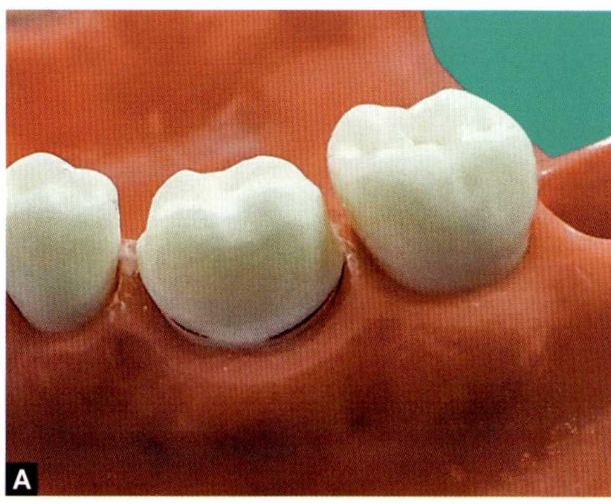

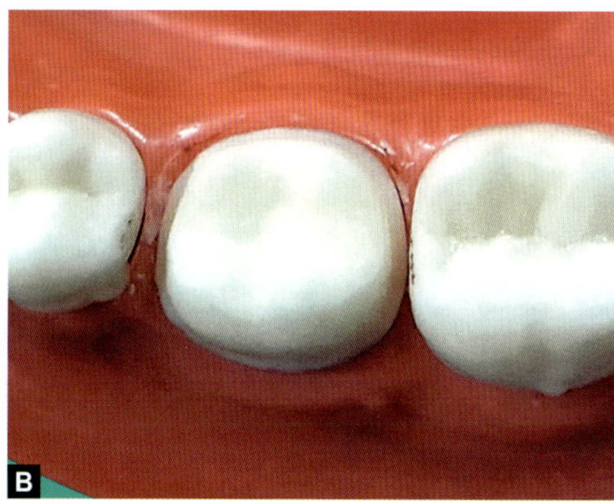

Figs. 43.8A and B: Tooth prepared to receive all metal full veneer crowns. Side view and top view.

Functional Cusp Bevel

Functional cusp bevel is prepared at 45° to axial surface. This is prepared to give extra bulk of material on functional cusp to prevent fracture of restoration and to increase structural durability. Functional cusp bevel is given by round-end tapering diamond placing at 45° to functional cusps **(Fig. 43.9)**.

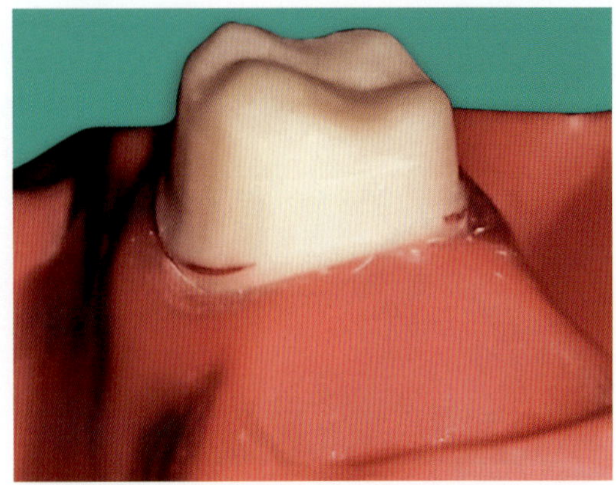

Fig. 43.9: Functional cusp bevel on buccal cusps.

FINISHING OF PREPARATION

Make all the point and line angles rounded. Axial surface can be finished with torpedo fine grit diamond.

CHAPTER 44

Fabrication of Three Unit Fixed Partial Denture

Paranjay Prajapati, Rajesh Sethuraman

INSTRUMENTS AND MATERIALS

- Inlay wax
- Sprue former
- Casting ring
- Ring liner
- Sprue base/investment material
- Distilled water
- Brush
- Furnace
- Crucible
- Tungsten carbide bur.

PROCEDURE

Tooth preparation is done and impression is made.

Die preparation is done after pouring the impression (**Fig. 44.1**).

Wax pattern is prepared on dies by indirect technique using inlay wax (type II) (**Figs. 44.2A and B**).

Sprue former is attached at maximum bulk of the wax pattern or on the nonfunctional cusp (**Figs. 44.3A and B**).

Casting ring liner is placed in casting ring. It should be 3 mm short at both the ends of the casting ring (**Figs. 44.4A and B**).

The ring is placed over the sprue base to which wax pattern is attached while the height is adjusted in such a way that wax pattern is one-fourth inch away for the open end of the ring (**Figs. 44.5A and B**).

Investment material is mixed with mixing liquid and is painted on the wax pattern with the help of the camel paint brush (**Fig. 44.6**). Sometimes dry investment material is sprinkled on it to eliminate excess water if any.

The ring is filled with remaining investment from the side of the ring allowing the material to flow uniformly against earlier investment painted over wax pattern, till the ring is completely filled with investment material (**Figs. 44.7A and B**).

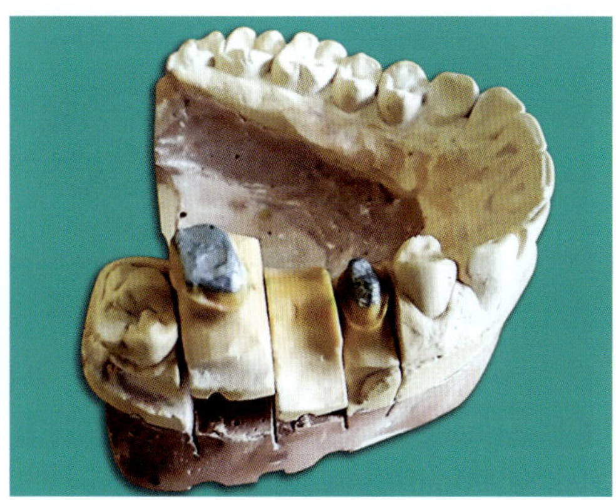

Fig. 44.1: Die preparation.

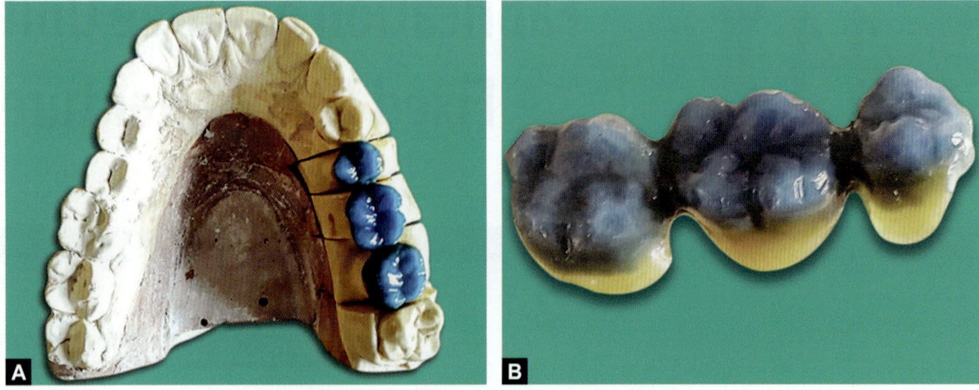

Figs. 44.2A and B: Preparation of wax pattern.

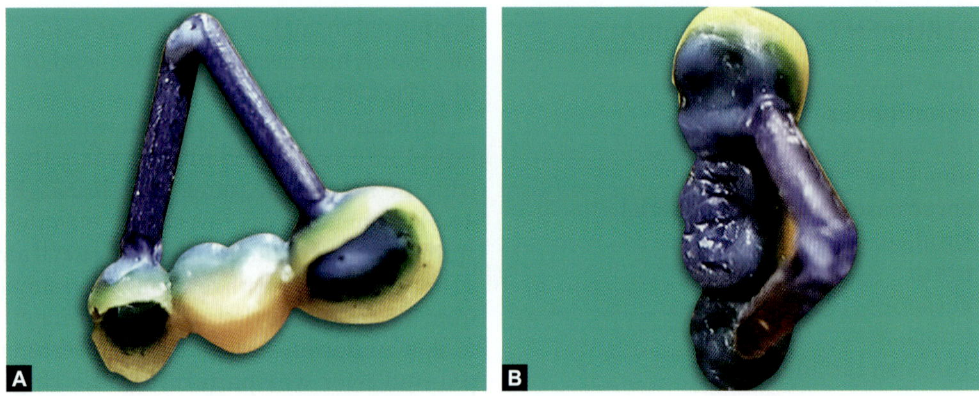

Figs. 44.3A and B: Attachment of sprue former on wax pattern.

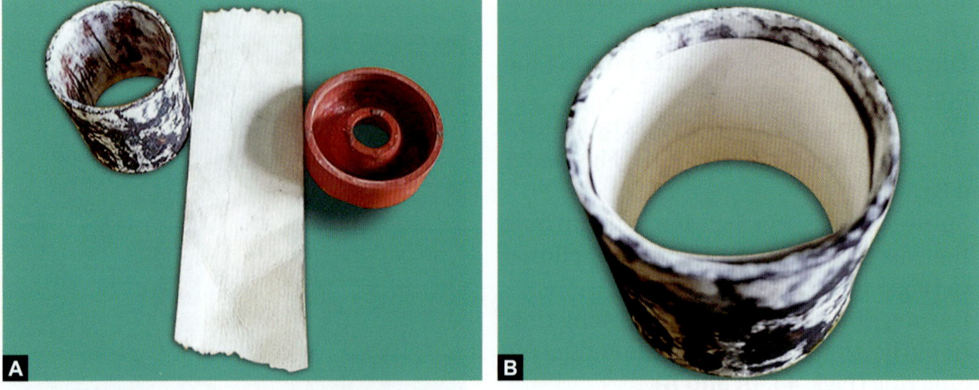

Figs. 44.4A and B: (A) Casting ring, ring liner, and sprue base; and (B) Ring liner 3 mm short of open end of ring.

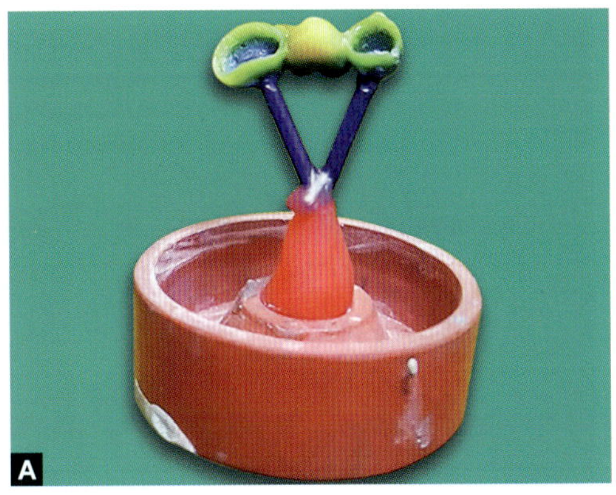
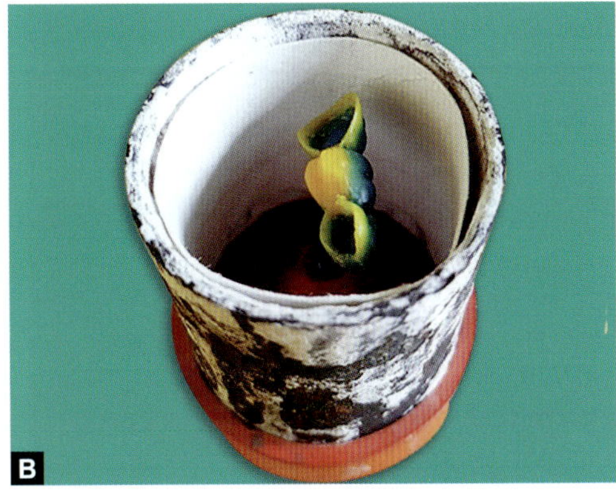

Figs. 44.5A and B: Wax pattern should be one-fourth inch away from open end of the ring.

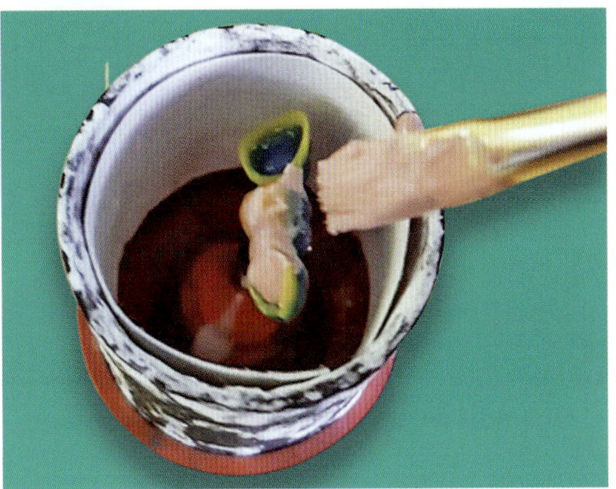

Fig. 44.6: Painting of investment material on wax pattern.

After investment has set, the ring is placed in the furnace and gradually heated at 650°C for an hour for wax pattern burn out **(Fig. 44.8)**.

Alloy is melted in casting crucible and allowed to flow in the mould formed after burn out procedure **(Figs. 44.9A and B)**.

The melted metal is flown to the casting ring to take shape of the restoration **(Figs. 44.10A and B)**.

Once the casting ring is cooled down to the room temperature, divestment is done to remove casting from the ring **(Fig. 44.11)**. Sprue is cut and casting is checked on the tooth fitting surfaces for any irregularities which will

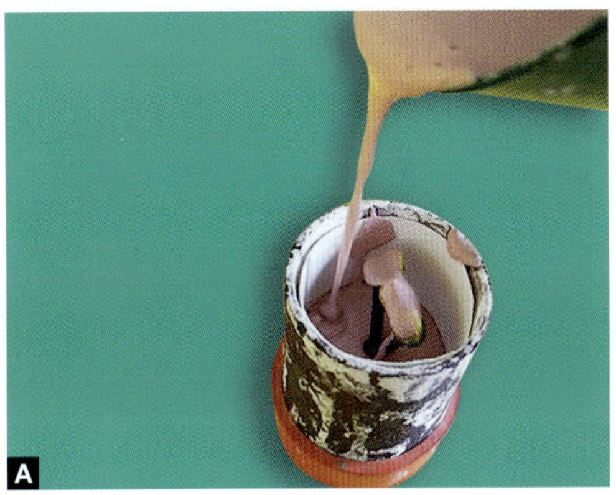
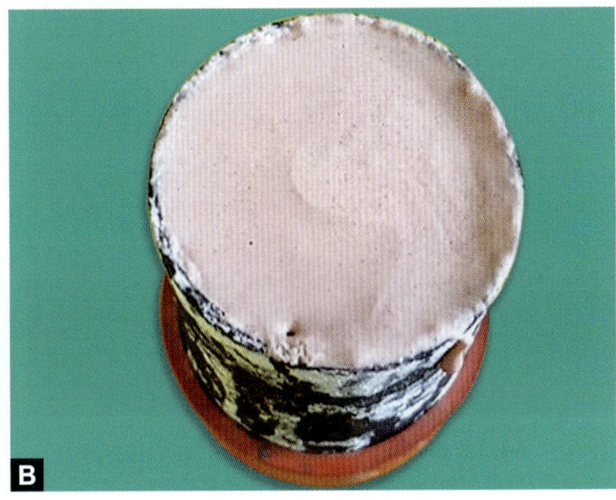

Figs. 44.7A and B: Pouring the investment material to fill the casting ring completely.

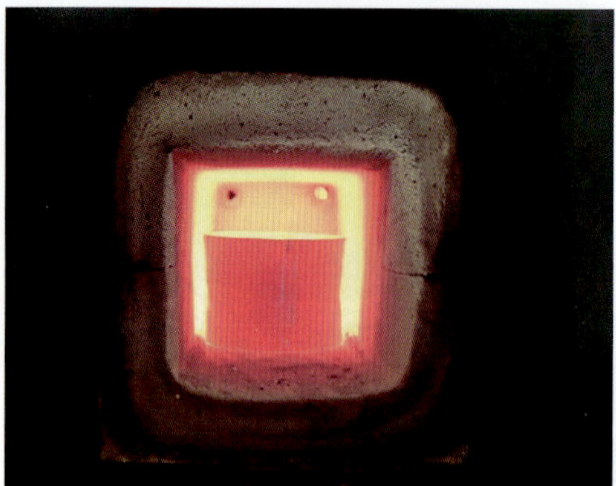

Fig. 44.8: Casting ring is placed in burn out furnace.

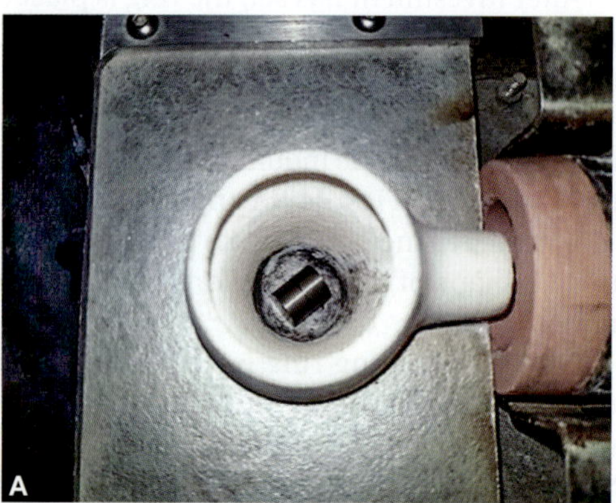

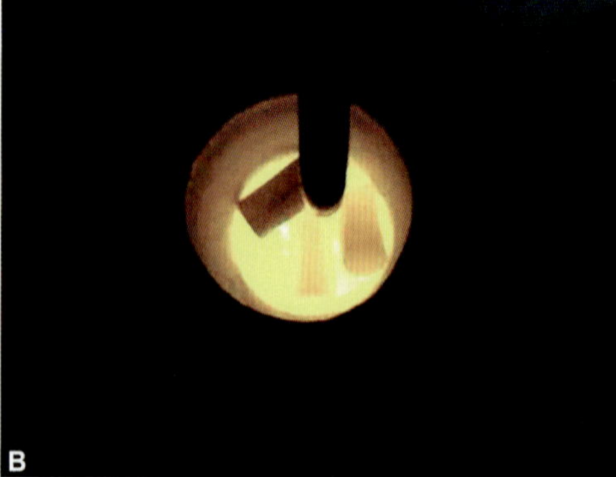

Figs. 44.9A and B: (A) Metal in crucible; and (B) Melted metal inserted in casting ring.

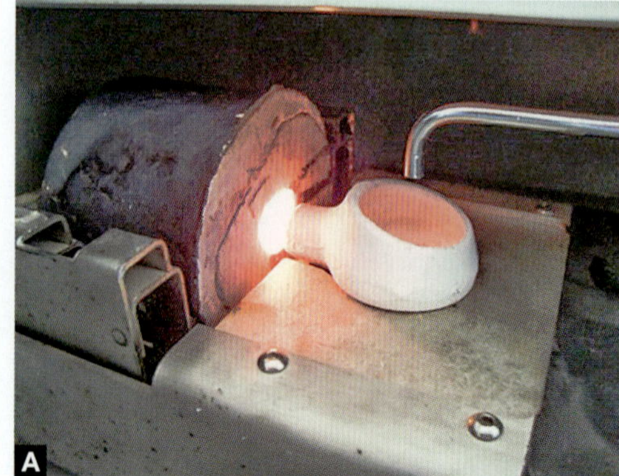

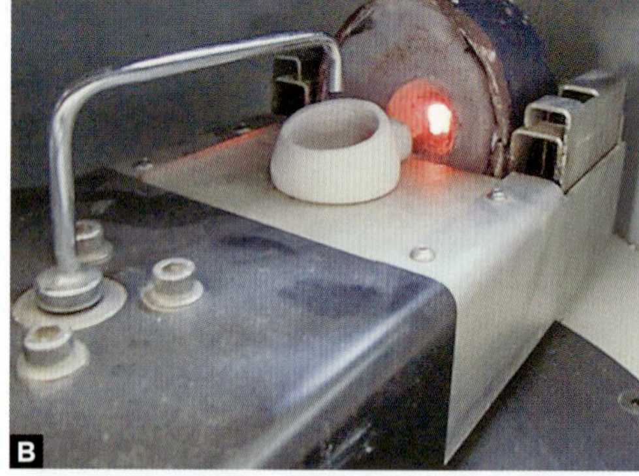

Figs. 44.10A and B: Metal flown into casting mould.

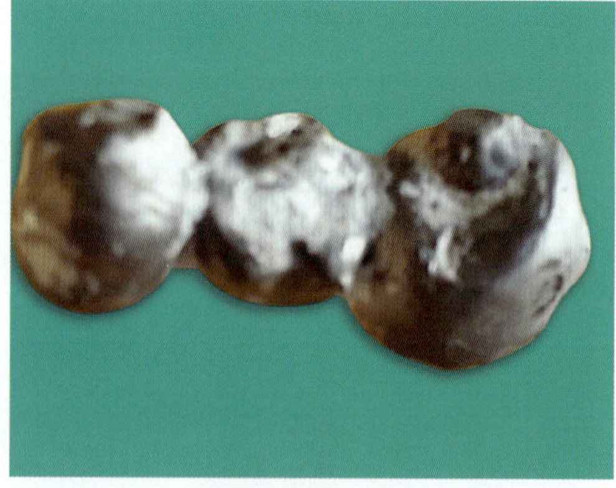

Fig. 44.11: Casting after cutting the sprues.

be eliminated using tungsten carbide burs **(Figs. 44.12A and B)**.

Opaque layer is applied on the casting coping to hide the metallic color of metal alloys and to improve esthetic **(Fig. 44.13)**.

After opaque layer dentine and enamel layers of porcelain are applied and occlusal anatomy is created **(Fig. 44.14)**.

Finally glazing is done to give final finish and luster to the prosthesis **(Fig. 44.15)**.

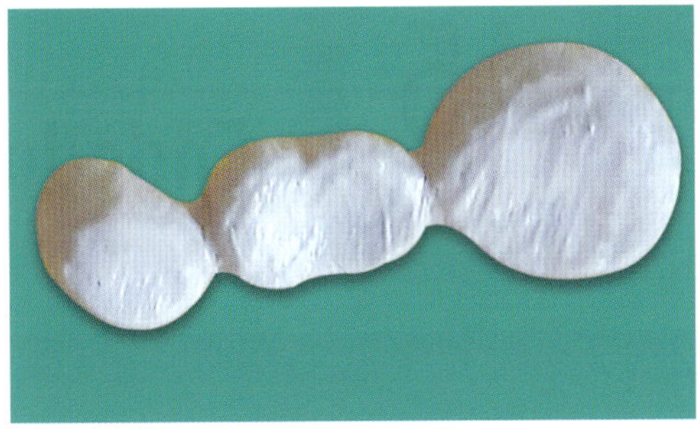

Fig. 44.13: Application of opaque layer to hide metallic hue.

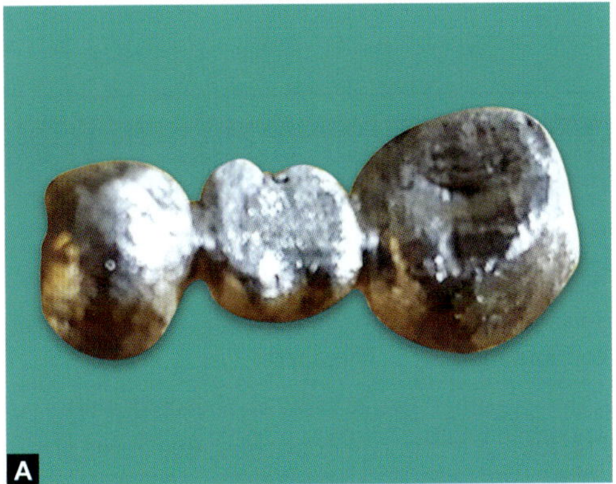

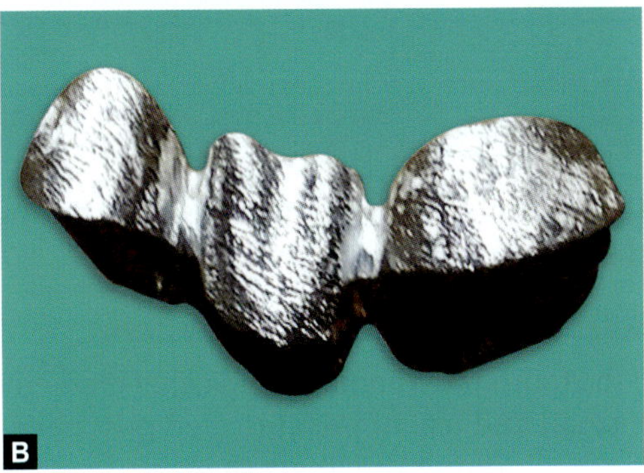

Figs. 44.12A and B: Cleaning of casting (removal of investment material from all surfaces).

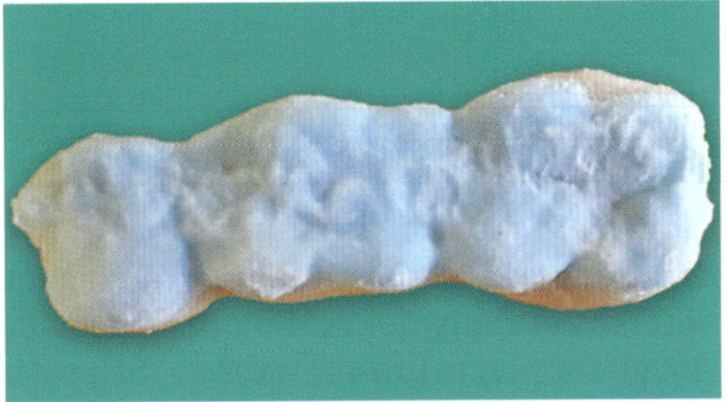

Fig. 44.14: Application of dentine and enamel layer of porcelain.

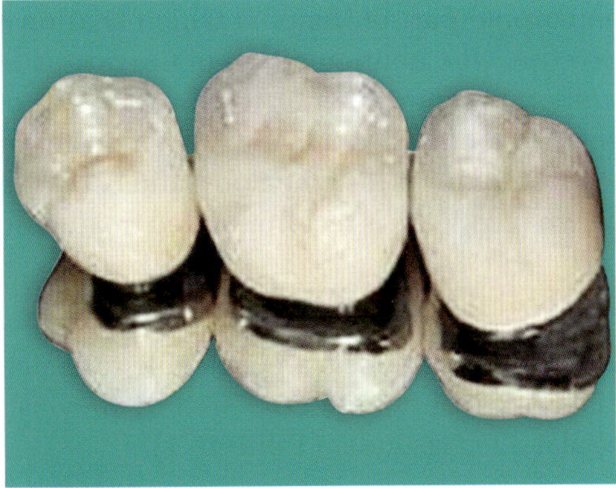

Fig. 44.15: Three units PFM bridge after glazing. *Note:* The metallic cementation surface and porcelain occlusal surface.

CHAPTER 45

Restoration of Endodontically Treated Tooth

Rajesh Sethuraman, Paranjay Prajapati

RATIONALE FOR USE OF POST

If the coronal tooth structure is lost due to fracture or severe carious lesion and remaining tooth structure is not sufficient to provide enough support to prosthesis, then the post is used to achieve additional support from root. Post is inserted into root canal to get support from root and restorative material is supported on coronal part of the post which is known as "core." The main function of the post is to support the core material. If more than 25% of anterior tooth structure and 50% of posterior tooth structure is lost, then post and core with crown prosthesis is recommended treatment.

CLASSIFICATION OF POST

Various types of posts are available to match different treatment needs. Broadly they can be classified as under **(Table 45.1)**.

Table 45.1: Different types of posts.

Characteristics	*Types*
Shape	(A) Parallel, (B) Tapered
Rigidity	(A) Rigid, (B) Nonrigid
Surface configuration	(A) Smooth, (B) Serrated, and (C) Threaded
Color	(A) Esthetic, (B) Nonesthetic
Pressure on tooth	(A) Active post, (B) Passive post
Availability	(A) Prefabricated, (B) Custom made
Material of post	(A) Metal, (B) Fiber reinforced composite post, and (C) Zirconia

PROCEDURE FOR POST AND CORE TREATMENT

Evaluation of Endodontically Treated Tooth

Once the root canal treatment is completed, the operator should observe the endodontically treated tooth for sometime. The tooth should be asymptomatic after root canal treatment. There should be no pain or sensitivity during chewing or any other function.

Selection of Post and Core System

If the tooth root diameter and canal diameter is small and use of prefabricated post needs more widening of canals then it results in additional loss of tooth structure. In such cases custom made post and core is used. Where wider canals are available prefabricated posts are used.

Preparation of Post Space

After endodontic treatment, the root canals are filled with restorative materials, most commonly the gutta-percha. For post space preparation, the gutta-percha is removed from the filled canals using Peeso Reamers or Gates Glidden drills. The apical seal of filled root canals should be kept intact. Minimum 5 mm of gutta-percha are kept in the root canals to maintain apical seal. Post space is modified after removal of gutta-percha from the canals.

- **Use of prefabricated post:** Prefabricated post is used when root canal diameter is wider and needs less canal preparation to accommodate prefabricated post.
- **Use of custom post:** When canal diameter is smaller and needs more canal preparation for receiving prefabricated post, in such cases custom post is fabricated after making impression of narrow post space (canal space). In such cases usually post and core is single unit.

Ferrule

When part of coronal tooth structure is lost, the remaining tooth structure is encircled with part of crown prosthesis. This remaining natural crown structure encircled by crown prosthesis is known as "ferrule". Minimum 2 mm of ferrule is indicated for longevity of prosthesis.

PROCEDURE AND PICTORIAL REPRESENTATION OF POST AND CORE TREATMENT

Fractured tooth or grossly carious tooth with more than 25% tooth structure loss is recommended for post and core treatment **(Fig. 45.1)**.

Endodontic treatment is recommended in such cases where pulp is exposed due to fracture of tooth structure or carious lesion. After removing the pulp tissue, the root canals are widens and shaped to receive the inert restorative material in place of pulpal tissue **(Fig. 45.2)**.

The coronal gutta-percha is removed keeping the apical seal intact to prevent infection **(Fig. 45.3)**. Apical gutta-percha of 3–5 mm is kept in the root canal to preserve the apical seal.

Appropriate inlay wax or pattern resin is inserted into root canal and wax pattern/resin pattern is made of the canal. The same material is extended on crown portion to shape it like prepared tooth. The extended material forming crown-like portion is called core.

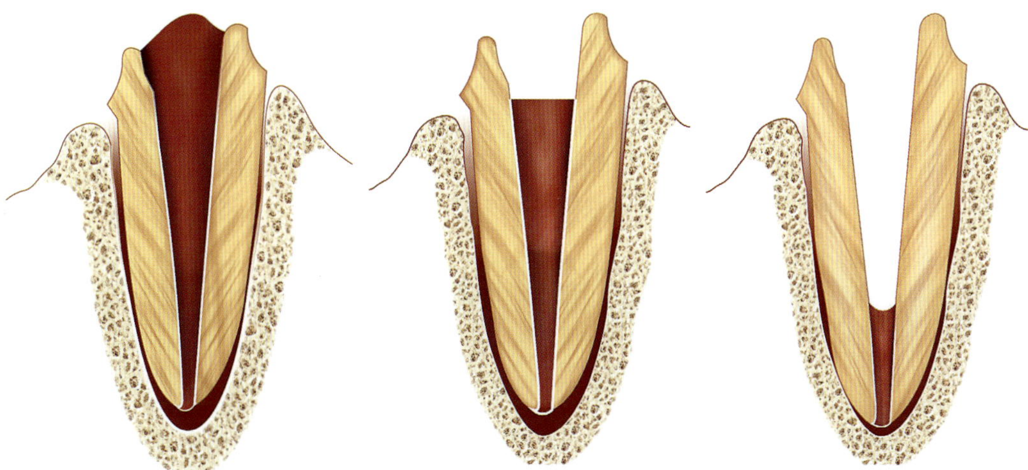

Fig. 45.1: A vital tooth with fractured crown.

Fig. 45.2: Endodontic restoration with gutta-percha.

Fig. 45.3: Removal of gutta-percha to make post space.

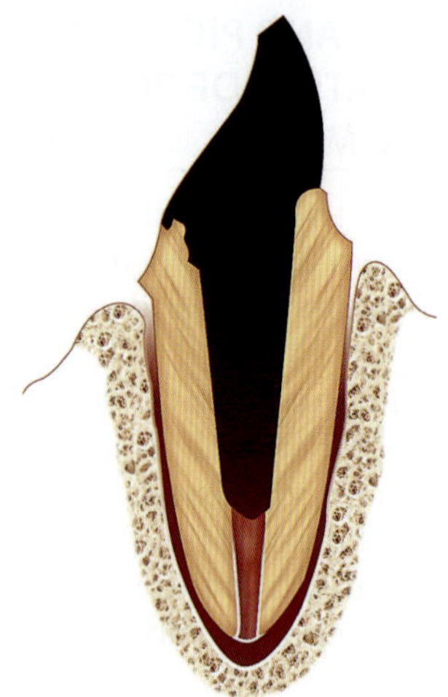

Fig. 45.4: Cementation of custom post and core in root canal space.

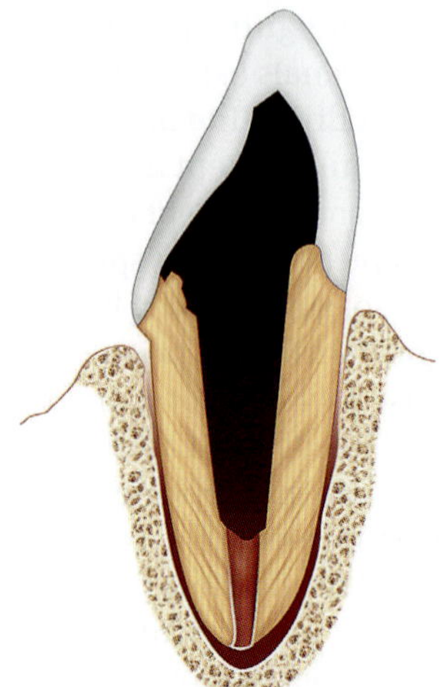

Fig. 45.5: Crown prosthesis cemented on core portion of cast post and core.

The post and core wax pattern is casted and converted to custom post and core and cemented into post space **(Fig. 45.4)**. Impression is made after cementation and crown prosthesis is prepared. Prepared crown prosthesis is cemented over core to restore the fractured tooth **(Fig. 45.5)**.

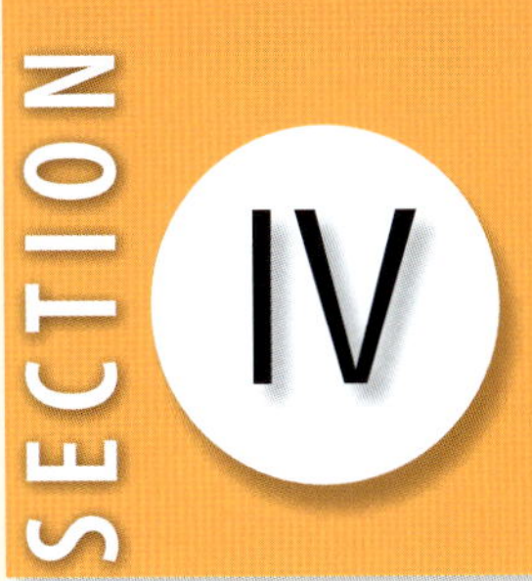

Maxillofacial Prosthodontics

Section Outline

CHAPTER 46

Introduction to Maxillofacial Prosthesis

Paranjay Prajapati, Rajesh Sethuraman

MAXILLOFACIAL PROSTHETICS/ PROSTHODONTICS

The branch of prosthodontics concerned with the restoration and/or replacement of the stomatognathic and craniofacial structures with prostheses that may or may not be removed on a regular or elective basis.

This branch of prosthodontics deals with replacement and rehabilitation of missing structures of face and stomatognathic system.

The intraoral maxillofacial prosthesis are obturator, mandibular resection prosthesis, and nasoalveolar molding prosthesis and extraoral maxillofacial prosthesis are nasal prosthesis, auricular prosthesis, cranial prosthesis, orbital prosthesis, and facial prosthesis.

CLASSIFICATION OF MAXILLOFACIAL PROSTHESIS

The classification of maxillofacial prosthesis is given in **Flowchart 46.1**.

OBJECTIVES OF MAXILLOFACIAL PROSTHESIS

- Restoration of defects to improve esthetic or cosmetic appearance
- Restoration of function
- Protection of tissue
- Therapeutic or healing effect
- Psychologic therapy.

Flowchart 46.1: Classification of maxillofacial prosthesis.

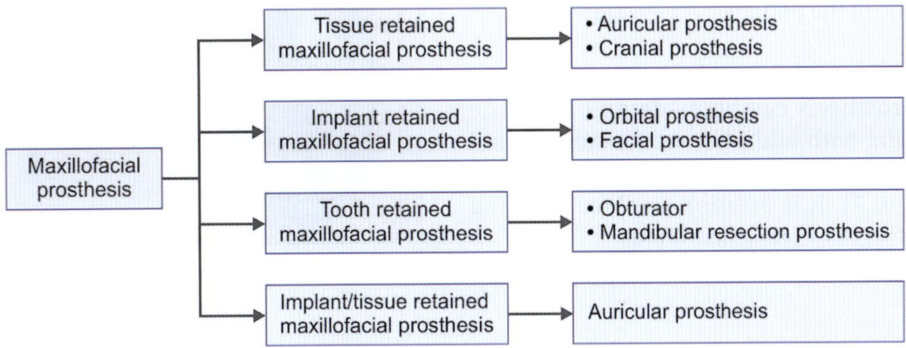

MATERIALS USED FOR FABRICATION OF MAXILLOFACIAL PROSTHESIS

- Acrylic resin
- Vinyl plastisols (realistic, mediplast)
- Acrylic copolymers—Palamed
- Chlorinated polyethylene
- Latex
- Heat vulcanizing silicone
- Room temperature silicone (Silastic)
- Polyphosthazines.

TYPES OF MAXILLOFACIAL PROSTHESIS

Obturator

Obturator prosthesis is used to prevent the communication between the nasal cavity and oral cavity. This communication is may be due to congenital or acquired **(Figs. 46.1 to 46.3)**.

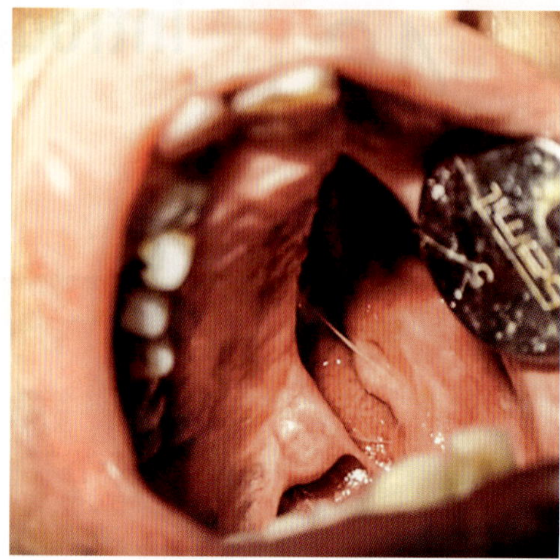

Fig. 46.1: Surgical site.

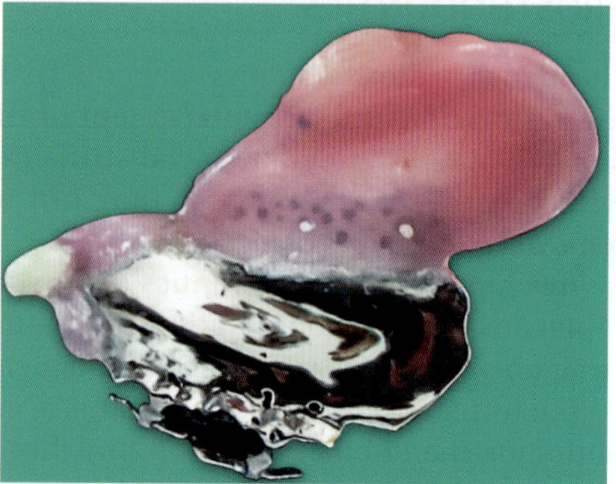

Fig. 46.2: Obturator.

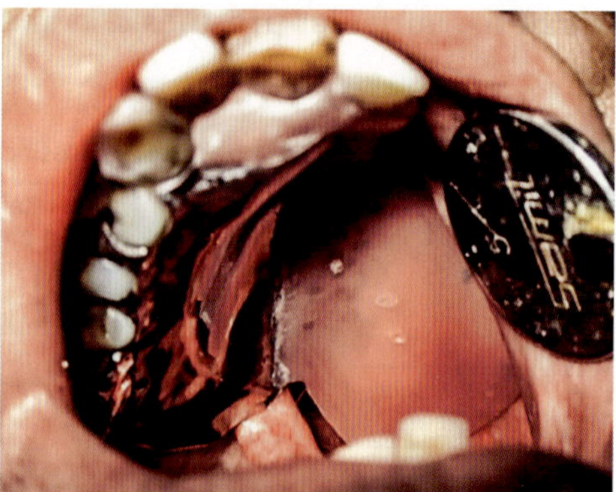

Fig. 46.3: Obturator in oral cavity.

Gunning Splint

Gunning splint is stabilizing device used for reduction and stabilization in case of jaw fracture in edentulous patient. Special features are added to fix the upper and lower part of gunning splint to stabilize fractured jawbone **(Figs. 46.4A to C)**.

Nasal Prosthesis

Nasal prosthesis is artificial nose made up of silicone material with internal stains/pigments added to material to match patient's skin color **(Figs. 46.5 and 46.6)**. It improves the facial esthetic of the patient.

Ear Prosthesis

Ear prosthesis can be made up of silicone material with added internal and external pigments to match with facial skin color **(Fig. 46.7)**. It is position in place by using adhesive or by using hair band.

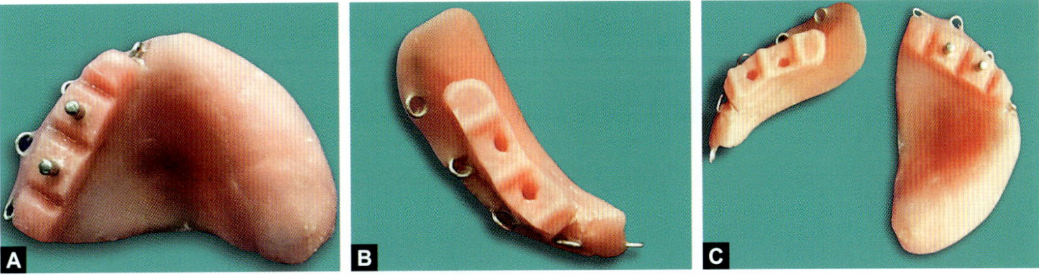

Figs. 46.4A to C: Gunning splint. Note the fixation provision provided in terms of wire loops and metallic inserts.

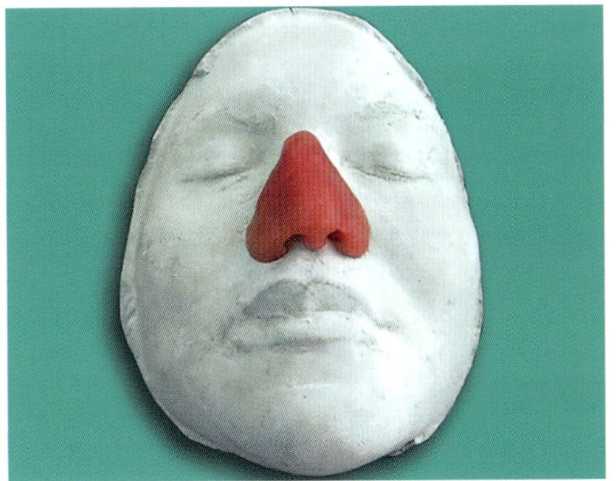

Fig. 46.5: Wax pattern of nasal prosthesis.

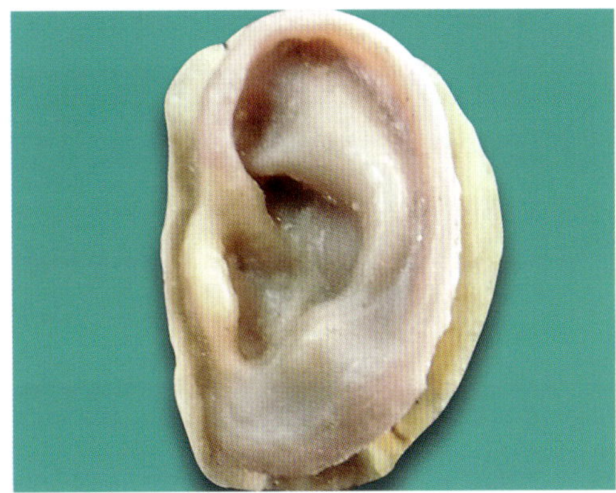

Fig. 46.7: Ear prosthesis.

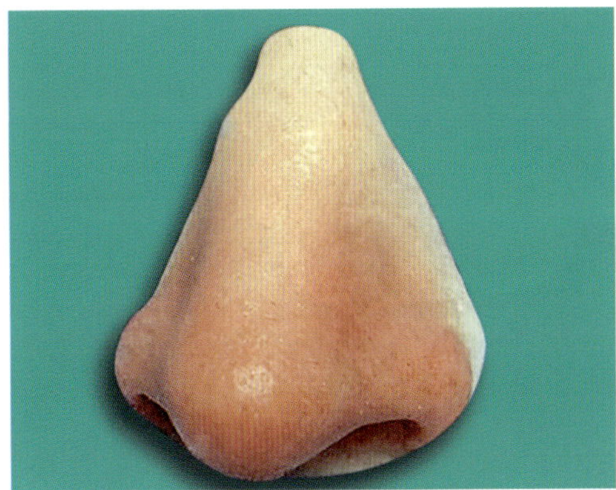

Fig. 46.6: Nasal prosthesis.

Orbital Prosthesis

Orbital prosthesis replaces eye and part of the orbit. The sclera and iris should match exactly with patient eye to impersonate the natural color of eye **(Figs. 46.8 and 46.9)**.

Finger Prosthesis

Replaces lost fingers either congenitally or due to some accidents **(Fig. 46.10)**.

Nasoalveolar Molding Prosthesis/Plate

The nasoalveolar molding prosthesis/plate is described in **Figures 46.11A and B**.

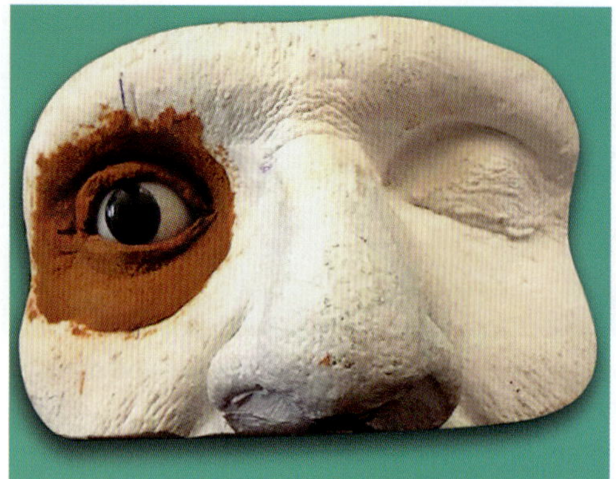

Fig. 46.8: Carving the orbital prosthesis.

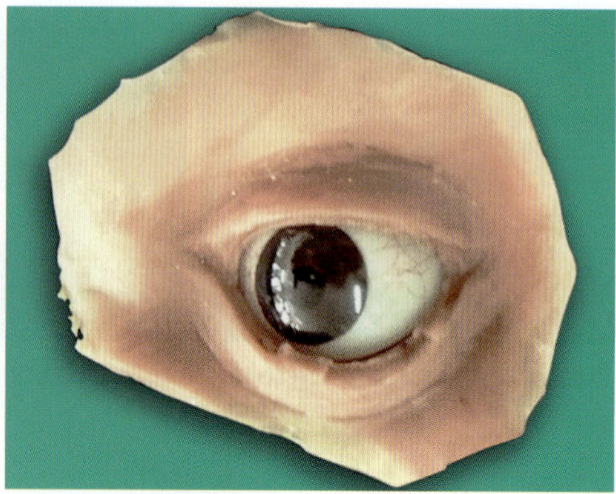

Fig. 46.9: Orbital prosthesis.

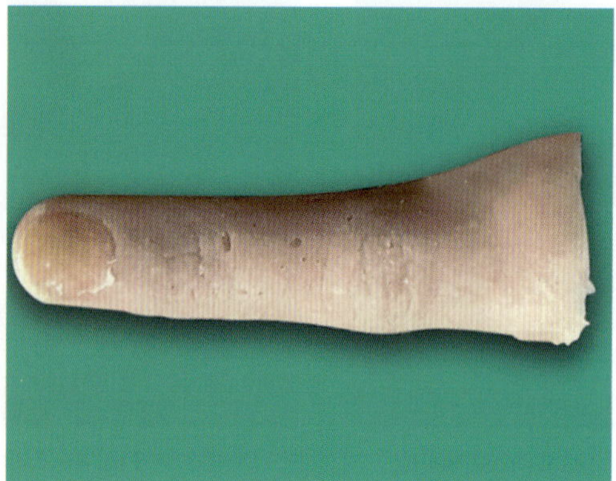

Fig. 46.10: Finger prosthesis.

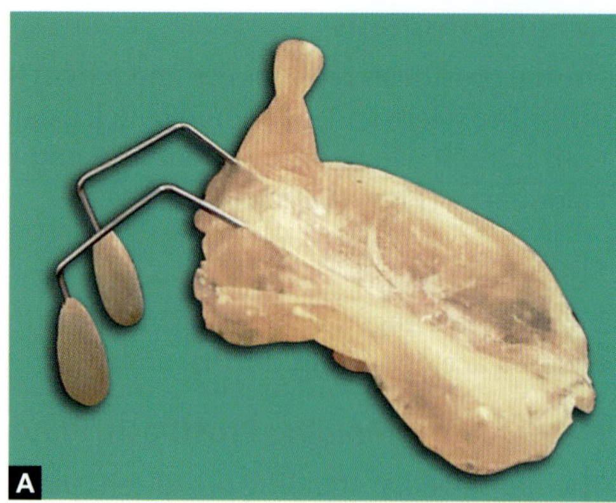

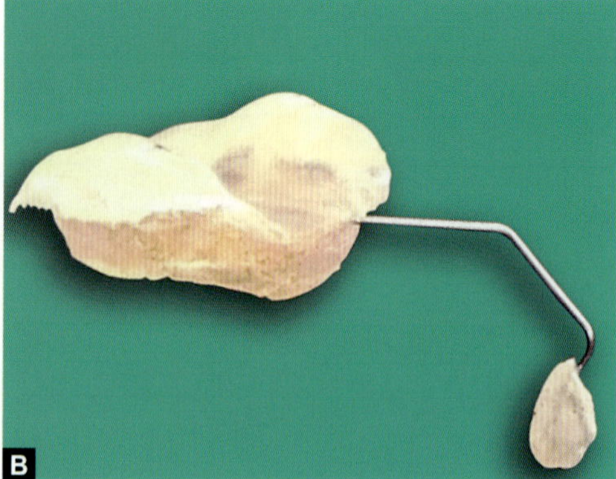

Figs. 46.11A and B: Nasoalveolar molding.

CHAPTER 47

Introduction to Implant Prosthesis

Rajesh Sethuraman, YG Naveen

DEFINITION

Dental implant is defined as "a prosthetic device made of alloplastic material implanted into oral tissues beneath the mucosal or/and periosteal layer, and on/or within the bone to provide retention and support for a fixed or removable dental prosthesis."

A substance that is placed into or/and upon the jawbone to support a fixed or removable dental prosthesis.

Dental implants are basically root form of some metallic alloy mainly containing medical grade pure titanium. These implants are inserted into alveolar bone or jawbone to fix with bone tissue by process known as osseointegration. See photographs of transparent model here to understand the process of implant placement in the bone **(Figs. 47.1 and 47.2)**.

INDICATIONS

Dental implant can be used to support any kind of dental prosthesis. Implants can be used for retention and support of extraoral prosthesis.

Implants are indicated for:

- Partial edentulous conditions
- Complete edentulism
- Implant supported fixed dental prosthesis
- Rehabilitation of maxillofacial defects with implant supported prosthesis.

IMPLANT PROSTHETIC COMPONENTS

The implantation of prosthetic components is described in **Figure 47.3**.

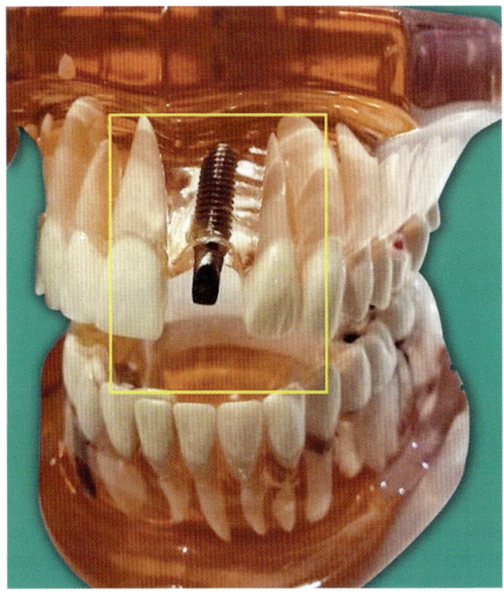

Fig. 47.1: Model showing single tooth replacement with implant.

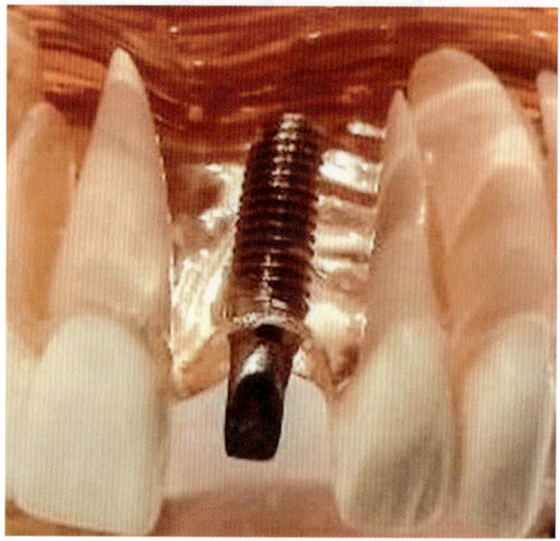

Fig. 47.2: Dental implant replaces the root of the tooth and provides foundation to put abutment and artificial tooth over it.

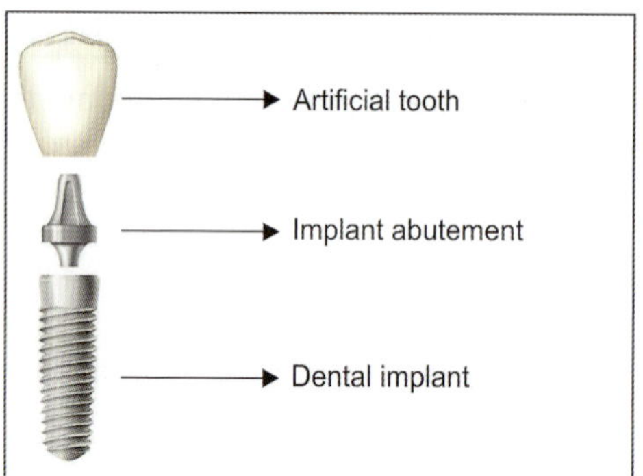

Fig. 47.3: Root form dental implant is placed in alveolar bone. On the dental implant an implant abutment is fixed. The artificial tooth is cemented or fixed with screw on the implant abutment.

SINGLE TOOTH REPLACEMENT

To replace single missing tooth implant is widely used. A single root form implant is placed in place of missing tooth **(Figs. 47.3 and 47.4)**. Once the osseointegration is done, an implant abutment is fixed on the implant with screw. The artificial tooth (crown) is then cemented or fixed on abutment with screw **(Fig. 47.5)**. Also see **Figures 47.6A and B** for clinical case representation.

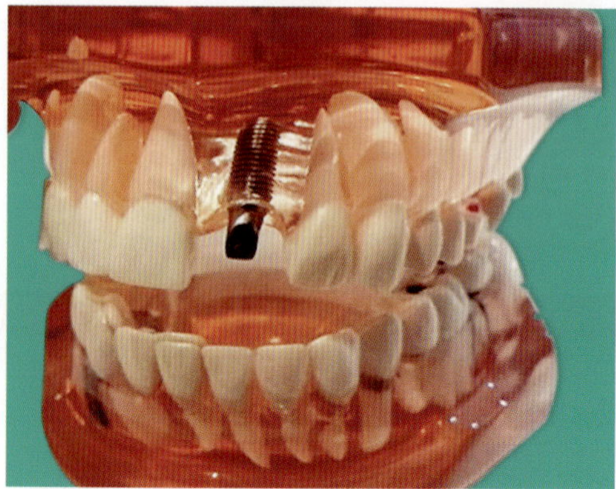

Fig. 47.4: Placements of implant and implant abutment on it.

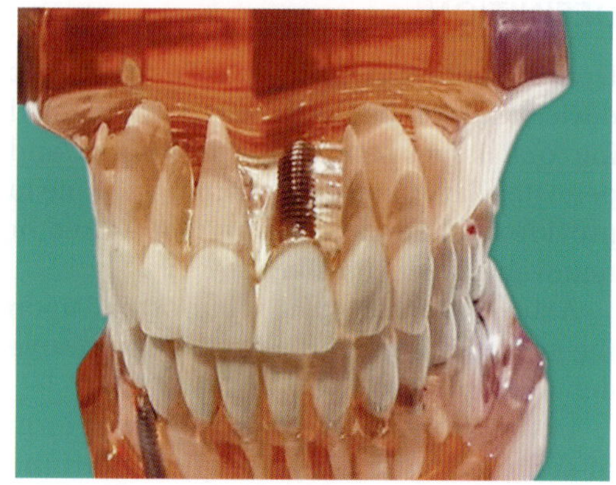

Fig. 47.5: Crown prosthesis is fixed on implant abutment.

REPLACEMENT OF MULTIPLE MISSING TEETH

Dental implants can be used for replacement of more than one missing teeth. Prosthesis (bridge) can be fixed on implants to replace multiple missing teeth. Model showing two implants placed to replace three missing teeth **(Fig. 47.7)**. Three-unit prosthesis is fixed on implant abutments to replace three missing teeth **(Fig. 47.8)**.

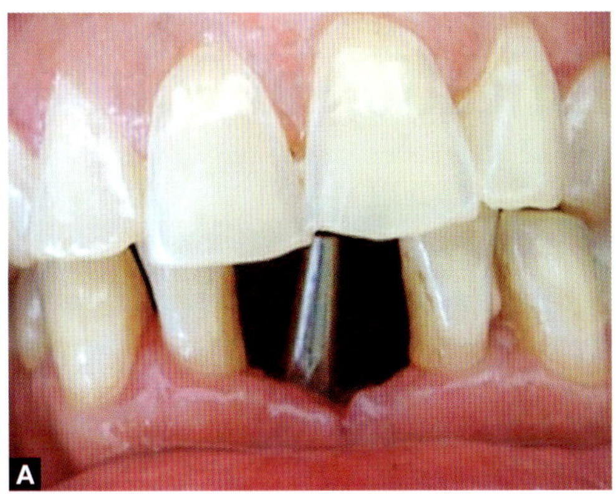

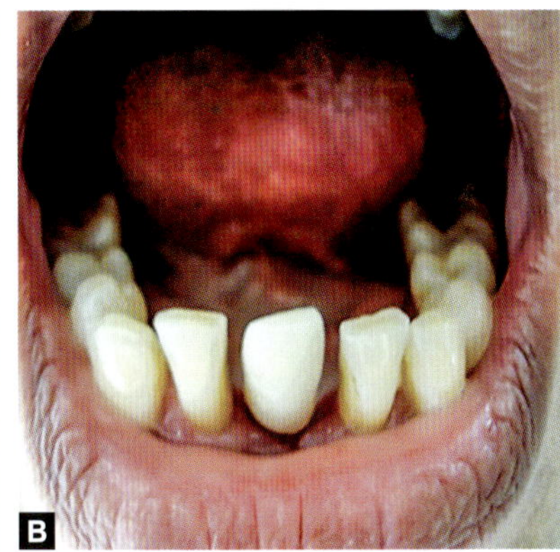

Figs. 47.6A and B: Replacement of single missing tooth in mandibular anterior region.

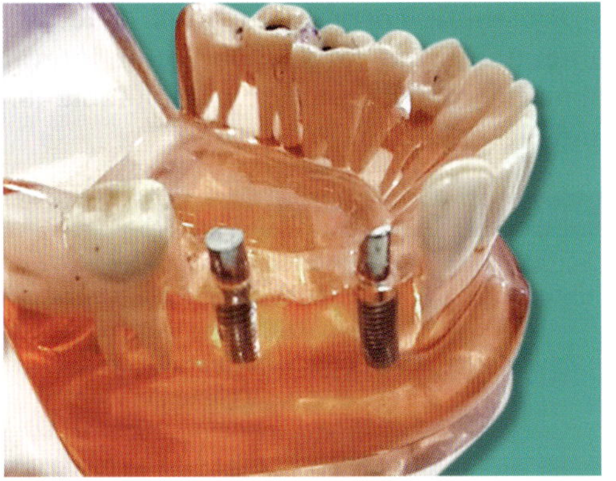

Fig. 47.7: Two implants in position with abutments on them.

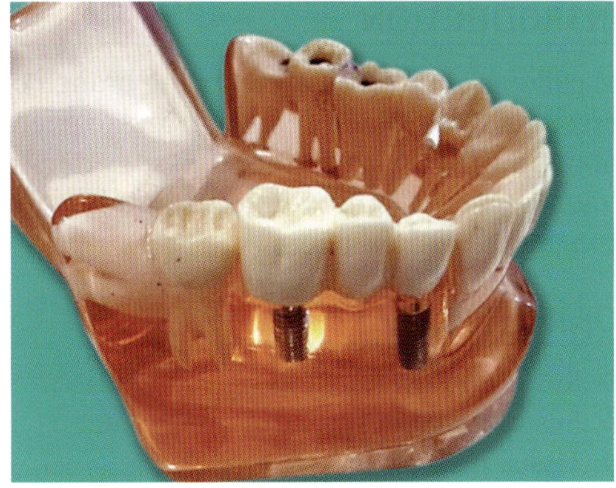

Fig. 47.8: Three units bridge prosthesis fixed on implant abutments.

CHAPTER 48

Fabrication of Obturator

Rajesh Sethuraman, Paranjay Prajapati

INTRODUCTION

Maxillofacial prosthodontics is the branch of prosthodontics which deals with replacement of missing oral and extraoral tissues due to trauma, surgical intervention, pathology, or congenital malformation.

OBJECTIVES

- ❖ Restoration of function
- ❖ Restoration of esthetic or appearance
- ❖ Tissue protection
- ❖ Psychologically beneficial
- ❖ Improvement in quality of life.

TYPES

- ❖ Obturator
- ❖ Nasal prosthesis
- ❖ Ear prosthesis
- ❖ Eye prosthesis
- ❖ Orbital prosthesis
- ❖ Auricular prosthesis
- ❖ Facial prosthesis
- ❖ Mandibular resection prosthesis.

OBTURATOR

Obturator is prosthesis used to close a defect (tissue opening) mainly of the hard palate or contiguous alveolar structures.

Prosthetic correction of such defects is often done with surgical obturator, interim obturator, and definitive obturator (**Table 48.1 and Figs. 48.1A to C**).

Table 48.1: Different types of obturator.

Surgical obturator	It is inserted at the time of surgery or within short period after surgery. Usually no teeth present on surgical obturator. It reduces oral and nasal contamination. Helps in deglutition and eliminate nasogastric tube. Usually made up of heat cure acrylic resin. Retention is achieved by clasp and tags
Interim obturator	It is usually inserted 3–4 weeks postsurgically. It helps in minimizing wound contraction. It contains teeth and bulb. It improves speech, deglutition, and function. Clasps and tags are given to provide retention
Definitive obturator	This type of obturator is made when the surgical wound is fully healed. Necessary mouth preparation like caries removal, restoration tooth extraction should be carried out before fabrication of definitive obturator. It is fabricated using cast metals, however, can be fabricated with heat cured acrylic resin. Retention achieved by cast clasps

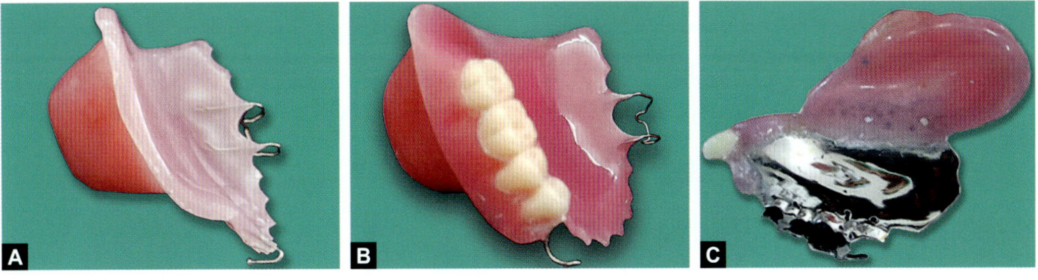

Figs. 48.1A to C: (A) Surgical obturator; (B) Interim obturator; (C) Definitive obturator.

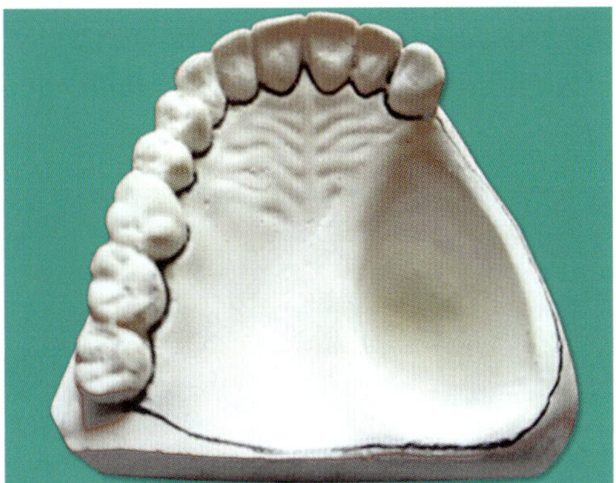

Fig. 48.2: Final cast of maxillary defect.

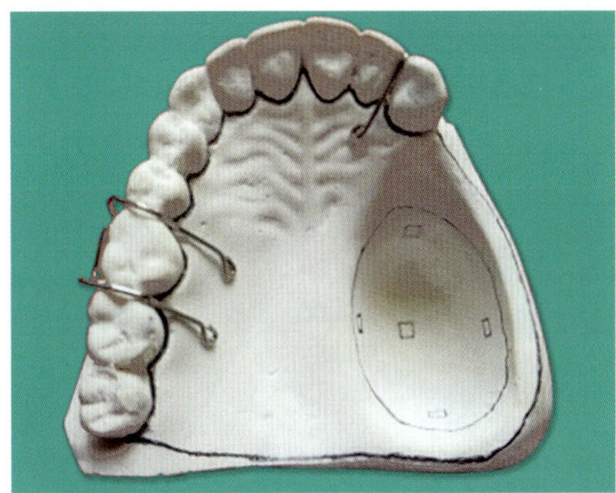

Fig. 48.3: Clasps and tags fabricated.

Fabrication of Hollow Bulb Obturator

Observe the final cast for any pouring defects and correct it if any **(Fig. 48.2)**. Mark the outline for the obturator.

Prepare clasp for retention on two abutments which are widely separated from each other **(Fig. 48.3)**. Clasps are made on molar and canine region for retention. Mark tissue stops in defect area of cast.

Adapt a sheet of modeling wax into defect and cut the windows for tissue stops **(Fig. 48.4)**.

Adapt a sheet of self-cure acrylic over the wax sheet to make outer part of the bulb **(Fig. 48.5)**. This part of the bulb is covered with another sheet of the acrylic resin to make it hollow **(Fig. 48.6)**.

Once the self-cure resin is set, remove the bulb from the cast and examine that the resin is in contact with cast through all the tissue stop windows and tissue stops are formed properly.

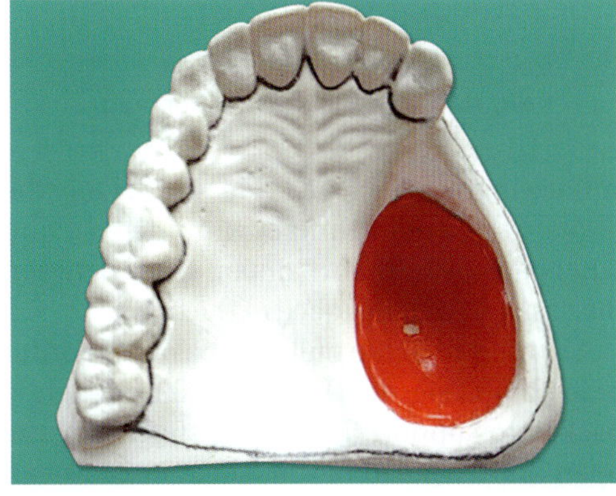

Fig. 48.4: Adaptation of spacer wax.

Remove the wax sheet from outer surface of the bulb and place the bulb in the cast. Check that all the tissue stops are in contact with cast

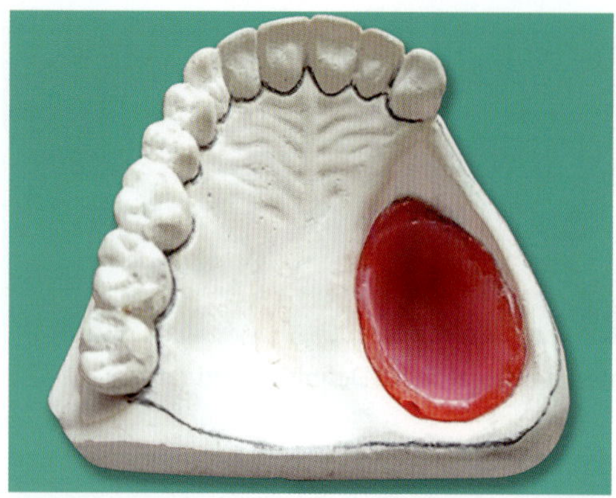

Fig. 48.5: Making bulb for obturator.

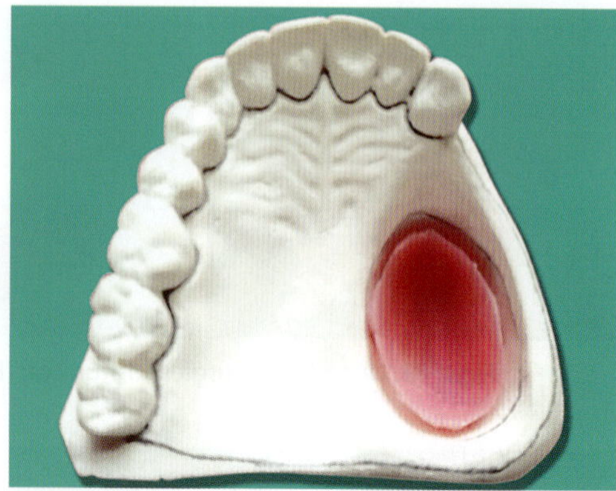

Fig. 48.7: Checking contact of tissue stops with cast surface.

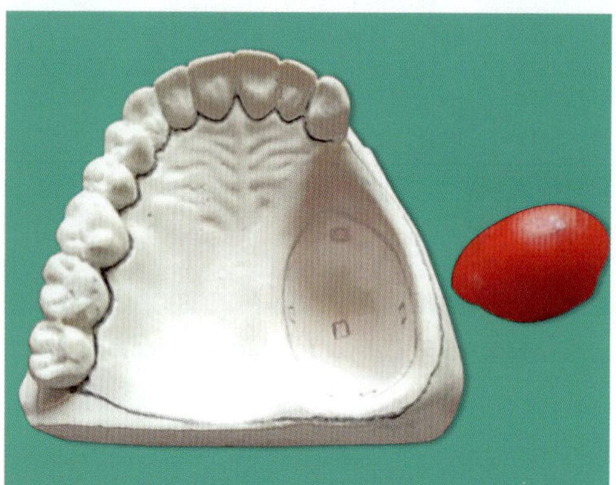

Fig. 48.6: Making of obturator bulb.

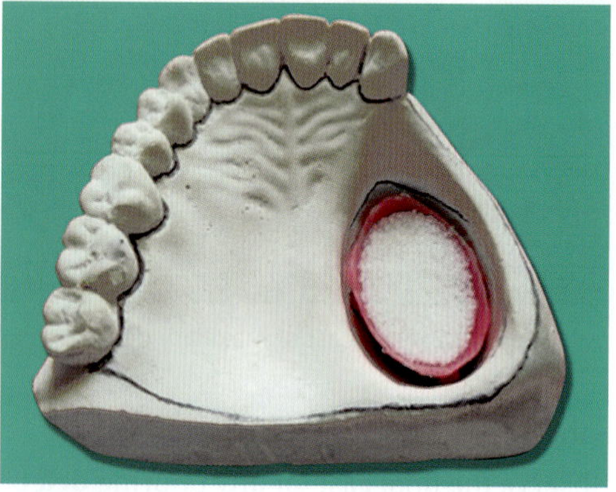

Fig. 48.8: Use of salt for hollowing the bulb.

surface in the defect area **(Fig. 48.7)**. Only the tissue stops are in contact with the cast and other parts of the bulb maintain space between the cast and outer surface of the bulb.

Fill the salt in the bulb till the outer border of the bulb **(Fig. 48.8)**. The salt should tightly packed to support the closing sheet over the open bulb. Instead of salt, sugar crystals can also be used for the same purpose.

Mix little quantity of self-cure acrylic resin and make a small sheet of it. Place it over the salt packed bulb to close the bulb **(Fig. 48.9)**.

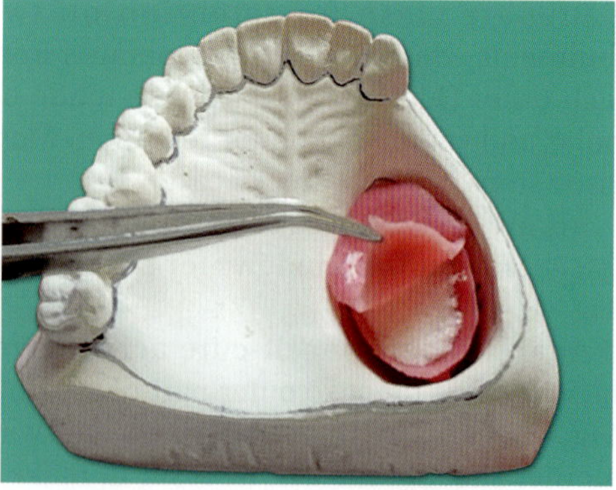

Fig. 48.9: Closing the open bulb.

Apply material as needed and close the bulb from all the surfaces.

Make one or two small holes on the surface of the bulb. Use thin needle to insert water from one hole and let it come out from the other hole. Repeat this exercise till full quantity of salt is melt and removed with water **(Fig. 48.10)**.

Once the salt is removed close holes made for removal of salt using self-cure acrylic. Put the hollow bulb in bowl or glass of water and check for hollowness **(Fig. 48.11)**.

> The hollow bulb is tied with floss and inserted in glass full of water to check the hollowness; the hollow bulb is floating and not sinking in the water. This is because the bulb is hollow and air is entrapped in hollow space which makes it light weight and empty inside.

Place the clasps on abutment and secure them on the cast using small quantity of dental plaster **(Figs. 48.12A and B)**. Cover the clasp with plaster to keep them in place during dewaxing and packing procedures.

Remove the bulb from the defect area and fill the area with modeling wax. Put the clasp and on the abutments and do the wax up as shown in the photograph **(Fig. 48.13)**. Make sure that wax is properly carved and inserted in the interdental area for additional retention. Teeth can be arranged if needed and according to type of obturator.

Conventional flasking procedure is followed for flasking of obturator **(Fig. 48.14)**.

Follow conventional dewaxing procedure and make sure that there is no trace of modeling wax left in the mould **(Fig. 48.15)**.

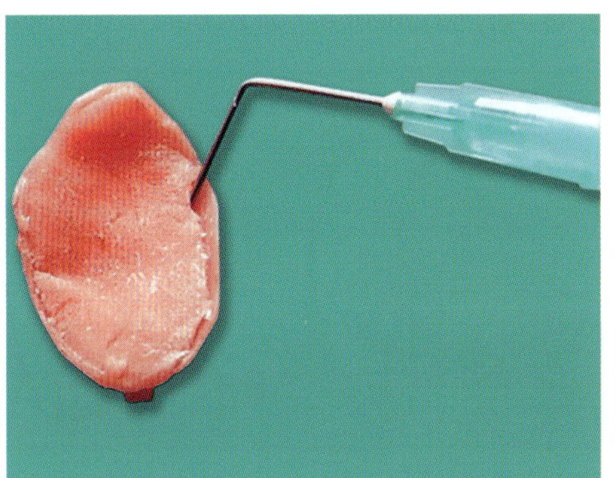

Fig. 48.10: Removal of salt.

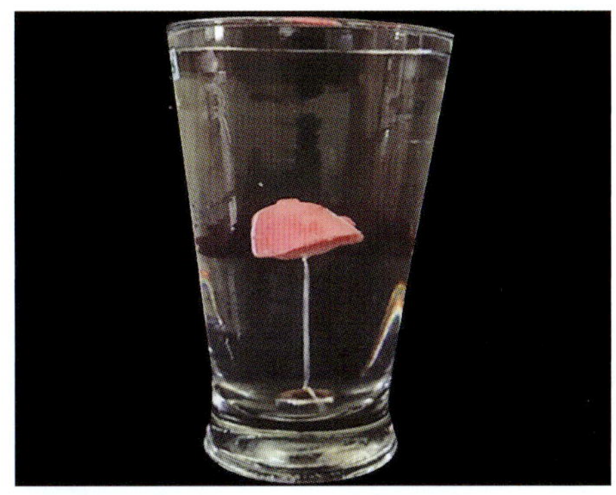

Fig. 48.11: Checking hollow bulb.

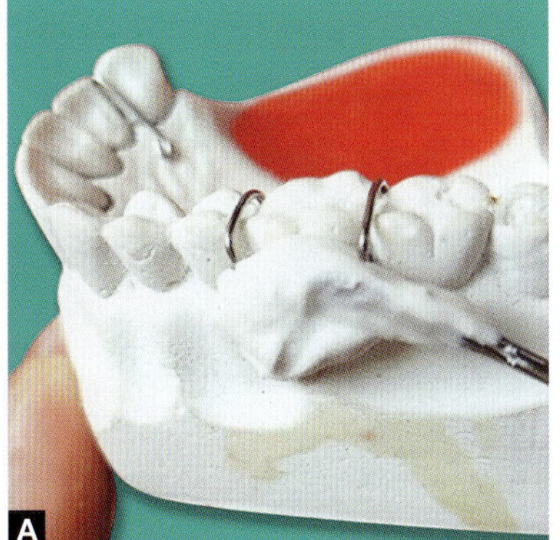

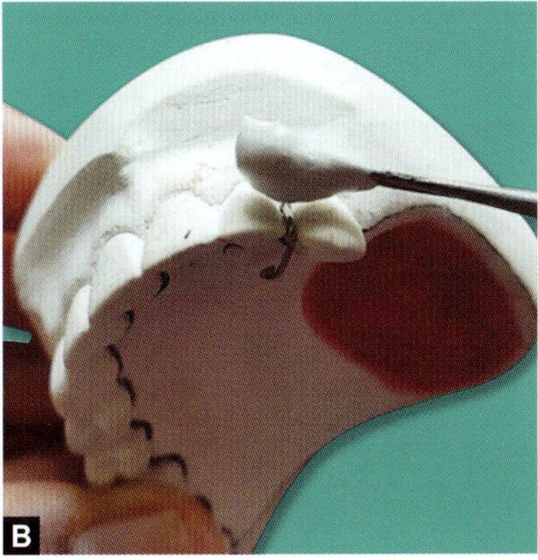

Figs. 48.12A and B: Securing the clasps on the cast.

Place the hollow bulb in position and make sure that all tissue stops are contact with cast **(Fig. 48.16)**.

Mix heat-cure acrylic resin and pack for making obturator **(Fig. 48.17)**. Cure it for long curing cycle.

After curing, open the flask and retrieve the obturator. Trim the excess material if any. Do finishing with sandpapers of different grit size. Polish it till it get shiny surface **(Fig. 48.18)**. Obturator is ready to use.

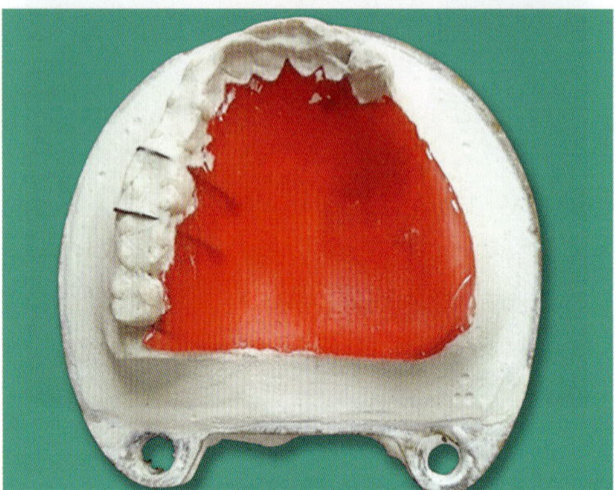

Fig. 48.13: Closing the defect and wax up.

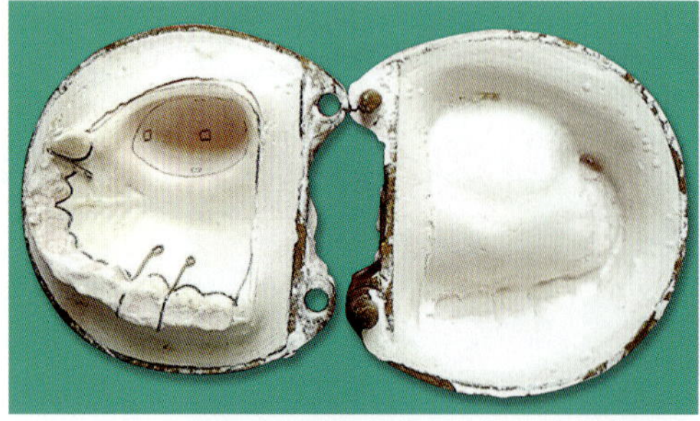

Fig. 48.14: Flasking of obturator.

Fig. 48.15: Base and counter of flask after dewaxing.

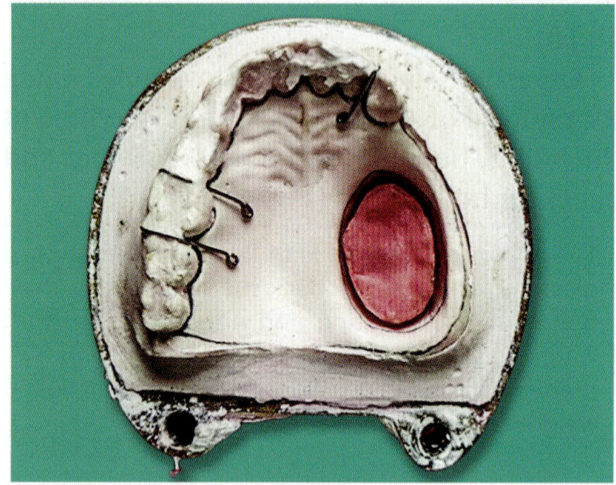

Fig. 48.16: Placement of hollow bulb in the mould.

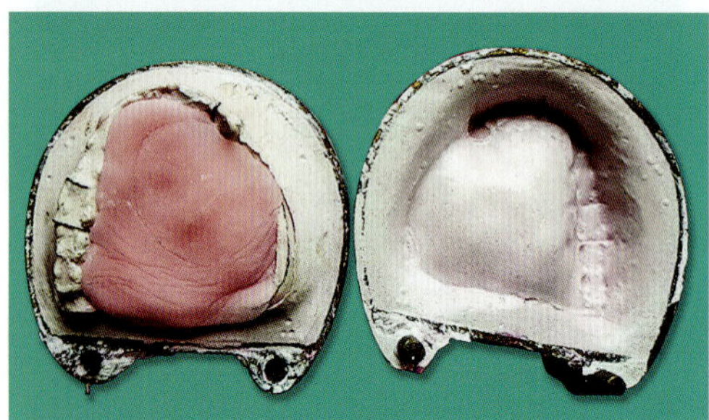

Fig. 48.17: Packing of heat cure acrylic for making obturator.

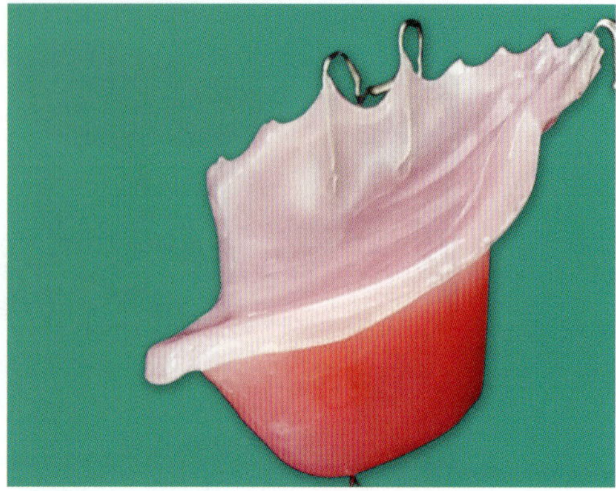

Fig. 48.18: Obturator after finishing and polishing.

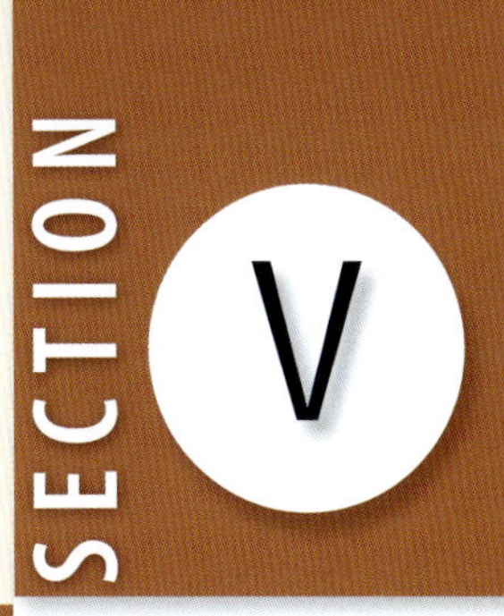

Instruments and Equipment

Section Outline

CHAPTER 49

Instruments for Removable Prosthodontics

Paranjay Prajapati, Rajesh Sethuraman

RUBBER BOWL (FIG. 49.1)

It is used to mix gypsum products (dental plaster, dental stone, die stone, and investment material) and alginate. It is available in various sizes and colors. It is made up of stiff and flexible rubber. It can also be used to carry hot water during manipulation of impression compound and green stick material. Usually, separate rubber bowls are kept for gypsum and alginate.

> Use separate rubber bowl for mixing gypsum products and alginate. If alginate is mixed in the same bowl in which gypsum was mixed then traces of gypsum may accelerate alginate setting.

MIXING SPATULA (FIG. 49.2)

Straight-bladed Mixing Spatula

This type of spatula is used for mixing of gypsum products like dental stone, dental plaster, die stone, investment material, etc. It has handle made up of either hard plastic or wood and available in various lengths. Mixing blade is made up of metal with rounded end.

Curved-bladed Mixing Spatula

This spatula is used for mixing alginate impression material. Curve blade confines with inner walls of flexible rubber bowl and material is pressed in between to mix properly. Mixing blade is curved with rounded end.

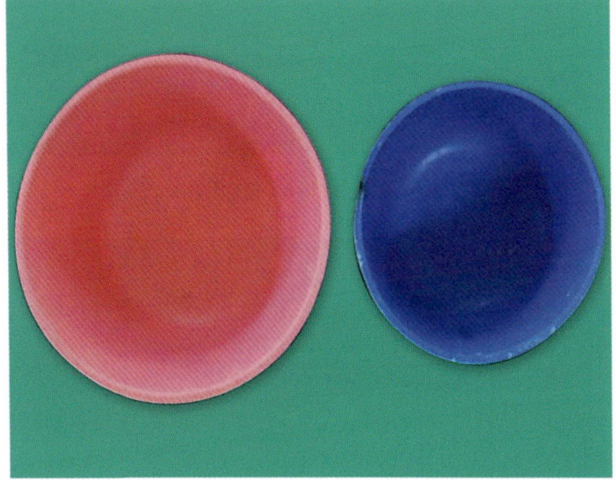

Fig. 49.1: Rubber bowl.

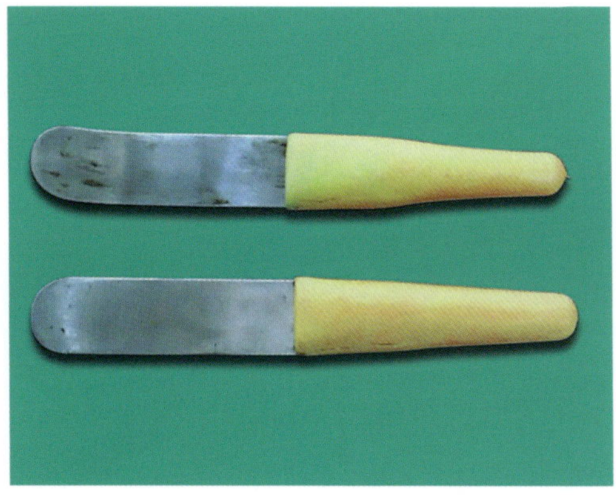

Fig. 49.2: Mixing spatula.

WAX KNIFE (FIG. 49.3)

This instrument has two working ends. One end is straight with pointed termination and sharp working edge. The other end is slightly curved with rounded termination.

Straight end is used for cutting/manipulation of wax and making wax rims. Curved end used to carry molten wax and for manipulation of curved surfaces like palatal surface of maxillary wax rim. Wax knife is used for making occlusion rims, teeth arrangement, and wax-up procedure. It can also be used for manipulation of plaster during flasking and mounting procedures. The curved end can be used to carry mixed acrylic resin from mixing jar.

PLASTER KNIFE

It is knife-like instrument used for manual trimming of casts **(Fig. 49.4)**. Its working edge is sharp for easy trimming of gypsum products. Handle is made up of wood or plastic.

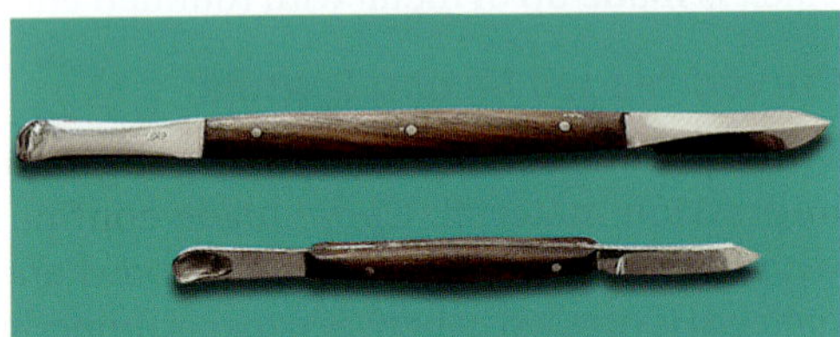

Fig. 49.3: Wax knife.

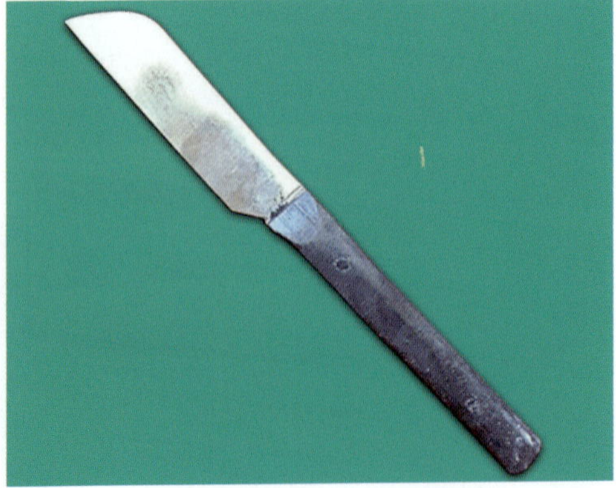

Fig. 49.4: Plaster knife.

WAX SPATULA

This instrument has two working ends **(Fig. 49.5)**. One end is spoon-shaped to carry molten wax for wax-up procedure and the other end is pointed diamond-shaped which is used for removal of wax from interdental area during carving procedure. Wax spatula can be used for cervical and root carving after teeth arrangement.

WAX CARVER

It is two-ended instrument **(Fig. 49.6)**. One end is scoop shape and the other one is sharp blade. Mainly used for wax carving. Used for tooth carving, pattern carving, and scooping extra wax during denture wax-up procedure. Carver should not be heated over flame otherwise it will become blunt.

SCISSORS (FIG. 49.7)

Straight Scissors

It has straight beak end. It is used for cutting gauge cloth and sticking plaster.

Curved Scissors

It has curved beak. It is usually used for cutting shellac baseplate or light cured resin material

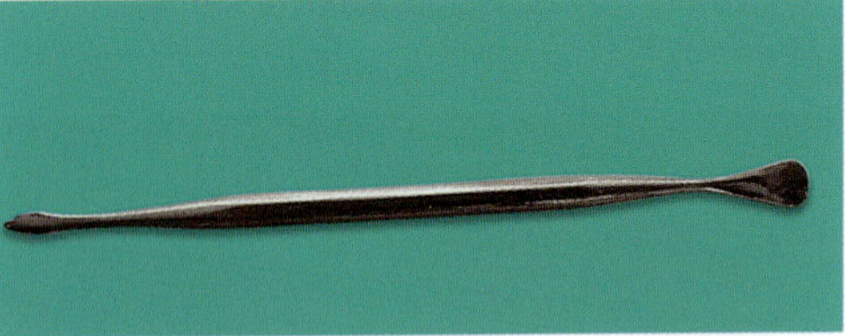

Fig. 49.5: Wax spatula.

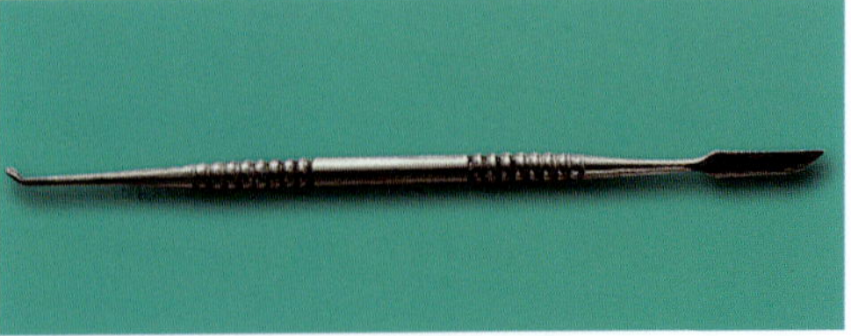

Fig. 49.6: Wax carver.

during their manipulation for making denture base.

DAPPEN DISH

It can be used either side. One side is dipper than the other side. It is used to carry small amount of material like cold mould seal, tooth colored acrylic, self-cure acrylic, and monomer liquid. It can be used as standard to mix heat cure acrylic resin by volume. It is available in various colors. It is made up of glass or ceramic **(Fig. 49.8)**.

SPIRIT LAMP

This is metallic lamp with wick and cover for it. Spirit is poured into the lamp container as fuel to light the wick. It gives noncarbon flame with good temperature. Mainly used during clinical procedure for heating instruments like wax spatula and knife **(Fig. 49.9)**.

BUNSEN BURNER

Bunsen burner can be used as substitute for spirit lamp. It gives continuous noncarbon flame **(Fig. 49.10)**. Used for various clinical procedures like heating the wax instruments, manipulation of wax, greenstick compound, impression compound, etc.

CHIP BLOWER (FIG. 49.11)

It is miniair blower. It is made up of a rubber blower and hollow metal tube curved at

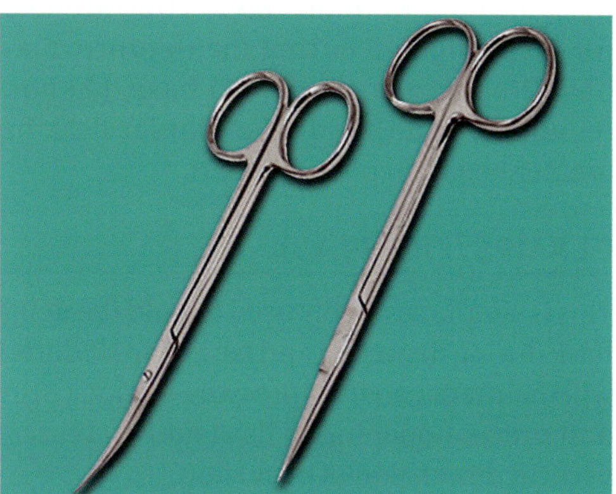

Fig. 49.7: Scissors.

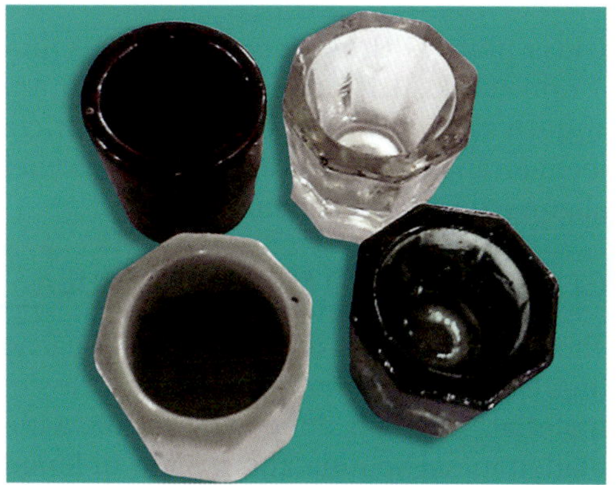

Fig. 49.8: Dappen dish.

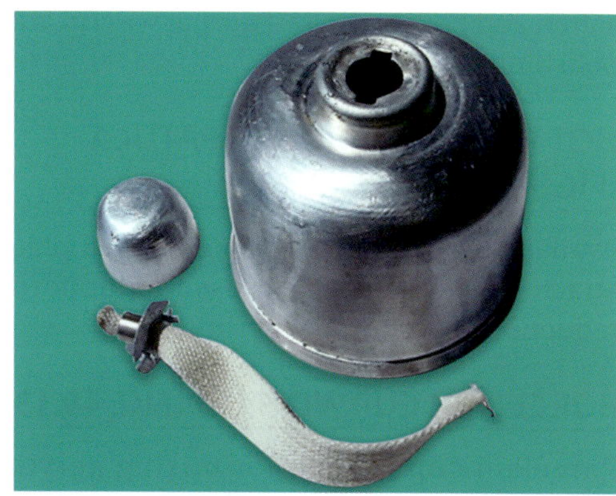

Fig. 49.9: Spirit lamp.

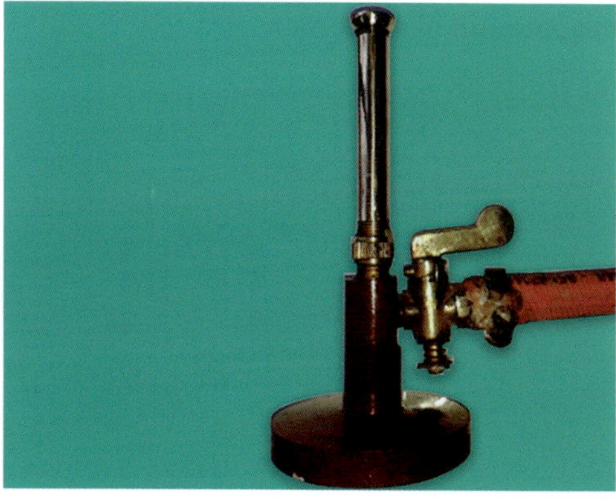

Fig. 49.10: Bunsen burner.

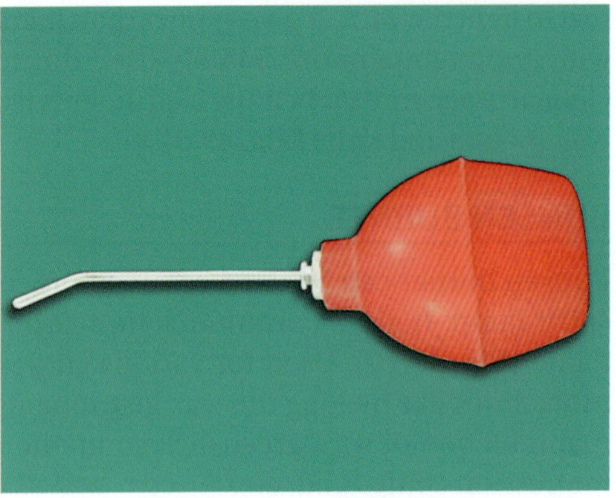

Fig. 49.11: Chip blower.

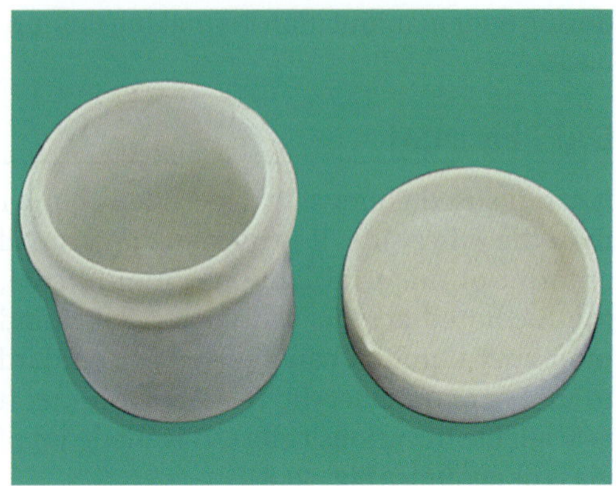

Fig. 49.13: Porcelain cup with lid.

working end. Metal tube is attached with rubber blower. This is used to direct the burner flame in particular area where wax needs to soften and polished. Used during wax up and polishing procedure.

HOT PLATE/HOT PLATE SPATULA (FIG. 49.12)

Available as triangle or square-shaped plate attached with handle. It is used for uniform reduction of occlusion wax rims.

PORCELAIN CUP WITH LID (FIG. 49.13)

Porcelain cup is used for mixing acrylic resin. When polymer and monomer are mixed in cup, it is covered with lid to prevent evaporation of monomer.

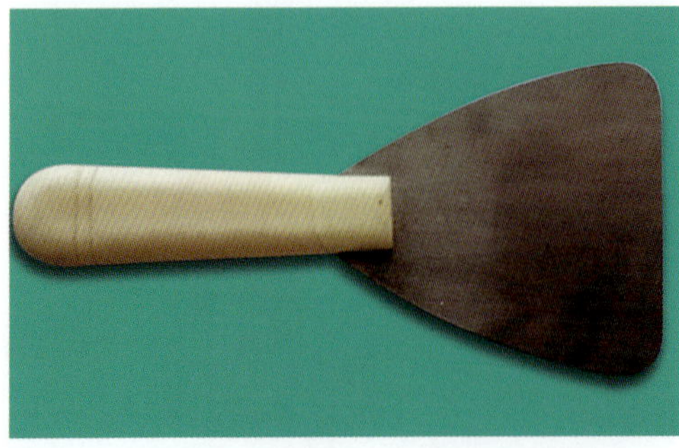

Fig. 49.12: Hot plate/hot plate spatula.

DENTAL FLASKS (FIGS. 49.14A AND B)

Dental flasks are available in pair as maxillary flask and mandibular flask. They are used for investing and curing the denture. Flask has three parts namely: (1) base, (2) body (counter), and (3) lid. Mandibular flask has greater height in posterior part.

CLAMPS (FIG. 49.15)

This is simple assembly used to hold the dental flask during dewaxing and curing procedure. It will maintain constant pressure during curing and prevent opening of flask and increase of vertical dimension of occlusion.

GLASS PLATE (FIG. 49.16)

Glass plate is thin piece of glass around 5 mm thick. It is available in round and square shapes. It is used during artificial teeth arrangement on wax rim to check their alignment and inclination.

GLASS SLAB AND MIXING SPATULA

These are used for mixing of zinc oxide eugenol impression paste and light body impression material. Mixing is done with flexible wide-bladed metal spatula about 5 cm in length **(Fig. 49.17)**.

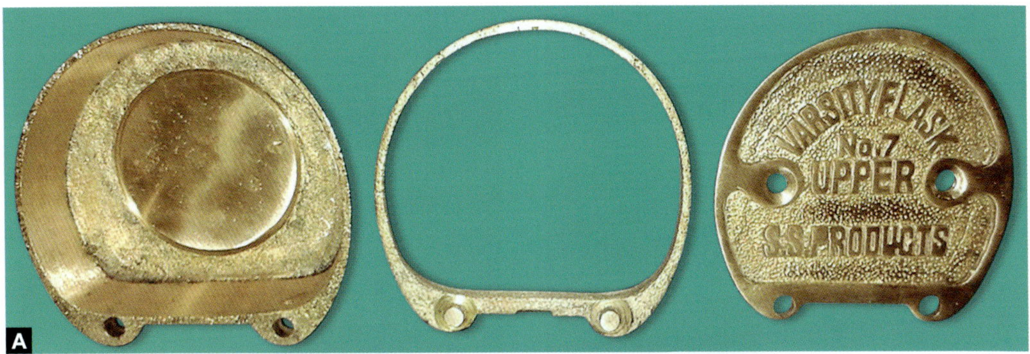

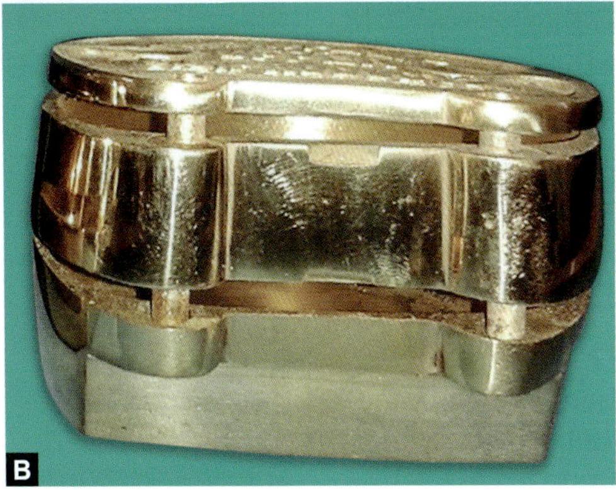

Figs. 49.14A and B: Dental flasks.

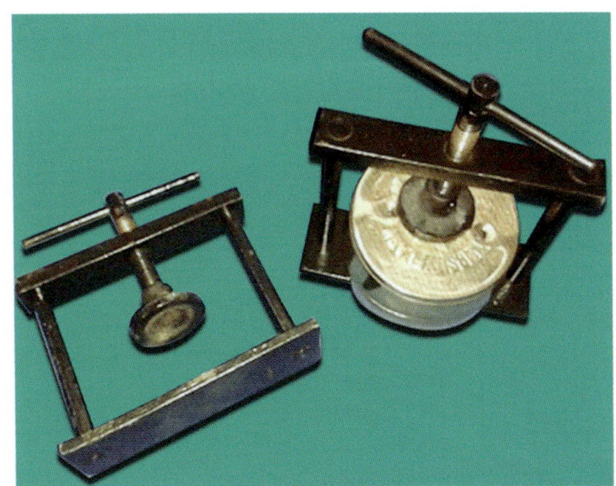

Fig. 49.15: Clamps.

Fig. 49.16: Glass plate.

MIXING PAD AND SPATULA

This pad is made of oil impervious paper **(Fig. 49.18)**. It is used for mixing light body elastomeric impression material or zinc oxide eugenol impression paste. Mixing pad has two lines drawn on it with numbers indicating length which serves as guide to take equal length of base paste and reactor paste. Mixing

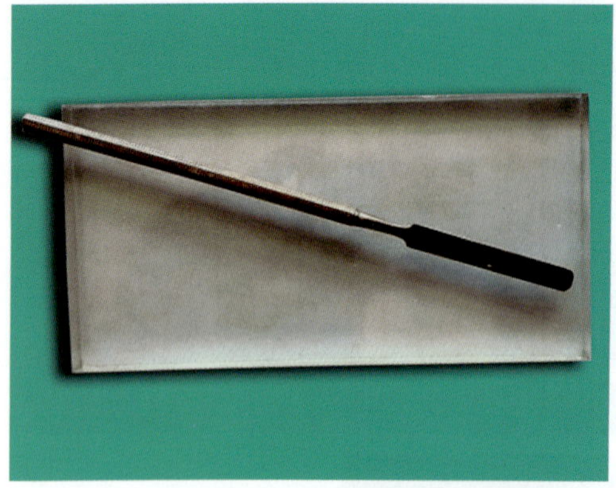

Fig. 49.17: Glass slab and mixing spatula.

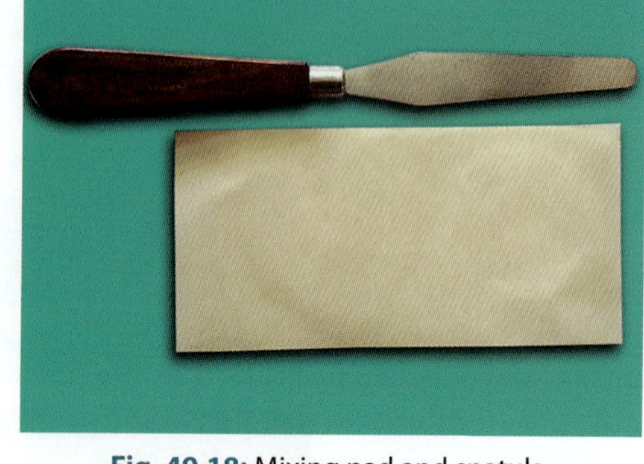

Fig. 49.18: Mixing pad and spatula.

spatula for mixing has stiff wide blade and plastic or wooden handle.

ACRYLIC TRIMMER (FIG. 49.19)

Mounted Stone

It is motor driven tool. Used with laboratory hand motor. It can be mounted on laboratory lathe. It is used for trimming excess acrylic material and finishing of denture prior to polishing. It is available in various shapes and grits. They are available as extra coarse, coarse, medium, and fine grit.

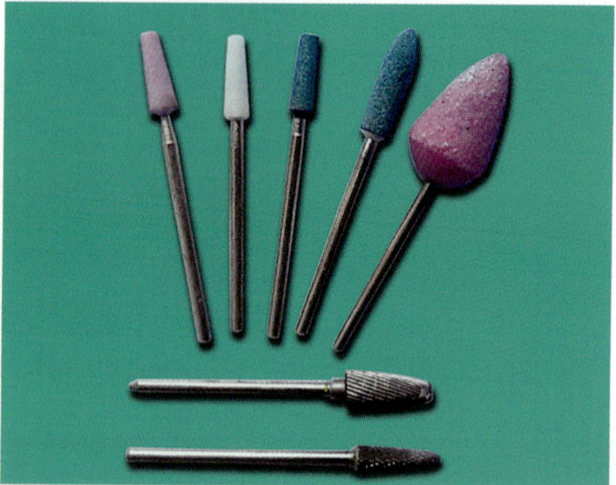

Fig. 49.19: Acrylic trimmer.

Tungsten Carbide Trimmer (TC Trimmer)

It is also motor driven tool. Usually, attached with laboratory micromotor handpiece. It is available in various sizes and shapes. Used for trimming and finishing of acrylic prosthesis after processing. Available for gross trimming to fine finishing.

SANDPAPER MANDREL

It is motor driven tool. It has fragmented working end which is used to hold sandpaper for finishing the acrylic **(Fig. 49.20)**.

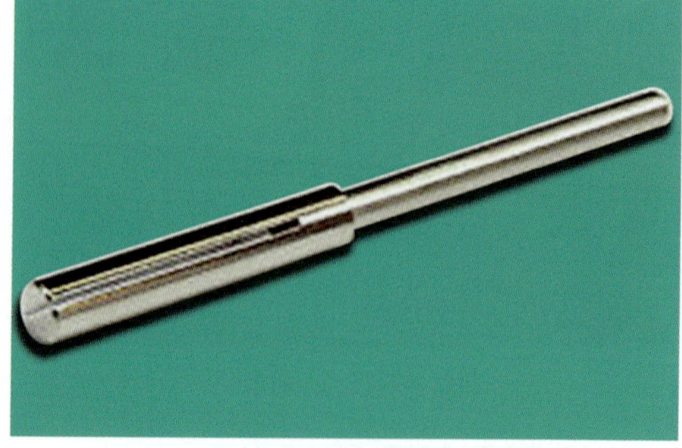

Fig. 49.20: Sandpaper mandrel.

BP BLADE (BARD-PARKER BLADE) AND HANDLE (FIG. 49.21)

It is available in various shapes. Handle is available for mounting blades on it for easy use. It is used for trimming impression compound and green stick compound during clinical procedures.

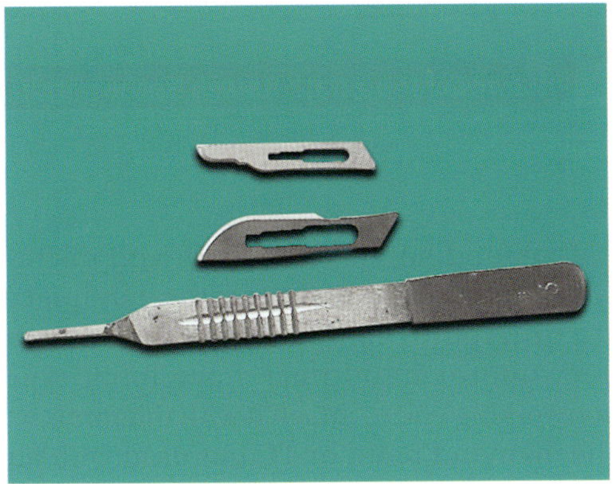

Fig. 49.21: BP blade (Bard-Parker blade) and handle.

RAG WHEEL (FIG. 49.22)

It is made with cotton or polyester cloth and attached to lathe machine. It is used for polishing of acrylic and metal. Polishing agents like pumice, rouge, and tin oxide are applied on it for polishing procedure.

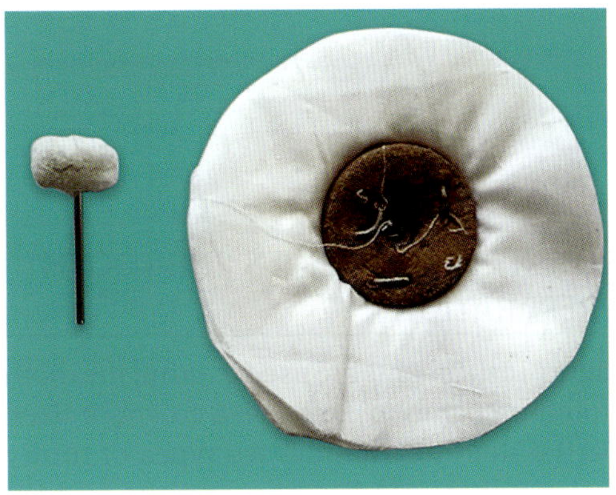

Fig. 49.22: Rag wheel.

CHAPTER 50 Instruments for Fixed Prosthodontics

Paranjay Prajapati, Rajesh Sethuraman

ROTARY INSTRUMENTS FOR TOOTH PREPARATION

Rotary instruments are used to grind the tooth (tooth preparation) to receive crown or fixed partial denture. Mainly two types of rotary instruments—(1) Diamond points and (2) Tungsten carbide (TC) burs are used for tooth preparation **(Figs. 50.1 and 50.2)**.

They are available in various shapes and grits. The diamond points are classified as coarse, medium course, medium fine, and super fine and color coded as red, green, blue, and yellow, respectively. They are rotary instruments used with contra-angled handpiece. Diamond points are widely used for tooth preparation.

Diamond points to be used with micromotor handpiece and air-rotor handpiece are different. Diamond points used with micromotor handpiece have latch type nonworking end to attach it with micromotor. The diamond point or TC bur used with air rotor has straight nonworking end which is attached to air rotor due to friction grip **(Fig. 50.3)**.

DIAMOND POINTS (FIG. 50.4)

These are commonly used rotary instruments for tooth preparation. The basic tooth preparation kit includes straight fissure diamond, flat-end tapering diamond, round-end tapering diamond, torpedo-shaped

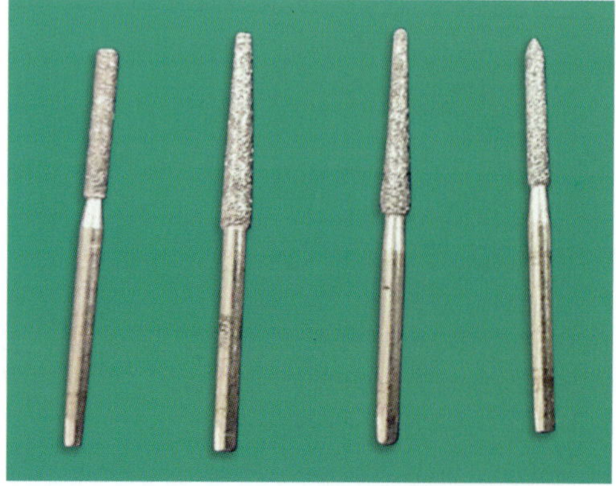

Fig. 50.1: Diamond points.

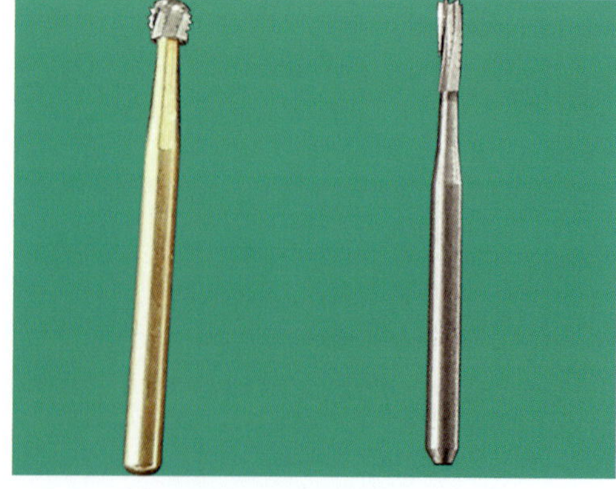

Fig. 50.2: Tungsten carbide burs.

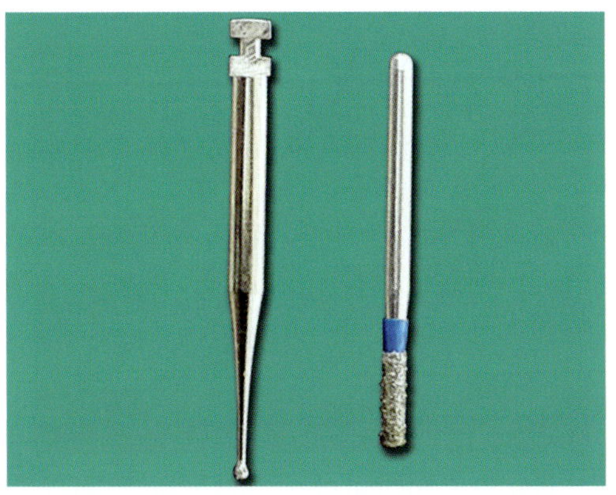

Fig. 50.3: Latch type and friction type nonworking ends of diamond points.

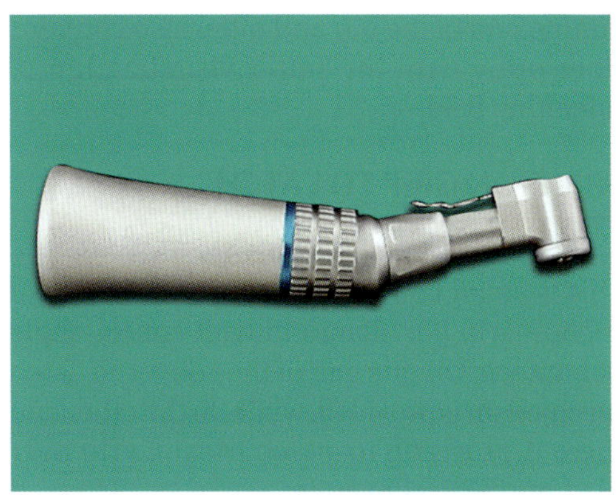

Fig. 50.5: Contra-angle handpiece.

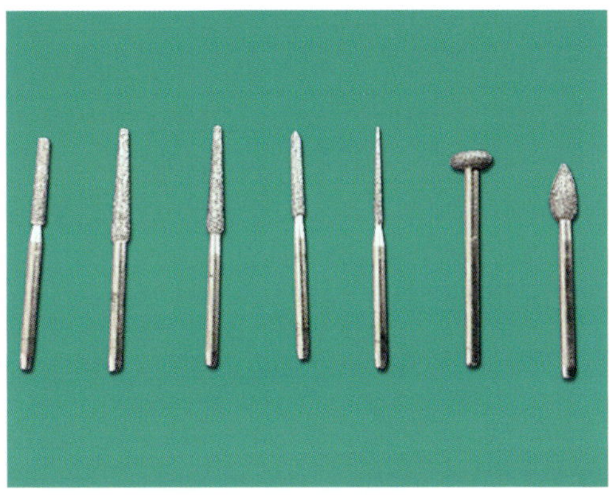

Fig. 50.4: Diamond points.

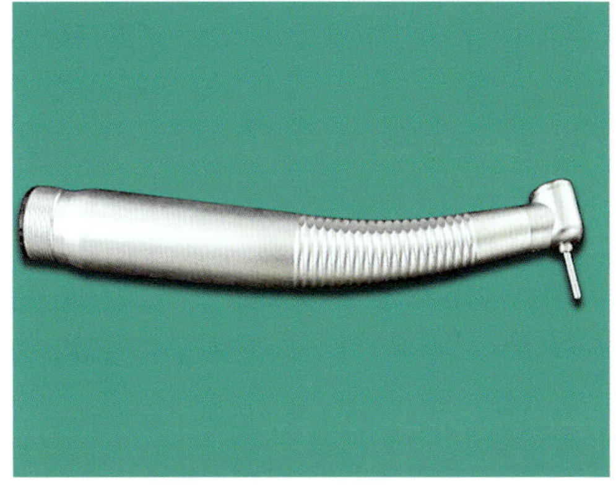

Fig. 50.6: Air rotor handpiece.

diamond, long needle diamond, wheel-shaped diamond, and flame-shaped diamond (right to left shown in **Fig. 50.4**).

CONTRA-ANGLE HANDPIECE (FIG. 50.5)

This is motor driven handpiece. It gets power from electric micromotor. This handpiece has high torque and low speed. In contra-angle handpiece the head of handpiece is first angled away from the long axis and then back toward the long axis of the handle. Because of such design, bur head lies close to long axis of the handle of handpiece which improves visibility and accessibility to working field. This design also improves stability while working. Bur or diamond points with latch type attachment/ nonworking ends are used with contra-angle micromotor handpiece.

AIR ROTOR HANDPIECE (FIG. 50.6)

This handpiece gives very high speed but with lower torque than low speed handpieces. It has speed of 250,000–500,000 revolutions per minute (RPM). The high speed is achieved by small air driven turbine or rotor mounted in bearing the head of handpiece. The sank of the bur is inserted into the rotor of handpiece and revolves with it. The handpiece always contains a system which directs water spray at cutting end of the bur and often also contains fiber optic light for better visualization of operating field.

FRICTION GRIP TO LATCH CONVERTER (FIG. 50.7)

This is small converter that facilitates use of friction grip bur/diamond with contra-angle handpiece. On one end of the converter, latch mechanism is provided, while on the other end there is provision to attach friction grip bur/diamond with converter.

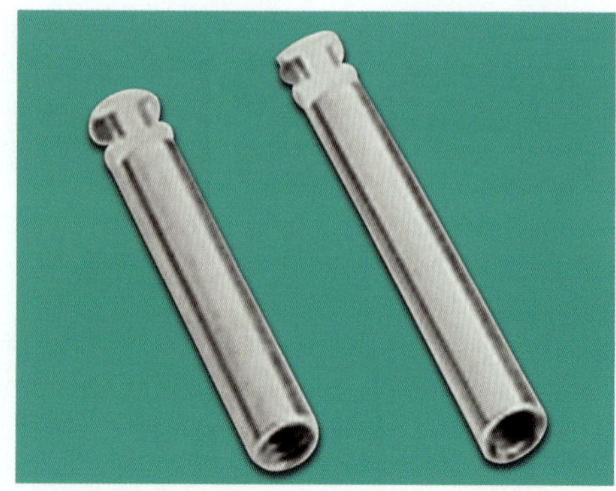

Fig. 50.7: Friction grip to latch converter.

CHAPTER 51

Equipments Used in Prosthodontic Laboratory

Paranjay Prajapati, Rajesh Sethuraman

PLASTER DISPENSER

This is storage cum dispensing equipment for gypsum products mainly dental plaster and dental stone. This is wall mounted equipment which has vibrator mechanism to dispense dental stone or plaster in desired quantity. It prevents contamination of gypsum products (**Fig. 51.1**).

BUNSEN BURNER

It is a gas burner. The fuel for the burner is liquefied petroleum gas (LPG). It produces clean blue flame when gas and air is available in balance. It is made up of metal and has provision for gas inlet and gas outlet valve. It has air collar to adjust the available air while burning. It is used to heat the instrument used for wax manipulation and carving. It should give blue flame when burning (**Fig. 51.2**).

MODEL TRIMMER

Model trimmer (**Fig. 51.3**) is electric equipment used to trim and contour the dental casts. The model trimmer has abrasive wheel which rotates to trim the cast. It has cast holding stand or work table.

The model trimmer has provision for water inlet. Water is sprayed on abrasive wheel to prevent clogging and keep it clean of dental

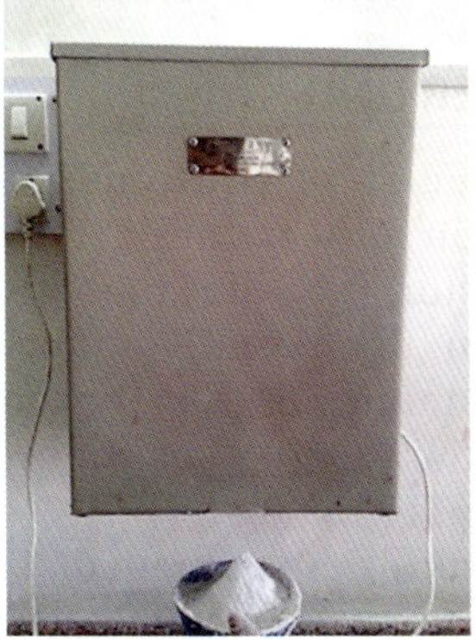

Fig. 51.1: Plaster dispenser.

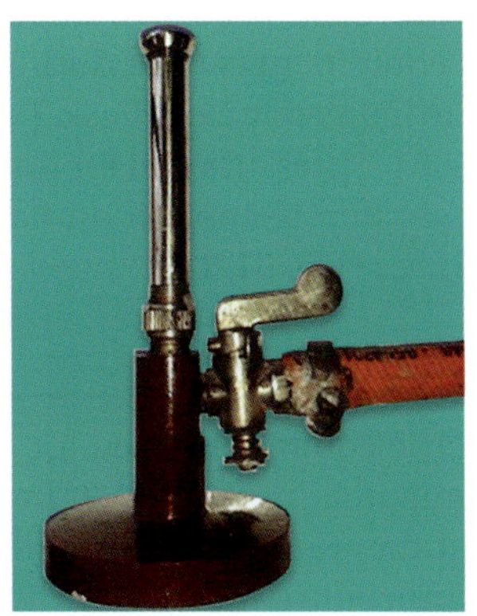

Fig. 51.2: Bunsen burner.

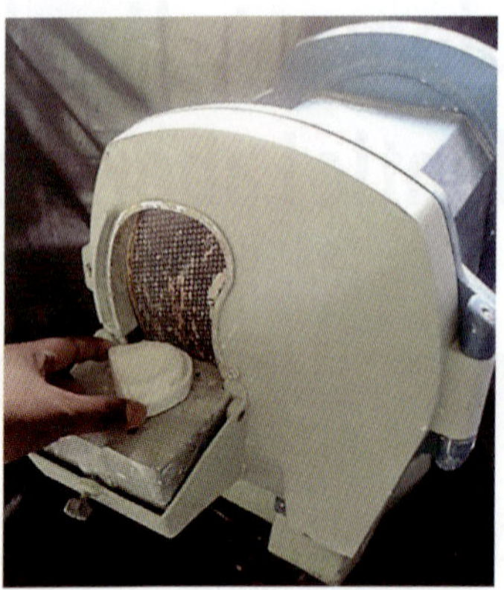

Fig. 51.3: Model trimmer.

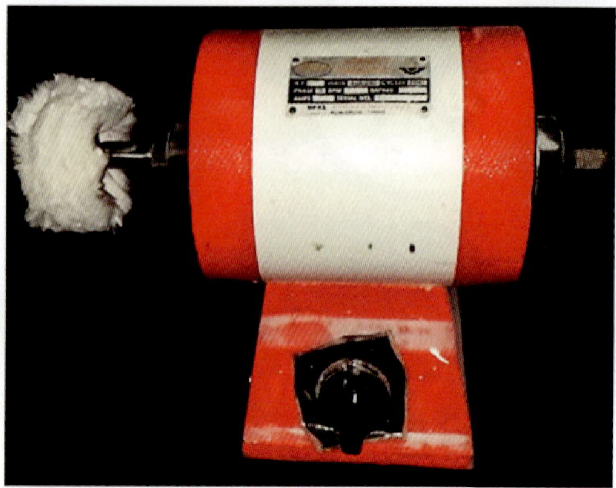

Fig. 51.4: Bench lathe.

plaster or stone. Water supply is maintained for at least 1 minute after trimming is over. This is done to flush out the dental stone/plaster and to prevent clogging.

BENCH LATHE

This equipment is used for variety of laboratory procedures. It is used for gross trimming, grinding, finishing, and polishing procedures. The abrasive grinding wheel is attached at one end and the other end has provision for attachment of rag wheel, trimming burs, or stones **(Fig. 51.4)**.

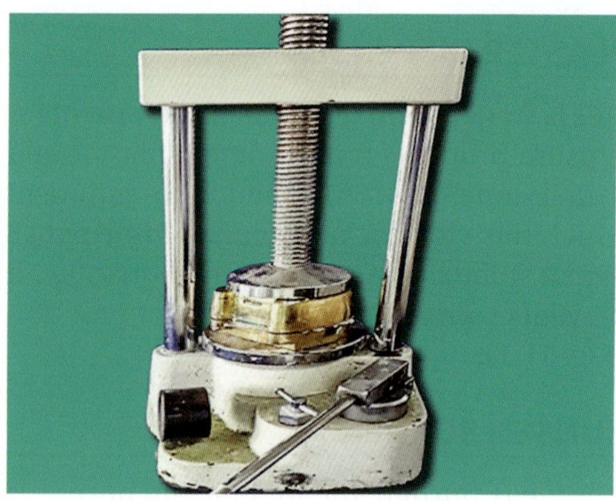

Fig. 51.5: Hydraulic press.

HYDRAULIC PRESS

It is a hydraulic equipment. It has provision to slowly increase pressure according to need. This equipment is used during packing procedure to intimately close flask. During trial closure 1,500 psi pressure and for final closure 3,500 psi pressure is applied on flask under hydraulic press **(Fig. 51.5)**.

DEWAXING UNIT

This is electric equipment used for dewaxing or wax elimination procedure. It has heating coil to heat the water in water bath. During dewaxing procedure molten wax may come out through the flask and mix with water, to discard this water tap is provided. Flask and clamp assembly are placed in boiling water for 5 minutes for dewaxing procedure.

ACRYLIZER UNIT

It is a electrical equipment used for acrylization of heat cure acrylic resin. It has provision for water bath and special mechanism (thermostat) for providing time and temperature control. The temperature and time duration can be set by provided mechanism **(Fig. 51.6)**.

If long curing cycle is required for curing the acrylic resin, the temperature can be set at 74°C using temperature control and time

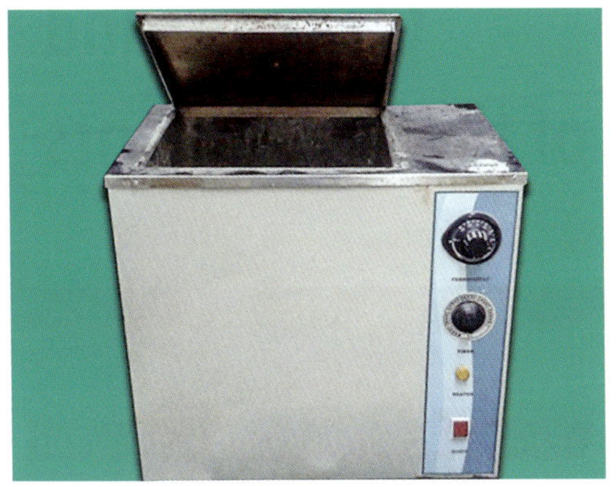

Fig. 51.6: Acrylizer unit.

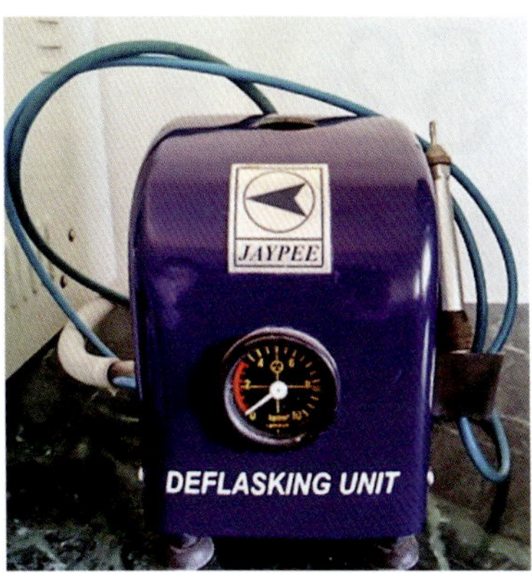

Fig. 51.7: Deflasking unit.

can be set for 8 hours using time control, so the same temperature will be maintained for required time interval.

DEFLASKING UNIT

This is pneumatic equipment. It is used for separation of two halves of flask after polymerization of complete denture. Some equipment has provision of pneumatic chisel to separate cured denture from investment plaster **(Fig. 51.7)**.

CHAPTER 52

Cleaning and Caring of the Instruments

Paranjay Prajapati, Rajesh Sethuraman

RUBBER BOWLS

Usually, in preclinical exercises, two rubber bowls are used. Rubber bowls are used for the manipulation of gypsum products and alginate impression material. Keep separate bowls for gypsum product manipulation and alginate manipulation.

After manipulation of gypsum products, rubber bowl can be cleaned with water. After manipulation of alginate, rubber bowl can be cleaned first with small piece of cotton or gauze and finally with water.

WAX MANIPULATION INSTRUMENTS

Bunsen burner or spirit lamp is used as heat source to heat the instruments in dental laboratory and clinic. Due to heating, the instruments over fire flame, working ends of instruments become black due to carbon deposition over them. The working ends should be clean and free of carbon deposits on it.

At the end of every laboratory session, clean the instruments with cotton to remove wax from the working end. These instruments can be cleaned with sand papering when the working end becomes black due to carbon deposits.

GLASS SLAB

Glass slab used for manipulation of various impression materials like zinc oxide eugenol (ZOE) paste, light body consistency elastomers, etc. The glass slab can be cleaned with piece of cotton or gauze. If dental cements are manipulated over glass slab, it can be cleaned with piece of cotton or gauze soaked with drop of spirit.

After manipulation of ZOE paste, glass slab is cleaned with carbon tetrachloride. If the paste hardened over the spatula, hold it over a flame to soften and then wipe out the spatula.

GLASS PLATE

Glass plate is used as template while teeth arrangement. Wax usually sticks to the glass plate. Glass plate can be cleaned by slightly and very carefully heating over the flame and cleaning it with dry cotton piece. *Do not heat it excessively otherwise it will break.*

MODEL TRIMMER

It is used to trim the dental casts. Water supply should be ensured while trimming the casts. Allow the water to run for at least 1–2 minutes after trimming is over. This will flush all of the gypsum particles from the trimmer and prevents clogging.

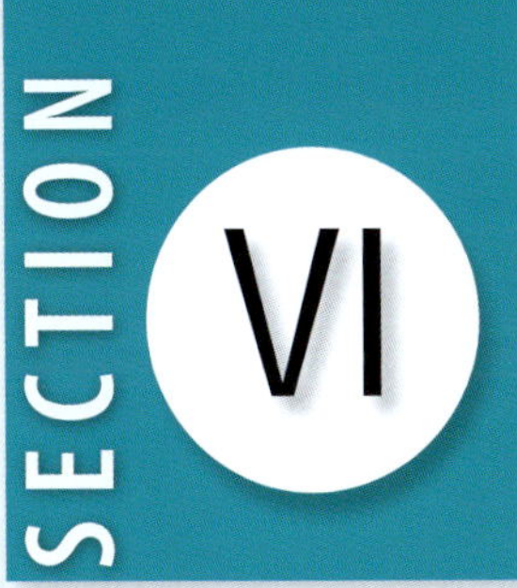

Dental Materials

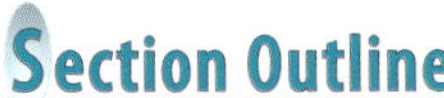

CHAPTER 53

Dental Materials Used in Prosthodontics

Paranjay Prajapati, Rajesh Sethuraman, Sneha Kulkarni

GYPSUM PRODUCTS

INTRODUCTION

Various dental biomaterials are used in prosthodontic procedures. One should identify and know their use as dental material. This chapter gives brief idea about various dental biomaterials used in prosthodontic clinical and laboratory procedures. Dental materials are broadly divided here into three categories for easy understanding as gypsum products, impression materials, processing materials, etc.

DENTAL BIOMATERIALS

Dental Plaster (Type-I Gypsum Product)

Impression plaster is modified dental plaster used for making impression of edentulous arch. Not in used widely. It has low strength. Water-powder ratio is 0.50–0.75.

Dental Plaster (Type-II Gypsum Product) (Fig. 53.1)

Dental plaster is used for making primary cast/diagnostic cast. It is used for mounting casts on articulator and also used for flasking procedure. It consists of irregular, porous beta hemihydrate particles of calcium sulfate. It has low strength compared to dental stone. Usually white in color. Water-powder ratio is 0.45–0.50.

Dental Stone (Type-III Gypsum Product) (Fig. 53.2)

It is used for making master casts and for flasking procedures. It consists of regular, crystalline alpha hemihydrate particles of

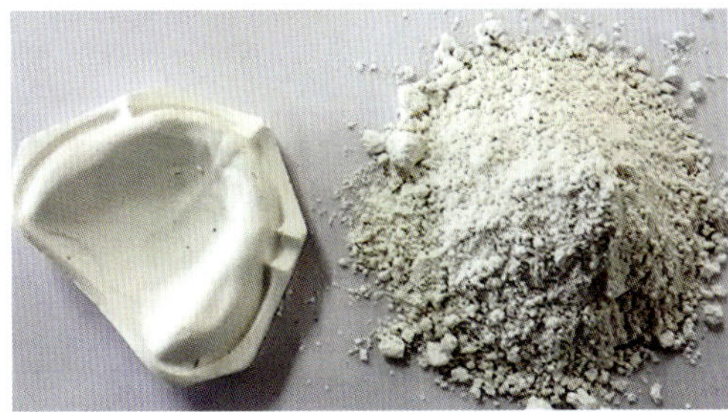

Fig. 53.1: Dental plaster (Type-II gypsum product).

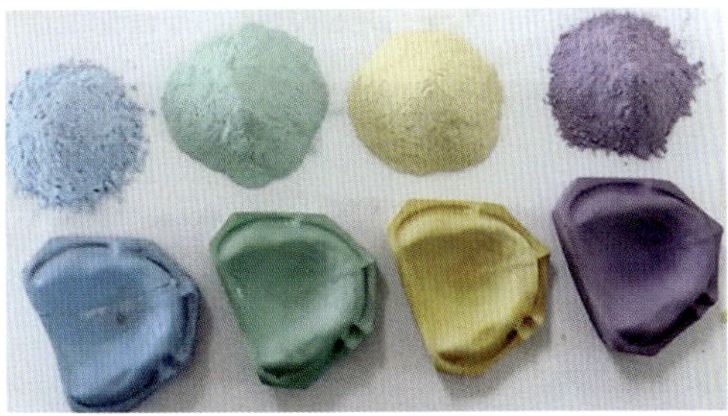

Fig. 53.2: Dental stone (Type-III gypsum product).

calcium sulfate. It is available in various colors. Water-powder ratio is 0.28–0.30.

Die Stone (Type-IV Gypsum Product) (Fig. 53.3)

It is widely used die material. Used for making die of prepared tooth/teeth. It has high strength and abrasion resistance. It has finer particle size. It is available in various colors. Water-powder ratio is 0.22–0.24.

Investment Material (Type-V Gypsum Product) (Fig. 53.4)

It is used for investment of wax pattern and casting them into metal. It consists of powder and silica suspension. It has high strength and high expansion. It can withstand high temperature. Water-powder ratio is 0.18–0.20.

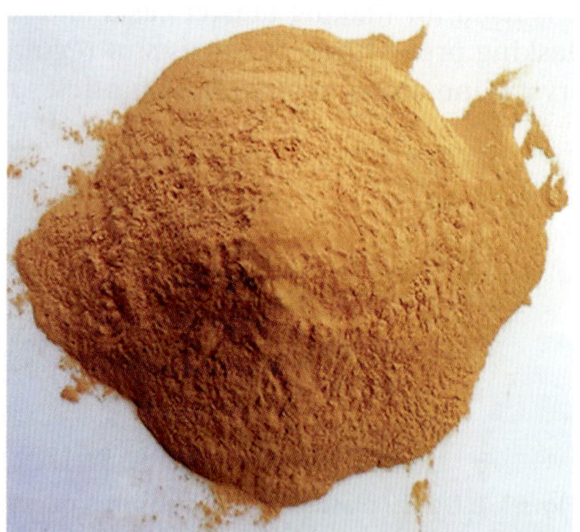

Fig. 53.3: Die stone (Type-IV gypsum product).

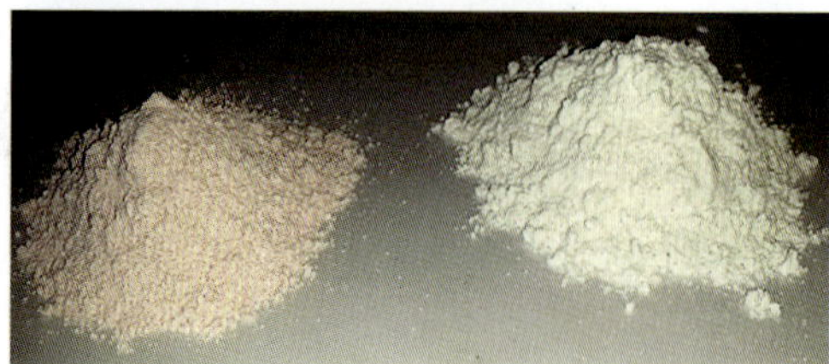

Fig. 53.4: Investment material (Type-V gypsum product).

> Water-powder ratio: This indicates recommended proportion of gypsum product to be mixed with water. It indicate required amount of water per 100 g of powder (gypsum product). For dental plaster, it is 0.45–0.50. This means 45–50 mL of water is needed to mix 100 g of dental plaster to achieve optimum mix and properties.

IMPRESSION MATERIALS

IMPRESSION MATERIALS IN DENTISTRY

Variety of impression materials are available to be used in dentistry.

Impression Compound (Fig. 53.5)

It is used for making primary impression of edentulous arches. It is rigid impression material. It is thermoplastic in nature, changes consistency according to change in temperature. It consists of wax, resin, fillers, and coloring agent. It is available in various colors. The American Dental Association (ADA) specification number is 3.

Zinc Oxide Eugenol Paste (Fig. 53.6)

It becomes rigid after set. It is used for making final impression of edentulous arches. It is also used for bite registration. Thermosetting in nature, there is no effect of temperature once

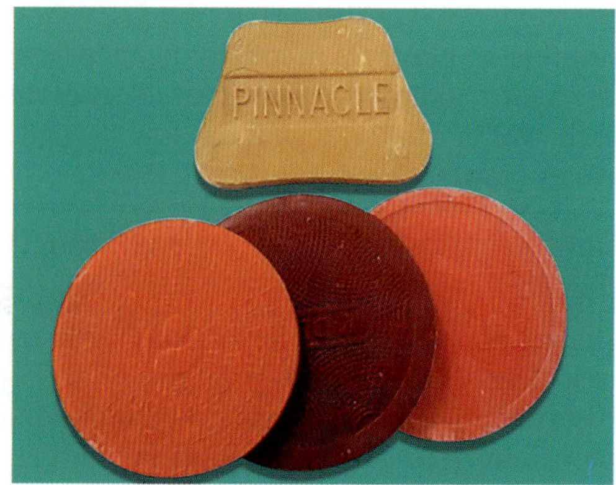

Fig. 53.5: Impression compound.

it is set. It is available in two pastes system. It sets by chelation reaction and forms chelate as zinc eugenolate. It contains eugenol which causes burning sensation and allergic reaction in some patients. ADA specification number is 16.

Agar-agar (Reversible Hydrocolloid) (Fig. 53.7)

It is elastic impression material. It is reversible hydrocolloid. For making impression of dentulous and partially edentulous arches. It is also used for duplication of cast. Specially designed trays called rim locked water-cooled tray are used for agar impression. Special equipment called as "conditioning unit" is required for manipulation of agar.

Alginate (Irreversible Hydrocolloid) (Figs. 53.8A and B)

It is elastic impression material. It is irreversible hydrocolloid. For making impression of dentulous, partially edentulous, and complete edentulous arches. It is natural product generated from seaweed. Main ingredient is sodium alginate, potassium alginate, or triethanolamine alginate. Manipulation is done with rubber bowl and curved spatula. Chromatic alginate is also available which indicates color changes at different working

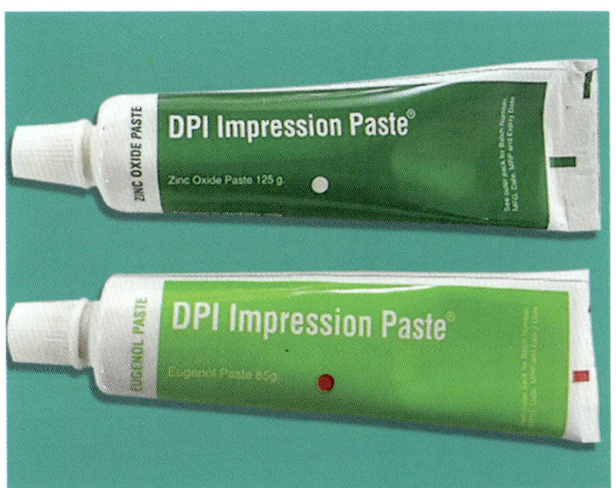

Fig. 53.6: Zinc oxide eugenol paste.

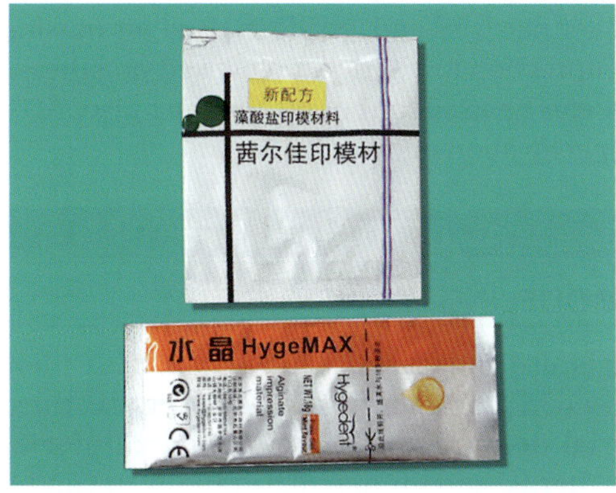

Fig. 53.8A: Alginate pouches for single impression.

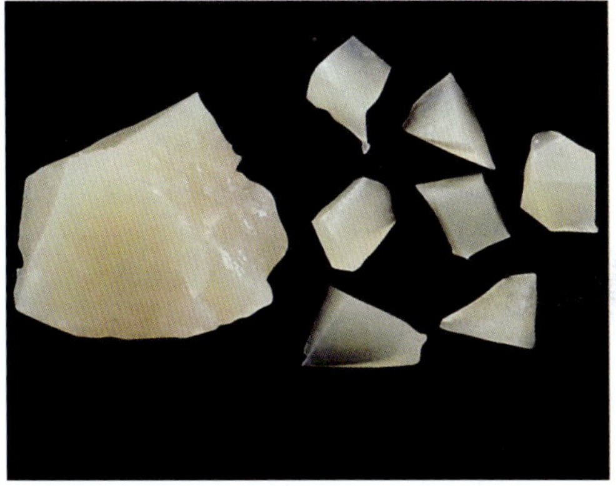

Fig. 53.7: Agar-agar (reversible hydrocolloid).

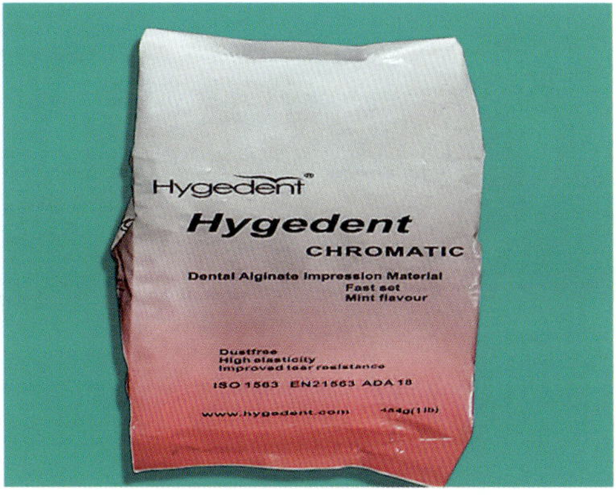

Fig. 53.8B: Chromatic alginate.

and setting stages. Water-powder ratio is 16 mL water and 38 g of powder. ADA specification number is 18.

Addition Silicone Impression Material (Fig. 53.9)

It is nonaqueous elastomeric material. It is hydrophobic in nature but can be converted in hydrophilic by adding surfactants. It is also known as polyvinyl siloxane or vinyl polysiloxane. It is available as reactor and base. It reacts by addition reaction. It gives most accurate surface reproduction. It is available in various consistencies like putty consistency, light body consistency, etc. Light body consistency has less filler particles and more flow. Putty consistency has more filler particles and less flow. Used for making impression for fabrication of fixed prosthesis. It can be used for border molding also. ADA specification number is 19.

DENTAL WAXES

MODELING WAX (FIG. 53.10)

It is also known as baseplate wax. It is widely used in prosthetic work for making wax rims, trial denture bases, making maxillofacial patterns, and for bite registrations. It can be used for spacer and blocking the undercut on the cast. It is available in three types as type-I soft, type-II medium, and type-III hard. Consist of paraffin wax, resins, and carnauba wax. ADA specification number is 24.

STICKY WAX (FIG. 53.11)

It is made up of beeswax, paraffin wax, and resin. The resin gives the sticky wax its adhesiveness and hardness. It is very sticky when heated. It is used to join broken parts of prosthesis before repair. Become firm and brittle when cooled. It is also used to stabilize components while soldering. It should break under pressure rather than bending or distort.

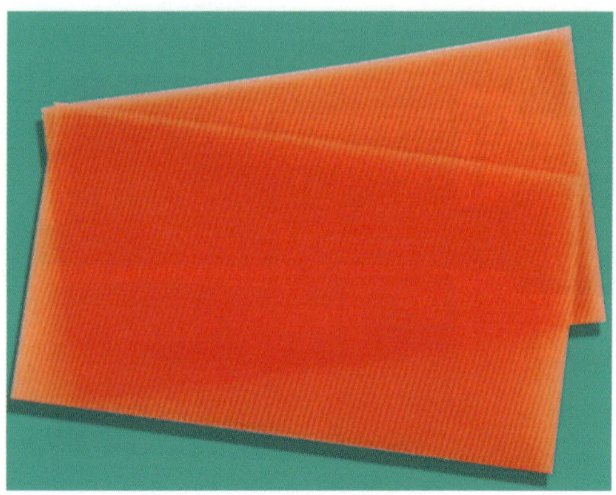

Fig. 53.10: Modeling wax.

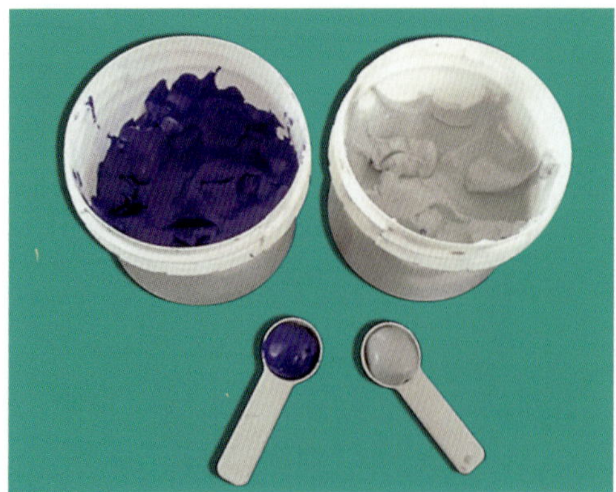

Fig. 53.9: Addition silicone impression material.

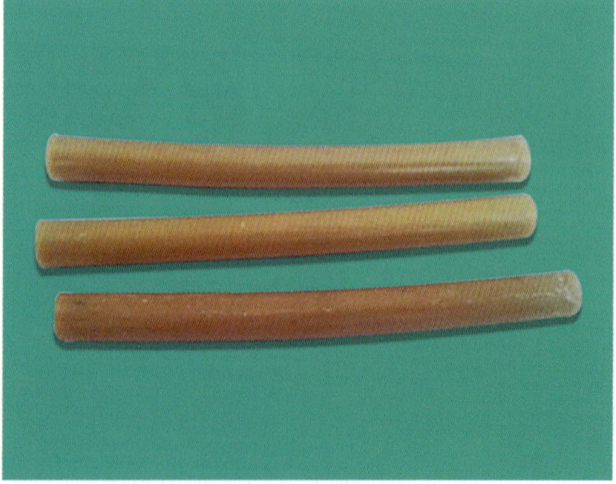

Fig. 53.11: Sticky wax.

PREFABRICATED PATTERNS FOR CAST PARTIAL DENTURE (FIG. 53.12)

Wax patterns in preformed shapes are available as ready to use for making pattern of cast partial dentures. Available as various component patterns as major connector, minor connector, circumferential clasps, and bar clasp.

INLAY WAX (FIG. 53.13)

It is available as type-I medium wax and type-II soft wax. Used for making inlay pattern by direct and indirect method. Medium wax is used for direct technique and soft wax is used for indirect technique.

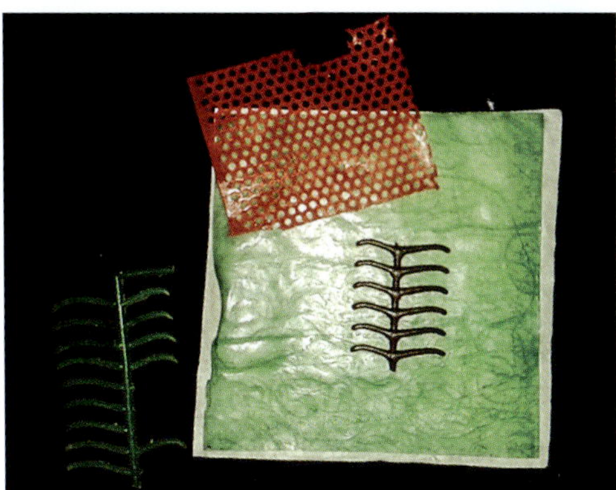

Fig. 53.12: Prefabricated patterns for cast partial denture.

PATTERN WAX (FIG. 53.14)

Available as body wax, margin wax, and occlusal wax, all three have different flow and consistency. It is used to make wax patterns for crown and bridge. Margin wax is usually red in color with good flow and hard in consistency. Body wax has medium flow and occlusal wax is soft that is desired property to carve occlusal anatomy.

DENTURE BASE RESIN

INTRODUCTION

The acrylic resins used in prosthodontics are polymers. The process by which they are processed is known as "polymerization." Acrylic resin can be classified by its method of processing or curing. According to processing/curing method, they are classified as heat-cured acrylic, self-cured acrylic, and light-activated acrylic resin.

SELF-CURE ACRYLIC RESIN

It is available as powder and liquid. It is also known as cold cure or autopolymerizing resin. It is used to make denture base, custom tray, relining, temporization, denture repair, and orthodontic appliance. Activator is dimethyl-para-toluidine **(Fig. 53.15)**.

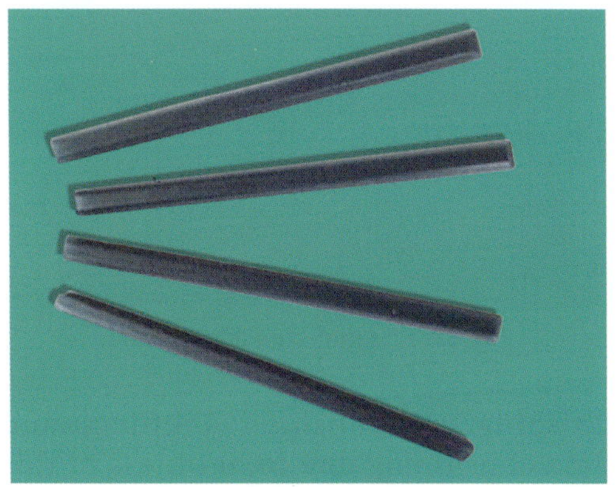

Fig. 53.13: Inlay wax.

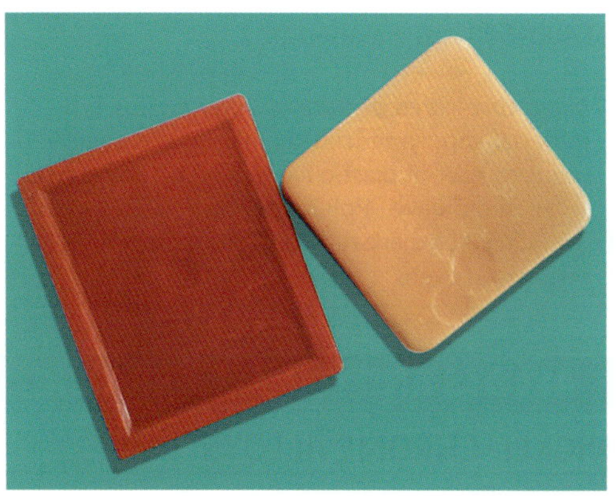

Fig. 53.14: Pattern wax.

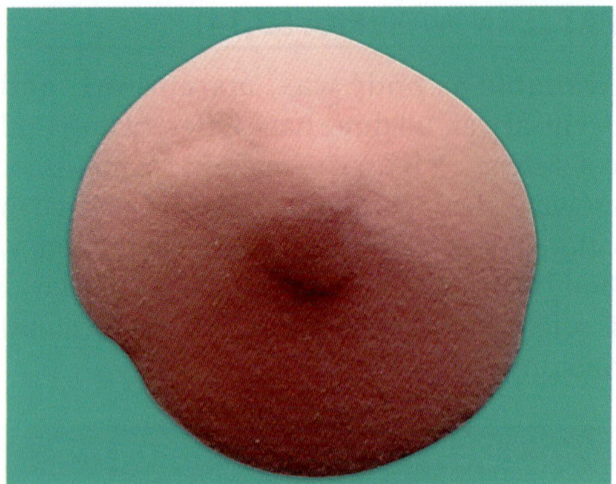

Fig. 53.15: Self-cure acrylic resin.

HEAT-CURE ACRYLIC RESIN

It is available as powder and liquid. Activator is heat supplied in water bath **(Figs. 53.16A and B)**. Mainly used for making removable prosthesis. Available as clear, pink, fiber reinforced, and high impact material. Appreciate fibers in fiber reinforced acrylic in **Figure 53.16**B.

LIGHT-CURE ACRYLIC RESIN

It consists of urethane dimethacrylate matrix with an acrylic copolymer, silica filler, and camphorquinone-amine photoinitiator system **(Fig. 53.17)**. It is supplied as premixed sheets. Unpolymerized material has clay-like consistency. It is supplied in tight opaque packages. Polymerization is done by blue light of 400–500 nm wavelengths.

Microwave-cured denture base resin: This type of material is polymerized by microwave energy. It requires special plastic flasks which can be used with microwave. Polymerization time is only 3 minutes. Polymerization can be done in household microwave ovens.

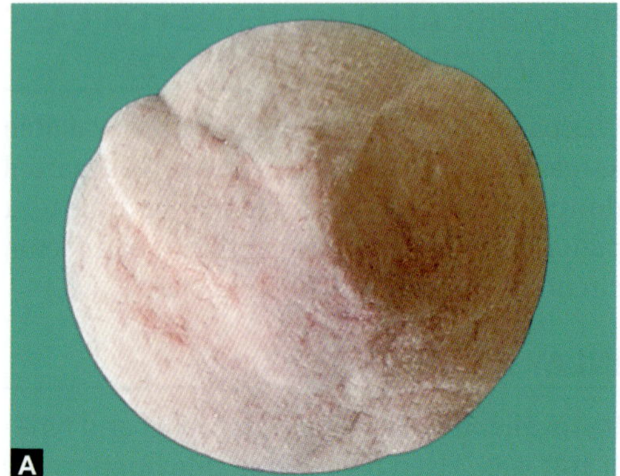

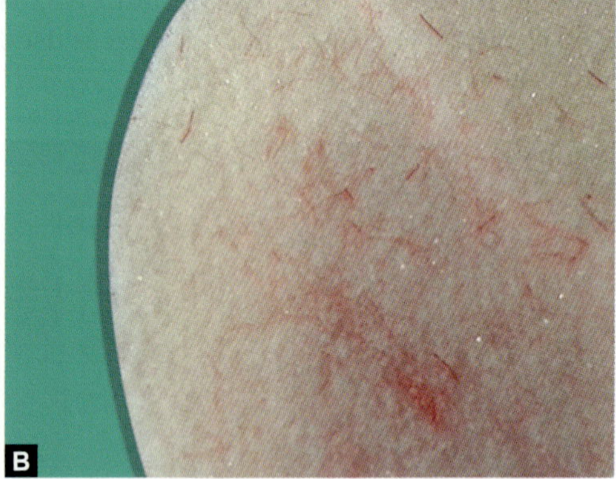

Figs. 53.16A and B: Heat-cure acrylic resin.

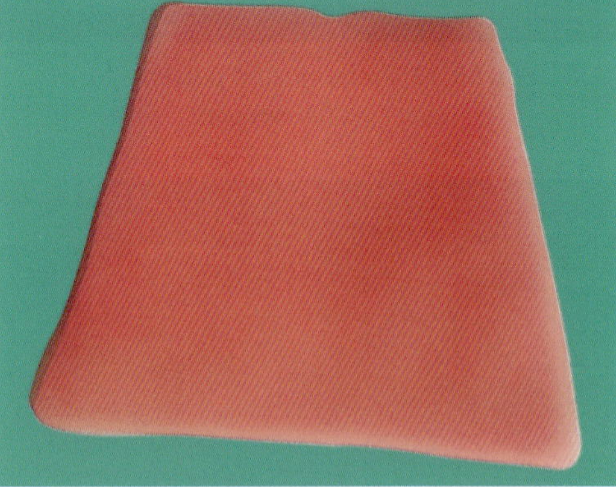

Fig. 53.17: Light-cure acrylic resin.

ALLOYS AND DENTAL CERAMIC

NICKEL-CHROME ALLOYS

These are used for making all metal restorations. Altering the metal, like cutting, finishing, and polishing is difficult and time consuming due to hardness of this alloy. It has passivation property making it resistance to tarnish and corrosion.

Melting temperature range is 1,100–1,304°C. Nickel-chrome alloys are available as pellets as shown in **Figure 53.18**.

COBALT-CHROMIUM ALLOYS

It has excellent corrosion resistance. Used for porcelain fused to metal restorations **(Fig. 53.19)**. It is also used for fabrication of framework of cast partial dentures. White in color. The fusion temperature range is 1,250–1,450°C.

DENTAL PORCELAIN OR CERAMIC

This is material of earthen origin with added material to achieve strength and shade **(Fig. 53.20)**. It is used for porcelain denture teeth, inlay, onlays, laminates veneers, all ceramic crown and bridge, and porcelain fused to metal restoration. It is available in various types and shades. According to fusion temperature, it can be classified as high fusing (more than 1,300°C), medium fusing (1,100–1,300°C), low fusing (850–1,100°C), and ultra-low fusing (less than 850°C).

FINISHING AND POLISHING AGENTS

SAND PAPER

Sand or any other form of quartz is used for finishing purpose. It is available in various particle size (grit) **(Fig. 53.21)**. Sand is bonded to paper to use as finishing agent. It can be

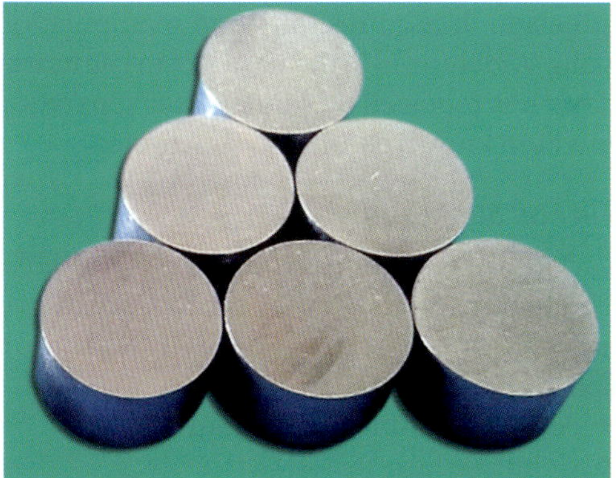

Fig. 53.18: Nickel-chrome alloys.

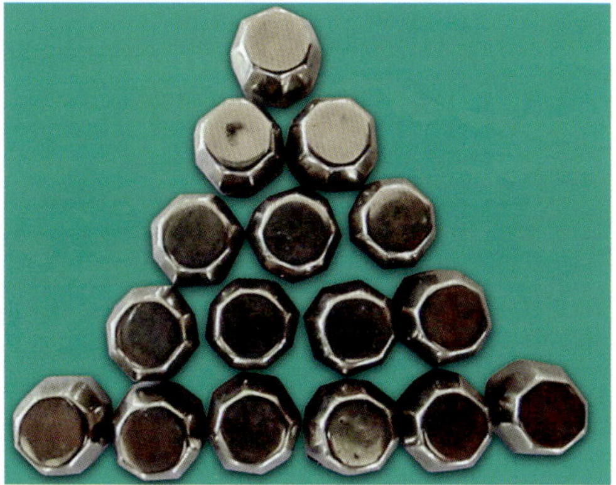

Fig. 53.19: Cobalt-chromium alloys.

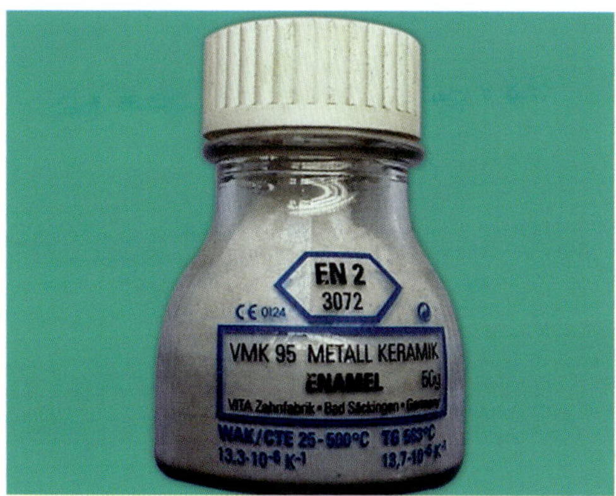

Fig. 53.20: Dental porcelain or ceramic.

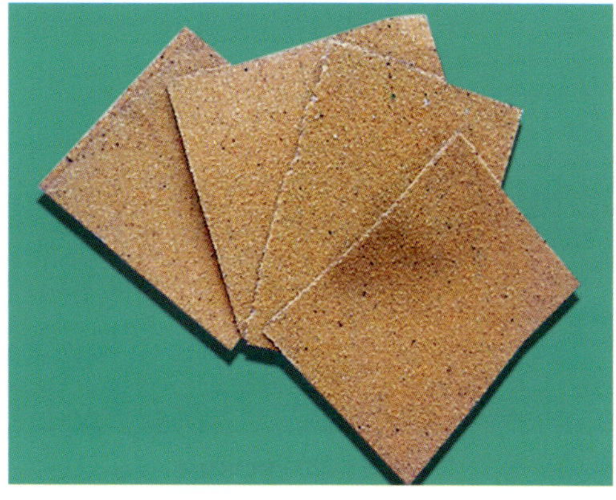

Fig. 53.21: Sandpaper.

used manually or with sandpaper mandrel. Available in different grit sizes.

EMERY PAPER

It consists of natural oxide or corundum. It is bonded with paper to make emery paper. It is used manually or with mandrel for finishing the acrylic resins as well as for metal surface **(Fig. 53.22)**.

PUMICE

Pumice is siliceous material of volcanic origin **(Fig. 53.23)**. It can be used as abrasive or polishing agent depending on its practical size. It is available as powder form and cake.

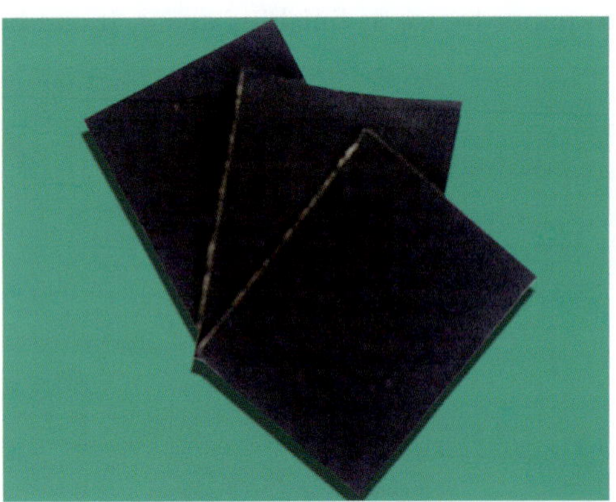

Fig. 53.22: Emery paper.

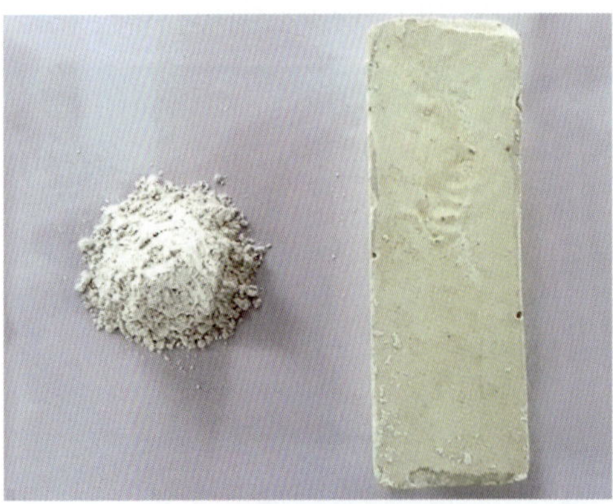

Fig. 53.23: Pumice.

Pumice can also be used for polishing of enamel, amalgam.

SEPARATING MEDIUM

INTRODUCTION

A coating applied to a surface and serving to prevent a second surface from adhering to the first surface **(Fig. 53.24)**.

It is used for easy separation of two surfaces.

It prevents seepage of monomer from resin when packed in mould and also prevent water to integrate with the resin.

TYPES

Tin Foil

It is adapted on surface of object to prevent adhesion. It requires time and manipulation skills. Widely used in the past. Not in use nowadays. It is replaced by some newer separating medium known as "tin foil substitutes".

Tin Foil Substitutes

Variety of separating materials are available. They are used instead of tin foil, so known as tin foil substitutes. Some of the tin foil substitutes are listed here.

- Aqueous solution of sodium silicate
- Cellulose lacquers

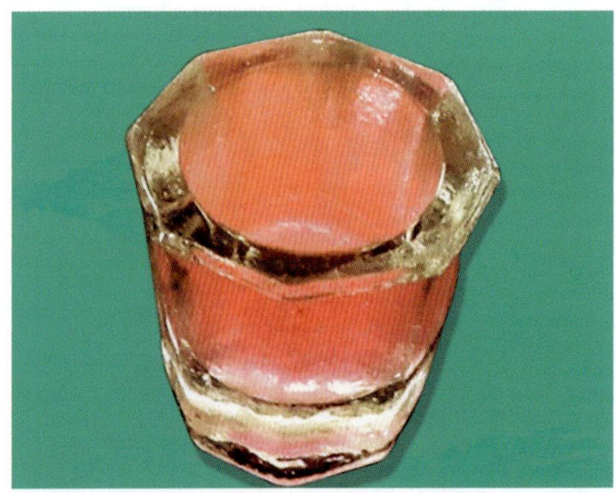

Fig. 53.24: Cold mould seal.

- Soap solutions
- Starch
- Calcium oleate
- Water soluble alginate (sodium alginate solution)
- Petroleum jelly.

Sodium alginate solution is most popular and widely used separating medium. It is also known as "cold mould seal."

Composition: 2% sodium alginate, water, glycerin, sodium phosphate, and alcohol preservatives.

Mode of action: When cold mould seal is applied on surface of gypsum products, sodium alginate of cold mould seal reacts with calcium sulfate of gypsum products and forms insoluble film of calcium alginate. This thin film will act as separating film between two surfaces.

Sodium alginate + Calcium sulfate → Calcium alginate

Application: It is applied with soft bristle brush in single direction. One or more coats can be applied. Cold mould seal should be applied in unidirectional only otherwise it may disturb the formation of thin film. It should be applied in even coating.

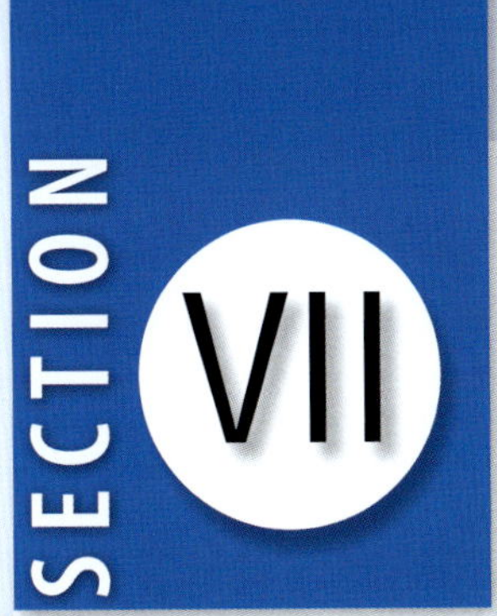

OSCE/OSPE/ Spotter Section

Section Outline

CHAPTER 54

OSCE/OSPE/Spotter Section

Objectively structured clinical examination (OSCE) which was later expanded to practical examination (OSPE). The OSCE-OSPE method can be used for both as an evaluation as well as a teaching tool.

Students move from one setup to the other setup; this setup is commonly known as "STATION".

Stations are of multiple types but the best known are of three types; procedure or skill station, observer station, and questions station. Most of the skill or procedural station has an observer stationed who is provided with objectively structured checklist to score the student performance.

At the procedure station student are given tasks to perform on volunteers, patients, casts or models, simulators.

At questions station students provide answer to objective questions or interpret lab data, or radiographs. These stations usually present clinical photographs, patient data, models with set of knowledge-based questions. Usually, OSCE-OSPE setup consist of equal number of procedural and question station, however the number may be modified to suit a specific examination model.

Types of OSCE-OSPE stations		
Question station	***Procedure station***	***Rest station***
Question–answer station	Procedure station	Nonscoring station
At questions station students provide answer to objective questions or interpret lab data, or radiographs, etc.	At the procedure station student are given tasks to perform on volunteers, patients, casts or models, or on simulators	Required to give time between subsequent stations to complete back log of previous station and taking washroom and water break

OSCE-OSPE setup	
Score	5 marks/station
Time duration	3–5 minutes for each station (equal time distribution)
Observer/Instructor	*Question station—observer not required *Procedure station—observer required

Example of station set up:

MARKS: 05	One mark per answer	Time allotted for station: 05 Minutes
Specimen	*Questions*	*Answers*
	Identify the specimen	Map of India
	Name any one country located north to it	China
	Name any one neighboring country located south to it	Sri Lanka
	Name any two ocean/sea bordering it	1. Indian ocean 2. Arabian sea
	Name any one island of it	Andaman and Nicobar Islands

In above example you can see Marks/Time given for this station/Mark per question/specimen and related questions. After observing the specimen student will answer the question. Once the time for this station is over the student will move to the other station and so on.

With this very brief introduction to the OSCE/OSPE type examination methodology you can go through following subject related stations.

MARKS: 05	One mark per answer	Time allotted for station: 05 Minutes
Specimen	*Questions*	*Answers*
	Identify the marked area	Incisive papilla
	Which type of landmark is it?	Relieving structure
	Its position with reference to central incisors	It is 6–8 mm away from maxillary central incisors
	What bony foramen is covered by this structure?	It covers incisive foramen
	What nerve and vessels are associated with this area?	Nasopalatine nerve and vessels

MARKS: 05	One mark per answer	Time allotted for station: 05 Minutes
Specimen	*Questions*	*Answers*
	Identify the marked area	Mid palatine raphe
	Which type of landmark is it?	Relieving structure
	Write its extension	It extends from incisive papilla to posterior part of hard palate
	What bony structure is covered by this structure? How it is formed	It covers bony suture at midline of palate formed due to fusion of two palatine bones
	Write characteristic of mucosa in this area	It is covered by thin mucosa. Submucosa in this area is absent or very thin. Thus, this area is sensitive to pressure

MARKS: 05	One mark per Answer	Time allotted for station: 05 Minutes
Specimen	*Questions*	*Answers*
	Identify the marked area	It is palatine rugae
	Which type of landmark is it?	It is secondary supporting area
	Write about its position	Located in anterior part of palate
	Write its importance	The folds of rugae helps in speech articulation and also prevents anterior displacement of maxillary denture
	Write characteristic of mucosa in this area	It is mucosal folds. Mucosa is firmly attached to bone and it is keratinized

MARKS: 05	One mark per answer	Total time allotted for station: 05 Minutes
Specimen	*Questions*	*Answers*
	Identify the marked area	It is maxillary tuberosity
	Which type of landmark is it?	It is secondary supporting area
	Write about its position	Located bilaterally posterior to last molar tooth
	Write about mucosa in this area	Mucosa is firmly attached to bone and it is keratinized
	Write characteristic of this area	It shows no or very less bone resorption

MARKS: 05	One mark per answer	Total time allotted for station: 05 Minutes
Specimen	*Questions*	*Answers*
	Identify the marked area	It is torus palatinus
	Which type of landmark is it?	It is relieving structure
	Its position with special characteristic	It is located on midline of the palate and it is bony enlargement
	Any special care required before fabrication of denture	If it is large in size, surgical removal is required and for smaller size relief should be provided
	What challenge is encountered due to this structure?	It causes discomfort to the denture wearer. Excess relief in this area may compromise the support of denture

MARKS: 05	One mark per answer	Total time allotted for station: 05 Minutes
Specimen	*Questions*	*Answers*
	Identify the marked area	It is labial frenum
	Which type of landmark is it?	It is limiting structure
	Write about the position of the structure.	It is located labially on the midline between two maxillary central incisors
	Which muscles fibers it contains?	It contains no muscle fiber. It is only a mucosal fold
	What care will you take during denture insertion?	Maxillary denture should provide relief in the form of "V" shaped notch for housing the labial frenum

MARKS: 05	One mark per answer	Time allotted for station: 05 Minutes
Specimen	*Questions*	*Answers*
	Identify the marked area	It is buccal frenum
	Which type of landmark is it?	It is limiting structure
	Its position and number	Located in premolar area. May be one or two in number
	Which muscles fibers it contains?	It contains Orbicularis Oris, Levator Anguli Oris and Buccinator (OO, LAO, B) muscles fibers.
	What special care will you take during denture fabrication?	As it is active frenum, enough relief is provided otherwise it may compromise denture retention due to movement during speech and mastication.

MARKS: 05	One mark per answer	Time allotted for station: 05 Minutes
Specimen	*Questions*	*Answers*
	Identify the marked area	It is fovea palatine
	Which type of landmark is it?	It is limiting structure
	Write its position with reference to posterior part of palate	It is located on midline, 2–3 mm anterior to anterior vibrating line
	How is it formed?	It is formed by coalescence of ducts of several minor salivary glands
	What special care will you take during denture fabrication?	It is not covered by posterior border of maxillary denture in patient with ropy and thick saliva to prevent dislodgement.

MARKS: 05	One mark per answer	Time allotted for station: 05 Minutes	
Specimen	*Questions*	*Answers*	
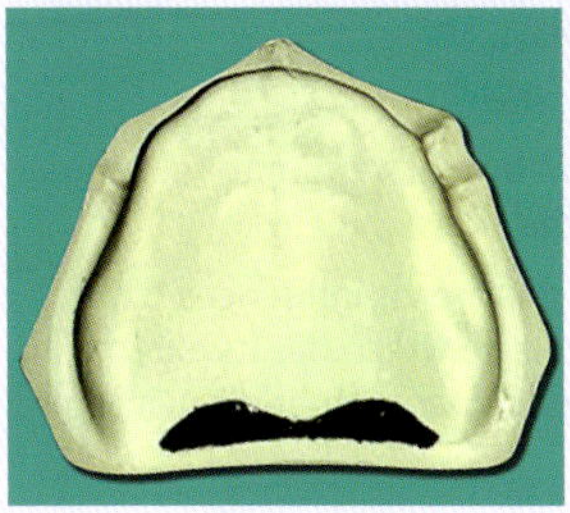	Identify the marked area	It is posterior palatal seal area	
	Which type of landmark is it?	It is limiting structure	
	Write boundaries of this area.	**Anteriorly**	By anterior vibrating line
		Posteriorly	By posterior vibrating line
		Medially	From one tuberosity to the other
		Laterally	Extends through the pterygomaxillary notch continuing for 3–4 mm anterolateral approximating the mucogingival junction.
	How will you locate anterior boundary of this area?	By performing the **VALSALVA MENUEVRE**	
	What special care will you take during denture fabrication?	Denture should place pressure within physiologic limits and compress this area to complete and maintain the peripheral seal. Thus, helps in achieving retention in maxillary denture	

MARKS: 05	One mark per answer	Time allotted for station: 05 Minutes
Specimen	*Questions*	*Answers*
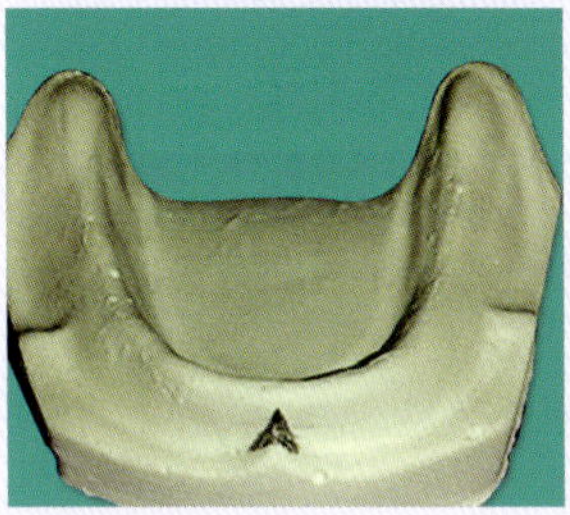	Identify the marked area	Labial frenum
	Which type of landmark is it?	Relieving structure
	What muscle is attached with it?	Orbicularis oris is associated with mandibular labial frenum
	What care is taken during making mandibular impression?	Relief should be given to labial frenum during making impression
	What care is taken during denture insertion?	If relief is not provided in denture, it may cause pain and dislodgement of denture

MARKS: 05	One mark per answer	Time allotted for station: 05 Minutes
Specimen	*Questions*	*Answers*
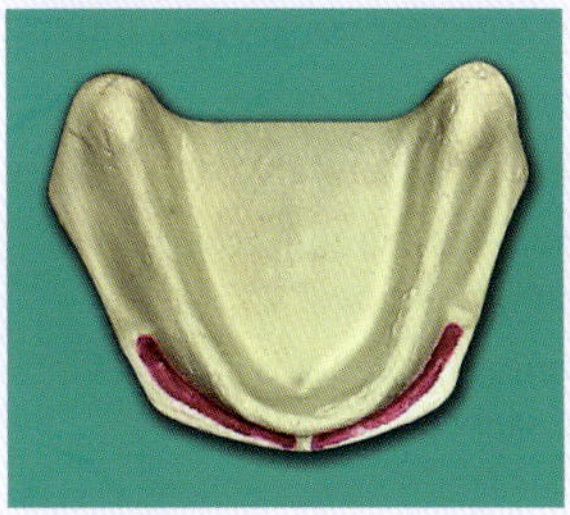	Identify the marked area	Labial vestibule
	Which type of landmark is it?	Limiting structure
	Write about extension/ boundary	It extends bilaterally from labial frenum to buccal frenum.
	What muscles are attached with it?	Fibers of orbicularis oris, incisivus and mentalis are active in this are near the crest of the ridge.
	What is the influence on mandibular denture?	This area limits the extension and width of the labial flange of mandibular denture.

MARKS: 05	One mark per answer	Time allotted for station: 05 Minutes
Specimen	*Questions*	*Answers*
	Identify the marked area	Buccal frenum
	Which type of landmark is it?	Limiting structure
	Write about extension/ boundary	It extends from buccal frenum to retromolar pad on both the sides.
	What influences the extent of the area?	The extent of this area is influences by buccinators muscle which has its extension from modiolus to pterygomandibular raphe posteriorly.
	What is the influence on mandibular denture?	It limits the extension of buccal flange of the mandibular denture

MARKS: 05	One mark per answer	Total time allotted for station: 05 Minutes
Specimen	*Questions*	*Answers*
	Identify the marked area	Lingual frenum
	Which type of landmark is it?	Relieving structure
	Write about its position	Located on the midline, lingually to the residual ridge, opposite to labial frenum
	Write about associated structures with it.	It covers the genioglossus muscle which is attached to superior genial tubercle.
	What is the influence on mandibular denture?	Relief should be provided in mandibular denture for lingual frenum to avoid displacement on elevation of tongue.

MARKS: 05	One mark per answer	Total time allotted for station: 05 Minutes	
Specimen	*Questions*	*Answers*	
	Identify the marked area	Retromolar pad	
	Which type of landmark is it?	Primary stress bearing area	
	Content of this area	Retromolar pad contains following;	
		Tissue	Loose alveolar tissue Glandular tissue
		Muscle	Fiber of buccinator muscle Fiber of superior constrictor muscle
		Raphe	Pterygomandibular raphe
		Tendon	Terminal part of tendon of temporalis
	Write about denture coverage of the area.	Distal part of mandibular denture covers the two-third of the retromolar pad	
	Which property of a complete denture does this area help to achieve?	Covering the retromolar pad helps in achieving stability of mandibular complete denture.	

MARKS: 05	One mark per answer	Total time allotted for station: 05 Minutes	
Specimen	*Questions*	*Answers*	
	Identify the marked area	Alveololingual sulcus	
	Which type of landmark is it?	Limiting structure	
	Write about the location of it.	It is space between tongue and residual alveolar ridge	
	Write its extension.	It extends from lingual frenum to retromylohyoid curtain posteriorly (Bilateraly)	
	Which muscle is attached in this area?	Mylohyoid is the main muscle attached in this area	
	Which bony structure divides this area into three parts?	Mylohyoid ridge divides the area into three parts	
	Different parts of this area	Three parts marked by the position of mylohyoid ridge are: 1. Premylohyoid fossa 2. Mylohyoid fossa 3. Retromylohyoid fossa	
	Write boundaries of different parts of this area.	***Area/part (Other name)***	***Boundary***
		Premylohyoid fossa (anterior region)	This part extends from lingual frenum to premylohyoid fossa
		Mylohyoid fossa (middle region)	From premylohyoid fossa to the distal end of the mylohyoid ridge.
		Retromylohyoid fossa (posterior part)	From distal end of the mylohyoid ridge till retromylohyoid curtain posteriorly.

MARKS: 05	One mark per answer	Time allotted for station: 05 Minutes	
Specimen	*Questions*	*Answers*	
	Identify the marked area	Buccal shelf area	
	Which type of landmark is it?	Primary stress bearing area	
	Mention its position/ location/boundary	**Anterior**	Buccal Frenum
		Posterior	Anterior aspect of retromolar pad
		Medially	Crest of residual alveolar ridge
		Laterally	External oblique ridge
	Quality of bone in this area	Dense and smooth cortical bone	
	Relative position with occlusal forces	Buccal shelf area lies at right angle to the vertical occlusal forces (which makes it suitable as primary stress bearing area)	

MARKS: 05	One mark per answer	Time allotted for station: 05 Minutes
Specimen	*Questions*	*Answers*
	Identify the marked structure	Torus mandibularis
	Which type of landmark is it?	It is a relief area
	Write about its position	It is located lingually near 1st and 2nd premolar area bilaterally
	What problem will it cause for denture patient?	If denture is fabricated without relief it may cause pain discomfort and dislodgement of denture
	Management for it during denture fabrication.	If smaller in size relief can be provided in denture and if it bigger is size it should be surgically removed before denture fabrication

MARKS: 05	One mark per answer	Time allotted for station: 05 Minutes
Specimen	*Questions*	*Answers*
	Identify the marked area	Mental foramen
	Which type of landmark is it?	Relieving structure (as and when required)
	Significance of it	In resorbed ridge case, mental foramen lie closer to crest of the ridge in such cases care should be taken while fabrication of denture
	Content of it	Mental nerve and vessels
	What special care will you take during denture fabrication?	The area in denture should be relieved to avoid pressure on this structure otherwise denture pressure on nerve leaving this foramen may cause pain and numbness of lower lip

MARKS: 05	One mark per answer	Time allotted for station: 05 Minutes
Specimen	*Questions*	*Answers*
	Identify the specimen	Beading of the Impression
	Which material is used for the procedure	Beading wax is used for the beading of the impression
	Objective of the procedure	It helps in forming land area on cast
	Write the location for the application for the wax	The beading wax should be placed 3 mm away from the impression border.
	Write about availability of wax required for this procedure.	Beading wax is available in round, square and rectangle shape in rope form

MARKS: 05	One mark per answer	Time allotted for station: 05 Minutes
Specimen	*Questions*	*Answers*
	Identify the specimen	It is boxed maxillary impression.
	Which material is used for the procedure	Boxing wax is used for the boxing of the impression
	Objective of the procedure	It helps in forming base of the cast
	Advantage of this procedure	Boxing of the impression helps controlling the height (thickness) of the base of the cast and give cast which requires minimum or no adjustment.
	When do you use this technique?	This technique is used for cast pouring of final impression.

MARKS: 05	One mark per answer	Time allotted for station: 05 Minutes
Specimen	*Questions*	*Answers*
	Identify the specimen	It is maxillary complete edentulous cast
	Write the parts of the same	1. Anatomical part of the cast 2. Base of the cast 3. Land area of the cast
	Write three uses of the specimen	1. Diagnosis 2. Fabrication of prosthesis on it 3. Fabrication of record base 4. Fabrication of custom tray
	Which materials can be used for fabrication of the same	1. Dental plaster 2. Dental stone

MARKS: 05	One mark per answer	Time allotted for station: 05 Minutes
Specimen	*Questions*	*Answers*
	Identify the specimen	It is complete edentulous maxillary cast
	Write the ideal thickness of the base	It should be 15 mm
	Write different methods of pouring/making it	1. Beading boxing method 2. Inversion pouring methods
	Mention the dimension of land area	Land are should be have 2–3 mm height and 3 mm width
	What should be angle of land area	Land area is sloped at 45° angle

MARKS: 05	One mark per answer	Time allotted for station: 05 Minutes	
Specimen	*Questions*	*Answers*	
	Identify the specimen	Maxillary edentulous cast	
	Name different parts of it.	1. Anatomical portion	
		2. Art portion	Base of the cast
			Land area of the cast
	Mention dimension of different parts of the cast	1. Anatomical part	As per intraoral dimension
		2. Base of the cast	15 mm thickness
		3. Land area	2–3 mm in height and width
			Slopped at 45°
	The specimen is: 1. Positive replica of....... 2. Negative replica of...........	1. Positive replica of edentulous arch 2. Negative replica of impression of arch	

MARKS: 05	One mark per answer	Time allotted for station: 05 Minutes
Specimen	*Questions*	*Answers*
	Identify the specimen	It is indexing (on the cast)
	Mention different types of it	**Indexing:** a. Notch Indexing b. Groove indexing
	Ideal requirement of it	❑ It should not weaken the cast ❑ It should be free of undercut ❑ Easy to perform ❑ Should permit easy removal and remounting
	Objective/use of it	Indexing is done on master cast. Indexing helps in remounting the casts in the same position on articulator after processing to do selective grinding.

MARKS: 05	One mark per answer	Time allotted for station: 05 Minutes	
Specimen	*Questions*	*Answers*	
	Identify the specimen	Maxillary occlusal rim	
	Position of it on edentulous alveolar ridge	In anterior region	Labial to the ridge
		In premolar region	On the ridge
		In posterior region	Buccal to the ridge
	Height at anterior region	20–22 mm from deepest part of the sulcus	
	Height at posterior region	16–18 mm from deepest part of buccal sulcus at molar area	
	Material used for fabrication	Modeling wax	
	Width in anterior region	5–6 mm	
	Width in posterior region	8–10 mm	
	Angulations in anterior region	Angulated labially to support the upper lip	

MARKS: 05	One mark per answer	Time allotted for station: 05 Minutes	
Specimen	*Questions*	*Answers*	
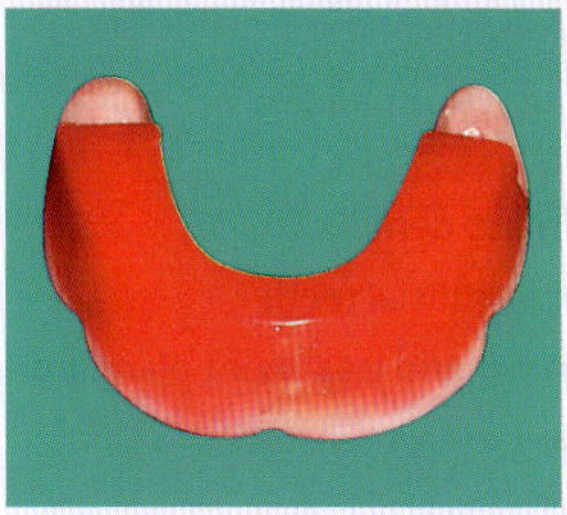	Identify the specimen	Mandibular occlusal rim	
	Position of it on edentulous alveolar ridge	In anterior region	Labial to the ridge
		In premolar region	On the ridge
		In posterior region	Lingual to the ridge
	Height at anterior region	16–18 mm from deepest part of sulcus	
	Height at posterior region	At the level of 2/3 of retromolar pad	
	Material used for fabrication	Modeling wax	
	Width in anterior region	3–5 mm	
	Width in posterior region	8–10 mm	
	Angulations in anterior region	Straight, no angulations given	

MARKS: 05	One mark per answer	Time allotted for station: 05 Minutes
Specimen	*Questions*	*Answers*
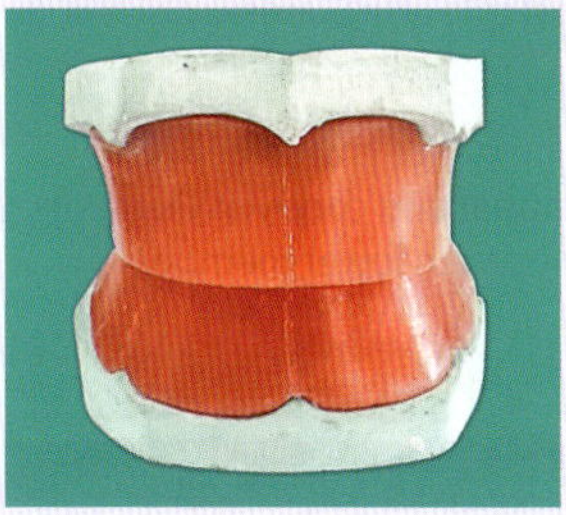	Identify the specimen	Maxillary and mandibular occlusal rims
	Material used for fabrication	Modeling wax
	Write uses of the specimen (minimum three uses)	To establish occlusal plane
		To record maxillomandibular relation
		To record midline, canine line high and low lip line for teeth arrangement
		Used for artificial teeth arrangement

MARKS: 05	One mark per Answer	Time allotted for station: 05 Minutes
Specimen	*Questions*	*Answers*
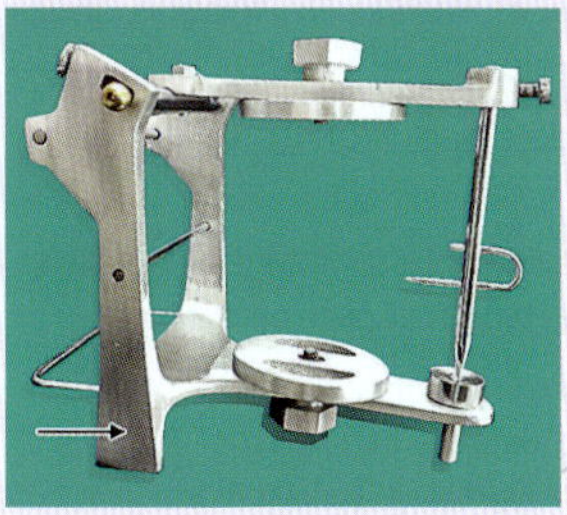	Identify the specimen	Articulator
	Type of instrument/ classification	Mean value articulator
	Based on which theory of articulator	Theory of equilateral triangle
	Who proposed the theory on which this instrument is designed?	WGA Bonwill
	How much is intercondylar distance?	4 inch
	How much is condylar guidance?	33 degrees
	How much is incisal guidance?	15 degrees

MARKS: 05	One mark per answer	Time allotted for station: 05 Minutes
Specimen	*Questions*	*Answers*
	Identify the specimen	Mean value articulator
	Mention any three uses	To simulate TMJ/mandibular movements
		For mounting dental casts
		To arrange artificial teeth
		For diagnosis and treatment planning
	Classify as per arcon concept	Nonarcon type articulator
	Classify as per adjustability	Nonadjustable articulator

MARKS: 05	One mark per answer	Time allotted for station: 05 Minutes
Specimen	*Questions*	*Answers*
	Identify the specimen	Hanau articulator
	Classify as per arcon concept	Arcon type articulator
	Classify as per adjustability	Semi adjustable articulator
	Which face-bow is used with it	Spring bow is used with it
	Write arrangement of condylar guidance and condylar element with reference to member of articulator	Condylar guidance is attached with upper member and condylar elements are attached with lower member

MARKS: 05	One mark per answer	Time allotted for station: 05 Minutes
Specimen	*Questions*	*Answers*
	Identify the specimen	Articulator
	Write any four advantages of it	Reduce chair time with patient
		Disturbances from saliva, tongue, cheek can be avoided
		Used to view occlusion from lingual side
		More comfortable to work on mounted casts on articulator compared to patient
	Write classification based on adjustability	a. Nonadjustable articulator b. Semi-adjustable articulator c. Fully-adjustable articulator

MARKS: 05	One mark per answer	Time allotted for station: 05 Minutes
Specimen	*Questions*	*Answers*
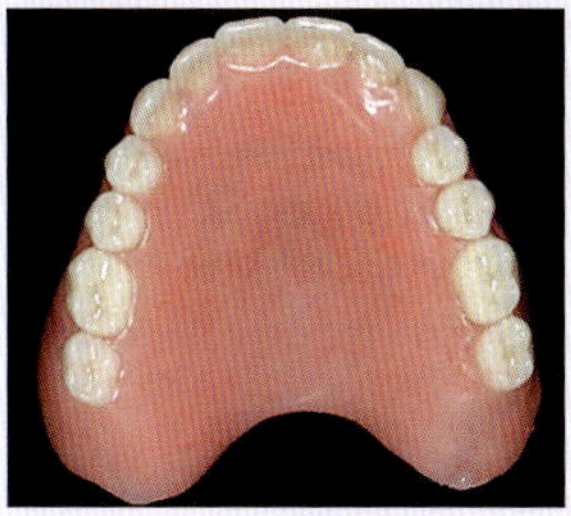	Identify the specimen	Maxillary complete denture
	Write different parts of it	Denture base
		Artificial teeth
		Denture flanges
	Write different surfaces of the specimen.	Occlusal surface
		Tissue surface
		Polished surface
	From which material it is fabricated?	Heat cured poly methylmethacrylate

MARKS: 05	One mark per answer	Time allotted for station: 05 Minutes
Specimen	*Questions*	*Answers*
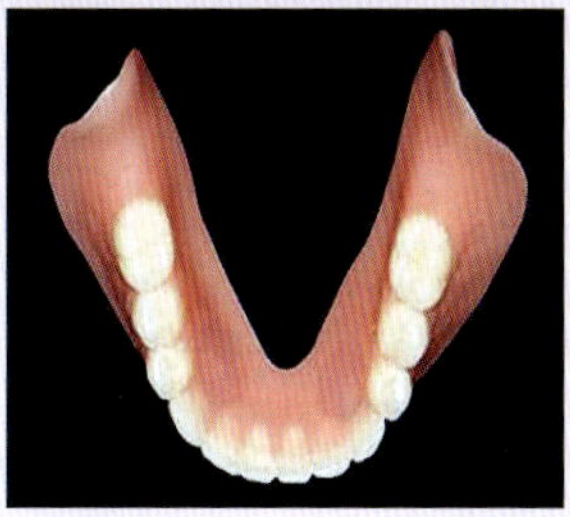	Identify the marked area	Mandibular complete denture
	Mention the types of flanges	Labial flange
		Buccal flange
		Lingual flange
	Write different surfaces of the specimen.	Occlusal surface
		Tissue surface
		Polished surface
	From which material it is fabricated?	Heat cured polymethyl methacrylate
	From which material it is fabricated?	Heat cured poly polymethyl methacrylate

MARKS: 05	One mark per answer	Time allotted for station: 05 Minutes
Specimen	*Questions*	*Answers*
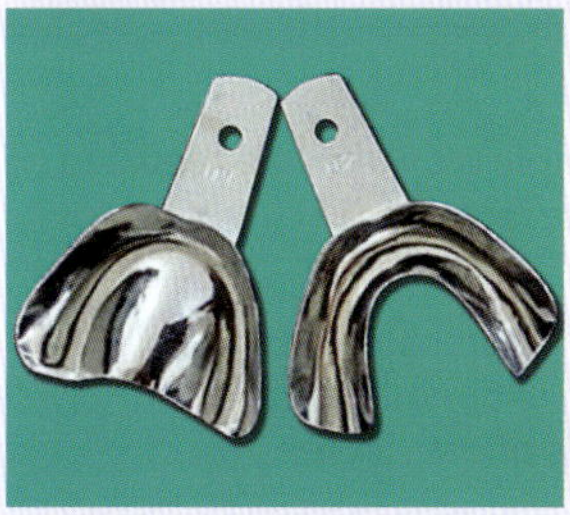	Identify the specimen	Maxillary and mandibular edentulous stock trays
	Which impression material is recommended to be used with it?	Impression compound
	Purpose/Use of the specimen	For making primary impression of edentulous arch
	From which material it is fabricated?	Stainless steel
	Write three advantages of it	It is rigid.
		It is dimensionally stable
		It can be used several times

MARKS: 05	One mark per answer	Time allotted for station: 05 Minutes
Specimen	*Questions*	*Answers*
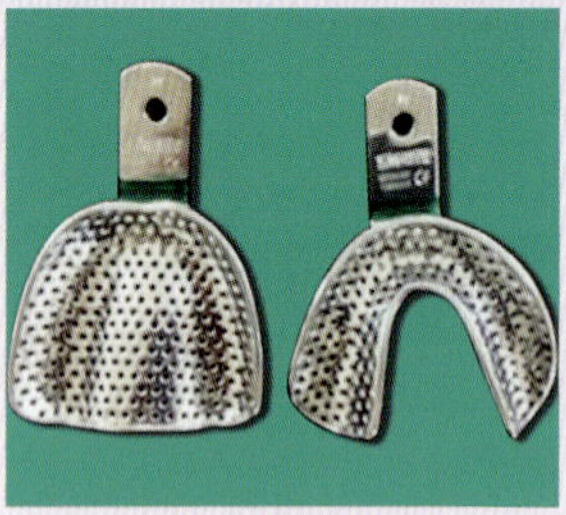	Identify the specimen	Maxillary and mandibular edentulous perforated stock trays
	Which impression material is recommended to be used with it?	Alginate impression material/elastomeric impression materials (polyether, polysulfide, A-silicone, C-silicone)
	Purpose/Use of the specimen	For making Impression of dentulous arch
	From which material it is fabricated?	Stainless steel
	What is objective/use/advantage of perforations	They act as escape holes for excess material and also provides mechanical retention to impression material with the impression tray

MARKS: 05	One mark per answer	Time allotted for station: 05 Minutes	
Specimen	*Questions*	*Answers*	
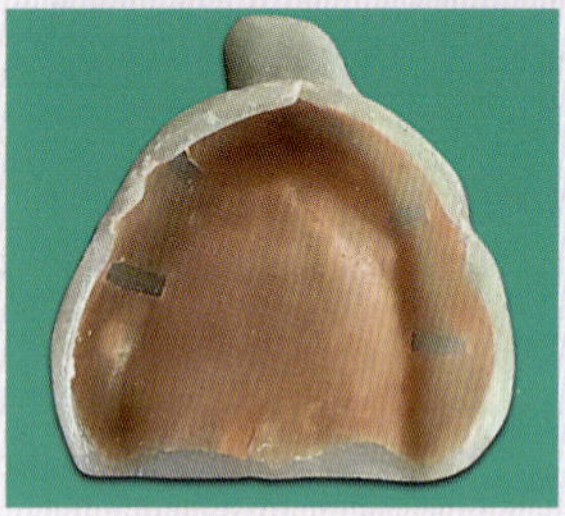	Identify the specimen	Maxillary custom tray	
	Mention different parts of the specimen.	Different parts are....	
		1. Tray Body 2. Tray handle	3. Spacer 4. Tissue stops
	Purpose/Use of the specimen	Making final impression of edentulous arch	
	Write its border relation with sulcus depth.	The border of the custom tray is 2 mm short of the sulcus depth.	
	Write any three materials used for fabrication of it.	1. Tray compound 2. Tray acrylic 3. Vacuum formed sheet	3. Shellac base plate 4. Light cured acrylic 5. Heat cured acrylic

MARKS: 05	One mark per answer	Time allotted for station: 05 Minutes
Specimen	*Questions*	*Answers*
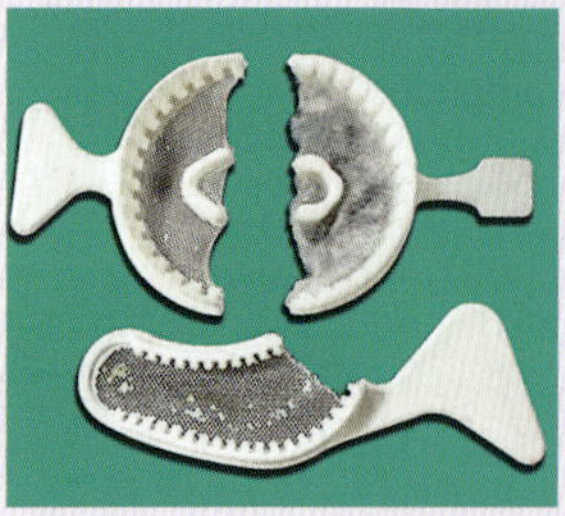	Identify the specimen	It is triple tray
	Write use of the shown specimen	For making impression of single prepared tooth with bite record
	Advantages of it	It records...... 1. Impression of prepared tooth 2. Impression of opposite tooth 3. Bite records of both arches
	From which material it is fabricated?	The frame is made up of plastic or metal and it is covered with plastic or cloth mesh/net
	Which material is recommended to be used with this tray?	Any elastic material can be used with triple tray. Most commonly elastomeric impression material is used with it (addition silicone/condensation silicone)

MARKS: 05	One mark per answer	Time allotted for station: 05 Minutes
Specimen	*Questions*	*Answers*
	Identify the specimen	Maxillary edentulous primary impression
	Write the material and device used for making it	Material: Impression compound Device: Nonperforated edentulous maxillary stock tray
	Objectives of it	1. Retention 2. Stability 3. Support 4. Preservation of residual alveolar ridge 5. Aesthetic
	Which theory of impression making is applied here	Mucocompressive
	Clinical condition where this material cannot be used for making primary impression.	If undercuts (specifically bilateral) are present in edentulous foundation impression can not be made with impression compound as it is rigid impression material, (as it cannot come from undercut after set as it is rigid)
	How will you disinfect this specimen?	Immersion in sodium hypochloride

MARKS: 05	One mark per answer	Time allotted for station: 05 Minutes
Specimen	*Questions*	*Answers*
	Identify the specimen	Maxillary edentulous primary impression
	Write the material and device used for making it	**Material:** Reversible hydrocolloid/alginate **Device:** Perforated edentulous maxillary stock tray
	Objectives of it	1. Retention 2. Stability 3. Support 4. Preservation of residual alveolar ridge 5. Aesthetic
	Which theory of impression making is applied here	Mucocompressive
	Clinical condition where this material is recommended to be used for making primary impression	If undercuts (specifically bilateral) are present in edentulous foundation impression is made with elastic impression material which can easily come out after setting. So, in such condition primary impression is made with alginate impression material

MARKS: 05	One mark per answer	Time allotted for station: 05 Minutes
Specimen	*Questions*	*Answers*
	Identify the specimen	Maxillary edentulous final impression
	Write the material and device used for making it	**Material:** ZOE impression paste **Device:** Custom tray/special tray
	Which theory of impression making is applied here	Selective pressure technique
	Clinical condition where this material is not recommended to be used for making primary impression.	1. Edentulous foundation with undercuts 2. Patient allergic to eugenol 3. Burning sensation 4. Smokers palate
	Alternative/modification to this impression material	Eugenol free zinc oxide impression paste (Eugenol is replaced with EBA)

MARKS: 05	One mark per answer	Time allotted for station: 05 Minutes
Specimen	*Questions*	*Answers*
	Identify the specimen	Maxillary edentulous final impression
	Write the material and device used for making it	**Material** Elastomeric impression material (light body consistency) **Device** Custom tray/special tray
	Which theory of impression making is applied here	Selective pressure technique
	Clinical condition where this material is recommended to be used for making primary impression.	1. Edentulous foundation with undercuts 2. Patient allergic to eugenol
	Name any other material of this type/class	Polyether, polysulfide, addition silicone, condensation silicone

MARKS: 05	One mark per answer	Time allotted for station: 05 Minutes
Specimen	*Questions*	*Answers*
	Identify the specimen	It is impression compound impression material
	Use of the specimen	It is used for making primary impression of complete edentulous arch
	Mention temperature of water required for its manipulation.	Hot water of temperature range of 50–55° is used for its manipulation
	Mention the tray used with this material	Complete edentulous non perforated trays are used with this material
	What kind of material it is in term of rigidity.	It is rigid impression material

MARKS: 05	One mark per answer	Time allotted for station: 05 Minutes
Specimen	*Questions*	*Answers*
Camper's line Ala-tragus line	Identify the specimen	It is Ala-Tragus line/plane
	What is the use of it?	It is used to establish occlusal plane during jaw relation
	Write the extension of the same	It extends from inferior border of the ala of the nose to superior border of the tragus of the ear
	Write other name(s) for the specimen	1. Campers line 2. Bromell's plane
	How to check its parallelism with occlusal plane?	When fox plane is attached on maxillary occlusal rim, the ala-tragus line should be parallel to fox plane

MARKS: 05	One mark per answer	Time allotted for station: 05 Minutes
Specimen	*Questions*	*Answers*
	Identify the specimen	It is curve of spee
	Who proposed/described this?	It was proposed/described by Ferdinand Graf Spee in 1890
	Describe the same?	"Anatomical curve established by the occlusal alignment of the teeth, as projected onto mesial plane, beginning with the cusp tip of mandibular canine and following the buccal cusp tips of premolars and molar teeth, continuing through the anterior border of the mandibular ramus, ending with the anterior most portion of the mandibular condyle."
	How is it formed?	It is imaginary curve. It is formed due to occlusal alignment of the teeth
	Write the importance of it.	It is used to achieve balanced occlusion in complete denture by providing required occlusal alignment

MARKS: 05	One mark per answer	Time allotted for station: 05 Minutes
Specimen	***Questions***	***Answers***
	Identify the specimen	It is curve of wilson
	Who proposed/described this?	It was proposed/described by George. H. Wilson in 1855
	Describe the same?	"It is mediolateral curve that contacts the buccal and lingual cusp tips on each side of the arch. It results from lingual inclination of mandibular molar, making the lingual cusp lower than the buccal cusps. (Accordingly, the buccal cusps of maxillary molar are placed higher than the palatal cusps resulting in buccal inclination of maxillary molar teeth)
	What is the shape of maxillary and mandibular curve ?	It is concave for maxillary arch and convex for mandibular arch
	Write the importance of it.	Curve of Wilson permits lateral mandibular excursions free from posterior interferences.

MARKS: 05	One mark per answer	Time allotted for station: 05 Minutes
Specimen	***Questions***	***Answers***
	Identify the specimen	It is curve of monson
	Who proposed/described this?	This curve is proposed by monson
	Describe the same?	Curve of occlusion in which each cusp and incisal edge touches or conforms to a segment of a sphere of 8 inch in diameter with its center in the region of glabella.
	This is based on which theory?	This curve is based on spherical theory of occlusion
	Write the importance of it.	It is used to achieve harmonious occlusal contact and movements. It is important to achieve lateral balance in occlusion.

MARKS: 05	One mark per answer	Time allotted for station: 05 Minutes
Specimen	***Questions***	***Answers***
	Identify the specimen	Artificial teeth set for denture
	Classify according to material used for fabrication	1. Acrylic teeth 2. Porcelain teeth 3. Composite teeth 4. Acrylic teeth with metal occlusion
	Classify according to occlusal anatomy	1. Anatomical teeth 2. Semi-anatomical teeth 3. Nonanatomical teeth
	Use of the specimen	Used in complete denture and removable partial denture
	Which is the most commonly used prosthetic teeth	Acrylic teeth are most commonly used prosthetic teeth

MARKS: 05	One mark per answer	Time allotted for station: 05 Minutes
Specimen	*Questions*	*Answers*
	Identify the specimen	Artificial prosthetic teeth-maxillary anterior teeth
	Indication for use	1. When opposite teeth are acrylic 2. When less interarch space is available 3. Opposite to natural teeth
	Contraindication for use	Opposite to porcelain teeth
	Write two advantages of it	1. Chemically bond with denture material 2. Can be trimmed very thin to fit in available space 3. Do not abrade opposing natural teeth
	Write two disadvantages of it	1. Wear with time 2. Stain and discoloration

MARKS: 05	One mark per answer	Time allotted for station: 05 Minutes
Specimen	*Questions*	*Answers*
	Identify the specimen	Porcelain teeth
	Indication for use	1. When opposing teeth is porcelain 2. When interarch space is sufficient 3. Well formed ridges 4. Requirement for high aesthetic
	Contraindication for use	1. Opposite to acrylic teeth 2. Less interarch space
	Write two advantages of it	1. More wear resistance 2. Good aesthetic 3. Does not stain or discolor easily
	Write two disadvantages of it	1. No chemical bond with acrylic material 2. If used opposite to natural teeth, they cause abrasion of natural teeth 3. Clicking noise

MARKS: 05	One mark per answer	Time allotted for station: 05 Minutes
Specimen	*Questions*	*Answers*
	Identify the specimen	Anatomical Prosthetic (Artificial) teeth -Molar
	How much is the cuspal angulation?	33° or more
	Mention its Indication for use	1. Well formed ridges 2. For balanced occlusion 3. Patient with good neuromuscular control
	Write two advantages of it	1. These teeth have better chewing efficiency 2. They have more natural appearance 3. They penetrate food more easily
	Write two disadvantages of it	1. More time consuming in arranging in balanced occlusion 2. Placement restricted by cusp and fossa relation

MARKS: 05	One mark per Answer	Time allotted for station: 05 Minutes
Specimen	*Questions*	*Answers*
	Identify the specimen	Semi-anatomical prosthetic (artificial) teeth
	How much is the cuspal angulation?	20 degree
	Mention its Indication for use	1. Fair or well formed ridges 2. Mild jaw discrepancy 3. To achieve balanced occlusion
	Write two advantages of it	1. Easy achievement of balanced occlusion 2. Good aesthetic 3. Shallow cuspal angulation generates less horizontal forces
	Write two disadvantages of it	1. Less aesthetic compared to anatomical teeth 2. Less aesthetic compared to anatomical teeth

MARKS: 05	One mark per answer	Time allotted for station: 05 Minutes
Specimen	*Questions*	*Answers*
	Identify the specimen	Nonanatomica prosthetic (artificial) teeth
	How much is the cuspal angulation?	Zero degree
	Mention its Indication for use	1. Patient with poor ridges 2. Patient with poor neuromuscular control 3. Patient with jaw discrepancy
	Write two advantages of it	1. Easy arrangement of teeth 2. Less force transferred to ridge 3. Freedom of occlusal movement
	Write two disadvantages of it	1. Less chewing efficiency 2. Least aesthetic 3. Difficult to achieve balance occlusion

MARKS: 05	One mark per answer	Time allotted for station: 05 Minutes
Specimen	*Questions*	*Answers*
	Identify the specimen	Leon–Williams theory/classification of face form
	Write different facial form shown in specimen picture	1. Square facial form 2. Tapering facial form 3. Ovoid facial form
	Write different facial landmarks used to get facial form	1. The forehead 2. Zygomatic arch 3. Angle of mandible
	Write its interpretation	It suggests that "Shape of maxillary anterior teeth should be inverse of the shape of face"
	Write use of the same	It can be used for anterior teeth selection

MARKS: 05	One mark per answer	Time allotted for station: 05 Minutes
Specimen	*Questions*	*Answers*
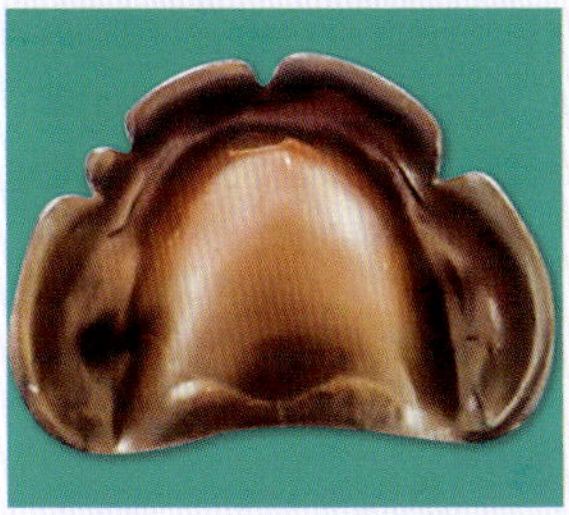	Identify the specimen	Maxillary shellac record base
	What is the use of it?	❑ Helps in recording jaw relation ❑ Allow setting of artificial teeth for trial ❑ Gives idea about extension of denture
	From which material it is made?	It is fabricated from shellac
	Mention two advantages of it	❑ Easy to fabricate ❑ Uniform thickness ❑ Easy to correct and low cost
	Mention two disadvantages of it	❑ Low strength ❑ Break at low force ❑ Distortion due to temperature change

MARKS: 05	One mark per answer	Time allotted for station: 05 Minutes
Specimen	*Questions*	*Answers*
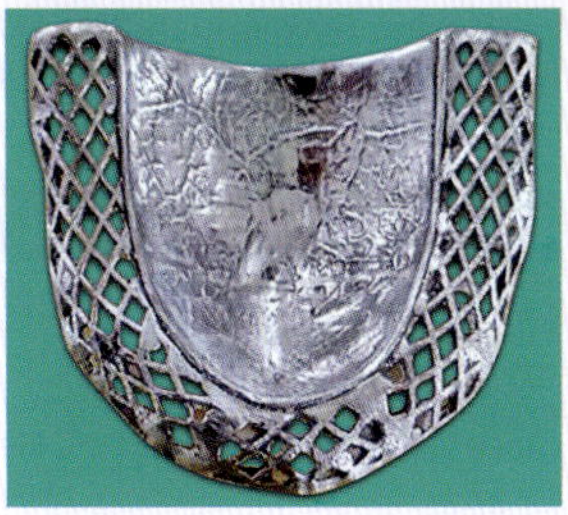	Identify the specimen	Metallic record base for maxillary arch
	What is the use of it?	❑ Helps in recording jaw relation ❑ Allow setting of artificial teeth for trial ❑ Gives idea about extension of denture
	From which material it is made?	It is fabricated from Co-Cr or Ni-Cr or Gold alloy
	Mention two advantages of it	❑ Dimensionally most stable ❑ Good conductor of heat ❑ For patient who encounters frequent fracture of denture
	Mention two disadvantages of it	❑ Fabrication is time consuming ❑ Relining is difficult

MARKS: 05	One mark per answer	Time allotted for station: 05 Minutes
Specimen	*Questions*	*Answers*
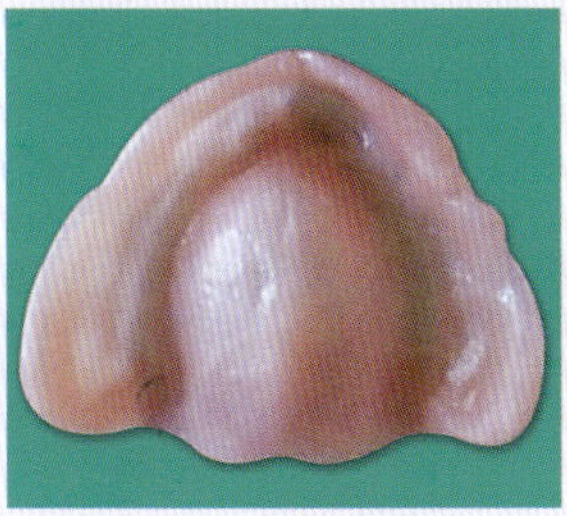	Identify the specimen	Record base
	Classify according to use	a. Temporary record base b. Permanent record base
	Classify based on material	a. Metallic record base b. Nonmetallic record base
	Mention three ideal requirements	1. Should be well adapted 2. Should be accurately formed 3. Rigid and dimensionally stable 4. Free of voids and surface irregularity 5. Should have rounded and smooth borders
	What is the use of it?	1. Helps in recording jaw relation 2. Allow setting of artificial teeth for trial 3. Gives idea about extension of denture

MARKS: 05	One mark per answer	Time allotted for station: 05 Minutes	
Specimen	***Questions***	***Answers***	
	Identify the specimen	Record base	
	Classify it	**Metallic record base**	**Nonmetallic record base**
		1. Co-Cr alloy 2. Ni-Cr alloy 3. Gold alloy	1. Self-cured acrylic resin 2. Heat cured acrylic resin 3. Shellac record base 4. Base plate wax 5. Vinyl and polystyrene
	Mention ideal requirements	1. Should be well adapted 2. Should be accurately formed 3. Rigid and dimensionally stable 4. Free of voids and surface irregularity 5. Should have rounded and smooth borders	
	What is the use of it?	1. Helps in recording jaw relation 2. Allow setting of artificial teeth for trial 3. Gives idea about extension of denture	
	Write definition of it	A material of device is representating the base of a denture. It is used for making maxillomandibular relation records and arranging teeth	

MARKS: 05	One mark per answer	Time allotted for station: 05 Minutes
Specimen	***Questions***	***Answers***
	Identify the specimen	Maxillary and mandibular spacer wax
	What is the use of it?	To make spacer for maxillary and mandibular arch
	Purpose/Use of the specimen	It provides space for impression material and also selectively relieve the relieving area
	From which material it is made?	It is made up of wax
	What is the thickness of it?	0.9–1.2 mm thickness

MARKS: 05	One mark per answer	Time allotted for station: 05 Minutes
Specimen	*Questions*	*Answers*
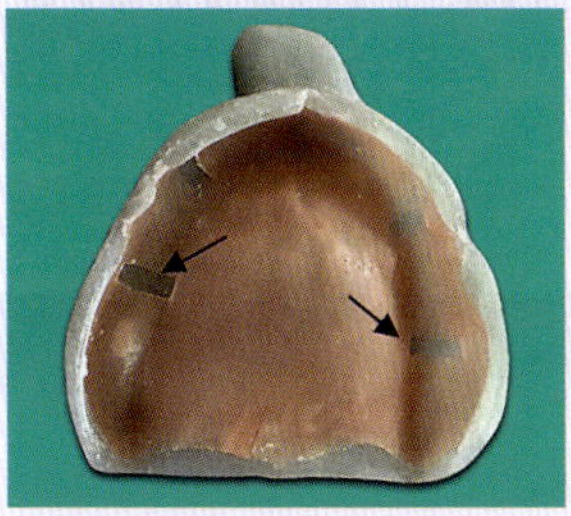	Identify the specimen	It is tissue stop(s)
	What is the use of it?	It helps in stabilizing and orienting the custom tray.
	Provide ideal location for it?	Two tissue stops on canine-premolar region on either side of the ridge and two tissue stops on molar region on either side of the ridge
	Write dimension of it.	Rectangular in shape. It should cover the edentulous ridge in buccolingual direction. **Dimension:** ❑ Mesiodistal: 2 mm ❑ Buccolingual: 4 mm
	What is the significance of this in final impression?	If all the tissue stops are exposed, that means all were in contact with denture foundation and equal pressure was applied while making final impression. If any one of them is not exposed that means less pressure was applied in that area.

CHAPTER 55 Viva Voce Questions-Answers

Question	*Answer*
What is anatomical landmark?	It is a recognizable anatomical structure used as a point of reference.
Classify anatomical landmarks.	They are classified as under: 1. Supporting structure (primary supporting and secondary supporting) 2. Limiting structure (also known as valve forming area) 3. Relief areas.
Mention primary stress bearing area of maxillary arch.	Primary stress bearing/supporting areas of maxillary arch are as follow: 1. Hard palate (on either side of palatal raphe) 2. Maxillary tuberosity.
List secondary supporting areas of maxillary arch.	Secondary stress bearing/supporting structures of maxillary arch are: 1. Palatine Rugae 2. Maxillary alveolar ridge.
Name valve forming structures (limiting areas) of maxillary arch.	The limiting structures are mentioned below: 1. Labial Frenum 2. Labial Vestibule 3. Buccal Frenum 4. Buccal Vestibule 5. Hamular Notch 6. Posterior palatal seal area 7. Coronomaxillary pouch (Area).
List out relief areas of maxillary arch.	Following is the list of relief areas of maxillary arch: 1. Mid Palatine raphae 2. Incisive Papilla 3. Torus palatinus/canine eminence or any bony protuberance.
Name muscles attached with buccal frenum.	Three muscles are attached with buccal frenum: 1. Orbicularis oris (OO) 2. Levator anguli oris (LAO) 3. Buccinator (B).

Question	*Answer*
Define posterior palatal seal area (PPS).	It is junction of hard and soft palate on which pressure within physiological limits can be applied by denture to aid in retention.
Write the boundaries of posterior palatal seal area.	**Anteriorly:** Anterior vibrating line **Posteriorly:** Posterior vibrating line **Medially:** One tuberosity to other **Laterally:** Extends through the pterygomaxillary notch continuing for 3–4 mm anterolateral approximating the mucogingival junction.
Which maneuver is performed to locate anterior vibrating line?	***Valsalva maneuver*** is performed by patient to locate anterior vibrating line.
Name primary stress bearing area of mandibular arch.	Primary stress bearing/supporting areas of mandibular arch are as follow: 1. Buccal shelf area 2. Retro-molar pad.
List secondary supporting areas of mandibular arch.	Secondary stress bearing/supporting structures of mandibular arch is: 1. Slopes of residual alveolar ridge.
Name valve forming structures (limiting areas) of mandibular arch.	The limiting structures are mentioned below: 1. Labial vestibule 2. Buccal frenum 3. Buccal vestibule 4. Alveololingual sulcus 5. Pterygomandibular raphae.
List out relief areas of mandibular arch.	Following is the list of relief areas of mandibular arch: 1. Crest of residual alveolar ridge (in case of sharp/knife edge ridge) 2. Mental foramen (in case of severely resorbed ridge) 3. Torus Mandibular is (if present, relief should be provided) 4. Sharp mylohyoid ridge.
Write boundary of buccal shelf area.	Boundary of buccal shelf area is as follows: **Anteriorly:** Buccal frenum **Posteriorly:** Retromolar pad **Medially:** Crest of residual alveolar ridge **Laterally:** External oblique ridge.
Write content of retromolar pad (RMP)	Retromolar pad contains following: 1. Loose areolar tissue 2. Glandular tissue 3. Fibers of buccinator muscle (buccal) 4. Fibers of superior constrictor muscle (lingual) 5. Pterygomandibular raphe 6. Tendon of temporalis
What is genial tubercle and its significance?	❑ They are small bony protrusions, two or three in number, located lingually near the inferior border of the mandible in the midline area. They provide attachment for the genioglossus and geniohyoid muscles. ❑ Relief should be provided in extremely resorbed ridge.

Question	*Answer*
Write about extent of alveololingual sulcus.	It is space between tongue and residual alveolar ridge. It extends from lingual frenum to retromylohyoid curtain (either side).
How can you divide alveololingual sulcus as per anatomic structure present in that region?	Alveololingual sulcus can be divided in three parts as follows: 1. Anterior region 2. Middle region 3. Posterior region.
Write about anterior region of alveololingual sulcus.	❑ It extends from lingual frenum to premylohyoid eminence. ❑ Anterior region of alveololingual sulcus is also known as sublingual crescent area or sublingual fold.
Write about middle region of alveololingual sulcus.	❑ It extends from premylohyoid fossa to distal end of mylohyoid ridge. ❑ It is also known as mylohyoid area.
Write the extends of posterior region of alveololingual sulcus.	❑ It is located posterior to the mylohyoid ridge. ❑ It is also known as retromylohyoid area.
What is posterior palatal seal (PPS)?	It is area located at or beyond the junction of hard palate and soft palate, on which pressure within physiologic limits can be applied by the prosthesis (complete denture) to aid in its (denture's) retention.
What are the functions of posterior palatal seal?	The functions of posterior palatal seal are: Primarily aids in retention. It prevents food entrapment beneath the denture. Reduces the patient's awareness of this area hence reduces gag reflex. It compensates for volumetric shrinkage of the acrylic resin.
What is impression?	A negative likeness or copy in reverse of the surface of an object; (an imprint of the teeth and adjacent structures for use in dentistry).
List the steps in manipulation of impression compound for making a primary impression.	The steps in manipulation of impression compound are breaking the compound in small pieces, softening, kneading, loading of tray, preforming, glazing, tempering, placing the tray in patient's mouth, moulding the material, removal of set material, and disinfection.
Enumerates the theories/techniques of impression making?	Theories of impression making are; (1) Mucostatic theory, (2) Mucocompressive theory and (3) Selective pressure technique.
What is tempering?	The heated and softened compound after glazing is at temperature around 55–60°C which is intolerable to oral tissue. It is tempered in a water bath to lower the temperature around 45°C which is well tolerated by oral tissue.
What is the purpose of kneading?	Kneading is done to uniformly mix all the constituents of the impression compound and improve the handling characteristic of material. It is kneaded under water because water acts as plasticizer.
What is the purpose of glazing?	Glazing is heating the preformed surface of a compound under a flame to record the minute surface details with minimum distortion of the bulk of material.
Why is custom tray required to be fabricated?	Custom tray is an individualized tray which closely adapts to the patient's arch. It provides even thickness of impression material and yields a more accurate impression.

Question	*Answer*
What should be the dimensions of custom tray handle?	The custom tray handle should be 8 mm in length, 8 mm in height and 3–4 mm in thickness. Maxillary custom tray handle is placed at 45° angulation and mandibular custom tray handle is placed at 90° angulation.
What is the need for a spacer in custom tray?	Spacer is placed on areas of relief where minimum pressure is to be applied while impression making. Thus, a space is created in custom tray and no pressure will be applied while making impression.
What spacer material is used for fabrication of shellac custom tray and for acrylic special tray?	For acrylic custom tray wax is used to make spacer. For shellac custom tray, shellac dusted with French chalk is used as spacer.
What are the drawbacks of the shellac custom tray?	Shellac is brittle and has less strength. The dimension stability is poor so easily distorts during border moulding procedure due to repeated temperature change.
What is dental cast?	A replica of the tooth surfaces, residual ridge areas and/or other parts of the dental arch and/or facial structures used to fabricate a dental restoration or prosthesis.
Mention types of dental cast.	Three types: 1. Diagnostic cast/primary cast 2. Final cast/master cast 3. Refractory cast.
Write parts of a dental cast.	Three parts: 1. Anatomical portion/part 2. Base of the cast 3. Land area of the cast.
List Ideal requirements of cast.	Ideal requirements are as follow: 1. It should be neat, clean and free of any voids and bubble 2. It should have proper thickness of base (15 mm) 3. Land area should be 2–3 mm in height and 3 mm in width 4. Land area is angulated at 45° 5. Denture foundation are is parallel to base of the cast.
Write uses of dental cast.	1. It is used for diagnosis purpose 2. Used for fabrication of prosthesis 3. Used for fabrication of special tray 4. Used for fabrication of record base 5. Used for casting (refractory cast).
Write various measurements related to dental cast.	1. It should have 15 mm thickness of base (15 mm) 2. Land area should be 2–3 mm in height and 3 mm in width 3. Land area is angulated at 45°.
Mention different methods of pouring cast.	There are two methods of pouring cast. 1. Beading–boxing method 2. Inversion pouring method.
Mention the objective of beading and boxing.	Beading of the cast gives properly formed land area and boxing is done to achieve desired thickness of base of the cast.

Question	*Answer*
Write the dimensions of maxillary occlusal rim.	Dimension for maxillary occlusal ridge should be: **Height:** ❑ **Anterior:** 20–22 mm from deepest part of the sulcus ❑ **Posterior:** 16–18 mm from deepest part of sulcus at molar area. **Width:** ❑ **Anterior:** 5–6 mm ❑ **Posterior:** 8–10 mm.
Write the dimensions of mandibular occlusal rim.	Dimensions for mandibular occlusal ridge should be: **Height:** ❑ **Anterior:** 16–18 mm from deepest part of sulcus ❑ **Posterior:** At the level of 2/3 of retromolar pad. **Width:** ❑ **Anterior:** 3–5 mm ❑ **Posterior:** 8–10 mm.
Write the uses of occlusal rims.	Uses of occlusal rim are mentioned below: 1. To establish occlusal plane 2. To record maxillomandibular relation 3. Used for artificial teeth arrangement 4. To record midline, canine line high and low lip line for teeth arrangement.
Define articulators	**Definition:** Articulator is a mechanical device that represent the TMJ and jaw members, to which maxillary and mandibular casts may be attached to simulate some or all the mandibular movements.
Why mean value articulator is called so?	The mean value articulator is called so because, the mean (average) values of Condylar guidance (33°), Anterior guidance (5°) and intercondylar distance (4 inch/110 mm) is taken for its designing and fabrication.
Write the mean values used in mean value articulator.	Following mean (average) values are used for mean value articulator: 1. Condylar guidance: 33° 2. Anterior guidance: 05° 3. Intercondylar distance: 110 mm (4 inch).
Mention the parts of articulator	Following is the list of parts of articulator: 1. Condylar guidance 2. Anterior guidance table 3. Mid Incisor pin/central pin 4. Incisal rod 5. Intercondylar rod 6. Upper member 7. Lower member 8. Mounting rings.
What is theory of equilateral triangle? OR What is Bonwill theory of articulator?	It states that: ❑ The distance between two condyles (centers) and distance from each condyle to mid incisal point (in mandible) is equal in dimension. ❑ Theoretically this distance is 4 inch (110 mm)

Question	*Answer*
Describe conical theory of articulator.	❑ This theory was proposed by RE Hall. ❑ It states that the lower teeth move over the surface of upper teeth as (if they move) over the surface of cone generating an angle of 45° with the central axis of cone tip.
What is spherical theory of articulator.	**It states that:** Lower teeth move over the surface of the sphere of 6 inch which has its center at the glabella. The surface of sphere passes through glenoid fossa along and articulating eminence.
What is ARCON articulator?	Any articulator which has Condylar guidance in upper member and condylar element in lower member is classified as ARCON articulator.
What is NON-ARCON articulator?	Any articulator which has condylar guidance in lower member and condylar element in upper member is classified as NON-ARCON articulator.
What is indexing of the cast?	It is done on master cast. It helps in remounting of the cast in the same position on articulator after processing.
What is remounting?	Remounting is positioning the master cast on articulator after processing to do selective grinding to eliminate processing errors.
Mention the types of indexing.	There are two types of indexing methods. 1. Groove indexing 2. Notch indexing.
Classify denture (artificial/prosthetic) teeth based on anatomy.	They are classified as: a. Anatomical teeth (33° or more cusp angulations) b. Semi-anatomical teeth (20° cusp angulations) c. Nonanatomical Teeth (zero-degree cusp angulations).
Classify denture (artificial/prosthetic) teeth based on material.	Based on material of teeth, they are classified as: 1. Acrylic teeth (most commonly used) 2. Porcelain teeth 3. Composite teeth 4. IPN resin teeth 5. Teeth with metallic stops/insert.
Mention advantages of acrylic teeth.	1. Chemical bond with denture base material 2. Can be trimmed very thin to fit in available space 3. They do not abrade opposite natural teeth if any 4. Easy to polish and modify.
Mention disadvantages of acrylic teeth.	1. They wear with time 2. Stain and discolor easily.
Mention disadvantages of porcelain denture teeth.	1. No chemical bond with denture base 2. Difficult to modify 3. More impact sound.
Mention advantages of porcelain denture teeth.	1. More aesthetic compared to acrylic teeth 2. More resistant to wear 3. Not easily stain or discolor.
What is indication for anatomical denture teeth?	Used for well-formed good ridges.
What is Indication for nonanatomical denture teeth?	Used for poor residual ridges (Resorbed ridges).

Question	*Answer*
What is indication for semi-anatomical denture teeth?	Used for fair residual ridges.
What is SPA concept?	SPA concept suggest selection of artificial teeth based on: a. Sex b. Personality c. Age of the patient.
What is curve of spee?	It is defined as the anatomical curve established by the occlusal alignment of the teeth, as projected onto the mesial plane, beginning with cusp tip of mandibular canine and following the buccal cusp tips of the premolar and molars teeth, continuing through the anterior border of the mandibular ramus, ending with the anterior most portion of the mandibular condyle.
What is curve of Wilson?	It is mediolateral curve that contacts the buccal and lingual cusp tips on each side of the arch. It results from lingual inclination of mandibular molar.
What is major connector in partial denture?	It is component of cast partial denture which connect different components located on one side of dental arch to those on the other side.
What is the purpose of making a record base?	It is used to support the occlusal rim material for recording maxillo-mandibular relation (Jaw relation) and for arranging the artificial teeth.
What are the requirements of temporary record bases?	It should be well adapted to the final cast, stable and retentive in the mouth, dimensionally stable, smooth and nonirritant to tissue.
What should be the ideal thickness of record bases?	The record base should be 01 mm. Thick on the ridge crest and facial slopes. It should be 02 mm. Thick in palatal and lingual flange region.
What is purpose of occlusal rim?	It is used to establish jaw relation, to determine lip support and aesthetic, aids in selecting teeth and to position and arrange them, determination of arch form, and determination of occlusal plane.
Which theory is mean value articulator based upon?	Mean value articulator is based upon Bonwill's theory of equilateral triangle.
What are the functions of Vertical pin?	It helps to maintain fixed distance between upper and lower member of articulator.
What is overjet?	The horizontal relationship of the incisal edges of the maxillary incisors to the mandibular incisors when the teeth are in maximum intercuspation.
What is vertical overlap or overbite?	The vertical relationship of the incisal edges of the maxillary incisors to the mandibular incisors when the teeth are in maximum intercuspation.
What is dentogenic concept?	According to this concept the Artificial teeth are selected according to sex, age and personality of patient. Teeth selected for female patient are rounded and whiter in color to give delicacy to the prosthesis. For male patient teeth with sharp edges and darker in color are selected. Attrition, abraded and gingival recession can be incorporated in denture to give natural look.

Question	*Answer*
What is Monson's spherical theory?	An arrangement of teeth that places their occlusal surfaces on the surface of an imaginary sphere (usually 8 inches in diameter) with its center above the level of the teeth.
What is antimonson curve or reverse curve?	In excessive wear of the teeth, the obliteration of the cusps and formation of either flat or cupped-out occlusal surfaces, associated with reversal of the occlusal plane of the premolar, first and second molar teeth (the third molars being generally unaffected), whereby the occlusal surfaces of the mandibular teeth slope facially instead of lingually and those of the maxillary teeth incline lingually.
What is mutually protected occlusion?	When posterior teeth are in occlusion there is gap between opposing anterior teeth and when anterior teeth are in contact there is disocclusion of posterior teeth. This phenomenon is called mutually protected occlusion or Christensen's phenomenon.
What is Leon Williams classification?	Leon Williams classification was based on matching tooth form to face form. Individual faces can be divided as square, Tapering and ovoid. The teeth for each type can be selected according to facial form.
What are the pre-extraction aids for teeth selection?	Pre-extraction aids for teeth selection are diagnostic casts, extracted teeth, photographs, and radiographs.
What is squint test?	This test is useful in selecting a color which is in harmony with the face. When different shades are compared with face color the shade that appears to be the best match according to the face color is selected.
What is buccal corridor or negative space?	It is the space between the buccal surface of posterior teeth and inner surface of cheeks. It is influence by buccolingual placement of posterior teeth.
What are the parts of flasks?	The parts of flasks are: 1. Base 2. Body/counter 3. Lid.
At what stage do you pack acrylic resin?	Acrylic resin is packed in the mould cavity in dough like stage
What is the purpose of trial closure?	To remove excess material (flash) as to minimize the processing errors such as increase of vertical dimension due to excess material.
What are processing errors?	They are warpage, fracture of denture, change in teeth position, polymerization shrinkage, internal or external porosity and increase in vertical dimension.
What are the components of acrylic partial denture?	The components of acrylic partial denture are artificial teeth, the denture base and wroght wire clasp.
Mention different types of maxillary major connectors.	a. Palatal bar b. Palatal strap c. Anterior-posterior strap d. Full arch palate e. Horseshoe shape.

Question	*Answer*
List different major connector for mandibular arch.	a. Lingual bar b. Lingual Plate c. Double lingual bar d. Labial bar.
Write types of minor connectors.	1. Minor connector joining clasp assembly to the major connector 2. Minor connector joining indirect retainer to major connector 3. Minor connector joining denture base to major connector 4. An approach arm of bar type clasp.
Write types of retainer (clasp) for cast partial denture.	Simple circlet clasp, multiple circulate clasp, embrasure clasp, ring clasp, fishhook clasp, onlay clasp.
Mention different types of bar clasp.	I bar, Y clasp, T clasp, Modified T clasp.
Mention the types of minor connector that joins the denture base to the major connector?	They are: 1. Lattice type/ladder type 2. Mesh work type 3. Neil bead/Neil head type.
What are the parts of the clasp?	The parts of clasps are: Rest, body of the clasp, shoulder, reciprocal clasp arm, retentive clasp arm, retentive terminal, minor connector, approach arm (in case of bar clasp).
What are the parts of a fixed partial denture?	Parts of fixed partial denture are pontic, connector and retainer.
What is an undercut?	The contour of a cross-sectional portion of a residual ridge or dental arch that prevents the insertion of a dental prosthesis or the portion of the surface of an object that is below the height of contour in relationship to the path of placement.
What is a height of contour?	A line encircling a tooth and designating its greatest circumference at a selected axial position determined by a dental surveyor or a line encircling a body designating its greatest circumference in a specified plane.
What are the forms of indirect retainer?	The indirect retainer can be an auxiliary rest (occlusal rest, cingulum rest or incisal rest). In some cases major connector provides indirect retention.
What is BULL'S law?	During selective grinding for alteration of occlusal surfaces the non functional cusp of maxillary teeth and mandibular teeth are altered. This is done according to BULL'S law. (**B**uccal-**U**pper and **L**ower-**L**ingual = BULL).
Classify finishlines according to location.	1. Supragingival finish line 2. Equigingival finish line 3. Sabgingival finish line.
Classify finishlines according to shape of finish line.	Chamfer, shoulder, beveled shoulder, heavy chamfer, knife edge.

Index

Page numbers followed by *b* refer to box, *f* refer to figure, *fc* refer to flowchart, and *t* refer to table.

A

Artificial tooth 67, 72, 201, 202, 236, 264, 264*f*

D

E

F

K

L

M

P

Q

R

S

T

U

V

W

Y

Z